Handbook of Peripheral Neuropathy

Handbook of Peripheral Neuropathy

edited by

Mark B. Bromberg
University of Utah
Salt Lake City, Utah, U.S.A.

A. Gordon Smith
University of Utah
Salt Lake City, Utah, U.S.A.

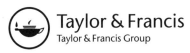

Taylor & Francis
Taylor & Francis Group

Boca Raton   London   New York   Singapore

Published in 2005 by
Taylor & Francis Group
6000 Broken Sound Parkway NW, Suite 300
Boca Raton, FL 33487-2742

International Standard Book Number-10: 0-8247-5432-8 (Hardcover)
International Standard Book Number-13: 978-0-8247-5432-7 (Hardcover)

Library of Congress Cataloging-in-Publication Data

Catalog record is available from the Library of Congress

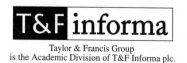

Taylor & Francis Group
is the Academic Division of T&F Informa plc.

Visit the Taylor & Francis Web site at
http://www.taylorandfrancis.com

To my wife, Diane, and my daughter, Katherine.

Mark

To Sam and Emily.

Gordon

Foreword

Writing a foreword to a new textbook is an act of faith. I do, however, have a considerable degree of faith since I know the editors and many of the authors. They are well trained, hard working, and expert.

Their intent has been to write a clinically useful handbook on the subject of peripheral neuropathy. Having edited (with others) four editions of another book on the same subject, I can understand the desire to produce a short and light book. The eminent neurologist Raymond Adams who reviewed our textbook on several occasions, complained about its weight, arguing that it was not a handbook and could not be read in bed.

The *Handbook of Peripheral Neuropathy* is to be a practical book that provides easy to understand information and which is light enough to hold in the hand, allowing it to be read in bed as well as at the bedside of a patient. The editors acknowledge the clinical expertise and mentorship of James Albers, MD, PhD, and his influence is perhaps reflected in the well ordered table of contents. The editors and contributors are experienced neurologists and electromyographers whose writings are worthy to be read. Now we await what they say about the subjects which they review—the proof of the pudding will be in the eating or in seeing the play ("to catch the conscience of the king"—Hamlet.). I hope this foreword whets your appetite so that you will read it.

Peter James Dyck, M.D.
Roy E. and Merle Meyer Professor of Neuroscience
The Peripheral Neuropathy Research Laboratory
Mayo Clinic College of Medicine, Rochester, Minnesota, U.S.A.

Preface

Peripheral neuropathies are common clinical problems. Foot numbness and pain are frequent complaints in the primary care setting. The complexity of nerve anatomy and pathology and the long list of causes of peripheral neuropathy may seem daunting and often lead primary care providers to refer patients to a neurologist. Even among neurologists, the evaluation can be challenging. All of these factors contribute to the general perception that the diagnosis and management of peripheral neuropathies is complex and mysterious. The goal of this text is to de-mystify the evaluation and treatment of peripheral neuropathies and to provide a practical guide to the management of common symptoms.

The diagnosis of peripheral neuropathy can be simplified by using a structured approach. One purpose of medical monographs is to bring order to apparent complexity. Accordingly, this book is designed around a diagnostic approach based on an understanding of the anatomy and pathophysiology of the peripheral nervous system. This approach involves asking a series of simple clinical and electrodiagnostic questions whose answers lead to a full characterization of the neuropathy. When knowledge of basic classes of neuropathies is added to this characterization, it can yield a reasonable differential diagnosis. At this point, a focused set of laboratory tests can be rationally selected that will maximize the diagnostic yield. Treatment and management of peripheral neuropathy also benefit from an approach that emphasizes an understanding of underlying pathophysiology of the neuropathy.

This book is divided into three broad sections. The first broad section provides an evaluation algorithm. This algorithm is based on the anatomy, physiology and pathology of peripheral nerves in the context of symptoms and signs. A similar algorithm is offered for designing and interpreting electrodiagnostic tests. The role of special diagnostic tests, including imaging, quantitative sensory testing, and nerve and skin biopsy is also reviewed in the first section. The second broad section presents classes of peripheral neuropathies. For each class, the clinical characteristics, electrodiagnostic features, examination findings, treatment options and outcome are reviewed. The third broad section discusses general treatment modalities and management issues which will improve the patient's well being.

We thank our many contributors who have provided their experience and expertise to make this a clinically useful book. The mechanics of editing a book on peripheral neuropathy are as daunting as the subject, and we could not have succeeded without the expertise of Ms. Becky Guertler. We also thank our publisher, especially Jinnie Kim the acquiring editor, for their patience, in preparing the book.

We want to acknowledge our mentor in neuromuscular diseases, James Albers M.D., Ph.D., who has provided an approach to the diagnosis and management of peripheral neuropathies that is reflected in the general outline of this book.

Mark B. Bromberg
A. Gordon Smith

Contents

Treatment of Peripheral Neuropathy

Contributors

James W. Albers, MD, PhD *Department of Neurology, University of Michigan, Ann Arbor, Michigan, USA*

Deborah T. Blumenthal, MD *Department of Neurology, University of Utah, Salt Lake City, Utah, USA*

Mark B. Bromberg, MD, PhD *Department of Neurology, University of Utah, Salt Lake City, Utah, USA*

Reem F. Bunyan, MD *Department of Neurology, King Faisal University, Al-Khobar, Saudi Arabia*

William W. Campbell, MD, MSHA *Department of Neurology, Walter Reed Army Medical Center, Washington DC, USA*

Lisa DiPonio, MD *Department of Physical Medicine & Rehabilitation, University of Michigan Medical Center, Ann Arbor, Michigan, USA*

Lydia Estanislao, MD *Department of Neurology and Clinical Neurophysiology, Mount Sinai Medical Center, New York, New York, USA*

Kevin J. Felice, DO *Department of Neurology, University of Connecticut Health Center, Farmington, Connecticut, USA*

John E. Greenlee, MD *Department of Neurology, University of Utah, Salt Lake City, Utah, USA*

Patrick M. Grogan, MD *Department of Neurology, Stanford University School of Medicine, Stanford, California, USA*

Estelle S. Harris, MD *Department of Pulmonary and Critical Care Medicine, University of Utah, Salt Lake City, Utah, USA*

David N. Herrmann, MB, BCh *Department of Neurology, University of Rochester Medical Center, Rochester, New York, USA*

Safwan S. Jaradeh, MD *Department of Neurology, Medical College of Wisconsin, Milwaukee, Wisconsin, USA*

Jonathan S. Katz, MD *Department of Neurology, Stanford University School of Medicine, Stanford, California, USA*

John C. Kincaid, MD *Department of Neurology, Indiana University School of Medicine, Indianapolis, Indiana, USA*

Mark E. Landau, MD *Department of Neurology, Walter Reed Army Medical Center, Washington DC, USA*

Victoria H. Lawson, MD *Department of Neurology, University of Utah, Salt Lake City, Utah, USA*

James A. Leonard Jr, MD *Department of Physical Medicine & Rehabilitation, University of Michigan Medical Center, Ann Arbor, Michigan, USA*

Richard A. Lewis, MD *Department of Neurology, Wayne State University School of Medicine, Detroit, Michigan, USA*

Jun Li, MD, PhD *Department of Neurology, Wayne State University School of Medicine, Detroit, Michigan, USA*

Patrick Luedtke, MD, MPH *Department of Family and Preventive Medicine, University of Utah, Salt Lake City, Utah, USA*

John E. McGillicuddy, MD *Department of Neurosurgery, University of Michigan Medical Center, Ann Arbor, Michigan, USA*

Kevin R. Moore, MD *Department of Neuroradiology, University of Utah, Salt Lake City, Utah, USA*

Rachel A. Nardin, MD *Department of Neurology, Beth Israel Hospital, Boston, Massachusetts, USA*

Sharon P. Nations, MD *Department of Neurology, University of Texas Southwestern Medical Center, Dallas, Texas, USA*

Hiroyuki Nodera, MD *Department of Neurology, University of Rochester Medical Center, Rochester, New York, USA*

Patrick C. Nolan, MD, PhD *Department of Neurology, University of Michigan, Ann Arbor, Michigan, USA*

Amanda C. Peltier, MD *Department of Neurology, University of Michigan and Veterans Affairs Medical Center, Ann Arbor, Michigan, USA*

Rahman Pourmand, MD *Department of Neurology, Stony Brook University Hospital, Stony Brook, New York, USA*

Thomas E. Prieto, PhD *Department of Neurology, Medical College of Wisconsin, Milwaukee, Wisconsin, USA*

David R. Renner, MD *Department of Neurology, University of Utah, Salt Lake City, Utah, USA*

James W. Russell, MD, MS, FRCP *Veterans Affairs Medical Center and Department of Neurology, University of Michigan, Ann Arbor, Michigan, USA*

Seward B. Rutkove, MD *Department of Neurology, Beth Israel Hospital, Boston, Massachusetts, USA*

Firas G. Saleh, MD *Department of Neurology, Stony Brook University Hospital, Stony Brook, New York, USA*

A. Mouaz Sbei, MD *Department of Neurology, University of Utah, Salt Lake City, Utah, USA*

J. Steven Schultz, MD *Department of Physical Medicine and Rehabilitation, University of Michigan Health System, Ann Arbor, Michigan, USA*

Michael E. Shy, MD *Department of Neurology, Wayne State University School of Medicine, Detroit, Michigan, USA*

Zachary Simmons, MD, FAAN *Department of Neurology, Penn State College of Medicine, Hershey, Pennsylvania, USA*

David Simpson, MD *Department of Neurology and Clinical Neurophysiology, Mount Sinai Medical Center, New York, New York, USA*

J. Robinson Singleton, MD *Department of Neurology, University of Utah, Salt Lake City, Utah, USA*

A. Gordon Smith, MD *Department of Neurology, University of Utah, Salt Lake City, Utah, USA*

Eric J. Sorenson, MD *Department of Neurology, University of Utah, Salt Lake City, Utah, USA*

M. Catherine Spires, MS, MD *Department of Physical Medicine and Rehabilitation, University of Michigan, Ann Arbor, Michigan, USA*

Michael Stanton, MD *Department of Neurology, University of Rochester Medical Center, Rochester, New York, USA*

John D. Steffens, MD *Department of Neurology, University of Utah, Salt Lake City, Utah, USA*

Jaya R. Trivedi, MD *Department of Neurology, University of Texas Southwestern Medical Center, Dallas, Texas, USA*

Orly Vardeny, Pharm.D. *Department of Pharmacy, University of Utah, Salt Lake City, Utah, USA*

Gil I. Wolfe, MD *Department of Neurology, University of Texas Southwestern Medical Center, Dallas, Texas, USA*

1

An Approach to the Evaluation of Peripheral Nerve Diseases

Mark B. Bromberg
University of Utah, Salt Lake City, Utah, USA

ABSTRACT

Neurologic diagnosis can be challenging, particularly for disorders of peripheral nerve. For many clinicians, basic nerve anatomy and physiology and the various patterns of pathology can be daunting. In general neurology, diagnostic efficiency is enhanced by first localizing the lesion within the nervous system followed by determination of the pathology, and then a consideration of cause. The same approach can be applied to peripheral nerve disorders. This chapter presents a structured approach to the evaluation of peripheral nerve diseases based on asking a series of questions during the history and examination, whose answers will lead to localization and characterization of the peripheral nerve lesion. Following this, a meaningful list of laboratory tests can be ordered.

1. INTRODUCTION

Numbness, tingling, and pain and weakness in the limbs are among the most common complaints voiced to clinicians. In the general population, the prevalence of peripheral neuropathy approaches 10% (1), that of median mononeuropathies 4% (2), and radiculopathies likely exceed median nerve mononeuropathies (carpal tunnel syndrome) (3). It can be challenging to separate, among these common symptoms, those that reflect peripheral nerve disorders from those that arise from the central nervous system and to identify underlying causes. Most experienced clinicians would likely agree that a structured approach to patient evaluation based on localization is more efficient than an unstructured or shotgun approach. Disadvantages of an unstructured approach are many. For the patient, there may be unnecessary false leads, hopes, and anxieties. Computed tomography (CT) and magnetic resonance imaging (MRI) scans are frequently relied upon to exclude lesion sites, but most lesions of the peripheral nervous system are not diagnosable by imaging studies. Further, unnecessary imaging studies are costly, and they may reveal coincident or irrelevant findings that can lead to unnecessary surgery. A shotgun approach to laboratory testing is expensive and unproductive (4). Batteries of blood tests are frequently ordered, but rarely informative because the majority of common tests are unrelated to disorders of peripheral nerves.

This chapter will outline a structured and efficient evaluation that leads to a full localization and characterization of the neuropathy. At this point, the scope of the differential diagnosis is reduced, and a rational list of laboratory tests can be ordered. Localization and characterization are discussed in terms of a series of layers (Table 1.1). The first layer is localization to the peripheral nervous system. Subsequent layers refine the localization within the peripheral nervous system and define underlying peripheral nerve pathology. The final layer includes a consideration of probability and epidemiology of peripheral nerve disorders that leads to an initial and reasonable differential diagnosis. Assigning layers and a sequence is somewhat artificial. The evaluation process is dynamic and layers will merge and the sequence will vary depending upon the clinician's experience and clinical situation.

The approach in this chapter can not only serve as a framework for evaluating patients, but also to be used to determine localizing features when reviewing the literature on specific disorders of peripheral nerve (including material presented in this book).

Table 1.1 Layers of Diagnostic Evaluation Leading to a Full Characterization of the Neuropathy and an Accurate Localization within the Peripheral Nervous System

First Layer	
Within the peripheral nervous system?	Exclude cortical, spinal, psychogenic loci
Second Layer	
What part of the peripheral nervous system?	Root, plexus, single nerve, multiple nerves, peripheral neuropathy
Third Layer	
What is the time course?	Acute, subacute, chronic, progressive, relapsing-remitting, event-linked
Fourth Layer	
What nerve fibers are involved?	Sensory, motor, autonomic, combinations
Fifth Layer	
What is the primary pathology?	Demyelination, axonal, mixed
Sixth Layer	
What are the other pertinent features?	Family, medical, social histories
Seventh Layer	
What are the epidemiologic features?	Probability, age of onset, rarity, gender

2. LAYER 1: LOCALIZATION TO THE PERIPHERAL NERVOUS SYSTEM

This level is usually assumed, but it deserves mention that not all symptoms of numbness, tingling, and pain and weakness are referable to the peripheral nervous system. Failure to localize can lead to diagnostic errors. Classic examples are strokes, tumors, central nervous system demyelinating disorders, and compressive myelopathies. Cortical origins of numbness and weakness frequently involve one side of the body, whereas spinal origins have bilateral leg symptoms with a truncal level of demarcation (5). Central demyelinating disorders can be challenging because they may include asymmetric and unusual symptom patterns, but associated features and examination findings such as pathologic tendon reflexes help localize the disorder to the central nervous system.

Some patterns of symptoms and signs may not be attributable to definable lesions within either the central or peripheral nervous systems (6). Under these circumstances, a somatoform disorder should be considered. Somatoform disorders represent distressful physical symptoms causing impaired social or occupational dysfunction with no diagnosable condition to account for them (7). Numbness, paresthesias, pain, weakness, and fatigue are among common peripheral nerve symptoms that are considered to be "pseudoneurological" when no neurological basis can be found. Whether a patient fulfills complete DSM-IV criteria for somatization or undifferentiated somatoform disorders is less important than recognition that further evaluation is unlikely to be diagnostic (7). Every patient deserves a considered evaluation, no matter how high the initial index of suspicion is that symptoms are not physiologic, because somatization can accompany true diseases (6). However, when reasonable localization cannot be achieved, the neurologic and laboratory examinations are normal, and the temporal pattern does not fit known pathologic processes, it is highly unlikely that the symptoms represent a definable pathology.

Under these circumstances, a discussion seeking other factors is appropriate. Leading such patients to understand that internal factors are causative or contributory should be taken slowly. Replacing long-standing symptoms with the "good news" of "good health" is rarely successful. Other psychiatric conditions such as depression, anxiety, and panic disorders may coexist (8). Many times, with long-standing symptoms, the family milieu has incorporated the patient's symptoms, and giving the patient a therapeutic way out of their dilemma, such as physical therapy, may be more successful for the patient and family.

3. LAYER 2: LOCALIZATION WITHIN THE PERIPHERAL NERVOUS SYSTEM

This layer is based on the anatomy of the peripheral nervous system. Symptoms expected from lesions at various sites along nerves, from root to plexus and peripheral nerve, can be queried during the history. The history should be taken as an active process, with the goal of understanding what the patient is experiencing to answer the question of localization. Neurologic findings during the examination should therefore be predicted from the history and represent a confirmatory step. Examples of symptoms that help localization to sites along peripheral nerves are considered below. At each site, issues addressed in layers 3 through 7 will be emphasized.

3.1. Radicular Pattern

Radicular patterns of shooting pain and paresthesias down one limb following a root distribution are rare compared with diffuse low back pain, and occur more frequently with lumbosacral than cervical spine or truncal movements (5,9). Diffuse back pain is not usually caused by focal radiculopathies. Degenerative disk and vertebral findings on MRI scanning are common, and unless marked in degree, are rarely the cause of focal radiculopathies (10). The frequency of root involvement is one-thirds cervical spine in the distribution of C7 ($\sim$70%), C6 ($\sim$20%), and C8 ($\sim$10%) and two-thirds lumbosacral spine in the distribution of L4–5 ($\sim$40%), S1 ($\sim$40%) and other roots ($\sim$10%). Sensory symptoms including pain are more common than weakness, and altered sensations and reduced tendon reflexes in the appropriate root distribution are supportive. Muscle atrophy and true weakness are rare examination findings (9). Diagnostically, acute disk herniation is less challenging than chronic disease due to degenerative foraminal narrowing. Spinal stenosis produces involvement of multiple roots and follows a chronic course with low back pain, leg pain, and paresthesias triggered or increased by walking (9).

3.2. Plexus Pattern

Plexopathies are rare. Trauma to the brachial plexus is the most common cause. Acute plexopathies associated with marked pain are frequently idiopathic when involving the brachial plexus (Parsonage–Turner syndrome) (11) and associated with diabetes when involving the lumbosacral plexus (12). Thoracic outlet syndrome is frequently queried, but the incidence of true neurogenic thoracic outlet syndrome is exceedingly rare, and is characterized by the pattern of axonal loss of ulnar sensory and motor and median motor nerve fibers caused by chronic pressure on the lower trunk (13). Plexopathies due to cancer are chronic in nature and may or may not include pain (14,15).

Differentiating radiculopathies from plexopathies may be difficult when symptoms are primarily vague pain. Radiculopathies more commonly include focal symptoms, whereas plexopathies produce more diffuse symptoms. Both conditions involve axonal pathology, and differentiating between them can be achieved by sensory nerve conduction studies and needle electromyography (EMG).

3.3. Mononeuropathy Pattern

Lesions involving individual nerves are characterized by loss of sensation and strength in the distribution of the affected nerve. There are multiple causes of mononeuropathies, but chronic pressure (entrapment neuropathies) with focal demyelinating pathology is most common. Mononeuropathy multiplex is a rare condition frequently caused by vasculitis associated with collagen vascular diseases. Another class of mononeuropathy multiplex pattern is multifocal motor neuropathy with conduction block caused by focal immune mediated demyelination.

3.4. Peripheral Neuropathy Pattern

Several patterns of peripheral nerve involvement can be recognized Table 1.2. The prototypic and most common pattern is length-dependent, with sensory loss and pain preceding distal weakness. As progressively shorter nerves are affected, symptoms and signs unroll as a stocking up the leg. The nerve length at the knee level approximately equals the length innervating the hand, and with further progression, symptoms and signs unroll as a long glove up the arm. The distribution is usually symmetric. In the extreme, a shield loss over the chest and abdomen can be observed when nerve length involvement reaches the circumference of the thorax. Most length-dependent peripheral neuropathies are chronic and involve axonal pathology (16). As a corollary, it is rare in polyneuropathy for there to be sensory involvement to the waist level, especially without marked sensory loss also to the elbows. Accordingly, isolated sensory loss to the upper thigh and waist levels suggests central nervous system localization (myelopathy). Causes of peripheral neuropathy are many, and are felt to reflect metabolic abnormalities. Diabetes mellitus is the most common underlying cause, followed by hereditary (genetic) neuropathies. The cause for many neuropathies is unknown, and idiopathic or cryptogenic neuropathies represent up to 25% of peripheral neuropathies.

When the pattern of symptoms and signs includes both proximal and distal limb involvement, the pathologic process is usually demyelination at multifocal sites along roots and nerves (inflammatory polyradiculoneuropathy). Acute and chronic forms occur (AIDP and CIDP).

Table 1.2 Patterns of Peripheral Neuropathy and Examples of Disorders and Causes

Sensory-motor symmetric (length-dependent pattern)	Diabetes, medications, toxins, metabolic disorders, hereditary
Sensory-motor symmetric (proximal and distal pattern)	Acute inflammatory demyelinating polyradiculopathy, chronic inflammatory demyelinating polyradiculopathy
Sensory-motor asymmetric (nerve or plexus pattern)	Diabetic amyotrophy, idiopathic plexopathy, vasculitic mononeuritis multiplex
Sensory-motor asymmetric	Porphyria, leprosy
Sensory symmetric or asymmetric	Paraneoplastic neuronopathy, Sjögren syndrome, idiopathic ganglionitis, vitamin B6 toxicity, leprosy
Motor symmetric or asymmetric	Amyotrophic lateral sclerosis, multifocal motor conduction block neuropathy, lower motor neuron syndrome, poliomyelitis, West Nile syndrome
Autonomic symmetric or asymmetric	With other neuropathies (diabetes, acute inflammatory demyelinating polyradiculopathy), isolated involvement (amyloidosis)

Asymmetric patterns are less common and include a number of different lesion sites and pathologic processes. It is useful to determine whether sensory or motor nerves are predominantly involved. Unilateral and focal symptoms and signs in a limb must be distinguished from radiculopathy, plexopathy, or mononeuropathy (mononeuritis multiplex). Atrophic weakness without sensory loss that does not follow radicular, plexopathy, or mononeuropathy pattern suggests motor neuron disease (amyotrophic lateral sclerosis).

4. LAYER 3: WHAT IS THE TIME COURSE?

The usual definitions of time course in neurology are somewhat blurred in diseases of the peripheral nerve, and Table 1.3 lists time courses with examples. True acute or apoplectic events are rare in atraumatic nerve injuries, and occur in the setting of vasculitis. More commonly, an acute onset is defined as days to several weeks, and suggests the Guillain–Barré syndrome or AIDP, a metabolic event, or a toxic exposure. Most chronic neuropathies are steadily progressive. A history of clear remissions and exacerbations suggests CIDP or other form of immune-mediated neuropathy. It can be challenging to accurately determine the start of a slowly progressive chronic neuropathy because patients may not appreciate an insidious onset. Querying patients about their functional performance during historic or calendar events can be helpful to identify the onset. When the time course clearly starts in adult life, an acquired neuropathy is more likely than a hereditary disorder. When the time course cannot be dated, a hereditary neuropathy should be considered. However, our understanding of hereditary neuropathies is expanding and a number of "idiopathic" neuropathies beginning in adulthood may represent mild forms of hereditary neuropathies.

5. LAYER 4: WHICH NERVE FIBERS ARE INVOLVED?

The peripheral nervous system can be divided into somatic and autonomic components, and somatic peripheral nerves can be further divided into sensory and motor functions. Within the somatic nervous system, sensory and motor fiber involvement can be accurately assessed and there are neuropathies affecting sensory, motor, or both types of fibers. In the autonomic nervous system, separating sensory (afferent) from motor (efferent) involvement is difficult and both are commonly affected. Neuropathies with isolated autonomic nervous system involvement are rare. Accordingly, it is practical to determine whether there is any involvement of autonomic nerve involvement.

Table 1.3 Peripheral Neuropathy Time Courses and Examples of Associated Neuropathies

Acute	
Apoplectic	Vasculitic mononeuritis multiplex, idiopathic plexopathy
Days to weeks	Acute inflammatory demyelinating polyradiculopathy, porphyria, acute toxic exposure, proximal diabetic neuropathy, paraneoplastic sensory neuronopathy
Chronic	
Years	Diabetic polyneuropathy, chronic inflammatory demyelinating polyradiculopathy, idiopathic
Insidious	Hereditary

5.1. Symptoms

From the chief complaint it may not be apparent which types of nerves are involved. Nerve dysfunction can be expressed as negative and positive symptoms (Table 1.4). Positive symptoms are felt to reflect inappropriate spontaneous nerve activity detected by the patient as uncomfortable and painful sensations, or other spontaneous phenomena. Negative symptoms reflect loss of nerve signaling. An important clinical difference between sensory and motor somatic nerves involves compensatory mechanisms. Following motor nerve loss, surviving motor nerves undergo collateral reinnervation to reinnervate orphaned muscle fibers. This compensatory process has the effect of blunting weakness due to mild motor nerve loss, and clinical weakness may not be apparent to the patient or on physical examination until 50% of motor nerve fibers are lost (80% in slowly progressive denervating disorders) (17). However, positive symptoms of cramps and fasciculations may be present early on as the only clinical indication of motor nerve involvement. The needle EMG is sensitive in detecting early motor fiber loss and will confirm motor nerve involvement.

5.2. Signs

The clinical neurologic examination is sensitive for peripheral nerve loss and dysfunction, and informative for localization. An appreciation of nerve physiology and pathology, and the limitations of clinical testing, are necessary to accurately interpret the clinical examination. It is important to emphasize that the sensory examination can be challenging and confusing because responses are indirect and represent a patient's interpretation of the testing questions. Accordingly, it is important that the patient fully understands the object of the test. Attention and co-operation are imperative. It is worthwhile having specific questions derived from the history to address on the neurologic examination. For example, does the sensory loss follow a stocking-glove (distal predominate), dermatomal, or radicular pattern?

The sensory examination frequently focuses on determining whether there is "large fiber" or "small fiber" involvement, based on a battery of simple clinical tests. However, psychophysical sensory perception testing suggests these distinctions are more apparent than real because of overlap between nociception, touch, and pressure stimulus properties. Although nociceptive information is conveyed by small diameter nerve fibers, some nociceptive receptors are innervated by myelinated fibers, and subjects can distinguish sharp from dull stimuli without feeling pain. Formal psychophysical testing of nociception is performed using hot stimuli, cold stimuli, and special equipment, which contrasts to clinical sensory testing performed using cool instruments (tuning fork and reflex

Table 1.4 Positive and Negative Symptoms Associated with Nerve Damage

	Positive symptoms	Negative symptoms
Somatic nerves		
Sensory	Pain, tingling	Numbness, lack of feeling
Motor	Cramps, fasciculations	Weakness, atrophy
Autonomic nerves		
	Hyperhydrosis, diarrhea	Orthostatic hypotension, impotence, anhydrosis, constipation

hammer) and sharp objects of varying shape (safety pin, broken wooden stick, and commercial pin probe).

Cutaneous mechanoreceptors are mainly innervated by large-diameter nerve fibers and are activated by a variety of moving stimuli. Touch stimulus threshold changes modestly with age. A comparison of quantitative sensory testing in neuropathy patients indicates that vibratory thresholds are well correlated with touch-pressure thresholds and vibratory thresholds are suitable indicators of large-diameter sensory nerve dysfunction (18).

With these principles and specific questions in mind, an informative battery of sensory tests can be performed. It is noteworthy that patients are generally able to determine the level of involvement on a limb by asking them to make a line of demarcation, below which sensations are abnormal and above which they are normal.

5.2.1. Touch Stimuli

Application of the lightest touch to the dorsum of the hand and foot represents a measure of low threshold mechanoreception. A series of monofilaments can be applied to grade the severity of touch loss. Ten-gram filaments are useful because lack of touch perception at this level of pressure is associated with risk for unappreciated trauma.

5.2.2. Vibration Stimuli

Tuning forks of 128 Hz assess larger diameter nerve fiber function. Various comparisons can be made, and it is very important that patients are fully attentive and understand the need to indicate complete disappearance of the vibration. Comparisons between patient and examiner for the disappearance of the vibration can be measured in seconds. Alternatively, the time for the vibration to disappear for the patient after the tuning is forcefully struck can be measured in seconds. Empiric data from the great toe indicate that young adults lose vibration perception after 15 s, with a loss of 1 s per decade of age, and a loss of vibratory perception in <10 s is abnormal at any age (4).

5.2.3. Sharp Stimuli

The goal is to apply a sharp stimulus without also applying undo pressure on the skin. A distinction between noxious and light pressure stimuli can be made by gently applying the two ends of a safety pin in association with a three-part question: "which is sharper, the first application, the second application, or are both the same?". Inability to distinguish between sharp and dull supports loss of nociceptive fibers relative to low-threshold mechanoreceptor fibers.

5.2.4. Position Sense

The ability to detect changes in digital joint position is normally exquisite (two degrees). It is important that patients understand the degree of sensitivity requested, and that they are blinded to the testing. Accordingly, misperception of joint movements (including falsely perceived position changes), and insensitivity to movements are significant for loss of large-diameter fibers. Profound joint position loss is unusual in peripheral nerve disorders, and often reflects central nervous system involvement.

5.2.5. Deep Tendon Reflexes

Tendon reflexes represent an objective measure of sensory nerve function. The myotatic reflex consists of a monosynaptic arc with large-diameter afferent (sensory) nerve fiber input from muscle spindle fibers and large-diameter efferent (motor) nerve fiber output

Table 1.5 NINDS Scale for Deep Tendon Reflexes

Grade	Reflex response
0	Reflex absent
1	Reflex small, less than normal; includes trace response, or response brought out only with reinforcement
2	Reflex in lower half of normal range
3	Reflex in upper half of normal range
4	Reflex enhanced, more than normal; includes clonus, which optionally can be noted in an added verbal description of the reflex

Source: Modified from Litvan et al. (19).

from alpha motor neuron fibers. The reflex is much more vulnerable to sensory nerve fiber than to motor nerve fiber damage. Accordingly, an absent reflex is an objective indication of significant dysfunction of large-diameter sensory fibers. However, assurance that the reflex is truly absent is essential, and reinforcing maneuvers, such as clinching the jaw or fists and the Jendrassic maneuver, should be used before the reflex is considered absent. Various grading systems for tendon reflexes have been proposed, and the National Institute of Neurological Disorders and Stroke (NINDS) scale has good intraobserver reliability (Table 1.5) (19). Tendon reflexes diminish with age, and although precise data are not available, an absent Achilles reflex after the age of 80 years may be normal.

5.2.6. Motor Signs

Detecting motor nerve involvement can be challenging due to the compensatory process of collateral innervation that obscures early effects of denervation. Muscle inspection for atrophy is useful, and the extensor digitorum brevis muscle will show the early changes in the feet and first dorsal interosseous muscles early changes in the hands. A certain degree of age-related motor fiber loss occurs above 65 years and must be taken into consideration. Inspection for contraction fasciculations is useful to detect motor fiber loss. Contraction fasciculations are visible twitches of a muscle during early activation, and represent the discharge of individual motor units (20). Such twitches are not visible in muscles with normal numbers of motor units, but enlarged motor units from denervation and collateral reinnervation are readily observed.

Strength testing can be optimized to detect mild degrees of weakness by assessing muscles that can be just overcome on manual muscle testing in normal individuals. Informative muscles in the legs include flexors and extensors of the lesser toes and extensors of the great toe, and in the arms include abductors of the second and fifth digits and extensors of the fingers. Ankle dorsiflexion weakness occurs in more severe neuropathies, but ankle plantar flexion weakness is evident only in the most severe neuropathies (21). Subtle weakness of ankle dorsiflexion and plantar flexion can be tested best during gait assessment by having patients walk on their heels and toes or hop on one leg at a time.

5.2.7. Orthopedic Signs

Limb inspection should include structural changes in the lower legs, feet and hands. The following changes may be encountered in normal individuals, but in the setting of a peripheral neuropathy evaluation, suggest a long-standing condition. The angle between the shin and the unsupported foot is normally about 130°, and a larger angle suggests weakness of ankle dorsiflexor muscles. High arches and hammertoe deformities suggest long-standing differences in the muscular forces exerted on the bones of the foot leading to foreshorten feet. Fallen arches can also be observed in severe neuropathies. Toe and foot injuries unnoticed by the patient suggest a marked degree of sensory loss. In the hands, flexion contractions of the fingers suggest weakness of finger extensor muscles. Inability to adduct the fifth digits suggests weakness of lumbrical muscles.

5.2.8. Other Signs

Mild dependent pedal edema, rubor, coolness and shininess of the lower leg and foot despite good distal arterial pulses, suggests decreased movements of distal leg muscles caused by mild muscle weakness, reducing the vascular return of blood and lymph.

5.2.9. Autonomic System Signs

The autonomic nervous system is involved in many peripheral neuropathies, but symptoms and signs of dysautonomia are uncommonly voiced by the patient and must queried. Orthostatic dizziness and changes in blood pressure (a drop of >30 mmHg systolic pressure and >15 mmHg diastolic pressure recorded $60-90$ s after standing following 5 min of supine rest) support autonomic involvement. Impotence has many causes, but is frequently associated with autonomic neuropathy. The sicca symptoms (dry eyes and mouth) are associated with the Sjögren syndrome and represent end organ failure of salivary and tear glands. Sjögren syndrome is associated with sensory neuropathies.

6. LAYER 5: WHAT IS THE PRIMARY PATHOLOGY?

Determining the primary pathologic process is important for diagnosis, treatment, and prognosis. The two basic pathologic processes are demyelination and axonal loss. They may occur together, especially when the primary process is demyelination because demyelination frequently involves immune attack and axons can be damaged as innocent bystanders.

Electrodiagnostic testing is most able to distinguish axonal from demyelinating primary pathology (discussed in Chapter 2). Nerve biopsy is less practical and informative in this regard for several reasons. Biopsies evaluate only a small segment of sensory nerves, and the relevant pathologic process may be missed. Biopsies are rarely repeated, and the time course of changes cannot be followed. A nerve biopsy leaves permanent dysfunction, and most biopsies are of sensory nerves because a localized area of numbness is tolerable whereas permanent weakness is not. Nerve biopsy is important when vasculitis is a consideration, and a biopsy can detect rare causes of neuropathy due to deposition of protein or other substance, such as amyloid, and abnormal cells such as sarcoid (granulomas) and malignant cells. The role of nerve biopsy is further discussed in other chapters.

7. LOCALIZATION SUMMARY

At this point in the evaluation, the neuropathy should be fully characterized. Table 1.6 summarizes the clinical, electrodiagnostic, and pathologic characteristics. The next two layers focus on factors unique to the patient under evaluation, and help refine diagnostic considerations and the order of laboratory testing.

Table 1.6   Clinical, Electrodiagnostic, and
Pathologic Characteristics of Peripheral
Neuropathies

Clinical characteristics
  Acute or chronic
  Symmetric or asymmetric
  Distal length-dependent or distal and proximal
Electrodiagnostic and pathologic characteristics
  Uniform demyelinating; sensory + motor
  Segmental demyelinating; motor > sensory
  Axonal; motor > sensory
  Axonal; sensory neuropathy or neuronopathy
  Axonal; motor neuropathy or neuronopathy
  Axonal and demyelinating; sensory + motor

---

8.   LAYER 6: WHAT ARE THE OTHER PERTINENT FEATURES?

Determining the underlying causes of peripheral neuropathies and other disorders of peripheral nerve is challenging, and a thorough review of the patient's medical and family history is valuable.

8.1.   Medical History

Past and current medical histories are obviously important, but the number of medical conditions associated with clinically significant peripheral nerve disorders is limited (4). The clear exceptions are diabetes mellitus, certain collagen vascular disorders, chronic renal failure, and HIV infection. Despite this, many laboratory tests are frequently ordered in the evaluation of a neuropathy that represent general medical tests that are not truly informative or pertinent to the evaluation of peripheral nerve disorders. Medical causes of peripheral neuropathy will be covered in other chapters.

8.2.   Medications and Other Compounds

Inquiring about medication use is important, and should include vitamins and other over the counter compounds. Although the list of drugs, compounds, and vitamins associated with peripheral neuropathies is limited, drug-induced neuropathies represent readily treatable causes. These will be discussed in other chapters.

8.3.   Family History

An important line of inquiry is the family history, seeking evidence to support a hereditary neuropathy. Although it may seem that a hereditary condition should be known within a family, the slow progression and variable expression masks detection. Interestingly, in large families with known Charcot–Marie–Tooth neuropathy, <30% of affected individuals seek medical attention for their symptoms (22). Therefore, a careful line of questions can be very informative when there are clinical features suggesting a very long-standing condition, such as insidious onset, high arches, and hammertoes. Table 1.7 lists useful questions that can be addressed to parents, siblings, and children.

Table 1.7 Questions Pertinent to Chronic Neuropathies

Difficulty with running, sports, or military activities?
High-arched feet?
Hammer or curled-up toes?
Claw hands?
Wasting of distal muscles?
Foot troubles, foot ulcers?
Use of braces?
Foot troubles attributed to "arthritis" or "poliomyelitis (incorrect diagnosis)?"
Difficulty with walking on heels?
Difficulty rising from a kneeled position?

---

9. LAYER 7: WHAT ARE PERTINENT EPIDEMIOLOGIC FACTORS?

Review of epidemiology and establishing disease probability in the context of the specific patient is the final step. The often recited maximum of hoof beats being more likely to be caused by horses than by zebras applies to peripheral neuropathies. Clinicians frequently express premature concern about zebras in the form of rare and unlikely diseases on the initial laboratory evaluation. The fear of "not missing something" overrides good epidemiologic sense. Knowledge about epidemiology patterns and disease probability, and comfort with these issues, comes from the literature on specific types of neuropathies. It is hoped that subsequent chapters in this book will be informative in this regard.

10. SUMMARY

The diagnostic process, in clinical practice, takes many forms. However, there is a core amount of information that is necessary to make an efficient and accurate differential diagnosis. This chapter identifies the major points to be covered during the history and examination. The clinical goal is the correct diagnosis, the art of achieving this goal is in making the process direct and efficient.

REFERENCES

1. The Italian General Practitioner Study Group. Chronic symmetric symptomatic polyneuropathy in the elderly: A field screening investigation in two Italian regions. I. Prevalence and general characteristics of the sample. Neurology 1995; 45:1832–1836.
2. Astroshi I, Gummersson C, Johnsson R, Ornstein E, Ranstam J, Rosén I. Prevalence of carpal tunnel syndrome in a general population. J Am Med Assoc 1999; 282:153–158.
3. Wilbourn A, Aminoff M. AAEM Minimonograph 32: The electrodiagnostic examination in patients with radiculopathies. Muscle Nerve 1998; 21:1612–1631.
4. Barohn R. Approach to peripheral neuropathy and neuronopathy. Semin Neurol 1998; 18:7–18.
5. Brazis P, Masdeu J, Biller J. Localization in Clinical Neurology. Boston: Little, Brown and Company, 1990.
6. Schiffer R. Psychiatric aspects of clinical neurology. Am J Psychiatry 1983; 140:205–207.

7. Task Force on DSM-IV. Diagnostic and Statistical Manual of Mental Disorders. Washington, DC: American Psychiartic Association, 1994.
8. Halloway K, Zerbe K. Simplified approach to somatization disorder. Postgrad Med 2000; 108:89–95.
9. Quebec Task Force on Spinal Disorders. Scientific approach to the assessment and management of activity-related spinal disorders. Spine 1987; 12 (suppl):S1–S54.
10. Jensen M, Brant-Zawadzki M, Obuchowski N, Modic M, Malkasian D, Ross J. Magnetic resonance imaging of the lumbar spine in people without back pain. N Engl J Med 1994; 331:69–71.
11. Tsairis P, Dyck P, Mulder D. Natural history of brachial plexus neuropathy. Arch Neurol 1972; 27:109–117.
12. Barohn R, Sahenk Z, Warmolts J, Mendell J. The Burns-Garland syndrome (diabetic amyotrophy). Revisited 100 years later. Arch Neurol 1991; 48:1130–1135.
13. Le Forestier N, Moulonguet A, Maisonobe T, Léger J-M, Bouche P. True neurogenic thoracic outlet syndrome: Electrophysiological diagnosis in six cases. Muscle Nerve 1998; 21:1129–1134.
14. Lederman R, Wilbourn A. Brachial plexopathy: recurrent cancer or radiation? Neurology 1984; 34:1331–1335.
15. Thomas J, Cascino T, Earle J. Differential diagnosis between radiation and tumor plexopathy of the pelvis. Neurology 1985; 35:1–7.
16. Sabin T. Classification of peripheral neuropathy: the long and the short of it. Muscle Nerve 1986; 9:711–719.
17. McComas A, Sica R, Campbell M, Upton A. Functional compensation in partially denervated muscles. J Neurol Neurosurg Psychiat 1971; 34:453–460.
18. Dyck P, Karnes J, O'Brien P, Zimmerman I. Detection thresholds of cutaneous sensation in humans. In: Dyck P, Thomas P, Lambert E, Bunge R, eds. Peripheral Neuropathy. Vol. 1. Philadelphia: WB Saunders Company, 1984:1103–1136.
19. Litvan I, Mangone C, Werden W et al. Reliability of the NINDS myotatic reflex scale. Neurology 1996; 47:969–972.
20. Denny-Brown D, Pennybacker J. Fibrillation and fasciculation in voluntary muscle. Brain 1938; 61:311–334.
21. Bourque P, Dyck P. Selective calf weakness suggests intraspinal pathology, not peripheral neuropathy. Arch Neurol 1990; 47:79–80.
22. Dyck P, Oviart K, Lambert E. Intensive evaluation of referral unclassified neuropathies yields improved diagnosis. Ann Neurol 1981; 10:222–226.

Laboratory Evaluation of Peripheral Neuropathy

2

Electrodiagnostic Evaluation

Mark B. Bromberg
University of Utah, Salt Lake City, Utah, USA

ABSTRACT

Electrodiagnosis plays a unique role in the evaluation of peripheral nerve disorders. The neurologic history and examination are essential first steps in neurologic localization, while electrodiagnostic testing can accurately determine which elements of the peripheral nervous system are involved, the distribution of involvement, and help delineate underlying pathology. Full use of electrodiagnostic information can narrow the differential diagnosis and lead to rational laboratory testing. This chapter presents an approach to the electrodiagnostic evaluation, using routine nerve conduction and needle EMG testing procedures. Technical issues are pointed out, and the clinically important features and limitations of these tests are discussed. Distinguishing between primary demyelinating and primary axonal neuropathies is discussed in detail. Finally, the electrodiagnostic features of major categories of peripheral nerve lesions are reviewed.

1. INTRODUCTION

The approach to evaluating disorders of peripheral nerves presented in Chapter 1 relies on the electrodiagnostic evaluation for information that cannot be fully obtained from the history and neurologic examination. The two most important components in neuro-diagnostic testing are nerve conduction studies (electroneurography) and needle electro-myography (EMG). Nerve conduction studies provide information on what types of nerves are involved, the distribution and severity of involvement, and the underlying pathology. Needle EMG provides information on motor nerve involvement, including the distribution and severity, and chronicity of the process. This chapter discusses how routine electrodiagnostic tools can be used to achieve these goals. Tests of autonomic fiber function are reviewed in another chapter.

2. APPROACH TO THE ELECTRODIAGNOSTIC EXAMINATION

A structured approach can be applied to electrodiagnosis to answer specific question about the pattern and distribution of nerve involvement and underlying pathology. Nerve conduction and needle EMG studies have the advantage of being conducted in "real time" by the clinician, with flexibility to make changes in testing sequences as data are acquired. Electrodiagnostic evaluations based on set protocols, such as a "peripheral neuropathy protocol," forfeit this advantage. The same diagnosis can result from different approaches, but the danger in following set protocols and analyzing data at the conclusion of the study is that important questions may be not be clearly asked and answered. This limitation may lead to potential bias in interpreting electrodiagnostic findings to fit impressions from the history and neurologic examination. Bias may be reduced by designing the electrodiagnostic study to answer a set of specific questions, but modifying the evaluation as initial results become available.

Questions that can be answered with electrodiagnostic testing include the following: (i) Which elements are involved (sensory nerves, motor nerves, or both)?, (ii) What is the underlying pathology (primary demyelination, primary axonal, or mixture)?, (iii) What is the distribution of nerve damage (single nerve, multiple nerves, length-dependent pattern, plexus, roots, symmetric, or asymmetric)?, and (iv) What is the time course (ongoing or chronic)?

Electrodiagnostic testing can be viewed from two perspectives; as an active process by the person designing and conducting the study or as a passive process by the person reviewing a study performed by someone else. The latter situation can be considered as an exercise in translating a document, from a sequence of testing that may be different than the reader would have chosen, to an order that matches the reader's approach. The reader can impose an order by posing the previous questions and searching the report for data to answer the questions.

3. TECHNICAL ISSUES

Operational principles of nerve conduction and needle EMG studies are well known and discussed elsewhere (1–4), but several points are worth reviewing. Temperature is the most important controlled variable. Limbs should be warm, with temperatures above 31°C. If cool, limbs should be thoroughly warmed with an external heat source. Use of conversion formulae to correct for cool temperatures are less desirable for distal latency and conduction velocity, and do not correct the response amplitude.

Supramaximal nerve stimulation must be obtained (defined as 120% of the current required to achieve a maximal response) to ensure a maximal nerve response, but overstimulation should be avoided because it may lead to activation of adjacent nerves. Attention to placement of stimulation electrodes over the appropriate nerve results in lower currents to achieve maximal responses. Identification of anomalous innervation in the forearm (Martin–Gruber) is essential because it can mimic ulnar nerve conduction block in the forearm.

Optimal placement of the active recording electrode to achieve the highest amplitude compound muscle action potential (CMAP) is important, especially if the amplitude is lower than expected (Fig. 2.1). Determination of the motor point cannot be made from anatomical landmarks and requires trial and error placements to determine which site yields the largest CMAP amplitude (5). Similar concerns apply to placement of recording electrodes for sensory nerve action potentials (SNAP) (6).

4. STATISTICAL ISSUES

Statistical issues are inherent to electrodiagnosis, and include sampling and setting normal values and limits. An appreciation of these issues is essential for accurate interpretation of electrodiagnostic data.

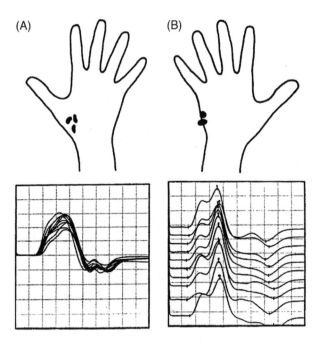

Figure 2.1 Effects of recording electrode placement on CMAP amplitude. (A) Figurine of 10 active electrode positions over thenar eminence and resultant waveforms (superimposed) following stimulation of the median nerve. Lowest CMAP amplitude was 60% of the highest. Note that steep waveform rise time is associated with higher CMAP amplitude. (B) Similar figurine for hypothenar eminence and resultant waveforms (rastered) following stimulation of the ulnar nerve. Lowest CMAP amplitude 71% of highest. Similar influence of active electrode position found for extensor digitorum and abductor hallucis muscles. [Adapted with permission from Bromberg and Spiegelberg (5).]

4.1. Nerve Conduction Limits of Normal

Nerve conduction values are delimited by statistically derived limits of normal, determined from data obtained from "normal" subjects. Few electrodiagnostic laboratories obtain their own normal nerve conduction data. When they do, subjects sampled may come from a variety of clinical backgrounds, and few normal groups represent true random samples from the general population. Common limits used in nerve conduction studies are; (i) lower limits of normal (LLN) for sensory and motor response amplitudes and conduction velocities and (ii) upper limits of normal (ULN) for distal latencies and F- and H-wave latencies. These limits vary somewhat between laboratories, and commonly represent 2–3 standard deviations from normally distributed data or 95% confidence limits from asymmetrical data. It follows that between 1.25% and 2.5% of normal individuals will have values outside (below or above) those statistically defined as normal. The use of standard deviations implies that nerve conduction data are normally distributed, but in fact distributions of many measures are skewed (7). These issues emphasize that LLN and ULN are not true limits of normal, but should be considered as "reference values" that provide information as to the probability that a particular set of nerve conduction values come from healthy or diseased nerves (8).

Erroneous classifications can easily occur. For example, patient height (limb length) is an important variable that influences distal latency, F-wave latency, and conduction velocity values, and should be incorporated in limits of normal for these values (9).

Conduction velocity values vary 3–5 m/s and F-wave latencies vary 6–8 ms over the common height range of 60 in. (~152 cm) to 72 in. (~183 cm) (9). Reporting values as "normal" or "abnormal" may be misleading, and the degree of the abnormality should be considered. A related issue is values just above or below the normal limits may not be the expected value for that individual. Thus, in a patient with normal extensor digitorum muscle bulk and strength, a CMAP value just at the LLN more likely represents suboptimal placement of the recording electrode than pathology because the expected value for a normal subject should be close to the mean value in the distribution. Similarly, in a young diabetic patient, a peroneal motor conduction velocity just above the LLN more likely reflects pathologically slowed conduction rather than normal conduction because the expected velocity should be close to the mean value.

4.2. Collateral Reinnervation

Collateral reinnervation is a compensatory process whereby surviving motor nerve terminals reinnervate denervated muscle fibers. The effect is to preserve both muscle strength and CMAP amplitude until further loss of motor nerve fibers exceeds the capacity of reinnervation to keep up, leading to fall of strength and CMAP amplitude. As a consequence of collateral reinnervation, CMAP amplitude values may remain above the LLN until ~50–80% or more of axons have degenerated, depending on the rate of denervation. Mild degrees of axonal loss occur with normal aging >65 years, affecting the LLN among the very elderly. Needle EMG is the most sensitive indicator of previous and active axonal loss.

4.3. Symmetry of Nerve Conduction Values

The peripheral nervous system can reasonably be considered symmetric, with the expectation that corresponding nerve conduction results from the right and left sides will be of similar value. Assessing for asymmetry can be diagnostically useful. However, practical aspects of nerve conduction studies can lead to some degree of asymmetry of values. Asymmetric limb temperatures can affect side-to-side measures of amplitude distal latency and conduction velocity. Suboptimal placement of recording electrodes can give false asymmetric CMAP amplitude values (5). Accordingly, side-to-side differences need to differ by fairly wide margins before concluding that there is an electrodiagnostically significant degree of axonal loss. Degrees of asymmetry, as encountered on routine nerve conduction studies, have been determined and vary among nerves and for the different measures (Table 2.1) (10).

4.4. Needle EMG Sampling

Needle EMG can answer two basic questions: (i) Is there evidence for denervation? (ii) what is the nature of the denervation? Evidence for denervation is the presence of abnormal spontaneous activity in the form of positive sharp waves and fibrillation potentials. These potentials are very sensitive for motor nerve damage, but cannot distinguish between pathologic causes (neuropathic vs. myopathic). Distinguishing among pathologic causes can be determined by assessment of motor unit action potentials (MUAPs) recorded at low levels of voluntary muscle activation.

Needle EMG samples a limited number of motor units from a much larger pool within a muscle (~10–20%), with a bias to those with low recruitment thresholds. Further, MUAP is limited to the summed activity from 7 to 15 muscle fibers out of a

Table 2.1 Limits of Asymmetry in Normal Nerve Conduction Studies

	Motor nerves				Sensory nerves		
	Median	Ulnar	Peroneal	Tibial	Median	Ulnar	Sural
Amplitude	0.5	0.7	0.2	0.4	0.6	0.5	0.4
Distal latency	1.3	1.3	1.4	1.4	1.2	1.2	1.2
Conduction velocity	0.8	0.9	0.8	0.8	0.8	0.8	0.8
F-wave latency	1.1	1.1	1.1	1.1			

Note: The side with the "worse" values was subtracted from the side with the "better" value. The values were plotted and the table displays 95% confidence limits. For example, for a median nerve, CMAP value on one side should be less than half the value on the other side, or the distal latency >130%, the conduction or the velocity slower than 80%, or the F-wave latency prolonged by >110% to be considered abnormal.
Source: With permission from Bromberg and Jaros (10).

total number of 100–2000 fibers comprising the whole motor unit (11,12). Despite these restrictions, it is possible to distinguish neuropathic MUAPs from myopathic MUAPs by their recruitment pattern and by assessment of their waveforms. This discussion will focus on neuropathic changes.

MUAP duration and area are normally distributed, but MUAP amplitude is skewed toward lower amplitude values (13). During the needle EMG study, the electromyographer is visually and aurally attuned to recognizing outlying motor units that have either high amplitude or greater complexity than normally expected (polyphasia and polyturns). Quantitative EMG studies show that normal muscles may include 10–15% polyphasic motor units (defined as greater than four phases). To strike a balance between overemphasizing isolated findings and missing abnormal motor units, ~20 MUAPs should be assessed in a given muscle (13). Finding one or two high amplitude or complex MUAPs does not necessarily designate a muscle as abnormal. The appropriate question to ask is, "what is the probability that the next motor unit is also large or complex?". If only one in 10 MUAPs is abnormal, the muscle is likely normal. Another test of normality is the presence of abnormal spontaneous activity, and an isolated MUAP abnormality is more often clinically insignificant, provided other abnormalities are absent.

5. NERVE CONDUCTION STUDIES

Nerve conduction studies are most useful for assessing the functional state of myelinated nerves. An understanding of the physiology, pathology, and principles of conduction measurements aids in designing and interpreting electrodiagnostic studies.

5.1. Normal Nerve Conduction

A whole nerve consists of hundreds of myelinated axons whose diameters range from ~7 to 12 μm. Nerve conduction studies are typically performed by percutaneous electrical stimulation of all axons in a nerve and recording the resultant evoked response. Sensory and motor nerves can be studied separately by varying the placement of the recording electrodes. The conduction velocity of a nerve fiber is proportional to its axon diameter, leading to a range of nerve fiber conduction velocities within a nerve, ~35–70 m/s for sensory nerves and ~35–55 m/s for motor nerves (14). For sensory nerves, recording electrodes are placed over the nerve, and the evoked response (SNAP) represents the summed activity of all sensory nerve fiber action potentials. For motor nerves, recording electrodes are placed over the muscle and the evoked response (CMAP) represents the summed activity of all muscle fiber action potentials. Accordingly, the CMAP includes synaptic delays across neuromuscular junctions. Following nerve stimulation, the volley of action potentials propagating down the nerve is led by the fastest conducting fibers. Although the rest of the volley contributes to SNAP or CMAP waveforms, measures of nerve conduction timing (distal latency, conduction velocity, and F- and H-wave latency) focus only on the fastest conducting fibers. In some EMG laboratories, the SNAP distal latency is measured from the negative peak (a hold over from a time when the signal-to-noise ratios of the amplifiers was poor and the onset latency difficult to define) and distal latency will represent conduction of slower conducting fibers. However, sensory nerve conduction velocity measurements are made from waveform onset, and reflect the fastest conducting fibers.

5.2. Temporal Dispersion

Measures reflecting slower conducting fibers in a nerve are less exact, but can be estimated from the waveform duration and shape. SNAP and CMAP waveforms differ in shape for several reasons (Fig. 2.2). Individual sensory nerve fiber action potentials are of low amplitude (microvolts) and short duration ($\sim$1 ms), whereas individual muscle fiber action potentials are of larger amplitude (millivolts) and longer duration ($\sim$4 ms). SNAP and CMAP waveforms represent the summed activity of individual nerve or muscle fiber waveforms, including temporal dispersion of their arrival times. The summation is algebraic. Nerve and muscle fiber action potentials are biphasic, leading to a degree of phase cancellation between positive components of early arriving potentials and negative components from later arriving action potentials. The short waveform duration of sensory nerve fiber action potentials compared with muscle fiber action potentials, leads to a greater degree of phase cancellation within the SNAP than within the CMAP waveforms (Fig. 2.2).

The effect of normal temporal dispersion of nerve fiber action potentials (based on their range of conduction velocities) becomes more evident with increasing conduction distance. This effect can be understood by analogy with the increase in arrival times of runners as race distances increase. For example, the arrival times of runners whose running paces range from 6 to 7 min/mile will be 1 min in a 1-mile race, but increases to 10 min in a 10-mile race. In a similar way, the duration of the negative waveform represents the spread of arrival times of individual action potentials and the duration will normally increase with greater conduction distances. The normal spread of arrival times of nerve action potentials are relatively broad for sensory nerves (25 m/s), but tight for motor nerves (13 m/s) (15). These distributions of arrival times combined with the durations of the sensory nerve and muscle action potentials lead to a greater increase in negative peak duration for SNAP than for CMAP with greater condition distance (Fig. 2.3). The clinical value of negative peak duration measurements is in recognizing when values are abnormally high, reflecting abnormal temporal dispersion.

5.3. Axonal Loss

Axonal loss reduces SNAP and CMAP amplitudes because they represent the summed activity of action potentials. SNAP amplitude is very sensitive to sensory axon loss because there is no compensatory collateral reinnervation. The SNAP originates from $\sim$2000 of the larger diameter nerve fibers ($>$9 μm in diameter) and amplitude falls

Compound Muscle Action Potentials

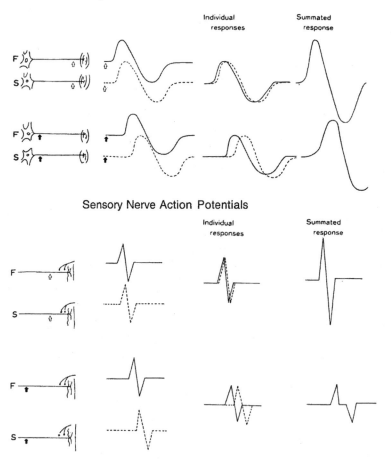

Sensory Nerve Action Potentials

Figure 2.2 Analysis of compound muscle action potential (CMAP) and sensory nerve action potential (SNAP) showing the effect of normal temporal dispersion and phase cancellation. For the CMAP, individual muscle fiber action potentials have relatively long durations (~4 ms) leading to relatively little phase cancellation and little effect on CMAP amplitude with greater conduction distances. For the SNAP, nerve fiber action potentials have relatively short durations (~1 ms) leading to larger degrees of phase cancellation and greater effects on SNAP amplitude with greater conduction distances. [Modified from Kimura et al. (96).]

rapidly with fiber loss (50% amplitude loss with 50% fiber loss) and is unobtainable with surface recording when ~75% of large fibers are lost (16). However, smaller diameter fibers may remain visible on nerve biopsy. CMAP will be insensitive to mild degrees of motor axon loss because of collateral reinnervation. In slowly progressive disorders, >50–80% of motor nerve fibers can be lost before CMAP amplitude falls below LLN (17).

Axonal pathology affects conduction velocity measurements (reflected in distal latency, F-wave latency, and conduction velocity) in proportion to the number of large fibers lost. Empiric data from axonal neuropathies (amyotrophic lateral sclerosis) shows a modest effect: distal latency ≤125% of the ULN, F-wave latency ≤125% of the ULN, and conduction velocity ≥70% of the LLN (18). Surviving axons will conduct at normal velocities and with normal temporal dispersion [Fig. 2.4(B)].

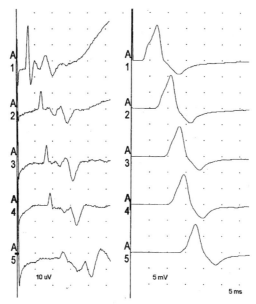

	SNAP		CMAP		
	Negative Peak Amplitude (µV)	Negative Peak Duration (msec)	Negative Peak Amplitude (mV)	Negative Peak Area (mV msec)	Negative Peak Duration (msec)
Wrist	27	1.2	11.2	33.3	5.9
Below Elbow	11	1.4	10.5	32.8	6.2
Above Elbow	10	1.7	9.5	29.2	6.3
Axilla	7	1.5	9.3	28.3	6.2
Erb's Point	4	2.0	8.9	27.1	6.6

Figure 2.3 Normal SNAP and CMAP waveforms for ulnar nerve stimulation at the wrist (A1), below the elbow (A2), above elbow (A3), axilla (A4), and at Erb's point (A5). Note the greater loss of SNAP amplitude than CMAP amplitude over the same distance.

5.4. Conduction Block

Conduction block represents failure of nerve fiber action potentials to conduct beyond a certain point along the axon. This implies that nerve conduction along the fiber is normal on either side of the block. Conduction block can be at a specific site along the nerve (focal conduction block) or at multiple sites along the nerve (multifocal conduction block) [Fig. 2.4(C) and (D)]. Not all fibers in a nerve may be affected (partial vs. complete conduction block). It should be noted that the term "multifocal conduction block" has taken on several different meanings. In the current discussion, it means conduction block in different nerve fibers distributed over the length of the nerve (19). The term has also been used for a specific syndrome, multifocal motor neuropathy, where one or more different nerves in the same patient may have discrete foci of conduction block (20).

Electrodiagnostic features of focal conduction block are normal conduction distal to the block (normal response amplitude), abnormal conduction across the block (reduced response amplitude), and normal conduction proximal to the block (no further reduction of response amplitude) [Fig. 2.4(D)]. The magnitude of these changes will vary depending upon how many fibers in the nerve are blocked, and the ability to demonstrate these features may vary depending upon anatomical access to nerve segments above the block. Electrodiagnostic features of multifocal conduction block are abnormal conduction

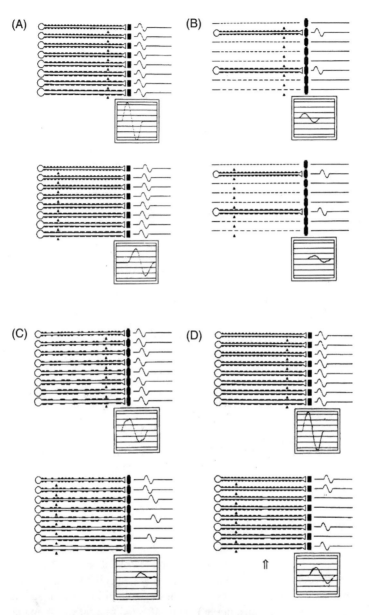

Figure 2.4 Computer simulation models of normal and abnormal motor nerve conduction showing the effects on CMAP waveforms when stimulating at distal (upper traces) and proximal (lower traces) sites along the nerve. (A) Normal nerve showing the effects of normal temporal dispersion on CMAP amplitude. (B) Axonal neuropathy showing loss of CMAP amplitude but normal temporal dispersion. (C) Multifocal slowing and conduction block showing marked CMAP amplitude loss due to conduction block and abnormal temporal dispersion with greater conduction distance. (D) Focal conduction block (at arrow) showing CMAP amplitude loss due to conduction block with normal temporal dispersion. [Modified from Albers and Kelly (38).]

along the nerve (reduced response amplitude) that becomes more marked (greater reduction of response amplitude) with greater conduction distances [Fig. 2.4(C)].

As the principles of the various forms of conduction block are clear, devising electrodiagnostic criteria to distinguish among them is challenging. The goal for focal conduction block is to show a focal loss of response amplitude above the site of block, while the goal for multifocal conduction block is to show an accumulation of nerve conduction abnormalities over longer nerve segments. In practice, the number of blocked fibers in either situation may be small, leading to small changes in response amplitude to stimulation along the nerve. Under these circumstances, issues of good nerve conduction recording technique become particularly important.

5.5. Abnormal Temporal Dispersion

The greatest issue in diagnosing either forms of conduction block relates to determining whether the reductions in response amplitude represent blocked nerve conduction or the effects of abnormal temporal dispersion. Abnormal temporal dispersion will spread out the arrival times of the action potentials that make up the SNAP and CMAP, leading to greater phase cancellation (Fig. 2.5). In model systems, amplitude reductions attributed solely to abnormal temporal dispersion may reach 50% (21). Accordingly, when the amplitude difference between the distal and proximal stimulation sites is <50%, caution must be exercised when attributing the amplitude loss solely to focal conduction block, because some amplitude loss may be due to phase cancellation.

Phase cancellation is more problematic with sensory nerves than motor nerves because of the short duration of individual nerve action potentials (~1 ms) compared

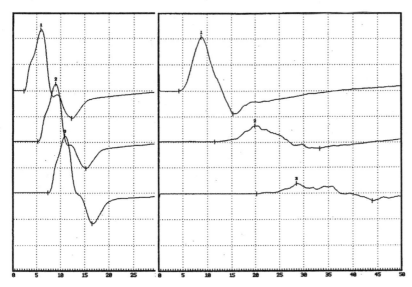

	Normal Conduction			Multifocal Demyelination		
	Negative Peak Amplitude (mV)	Negative Peak Area (mV ms)	Conduction Velocity (m/s)	Negative Peak Amplitude (mV)	Negative Peak Area (mV ms)	Conduction Velocity (m/s)
Wrist	11.8	35.7		4.1	16.8	
Below Elbow	11.2	34.6	60	1.3	8.6	30
Above Elbow	11.2	33.9	57	0.7	6.2	16

Figure 2.5 Motor nerve conduction studies in response to stimulation at the wrist, below the elbow, and above the elbow. Left: Normal change in CMAP waveforms. Right: Abnormal CMAP waveforms with amplitude reduction and abnormal temporal dispersion. CMAP values in table. Display settings: 5 ms/div and 5 mV/div.

with muscle action potentials (~4 ms). This leads to a greater reduction of the SNAP's small amplitude following to stimulation at more proximal sites than with the CMAP (Figs. 2.2 and 2.3). Very small proximal SNAP responses may be difficult to discern from baseline activity. As a consequence, most diagnostic nerve conduction tests for conduction block are carried out in motor nerves. Another reason for focusing on conduction block in motor nerves is that the clinical entity of multifocal motor neuropathy with conduction block is characterized by block of motor but not sensory fibers (20).

A measure of abnormal temporal dispersion is the duration of the negative CMAP waveform. Multifocal demyelination leads to both slowed conduction velocity of individual nerve fibers and conduction block (infinite slowing). With slowed conduction velocities, the arrival times of the action potentials are abnormally dispersed, and the waveform spread out (longer negative peak duration). Assessing conduction over longer distances of the nerve allows for the accumulative effects of multifocal demyelination to be more apparent. An increase in negative peak duration values by >20% supports the presence of abnormal temporal dispersion. Recent efforts to increase the sensitivity of detecting abnormalities of waveform duration have expanded the measurement of duration to include all negative components (phases) of the CMAP waveform (Fig. 2.6) (22).

Negative peak CMAP area is useful because it reflects the number of contributing fibers. Abnormal temporal dispersion leads to a reduction of negative peak amplitude due to phase cancellation, but should not affect negative peak area because the action potentials will eventually contribute to the waveform. In contrast, conduction block will result in fewer fibers contributing to the CMAP waveform, and negative peak area is reduced.

5.6. Electrodiagnostic Criteria

Distinguishing focal conduction block from multifocal conduction block with abnormal temporal dispersion is challenging. Sets of electrodiagnostic criteria have been proposed, but there is no clear consensus. Criteria are based on changes in CMAP amplitude, negative peak duration and negative peak area between distal and proximal stimulation sites. Some sets are complex with definite and probable diagnostic categories, reflecting research criteria. Among demyelinating neuropathies, many forms include combinations of focal conduction block, multifocal conduction block, and abnormal temporal dispersion. What is important diagnostically is recognition of demyelinating pathology. Accordingly, a combination of findings will be encountered more often than focal conduction block alone, and the combined abnormalities can be designated as "abnormal temporal dispersion/conduction block."

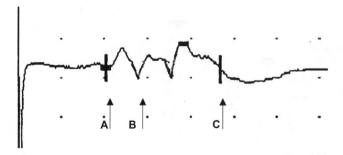

Figure 2.6 Motor nerve conduction studies showing markedly dispersed CMAP waveform. Customary marking of negative peak duration between A and B (4 ms), but more appropriate duration is between A and C (13 ms). Display settings: 5 ms/div and 0.2 mV/div.

Table 2.2 Electrodiagnostic Criteria to Distinguish Focal Conduction Block from Abnormal Temporal Dispersion in Motor Nerves

	CMAP negative peak amplitude	CMAP negative peak area	CMAP negative peak duration
Conduction block	<50%	<50%	≤30%
Conduction block and/or abnormal temporal dispersion	<50%	<50%	>30%
Abnormal temporal dispersion	<50%	>50%	>30%

Note: Percentage values represent proximal CMAP measures expressed as percentage of distal CMAP measures.
Source: From Lange et al. (23).

The principal nerve conduction changes that support focal conduction block at a single site are a reduction in CMAP amplitude and area >50% and a <10% prolongation of the negative peak duration to proximal stimulation (Table 2.2) (23). Multifocal conduction block along the length of a nerve is characterized by abnormal temporal dispersion, and the principal change will be a lesser percentage reductions in CMAP amplitude, a minimal reduction in negative peak area, and a >10% increase in duration to proximal stimulation.

6. NEEDLE EMG

Needle EMG is an adjunct to nerve conduction studies, and provides data on: (1) the presence of motor axon damage, (2) localization of lesions within the peripheral nervous system, and (3) an estimate of the chronicity of motor denervation.

6.1. Presence of Motor Axonal Damage

Motor axon damage may not be apparent from the clinical examination or from CMAP amplitude measures due to the effects of collateral reinnervation. The number of axons that need to be damaged before changes in the clinical examination or CMAP amplitude are apparent varies with the time course of axonal loss. In acute and ongoing disorders, the process of reinnervation will not be able to keep up with the rate of denervation, and clinical and CMAP changes will become apparent relatively early on. In very chronic disorders, the process of reinnervation has sufficient time to reach high capacity, and will be less apparent. An associated clinical factor for peripheral neuropathies is that weakness and atrophy of intrinsic foot muscles will likely escape notice by the patient.

Abnormal spontaneous activity (positive sharp waves and fibrillation potentials) represents discharges of single muscle fibers. These potentials represent muscle fiber membrane hypersensitivity due to denervation, and are very sensitive indicator of denervation. Although the presence of positive waves and fibrillation potentials does not distinguish between neuropathic and myopathic causes, the clinical context usually should be sufficient to distinguish between the two conditions. Other needle EMG findings focus on the MUAP, and in neuropathic conditions findings include reduced MUAP recruitment, increased amplitude, and increased number of phases and turns.

6.2. Localization of Axonal Damage

Nerve conduction studies are most suitable for the study of distal muscles, whereas needle EMG allows assessment of almost any muscle. This combined allows precise localization of axonal damage to nerve roots, the plexus or single nerves.

6.3. Chronicity

Needle EMG also can provide information on the rate of axonal loss. In acute and ongoing processes (recent denervation), fibrillation potentials tend to be large in amplitude (>500 μV). They become smaller as the period between the nerve lesion and the study increases, and may remain of vary small size (<100 μV) indefinitely (24). Accordingly, a pattern of large fibrillation potentials suggests a recent or ongoing process, whereas a pattern of small fibrillation potentials suggests an old or very slowly progressive (chronic) process. Denervated muscle fibers atrophy, and with recent reinnervation, the slower conduction velocity of small diameter muscle fibers contribute to the complexity of MUAPs (polyphasia and polyturns) (25). With time, reinnervated muscle fibers increase in diameter and motor units become simplified (fewer phases and turns) because of greater temporal dispersion of action potentials making up MUAPs. In static conditions, or slowly progressive conditions, motor unit recruitment will be reduced, MUAP amplitude will be high, but waveforms will be relatively simple (26).

7. APPROACH TO THE ELECTRODIAGNOSTIC EVALUATION, CONTINUED

The history and examination should lead to a close localization of peripheral nerve lesions. At this stage, refinement in localization and distribution, and determination of pathology and chronicity can be made with electrodiagnostic testing. The following sections review the general electrodiagnostic features of major classes of peripheral nerve lesions.

8. DEMYELINATING POLYNEUROPATHIES

Much has been written about the diagnostic distinction between primary demyelinating and primary axonal neuropathies. Identifying demyelinating pathology can be difficult, particularly with chronic neuropathies. Nerve biopsy is invasive and is not sensitive for primary demyelination, and electrodiagnostic testing, in particular nerve conduction studies, is the most useful diagnostic tool (27). Sets of nerve conduction criteria have been proposed to distinguish primary demyelinaiton, but even with acute inflammatory demyelinating polyradiculoneuropathy (AIDP), whose unique time course helps narrow the differential diagnosis, only 50% fulfilled criteria when studied within the first two weeks of symptoms (see following sections). The diagnosis of chronic demyelinating neuropathies has become more challenging as the clinical spectrum of these neuropathies has expanded (28–30). Classic chronic inflammatory demyelinating polyradiculoneuropathy (CIDP) is characterized by symmetric, proximal, and distal motor and sensory nerve involvement (31), but other forms of chronic demyelinating neuropathies are distinguished, including those with predominant distal nerve involvement (32), asymmetric nerve involvement (33), predominant sensory nerve involvement (34), predominant cranial nerve involvement (35), or focal motor nerve conduction block with and without sensory nerve involvement (20,36).

8.1. Electrodiagnostic Criteria for Demyelination

AIDP and CIDP are the most common examples of multifocal demyelinating polyneuropathies. Findings on motor nerve conduction studies supportive of demyelinating neuropathies include the following: (i) slowed conduction demonstrated by substantially prolonged distal latencies, reduced conduction velocities, and prolonged F- and H-wave latencies; (ii) greater degree of phase cancellation demonstrated by reduced CMAP amplitudes to stimulation at progressively more proximal stimulation sites with prolonged negative peak durations; and (iii) sites of focal conduction block (away from common entrapment sites) demonstrated by reduced CMAP amplitude to stimulation proximal to the block with no prolongation of the negative peak duration.

The probability of detecting these abnormalities increases if more nerves and longer lengths of nerve are studied. Long ulnar nerve segments can be assessed by stimulation in the axilla, but caution must be exercised with proximal stimulation of the median nerve because of the proximity of median and ulnar innervated thenar muscles. Therefore, care must be taken to prevent activation of the ulnar nerve caused by the close proximity of the two nerves in the axilla and Erb's point. Nerve root stimulation is technically difficult using percutaneous stimulation because of the need for high stimulation intensities, but needle stimulation can be used. In addition, to the commonly studied nerves (peroneal, tibial, ulnar, and median) can be added the musculocutaneous nerve if there is proximal weakness, and cranial nerves (blink reflex) if there is facial weakness. Secondary axonal damage also occurs with demyelinating pathology and needle EMG abnormalities are common in AIDP and CIDP (27,37).

Determining the magnitude of conduction slowing and phase cancellation necessary to distinguish primary demyelinating pathology from primary axonal pathology are the main issues. Empiric data from amyotrophic lateral sclerosis (pure axonal neuropathy) indicate limits due to loss of large diameter nerve fibers (18). Sets of electrodiagnostic criteria have been designed around these limits to aid in the diagnosis of AIDP (37–42) and CIDP (27,38,43–45). The sets of criteria differ in the limiting values and minimum number of nerves required to be abnormal.

Perhaps the most useful approach to diagnosing demyelinating neuropathies is to appreciate the underlying pathologic changes on nerve conduction, as reviewed earlier. It is not clear that one set of criteria for AIDP or CIDP is more sensitive than another. A basic set of electrodiagnostic criteria is offered for AIDP and CIDIP (Table 2.3). Whether a patient fulfills all criteria is less important than having an index of suspicion based on one or more abnormal responses (30). The electrodiagnostic features for major clinical examples of demyelinating neuropathies will be reviewed.

8.2. Electrodiagnostic Criteria for AIDP

Electrodiagnostic sensitivity for AIDP is dependent upon disease severity and when in the time course the studies are performed. A retrospective review of several sets of criteria reveals the following. For the initial electrodiagnostic test, sensitivities among the sets range from 37% to 72% (46). For serial studies, eventually 85% of patients fulfill criteria at an average of 3 weeks from symptom onset (37). The acute time course of AIDP is helpful in narrowing the differential diagnosis, and when the diagnosis is not clear, repeat nerve conduction studies are helpful in establishing the diagnosis.

8.3. Electrodiagnostic Criteria for CIDP

The range of disease severity and varied time points when studies are performed affect the sensitivity and specificity of electrodiagnostic criteria for chronic demyelinating neuropathies. In retrospective reviews of several sets of criteria, only 43–52% of patients with clinical CIDP fulfill strict electrodiagnostic criteria (44,47). Specificity for CIDP among

Table 2.3 Simplified Electrodiagnostic Criteria to Distinguish Primary Demyelinating Multifocal
Pathology from Primary Axonal Pathology in Motor Nerves

	Electrodiagnostic evidence supportive of primary demyelinating neuropathy	Electrodiagnostic evidence supportive of primary axonal neuropathy
Distal CMAP amplitude	Mild to moderate reduction	Normal to moderate reduction
Conduction block	Present (proximal-to-distal CMAP amplitude ratio <0.50)	Absent (proximal-to-distal CMAP amplitude ratio >0.50)
Temporal dispersion	Abnormal (proximal-to-distal CMAP negative duration ratio <0.75)	Normal (proximal-to-distal CMAP negative duration >0.75)
	Abnormal (distal negative CMAP duration >9 ms)	Normal (distal negative CMAP duration <9 ms)
Distal latency	Moderately to markedly prolonged (>125% ULN)	Normal to mildly prolonged (<125% ULN)
Conduction velocity	Moderately to markedly slowed (<75% LLN)	Normal to mildly slowed (>75% LLN)
F-wave latency	Moderately to markedly prolonged (>125% ULN)	Normal to mildly prolonged (<125% ULN)
Needle EMG	Mild to moderate denervation	Mild to severe denervation

other chronic polyneuropathies has been assessed by applying criteria to data from patients with diabetic polyneuropathy (mixed demyelination and axonal pathologies) and amyotrophic lateral sclerosis (pure axonal pathology), ranging from 91% to 100% (44,47). Modifications to the limiting values increases sensitivity for CIDP, but also reduces specificity because there is a considerable overlap in distal latencies, conduction velocities, and degree of phase cancellation among different forms of neuropathy (47). Measurement of the total duration of the negative distal CMAP waveform has been added to the criteria, leading to an increase in sensitivity for CIDP (Fig. 2.6) (44).

8.4. Sensory Nerve Conduction Studies in Demyelinating Neuropathies

Sensory nerve studies are less useful than motor nerve studies because responses are frequently absent, which do not distinguish between primary demyelination and axonal loss. However, a pattern of an abnormal median is more common in demyelinating neuropathies (39% in AIDP and in 28% in CIDP) than in mixed demyelinating and axonal neuropathies (14–23% in diabetic neuropathy) or axonal neuropathies (22% in amyotrophic lateral sclerosis) (37,48). The extreme pattern of an absent median sensory and present sural response was seen only in AIDP and CIDP patients. The preserved sural response is explained by the recording electrode arrangement for the sural nerve being more proximal along the nerve relative to ring recording electrodes over the digital branches of the median nerve (48).

9. AXONAL POLYNEUROPATHIES

Primary axonal neuropathies are common and generally follow a length dependent pattern (49). Findings expected on nerve conduction studies for axonal loss include the following: (i) reduced or absent motor and sensory responses, (ii) minimally slowed conduction, and (iii) evidence for neuropathic denervation on needle EMG (50). Abnormalities will be more severe in lower extremities, with SNAP responses more affected than CMAP responses (due to collateral reinnervation). Axonal loss may be severe, but will have a modest effect on nerve conduction velocity (Table 2.3). The pattern of an abnormal median sensory and normal sural response observed in demyelinating neuropathies is less frequently observed in primary axonal neuropathies due to the greater degree of lower extremity involvement (48). Needle EMG findings include abnormal spontaneous activity (positive waves and fibrillation potentials) and MUAPs show reduced recruitment and increased amplitude. The degree and extent of abnormalities will vary with the chronicity of the neuropathy.

10. MIXED AXONAL AND DEMYELINATING POLYNEUROPATHIES

CIDP will include secondary axonal loss, leading to reduced or absent CMAP responses and needle EMG abnormalities that can make the identification of demyelination difficult. Diabetes mellitus is the most common cause of distal symmetric polyneuropathies with mixed axonal and demyelinating features (51). Several other types of neuropathy can occur in the setting of diabetes mellitus, including polyradiculopathies, plexopathies, and CIDP (see following sections), complicating the electrodiagnostic interpretation (52). Clinically, the degree of neuropathy may bear no relation to the degree of glucose control or the duration of recognized diabetes (53,54).

10.1. Distal Diabetic Neuropathy

In some forms of primary sensory diabetic neuropathy, nerve conduction studies may be normal. With more severe diabetic neuropathies, sensory nerve studies show early involvement in the lower extremities with reduced SNAP amplitude, and some degree of slow conduction or absent responses, when severe (55). Motor nerve studies show mild to moderately slowed conduction velocities that are greater than can be attributed to axonal loss, suggesting a component of demyelination (51,55). F-wave latency prolongation may be an early finding (56). CMAP amplitude is less affected due to collateral reinnervation. However, the needle EMG shows evidence of denervation with abnormal spontaneous activity (positive waves and fibrillation potentials) and motor units with reduced recruitment, increased amplitude and greater complexity. Neurogenic findings occur in proportion to the severity of the neuropathy, with more prominent findings in distal than in proximal lower extremity muscles (52).

10.2. CIDP and Distal Diabetic Neuropathy

CIDP can occur in the setting of diabetes mellitus (both types I and II) (57,58), and diabetes may be a predisposing factor in the development of CIDP (59). Clinical features that lead to consideration of CIDP include rapid loss of strength in both upper and lower extremities, and greater proximal than distal weakness (59). Nerve conduction data from diabetic patients who developed CIDP indicate prolonged distal and F-wave latencies, slowed conduction, abnormal temporal dispersion, and conduction block that fulfill electrodiagnostic criteria (Table 2.3) (59). Responses to immunomodulating drugs provides clinical support for concurrent CIDP and diabetic neuropathies (57,58,60).

11. SMALL FIBER NEUROPATHIES

Small fiber neuropathies are clinically defined by symptoms of painful paresthesias in a
distal distribution (61,62). Sensory and motor responses in the legs are frequently
normal, and when abnormal, sensory responses are reduced or absent (63). The diagnosis
of small fiber involvement is confirmed by nerve biopsy showing reduced numbers of
unmyelinated fibers, or by skin biopsy showing reduced intraepidermal nerve fiber
density (discussed further in chapters 5 and 6). Among patients with no abnormalities
on electrodiagnostic testing or skin biopsy, other lesions localized to the central
nervous system such as multiple sclerosis have been identified (63).

12. FOCAL CONDUCTION BLOCK NEUROPATHIES

The term multifocal motor neuropathy with conduction block focuses on the clinical entity
of a primary motor neuropathy with foci of marked focal conduction block away from sites
of entrapment, suggesting multiple mononeuropathies (20). Electrodiagnostic studies
reveal conduction block over short nerve segments, as defined and discussed above
(Table 2.2). However, CMAP waveforms may show both focal conduction block, abnormal temporal dispersion (prolonged negative peak duration) and slowed conduction (prolonged distal and F-wave latencies) (Fig. 2.7) (64,65). There is predilection among nerves
for conduction block; ulnar > median > tibial > peroneal nerves (65). Although many
patients exhibit focal conduction block in limb nerve segments, a number have conduction
block at very proximal sites (plexus and root), and some may have the clinical features of
this type of neuropathy but no demonstrable block (66). Many, but not all, patients have

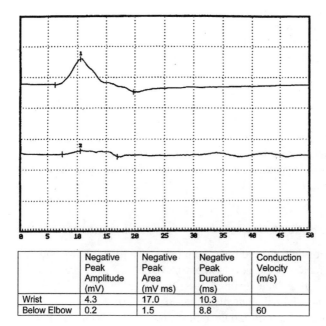

	Negative Peak Amplitude (mV)	Negative Peak Area (mV ms)	Negative Peak Duration (ms)	Conduction Velocity (m/s)
Wrist	4.3	17.0	10.3	
Below Elbow	0.2	1.5	8.8	60

Figure 2.7 Motor nerve conduction study showing focal conduction block across a 100 mm
segment with marked reduction of CMAP amplitude and area. CMAP values in table. Display
settings: 5 ms/div and 5 mV/div.

normal sensory nerve conduction across the segments of focal motor nerve conduction block (67).

13. HEREDITARY NEUROPATHIES

Hereditary neuropathies, from the electrodiagnostic perspective, represent a spectrum of neuropathic processes (68,69). They may be named by one of the two nomenclature systems; by the type of nerves involved (hereditary motor sensory neuropathies—HMSN) or by genetic mutations (Charcot–Marie–Tooth neuropathies—CMT). Each system has subtypes (1A, 1B, etc.; 2A, 2B, etc.). This discussion will focus on the more common hereditary neuropathies, with recognition that there are examples involving other combinations of nerves (sensory and autonomic nerves—HSN and HSAN).

13.1. CMT Types 1 and 2

Electrodiagnosis has a prominent historic role in dividing hereditary neuropathies into two broad types. Type 1 is traditionally characterized by slowed motor conduction velocities (empirically <38 m/s), and type 2 by normal or mildly slowed motor conduction velocities (>38 m/s) in legs and arms (70,71). Although type 1 is designated as demyelinating and type 2 as axonal, axonal loss occurs in both types and is responsible for clinical weakness (72). Accordingly, for both CMT types 1 and 2, SNAP and CMAP amplitudes in the legs will be reduced or absent, depending upon severity. Few needle EMG studies are reported, most patients show evidence for chronic and slowly progressive axonal loss indicated by abnormal spontaneous activity (positive waves and fibrillation potentials) and MUAPs with markedly reduced recruitment and very high amplitudes but with relatively simple waveforms.

Further division of CMT neuropathies into different genotypes has led to an appreciation for a spectrum of nerve conduction patterns. CMT1A, the most common form of hereditary neuropathy, is characterized by slowed conduction with normal temporal dispersion (Fig. 2.8) (73). However, there is overlap in electrodiagnostic features (conduction velocities) among the different mutations in CMT1 and 2 (68,69).

13.2. CMT-X

Nerve conduction velocities in affected males with X-linked CMT display a range of values, and some degree of slowing may be present in female carriers (74–76). Because a family history may not be appreciated, CMT-X should be included in the differential diagnosis of CIDP.

13.3. Hereditary Neuropathy with Predisposition to Pressure Palsies

This neuropathy is characterized electrodiagnostically by focal nerve conduction slowing and conduction block at common sites of entrapment (most common at the elbow) (77,78). Distal motor latencies are prolonged (median and peroneal > ulnar and tibial nerves) in the setting of normal or near normal conduction velocities and normal CMAP amplitudes. Sensory nerve studies show distal slowing or absent responses. These findings are often clinically unsuspected and are found during nerve conduction studies for focal neurologic symptoms.

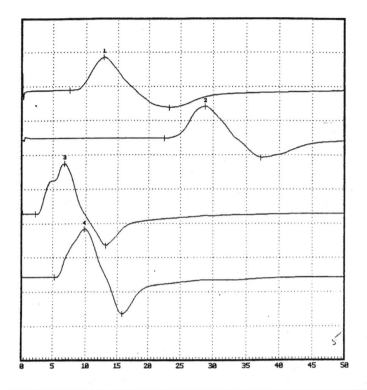

	CMT1A			Normal Conduction		
	Negative Peak Amplitude (mV)	Negative Peak Area (mV ms)	Conduction Velocity (m/s)	Negative Peak Amplitude (mV)	Negative Peak Area (mV ms)	Conduction Velocity (m/s)
Wrist	5.1	23.3		7.5	30.3	
Below Elbow	5.0	22.8	18	7.4	30.0	52

Figure 2.8 Motor nerve conduction studies in response to stimulation at the wrist and elbow. Top: Patient with CMT type 1A showing slowed conduction velocity with normal temporal dispersion. Bottom: Normal conduction velocity with normal temporal dispersion. CMAP values in table. Display settings: 5 ms/div and 5 mV/div.

13.4. Electrodiagnostic Approach to Hereditary Neuropathies

The growing complexity of hereditary neuropathies raises new challenges in both clinical diagnosis and electrodiagnosis (68). A family history may not be apparent. Type 1 is the most common hereditary neuropathy, and slowed conduction velocities (<38 m/s) without evidence for temporal dispersion (Fig. 2.8) is a strong clue that the neuropathy is not acquired. CMT-X includes mildly slowed conduction velocities with or without abnormal temporal dispersion, and should be considered along with CIDP. HNPP is also common, and is characterized by prolonged distal latencies with focal slowing with or without conduction block at common sites of entrapment. Needle EMG findings in all forms of CMT include reduced recruitment, very high amplitude but simple MUAP waveforms (chronic denervation). Chronic denervation may be the only clue to a very long-standing (hereditary) neuropathy. The most useful diagnostic procedure, when considering a hereditary neuropathy, is clinical and electrodiagnostic examination of other family members. Within a family with recognized CMT, only 20% of affected people seek medical attention for symptoms of their neuropathy (79). Finally, it is not possible to confidently exclude a hereditary neuropathy in the setting of a chronic peripheral neuropathy whose cause is unknown (69).

14. MONONEUROPATHIES

Mononeuropathies may be caused by focal pressure (entrapment and pressure neuropathy), trauma, tumor, or focal vascular compromise (ischemic neuropathy). Spontaneous entrapment syndromes along the course of nerves in the upper extremities occur but are very rare (80). Mononeuropathies due to ischemia can occur from vascular occulusion of vessels of all sizes (81). In the setting of small vessel vasculitis, several nerves may be involved in the form of mononeuritis multiplex.

14.1. Focal Entrapment Neuropathies

Entrapment neuropathies first affect myelin with redundancy of myelin layers and remyelination, and if prolonged, damage axons (82). Electrodiagnostic changes due to altered myelination are slowed or blocked conduction across entrapment site and normal conduction on either side of the site. This criterion may not be achievable for some entrapment sites do to limitations of access to stimulation sites. An alternative approach is demonstration of normal conduction in a neighboring nerve, or in comparison with the contralateral nerve. Sensory nerve studies may be more sensitive indicators of focal compression than motor nerve studies. Axonal damage is assessed by needle EMG showing abnormal spontaneous activity (positive waves and fibrillation potentials) and MUAP recruitment (reduced) and configuration (high amplitude).

14.2. Ischemic Neuropathies

Ischemic neuropathies due to vasculitis of small vessels that perfuse nerves cause axonal damage of varying degrees (81). Electrodiagnostic changes in ischemic mononeuropatheis and mononeuritis multiplex include reduced or absent sensory and motor responses. However, for 1–2 days after acute onset, the nerve segment distal to the lesion site will remain viable, and stimulation of the nerve distal to the site produces a normal response, while stimulation proximal to the site is abnormal, suggesting a focal conduction block (83). Needle EMG will show axonal pathology with abnormal spontaneous activity (positive waves and fibrillation potentials) and MUAPs with reduced recruitment and complexity (81). The needle EMG examination can be used to define the nerve distribution (mononeuropathy or mononeuropathy multiplex). Ischemic neuropathies are typically asymmetric, and side-to-side comparisons may be helpful. On occasion, the presence of a confluent mononeuritis multiples may mimic a diffuse, symmetric peripheral neuropathy.

15. PLEXOPATHIES

Diagnosing plexopathies is challenging because of the complex nerve anatomy and the varied pathologic causes. Discrete lesions affecting one plexus element are less common than diffuse lesions, making precise localization within the plexus difficult. Plexus lesions can mimic nerve root lesions, and vice versa, and traumatic injuries can produce both. MR imaging studies, especially neurography, can help localize the lesion in many situations. The underlying pathology causing plexopathies is most commonly axonal, although traction injuries and lesions involving pressure from a mass may include an element of conduction block (84).

Nerve conduction studies are of limited utility in localizing proximal lesions and stimulation at Erb's point assesses only the distal portion of the brachial plexus. The one exception is that sensory nerve conduction studies are the only study capable of localizing the lesion to the peripheral nervous system. Routine sensory nerve studies may show reduced or absent responses, and severe lesions may reduce CMAP amplitude with minimal slowing of conduction velocity. F-wave studies provide limited information on demyelinating pathology because rapidly conducting fibers are frequently spared and latencies are normal (84). A number of special sensory nerve conduction tests can be helpful in brachial plexopathies (85). Needle EMG is more useful and will show axonal damage with abnormal spontaneous activity (positive waves and fibrillation potentials) and MUAPs with reduced recruitment, increased amplitude, and greater complexity. The pattern of muscle involvement will be diagnostic, but distinguishing between radiculopathy and plexopathy can be difficult if sensory responses are normal because paraspinal muscle abnormalities are not always found in chronic radiculopathies (84).

Myokymic discharges occur in a number of clinical situations, but in the setting of a plexopathy in a patient with a history of radiation treatment that included the plexus, they are strongly associated with a radiation-induced plexopathy as opposed to direct infiltration of malignant cells (86,87).

16. RADICULOPATHIES

Nerve root compression from acute disk herniation may cause focal conduction block or axonal damage at the site of herniation. Focal block or slowing of motor nerve fibers could lead to prolongation of the F-wave latency, but small changes are more often than not diluted by long segments of normal nerve. H-waves are unique in their ability to assess proximal portions of both sensory and motor nerve fibers, but H-wave testing is practically restricted to S1 roots and experience in S1 radiculopathies indicates that they are inconsistent in their diagnostic utility because many rootlets make up the root and as long as any are uninvolved, the H-wave remains normal (88). Sensory nerve fibers may be more vulnerable to damage than motor fibers, but preganglionic root lesions will not affect the post ganglionic segment that is studied with routine sensory nerve conduction studies.

Needle EMG is diagnostically useful in the evaluation of suspected radiculopathy by its ability to sample many muscles and its sensitivity to mild degrees of denervation (88). However, there may be no electrodiagnostic evidence of denervation because root compression may affect sensory fibers to cause pain but not motor fibers. Most muscles, including paraspinal muscles, receive innervation from several roots, and the effect of axonal damage from one root may be mild and difficult to detect. Diagnosis of radiculopathy is based on finding neurogenic changes in several muscles innervated by the suspected root and excluding involvement of muscles innervated by one nerve. This may require sampling a large number of muscles and some root levels may be difficult to define (88,89). There may also be individual variation in the level of innervation (pre- or post fixed plexes) (90,91).

Needle EMG abnormalities vary with severity and duration of root damage, and abnormalities are more frequent in posterior myotomes (paraspinal muscles) than anterior myotomes (limb muscles) (92). Abnormal spontaneous activity (positive waves and fibrillation potentials) may be the only abnormality in a third of patients with known radiculopathy, and with more severe axonal damage, there are increased proportions of complex (polyphasic) MUAPs, followed by decreased recruitment. With acute radiculopathies, a centrifugal pattern of EMG abnormalities followed by a similar pattern of resolution of EMG abnormalities will be observed (88).

Paraspinal muscle abnormalities can separate radiculopathy from plexopathy. Superficial paraspinal muscles receive innervation from multiple levels, but the deep multifidus layer has single level innervation (93). Examination protocols have been developed for reproducible mapping of lumbosacral paraspinal muscles (94). In postsurgical paraspinal muscles, needle EMG study is informative for a new process when performed 3 months after surgery (to allow time for muscle fiber injury from retractor damage to resolve), when the electrode is 3 cm lateral to the scar, and is in the deeper portions of the muscles (3–5 cm deep) (95).

17. CONCLUSIONS

The goal of this chapter is to present an overview of the efficient use of routine electrodiagnostic testing for peripheral nerve disorders. The review has focused on an orderly approach designed to ask specific questions that may not be fully answered from the history and neurologic examination. At the conclusion of the electrodiagnostic study, the characterization of the nerve injury should be complete leading to a reasonable differential diagnosis and a rational selection of further laboratory tests. Other chapters will provide detailed clinical and electrodiagnostic information on specific neuropathies.

REFERENCES

1. Dumitru D, Amato A, Zwarts M. Electrodiagnostic Medicine. Philadelphia: Hanley and Belfus, Inc, 2002.
2. Kimura J. Electrodiagnosis in Diseases of Nerve and Muscle: Principles and Practice. Philadelphia: FA Davis Company, 2001.
3. Preston D, Shapiro B. Electromyography and Neuromuscular Disorders. Boston: Butterworth-Heinemann, 1998.
4. Oh S. Clinical Electromyography. Nerve Conduction Studies. Philadelphia: Lippincott Williams & Wilkins, 2003.
5. Bromberg M, Spiegelberg T. The influence of active electrode placement on CMAP amplitude. Electroencephalogr Clin Neurophysiol 1997; 105:385–389.
6. Raynor E, Preston D, Logigian E. Influence of surface recording electrode placement on nerve action potentials. Muscle Nerve 1997; 20:361–363.
7. Robinson L, Temkin N, Fujimoto W, Stolov W. Effects of statistical methodology on normal limits in nerve conduction studies. Muscle Nerve 1991; 14:1084–1090.
8. Campbell W, Robinson L. Deriving reference values in electrodiagnostic medicine. Muscle Nerve 1993; 16:424–428.
9. Rivner M, Swift T, Crout B, Rhodes K. Towards more rational nerve conduction interpretations: the effect of height. Muscle Nerve 1990; 13:232–239.
10. Bromberg M, Jaros L. Symmetry of normal motor and sensory nerve conduction measurement. Muscle Nerve 1998; 21:498–503.
11. Thiele B, Böhle A. Anzahl der Spike-Komponenten im Motor-Unit Potential. Zeit EEG-EMG 1978; 9:125–130.

12. Feinstein B, Lindegård B, Nyman E, Wohlfart G. Morphologic studies of motor units in normal human muscle. Acta Anat 1955; 23:127–143.
13. Engstrom J, Olney R. Quantitative motor unit analysis: The effect of sample size. Muscle Nerve 1992; 15:277–281.
14. Dorfman L. The distribution of conduction velocities (DCV) in peripheral nerves: a review. Muscle Nerve 1984; 7:2–11.
15. Olney R, Budingen H, Miller R. The effect of temporal dispersionon compound action potential area in human peripheral nerve. Muscle Nerve 1987; 10:728–733.
16. Rosenfalck A. Early recognition of nerve disorders by near-nerve recording of sensory action potentials. Muscle Nerve 1978; 1:360–367.
17. Carleton S, Brown W. Changes in motor unit populations in motor neurone disease. J Neurol Neurosurg Psychiat 1979; 42:42–51.
18. Cornblath D, Kuncl R, Mellits E et al. Nerve conduction studies in amyotrophic lateral sclerosis. Muscle Nerve 1992; 15:1111–1115.
19. van der Meché F, Meulstee J. Guillain–Barré syndrome: A model of random conduction block. J Neurol Neurosurg Psychiat 1988; 51:1158–1163.
20. Pestronk A, Cornblath D, Ilyas A et al. A treatable multifocal motor neuropathy with antibodies to GM1 ganglioside. Neurology 1988; 24:73–78.
21. Rhee E, England J, Sumner A. A computer simulation of conduction block: effects produced by actual block versus interphase cancellation. Ann Neurol 1990; 28:146–156.
22. Uncini A, Di Muzio A, Sabatelli M, Magi S, Tonali P, Gambi D. Sensitivity and specificity of diagnostic criteria for conduction block in chronic inflammatory demyelinating polyneuropathy. Electroencephalogr Clin Neurophysiol 1993; 89:161–169.
23. Lange D, Trojaborg W, Latov N et al. Multifocal motor neuropathy with conduction block: is it a distinct clinical entity? Neurology 1992; 42:497–505.
24. Kraft G. Fibrillation potential amplitude and muscle atrophy following peripheral nerve injury. Muscle Nerve 1990; 13:814–821.
25. Borenstein S, Desmedt J. Range of variations in motor unit potentials during reinnervation after traumatic nerve lesions in humans. Ann Neurol 1980; 8:460–467.
26. Zalewska E, Rowinska-Marcinska K, Hausmanowa-Petrusewicz I. Shape irregularity of motor unit potentials in some neuromuscular disorders. Muscle Nerve 1998; 21:1181–1187.
27. Barohn R, Kissel J, Warmolts J, Mendell J. Chronic inflammatory demyelinating polyradiculoneuropathy. Arch Neurol 1989; 46:878–884.
28. Parry G. Are multifocal motor neuropathy and Lewis–Sumner syndrome distinct nosologic entities? Muscle Nerve 1999; 22:557–559.
29. Lewis R. Multifocal motor neuropathy and Lewis–Sumner syndrome. Two distinct entities. Muscle Nerve 1999; 22:1738–1739.
30. Latov N. Diagnosis of CIDP. Neurology 2002; 59(suppl 6):S2–S6.
31. Dyck P, Lais A, Ohta M, Bastron J, Okazaki H, Groover R. Chronic inflammatory polyradiculoneuropathy. Mayo Clin Proc 1975; 50:621–636.
32. Katz J, Saperstein D, Gronseth G, Amato A, Barohn R. Distal acquired demyelinating symmetric neuropathy. Neurology 2000; 54:615–620.
33. Thomas P, Claus D, Jaspert A et al. Focal upper limb demyelinating neuropahty. Brain 1996; 119:765–774.
34. Oh S, Joy J, Kuruoglu R. Chronic sensory demyelinating neuropthy: chronic inflammatory demyelinating polyneuropathy presenting as a pure sensory neuropathy. J Neurol Neurosurg Psychiatry 1992; 55:677–680.
35. Rotta F, Sussman A, Bradley W, Ayyar D, Sharma K, Shebert R. The spectrum of chronic inflammatory demyelinating polyneuropathy. J Neurol Sci 2000; 173:129–139.
36. Saperstein D, Amato A, Wolfe G et al. Multifocal acquired demyelinating sensory and motor neuropathy: the Lewis–Sumner syndrome. Muscle Nerve 1999; 22:560–566.
37. Albers J, Donofrio P, McGonagle T. Sequential electrodiagnostic abnormalities in acute inflammatory demyelinating polyradiculoneuropathy. Muscle Nerve 1985; 8:528–539.
38. Albers J, Kelly J. Acquired inflammatory demyelinating polyneuropathies: clinical and electrodiagnostic features. Muscle Nerve 1989; 12:435–451.

39. Cornblath D. Electrophysiology in Guillain–Barré syndrome. Ann Neurol 1990; 27(suppl):S17–S20.

40. Ho R, Mishu B, Li C et al. Guillain–Barré syndrome in northern China. Relationship to Campylobacter jejuni infection and anti-glycolipid antibodies. Brain 1995; 118:597–605.

41. Meulstee J, Meché vd, Group DG-BS. Electrodiagnostic criteria for polyneuropathy and demyelination: application in 135 patients with Guillain–Barré syndrome. J Neurol Neurosurg Psychiatry 1995; 59:482–486.

42. The Italian Guillain–Barré Study Group. The prognosis and main prognostic indicators of Guillain–Barré syndrome. A multicentre prospective study of 297 patients. Brain 1996; 119:2053–2061.

43. Ad Hoc Subcommittee of the American Academy of Neurology ATF. Research criteria for diagnosis of chronic inflammatory demyelinating polyneuropathy (CIDP). Neurology 1991; 41:617–618.

44. Thaisetthawatkuo P, Logigian E, Herrmann D. Dispersion of the distal compound muscle action potential as a diagnostic criterion for chronic inflammatory demyelinating polyneuropathy. Neurology 2002; 59:1526–1532.

45. Nicolas G, Maisonobe T, Le Forestier N, Léger J-M, Bouche P. Proposed revised electrophysiological criteria for chronic inflammatory demyelinating polyradiculoneuropathy. Muscle Nerve 2002; 25:26–30.

46. Alam T, Chaudhry V, Cornblath D. Electrophysiological studies in the Guillain–Barré syndrome: distinguishing subtypes by published criteria. Muscle Nerve 1998; 21:1275–1279.

47. Bromberg M. Comparison of electrodiagnostic criteria for primary demyelination in chronic polyneuropathy. Muscle Nerve 1991; 14:968–976.

48. Bromberg M, Albers J. Patterns of sensory nerve conduction abnormalities in demyelinating and axonal peripheral nerve disorders. Muscle Nerve 1993; 16:262–266.

49. Sabin T. Classification of peripheral neuropathy: the long and the short of it. Muscle Nerve 1986; 9:711–719.

50. Donofrio P, Albers J. AAEM minimonograph no.34: polyneuropathy: classification by nerve conduction studies and electromyography. Muscle Nerve 1990; 13:889–903.

51. Herrmann D, Ferguson M, Logigian E. Conduction slowing in diabetic distal polyneuropathy. Muscle Nerve 2002; 26:232–237.

52. Wilbourn A. Diabetic neuropathies. In: Brown W, Bolton C, eds. Clinical Electromyography. Boston: Butterworth-Heinemann, 1993:477–515.

53. Said G, Goulon-Goeau C, Slama G, Tchobroutsky G. Severe early-onset polyneuropathy in insulin-dependent diabetes mellitus: a clinical and pathological study. N Engl J Med 1992; 326:1257–1263.

54. Said G, Bigo A, Améri A et al. Uncommon early-onset neuropathy in diabetic patients. J Neurol 1998; 245:61–68.

55. Albers J, Brown M, Sima A, Greene D, Trial TTSGatEDI. Nerve conduction measures in mild diabetic neuropathy in the Early Diabetes Intervention Trial: the effects of age, sex, type of diabetes, disease duration, and anthropometric factors. Neurology 1996; 46:85–91.

56. Andersen H, Stålberg E, Falck B. F-wave latency, the most sensitive nerve conduction parameter in patients with diabetes mellitus. Muscle Nerve 1997; 20:1296–1302.

57. Krendel D, Costigan D, Hopkins L. Successful treatment of neuropathies in patients with diabetes mellitus. Arch Neurol 1995; 52:1053–1061.

58. Stewart J, McKelvey R, Durcan L, Carpenter S, Karpati G. Chronic inflammatory demyelinating polyneuropathy (CIDP) in diabetes. J Neurol Sci 1996; 142:59–64.

59. Sharma K, Cross J, Farronay O, Ayyar D, Shebert R, Bradley W. Demyelinating neuropathy in diabetes mellitus. Arch Neurol 2002; 59:758–765.

60. Sharma K, Cross J, Ayyar D, Martinez-Arizala A, Bradley W. Diabetic demyelinating polyneuropathy responsive to intravenous immunoglobulin therapy. Arch Neurol 2002; 59:751–757.

61. Lacomis D. Small-fiber neuropathy. Muscle Nerve 2002; 26:173–188.

62. Mendell J, Sahenk Z. Clinical practice. Painful sensory neuropathy. N Engl J Med 2003; 348:1243–1255.

63. Periquet M, Novak V, Collins M et al. Painful sensory neuropathy. Prospective evaluation using skin biopsy. Neurology 1999; 53:1641–1647.

64. Chaudhry V, Corse A, Cornblath D, Kunck R, Freimer M, Griffin J. Multifocal motor neuropathy: electrodiagnostic features. Muscle Nerve 1994; 17:198–205.

65. Katz J, Wolfe G, Bryan W, Jackson C, Amato A, Barohn R. Electrophysiologic findings in multifocal motor neuropathy. Neurology 1997; 48:700–707.

66. Pakiam A, Parry G. Multifocal motor neuropathy without overt conduction block. Muscle Nerve 1998; 21:243–245.

67. Valls-Solé J, Cruz Martinez A, Graus F, Saiz A, Arpa J, Grau J. Abnormal sensory nerve conduction in multifocal demyelinating neuropathy with persistent conduction block. Neurology 1995; 45:2024–2028.

68. Lewis R, Sumner A, Shy M. Electrophysiological features of inherited demyelinating neuropathies: a reappraisal in the era of molecular diagnosis. Muscle Nerve 2000; 23:1472–1487.

69. Boerkoel C, Takashima H, Lupski J. The genetic convergence of Charcot–Marie–Tooth disease types 1 and 2 and the role of genetics in sporadic neuropathy. Curr Neurol Neurosci Rep 2002; 2:70–77.

70. Dyck P, Lambert E. Lower motor and primary sensory neuron diseases with peroneal muscular atrophy. I. Neurologic, genetic, and electrophysiologic findings in hereditary polyneuropathies. Arch Neurol 1968; 18:603–681.

71. Dyck P, Lambert E. Lower motor and primary sensory neuron diseases with peroneal muscular atrophy. II. Neurologic, genetic, and electrophysiologic findings in various neuronal degenerations. Arch Neurol 1968; 18:619–621.

72. Krajewski K, Lewis R, Fuerst D et al. Neurological dysfunction and axonal degeneration in Charcot-Marie-Tooth disease type 1A. Brain 2000; 123:1516–1527.

73. Lewis R, Sumner A. The electrodiagnostic distinctions between chronic familial and acquired demyelinative neuropathies. Neurology 1982; 32:592–596.

74. Birouk N, LeGuern E, Maisonobe T et al. X-linked Charcot–Marie–Tooth disease with connexin 32 mutations: clinical and electrophysiologic study. Neurology 1998; 50:1074–1082.

75. Tabaraud F, Lagrange E, Sindou P, Vandenberghe A, Levy N, Vallat J. Demyelinating X-linked Charcot–Marie–Tooth disease: unusual electrophysiological findings. Muscle Nerve 1999; 22:1442–1447.

76. Gutierrez EJD, Sumner A, Ferer S, Warner L, Supski J, Garcia C. Unusual electrophysiological findings in X-linked dominant Charcot–Marie–Tooth disease. Muscle Nerve 2000; 23:182–188.

77. Mouton P, Tardieu S, Gouider R et al. Spectrum of clinical and electrophysiologic features in HNPP patients with the 17p11.2 deletion. Neurology 1999; 52:1440–1446.

78. Li J, Krajewski K, Shy M, Lewis R. Hereditary neuropathy with liability to pressure palsy: the electrophysiology fits the name. Neurology 2002; 58:1769–1773.

79. Dyck P, Oviart K, Lambert E. Intensive evaluation of referral unclassified neuropathies yields improved diagnosis. Ann Neurol 1981; 10:222–226.

80. Stewart J. Focal Peripheral Neuropathies. New York: Raven Press, 1993.

81. Wilbourn A. Ischemic neuropathies. In: Brown W, Bolton C, eds. Clinical Electromyography. Boston: Butterworth-Heinemann, 1993:369–390.

82. Brown W. Pathophysiology of conduction in peripheral nerves. In: Brown W, Bolton C, Aminoff M, eds. Neuromuscular Function and Disease. Philadelphia: WB Saunders Company, 2002:56–95.

83. Cornblath D, Sumner A, Daube J et al. Conduction block in clinical practice. Muscle Nerve 1991; 14:869–871.

84. Wilbourn A. Electrodiagnosis of plexopathies. Neurol Clin 1985; 3:511–529.

85. Ferrante M, Wilbourn A. The utility of various sensory nerve conduction responses in assessing brachial plexopathies. Muscle Nerve 1995; 18:879–889.

86. Lederman R, Wilbourn A. Brachial plexopathy: recurrent cancer or radiation? Neurology 1984; 34:1331–1335.

87. Thomas J, Cascino T, Earle J. Differential diagnosis between radiation and tumor plexopathy of the pelvis. Neurology 1985; 35:1–7.
88. Wilbourn A, Aminoff M. AAEM Minimonograph 32: the electrodiagnostic examination in patients with radiculopathies. Muscle Nerve 1998; 21:1612–1631.
89. Levin K, Maggiano H, Wilbourn A. Cervical radiculopathies: comparison of surgical and EMG localization of single-root lesions. Neurology 1996; 46:1022–1025.
90. Kerr A. The brachial plexus of nerves in man, the variations in its formation and branches. The Am J Anat 1918; 23:285–395.
91. Phillips L, Park T. Electrophysiologic mapping of the segmental anatomy of the muscles of the lower extremity. Muscle Nerve 1991; 14:1213–1218.
92. Johnson E, Melvin J. Value of electromyography in lumbar radiculopaty. Arch Phys Med Rehabil 1971; 52:239–243.
93. Jonsson B. Morphology, innervation, and electromyographic study of erector spinae. Arch Phys Med Rehabil 1869; 50:638–641.
94. Haig A, Talley C, Grobler L, LeBreck D. Paraspinal mapping: quantified needle electromyography in lumbar radiculopathy. Muscle Nerve 1993; 16:477–484.
95. Weddell G, Feinstein B, Pattle R. The electrical activity of voluntary muscle in man under normal and pthological condictions. Brain 1967; 67:178–257.
96. Kimura J, Machida M, Ishida T et al. Relation between size of compound sensory or motor action potentials and length of nerve segment. Neurology 1986; 36:647–652.

3
Quantitative Sensory Testing

James W. Russell
Veterans Affairs Medical Center and University of Michigan, Ann Arbor, Michigan, USA

ABSTRACT

Quantitative sensory testing (QST) supports the clinical examination and more routine electrophysiological tests. A sensory testing system, the computer-assisted sensory examination (CASE IV) provides accurate and reproducible measures of sensory thresholds, for example the vibration detection threshold (VDT) and cold detection threshold (CDT). Warm detection thresholds are less reliable. Heat pain detection thresholds are normally used to assess C-fiber or unmyelinated fiber function, but are less reproducible than VDT and CDT. QST is useful in detecting sensory loss in mild distal neuropathy or where large fiber function is minimally affected. Newer testing algorithms, such as the 4, 2, and 1 stepping algorithm with null stimuli, allow CDT and VDT to be performed relatively rapidly and reproducibly and are useful clinically and in controlled clinical trials. However, QST requires careful interpretation in the context of the clinical evaluation, and despite computer algorithms to avoid patient bias, QST still relies on psychophysical tests that may be influenced intentionally or unintentionally by the subject. Accordingly, QST should be avoided in work-compensation or in medico-legal cases where there is potential bias toward a poor outcome.

1. INTRODUCTION

In traditional sensory testing, the examiner assesses light touch, pin prick, vibration, or joint position, and judgments are made based on the examiner's experience. Testing methods and techniques are not uniform between examiners and results are not compared with rigorously derived normative data. As a result, traditional sensory testing may include both false positive and false negative findings.

Quantitative sensory testing (QST) can provide information about pathology that may not be available from routine nerve conduction studies. QST can provide reliable and reproducible information about both large and small sensory fiber functions (1). QST is based on well-established psychophysical methods (2) that allow accurate characterization of responses from peripheral sensory receptors. Computer-based systems facilitate test and retest of sensory levels leading to normative data based on percentiles. This allows early detection of peripheral neuropathy in diseases where there may be minimal involvement of distal fibers or where small fiber loss predominates. QST also lends itself to epidemiological and clinical treatment trials.

Despite good sensitivity and reliability of QST, there are drawbacks. Unlike nerve conduction studies, QST is subjective. Response variability is reduced by repeatedly presenting the same sensory stimulus using a computer-based algorithm and determining whether the sensory response accurately represents the patient's sensory level. Patients with poor attention or cognitive deficits may struggle to complete the testing. Use of null stimuli coupled with repeated testing at threshold improves the accuracy in these subjects; however, if the deficit is severe it may not be possible to complete sensory testing. Methods of measuring sensory thresholds vary depending on the technical method and data may not be transferable from one testing device to another, in contrast to nerve conduction data. In QST, a subject's response to quantified natural occurring stimuli is specific to a particular modality, for example, cold detection threshold (CDT), warm detection threshold (WDT), heat pain detection threshold (HPDT), and vibration detection threshold (VDT). These stimuli test specific sensory organ modalities and do not necessarily reflect changes in afferent fiber function, although in general the VDT is a surrogate measure of large fiber sensory function, the CDT of small myelinated fibers (Aδ), and the HPDT of C-nociceptor fiber function.

2. TESTING STRATEGIES

QST techniques significantly affect testing outcome (1). Steep, linear, or exponential increases in temperature, where the patient experiences a change in temperature and signals by depressing a response key, overestimate the true sensory threshold. Furthermore, alternating the direction of thermal change and having subjects respond during heating or cooling also overestimates thresholds and provides poor discrimination for specific thresholds such as the CDT, WDT, and HPDT. A better method is a flat-topped pyramidal shaped stimulus ramp that provides a better range of defined levels of intensity (1,3,4). In the computer-assisted sensory examination (CASE IV) system, trapezoid stimuli are applied and range from baseline in a series of 25 steps called just noticeable differences (JND). From JND 1 through 21, heating pulses are pyramidal shaped. Temperature changes from baseline (34°C) to peak and returning to baseline are at 4°C/s. The highest temperature achieved is 48°C at step 21. At steps 22–25, 48°C is held for progressively longer periods of time. A similar technique is used for VDT. The thresholds obtained using these JND values can then be converted into normative curves based on age and sex, and ultimately converted to standard normal deviates.

3. METHODS

The CASE IV system consists of a personal computer that drives an electronic controller to shape and control stimulus characteristics (Fig. 3.1). There is a visual cueing device and response key. Prior to performing the QST, the patient is read specific instructions on the test. The same instructions are given each time the test is performed, and the technician avoids interpreting the test for the patient. This is important to ensure reproducibility of the test. The patient is presented with a visual cue indicating that a stimulus is being given. The technician must be convinced that the patient understood and was cooperating during the test. Furthermore, the patient should not be drowsy or under the influence of sedatives, pain medications, or other medications that would affect their concentration. At the end of the stimulus the patient responds to indicate whether or not they felt the stimulus. Among testing algorithms the two most common methods used in the CASE IV system are a forced choice method and a one-period 4, 2, and 1 stepping algorithm. In the forced choice method, the patient is given a stimulus during either period one or period two, and before proceeding to the next level of testing has to indicate which period they felt the stimulus in. The forced choice method has the advantage that it

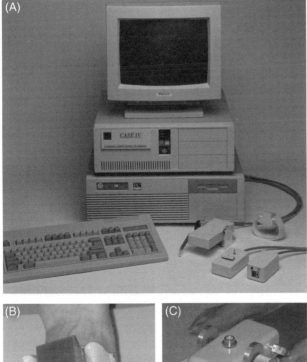

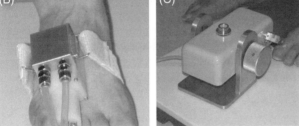

Figure 3.1 The computer-assisted sensory examination (Case IV) system (A), temperature thermode (B), and vibrometer (C). Figure (A) was kindly provided by WR Electronics (Stillwater, MN). Similar equipment is available from several different manufacturers.

requires a subject to provide a positive response comparing one stimulus to another. However, the forced choice method has the disadvantage that it is often very lengthy, particularly when the patient has minimal sensation and there is difficulty obtaining a sensory threshold. The one-period 4, 2, and 1 stepping algorithm with null stimuli can be used for detection of both the VDT and the CDT (5). The one-period algorithm uses the method of limits to detect temperature or vibration thresholds. The system begins at an intermediate level, level 13, and the stimulus is increased if not felt or decreased if felt, by four steps to the point of turn around. After the first computer generated reversal in the stimulus (turn), stepping occurs in steps of two, and after the second turn, stepping occurs in steps of one until the sensory threshold is determined. A total of 20 stimulus events are used, with five of them being randomly distributed null stimuli. If three consecutive failures are observed at level 25, the testing is terminated, and the subject is classified as being insensitive. If there is a positive response to more than one null stimulus, the program is aborted. The patient is then re-instructed and the test is re-run. The one-period 4, 2 and 1 stepping algorithm has proved to be as sensitive as the forced choice system, while permitting more rapid assessment of sensory levels.

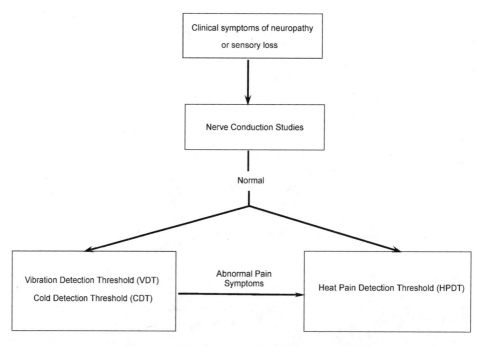

The specific methodology outlined in this section is that used by the CASE IV system. Similar methods are used in other commercially available quantitative sensory equipment. In general, it is important that reliable normative data for the specific sensory device are obtained from a sizable cohort of normal subjects using the specific sensory device. Furthermore, the equipment must allow for reproducible testing. Thus hand-held sensory devices generally produce less reproducible data than fixed positioned equipment.

3.1. VDT

The VDT is obtained using a computer-based system. Standard and calibrated 125 Hz vibratory mechanical oscillations are provided in 25 graded steps ranging in stimulus magnitude from 0.1 to 576.6 μm displacement. The cantilevered design provides a 30-gram preloading force and the objective is to determine the smallest mechanical displacement that can be detected. The vibration arm is usually placed on the dorsum of the great toe [Fig. 3.1(C)] or index finger immediately proximal to the nail, but may be used at other sites such as the dorsum of the foot or hand, volar forearm, lateral shoulder, anterior thigh, and lateral leg. During testing of the VDT, sound at 125 Hz is provided continuously by headphones to ensure that the vibration stimulus cannot be heard.

3.2. CDT and WDT

For detecting the CDT or WDT, a thermode is placed on the dorsum of the foot or hand, or at other specified sites as for VDT testing. The thermode works on the Peltier principle, and the standard thermode has a stimulating area of 10 cm^2. For these studies it is programmed to provide a trapezoid stimulus with an initial rise or fall of 4°C/s. The one-period 4, 2, and 1 stepping algorithm used for measuring VDT and CDT is shown in Fig. 3.2. The WDT is less reproducible than the CDT and is not used in our laboratory.

Thermal testing ramps may also be assessed using a continuous measuring system of thermal thresholds (6). This type of system is used on several types of commercially available equipments. The problem with this type of testing algorithm is that the heating or cooling ramp continues while the patient is deciding to press the response button. This system will thus overestimate the degree of heating or cooling. In addition, patients will improve the rate of response to the test with repeated testing. The net result of these defects in the testing method are that there will be an overestimate of heating or cooling, and lack of reproducibility with subsequent trials.

3.3. HPDT

Testing algorithms for heat pain are even more complicated. The rate of rise in temperature, frequency of testing, and the specific testing device all affect the perceived pain threshold. If a continuous linear ramp is used, the pain threshold will be inaccurate. Thus, a further algorithm, the nonrepeating ascending with null stimuli (NRA–NS) is used for heat pain responses and for measuring the HPDT (Fig. 3.3). The HPDT provides indirect information about C-nociceptor function. The initial skin temperature is taken with an infrared thermometer. If the temperature of the skin is <32°C, the limb is warmed in water. The thermode is calibrated for a range between 34°C and 50°C. Once the thermode is applied to the skin, it is set at 34°C and allowed to accommodate to the skin temperature. A series of software and hardware features in the system recognize excessive temperatures, or faulty operation and shut down the system if a fault is sensed. Although the test may induce erythema at the sight of testing, injury to the skin is extremely rare.

During heat pain testing, specific instructions are read and presented to the patient as for other types of QST. The patient is asked if they feel some degree of discomfort or pain, and if they do then the severity is graded by the patient from 1 to 10. Number 1 would correspond to the lowest level of discomfort or pain, number 10 would correspond to the most severe level of pain. Typically at a low stimulus magnitude nothing is felt. With a stronger stimulus, a pulse of warmth or heat is experienced. Occasionally, patients may not report warmth, but may report pain as the initial stimulus. This likely occurs at sites where warm receptors are not present. In the CASE IV system, the heating ramp uses a trapezoid stimulus to 49°C in order to try to avoid pain and skin temperature damage associated with higher temperatures. The measured HPDT is the thermal step

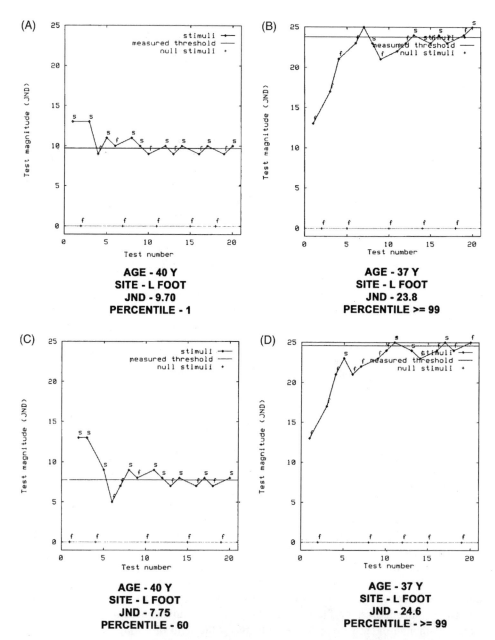

Figure 3.2 One-period 4, 2, and 1 stepping algorithm to determine VDT or CDT. Normal VDT response (A), subject of similar age with alcohol associated axonal neuropathy and an impaired VDT (B), normal CDT (C), same subject with an impaired CDT (D).

level at which the stimulus is felt as painful 50% of the time. In order to limit actual testing within the nociceptive range, an estimate is made of the 0.5 (HP:0.5) and 5.0 (HP:5.0) pain response level by testing all steps between the two response levels (7). The NRA–NS algorithm is superior to the 4, 2, and 1 algorithm and the forced choice algorithm for testing pain (7) because it avoids repeating pain stimuli at specific levels that may subsequently alter pain thresholds. The test can be completed in 8–15 min, which is important with limited testing time, or when patients have a poor attention span. Testing may be

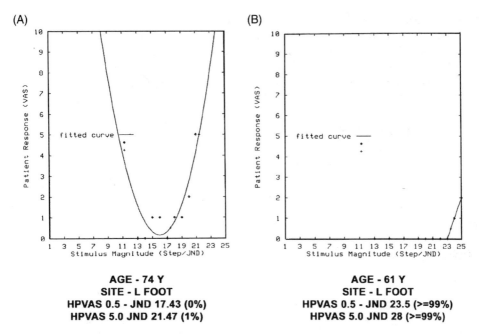

AGE - 74 Y
SITE - L FOOT
HPVAS 0.5 - JND 17.43 (0%)
HPVAS 5.0 JND 21.47 (1%)

AGE - 61 Y
SITE - L FOOT
HPVAS 0.5 - JND 23.5 (>=99%)
HPVAS 5.0 JND 28 (>=99%)

Figure 3.3 Measurement of the HPDT showing hypersensitivity to heat pain (A) in a patient with a cryptogenic "small fiber neuropathy," and hypersensitivity (B) heat pain in a patient with impaired glucose tolerance and neuropathy.

repeated in, as little as, 45 min without any significant difference in the second recorded response level (7).

4. CLINICAL USES OF QST

Potential uses for QST include (1) determination of the type of sensory modality affected in a peripheral neuropathy; (2) characterize the type of nerve fiber degeneration in a "small fiber neuropathy" where standard nerve conduction studies are normal (8); (3) characterize heat pain insensitivity or hypersensitivity in peripheral neuropathies, as well as in focal disorders such as trigeminal neuralgia; and (4) characterize response of sensory, or "small fiber neuropathies" to pharmacological agents.

There are concerns about using QST for workman's compensation or medico-legal claims. In psychophysical testing, a subject may have a bias toward a worse outcome, and therefore may consciously or unconsciously influence results of the test making QST unreliable (9,10). Furthermore, there is a concern about the reliability of QST in characterizing an entrapment neuropathy such as carpal tunnel syndrome. The diagnosis should not be made on the basis of a single test, but should rather correlate clinical findings, electrodiagnostic studies, QST findings, and the physician's judgment to determine the final assessment of the disorder.

5. CONCLUSIONS

QST using sensitive psychophysical methods attempts to evaluate subjective alterations in sensation such as hypo- or hyper-sensitivity. There are several indications for QST: (1) to quantify specific sensory system dysfunction and to evaluate ways of improvement in that function; (2) to evaluate the effects of treatment of a neuropathy or other sensory dysfunction; and (3) to evaluate small fiber dysfunction and elucidate the cause of hypersensitivity phenomena. QST may be of use where clinical methods or electrodiagnostic studies such as nerve conduction studies are too insensitive to characterize sensory loss.

ACKNOWLEDGMENTS

The author would like to thank Ms. Denice Janus for secretarial assistance. The author was supported in part by NIH NS42056, NS40458, The Juvenile Diabetes Research Foundation Center for the Study of Complications in Diabetes (JDRF), Office of Research Development (Medical Research Service), and Geriatric Research Educational and Clinical Center (GRECC), Department of Veterans Affairs.

REFERENCES

1. Dyck PJ, Zimmerman I, Gillen DA, Johnson D, Karnes JL, O'Brien PC. Cool, warm, and heat-pain detection thresholds: testing methods and inferences about anatomic distribution of receptors. Neurology 1993; 43(8):1500–1508.
2. Dyck PJ, Karnes JL, Gillen DA, O'Brien PC, Zimmerman IR, Johnson DM. Comparison of algorithms of testing for use in automated evaluation of sensation. Neurology 1990; 40(10):1607–1613.
3. Quantitative sensory testing: a consensus report from the Peripheral Neuropathy Association. Neurology 1993; 43(5):1050–1052.
4. Gruener G, Dyck PJ. Quantitative sensory testing: methodology, applications, and future directions. J Clin Neurophysiol 1994; 11(6):568–583.
5. Dyck PJ, O'Brien PC, Kosanke JL, Gillen DA, Karnes JL. A 4, 2, and 1 stepping algorithm for quick and accurate estimation of cutaneous sensation threshold. Neurology 1993; 43(8):1508–1512.
6. Yarnitsky D, Sprecher E. Thermal testing: normative data and repeatability for various test algorithms. J Neurol Sci 1994; 125(1):39–45.
7. Dyck PJ, Zimmerman IR, Johnson DM, Gillen D, Hokanson JL, Karnes JL, Gruener G, O'Brien PC. A standard test of heat-pain responses using CASE IV. J Neurol Sci 1996; 136:54–63.
8. Luciano CA, Russell JW, Banerjee TK, Quirk JM, Scott LJ, Dambrosia JM, Barton NW, Schiffmann R. Physiological characterization of neuropathy in Fabry's disease. Muscle Nerve 2002; 26(5):622–629.
9. Dyck PJ, Dyck PJ, Kennedy WR, Kesserwani H, Melanson M, Ochoa J, Shy M, Stevens JC, Suarez GA, O'Brien PC. Limitations of quantitative sensory testing when patients are biased toward a bad outcome. Neurology 1998; 50(5):1213.
10. Freeman R, Chase KP, Risk MR. Quantitative sensory testing cannot differentiate simulated sensory loss from sensory neuropathy. Neurology 2003; 60(3):465–470.

4
Evaluation of the Autonomic Nervous System

Safwan S. Jaradeh and Thomas E. Prieto
Medical College of Wisconsin, Milwaukee, Wisconsin, USA

ABSTRACT

The autonomic nervous system has diverse functions. Direct testing of autonomic nerves, as is performed with somatic nerves, is not readily available. Rather, the evaluation of the autonomic nervous system relies on indirect assessment of autonomic function. Accordingly, an understanding of the anatomy, physiology, and chemistry of autonomic nerves is essential. Individual tests are reviewed in this chapter. The final section includes common conditions encountered by the clinician that require neurophysiological testing.

1. OVERVIEW OF THE ANATOMY, PHYSIOLOGY, AND CHEMISTRY

The major autonomic centers in the brain are the ventral lateral medulla, the nucleus tractus solitarius (NTS), the parabrachial nucleus, the hypothalamus, the amygdala, and the insular cortex. These centers are sensitive to afferent impulses from end organs or to humoral mechanisms through the release of various substances. The NTS and the dorsal medulla receive afferent information from cardiovascular, respiratory, and gastrointestinal end organs. The NTS also receives information from afferent fibers from the viscera, as well as spinal information that integrates visceral and somatic stimuli. The NTS forwards signals to various brainstem and forebrain centers. Baroreceptor and chemoreceptor information is transmitted to the amygdala and paraventricular hypothalamic nucleus. The NTS projections to the nuclei of the vagus nerve are responsible for modifying the cardiac parasympathetic activity. The NTS projections to the ventral lateral medulla modify sympathetic cardiovascular responses. Important differences between the sympathetic and parasympathetic systems are summarized in Fig. 4.1 (1).

Postganglionic sympathetic fibers follow blood vessels. Those to the limbs and head emanate from paravertebral ganglia, while those to the viscera (cardiac, splanchnic) emanate from paravertebral and prevertebral ganglia. Postganglionic fibers do not exist in the adrenal medulla. Parasympathetic innervation is most important in the modulation of the enteric nervous system and in the innervation of the bladder. Sympathetic innervation to the arteries and veins is very important in the modulation of vasomotor reflexes. Both systems interact equally with cardiac responses. Sweat glands are innervated by sympathetic fibers that are cholinergic.

The neurotransmitters involved are mainly acetylcholine, norepinephrine, and epinephrine. Acetylcholine is the universal ganglionic transmitter (nicotinic receptors). It is also the postganglionic transmitter for parasympathetic and sympathetic sudomotor fibers (muscarinic receptors). Norepinephrine is the postganglionic transmitter for the remaining sympathetic fibers. Epinephrine is mainly formed at the adrenal medulla and following its release, stimulates the adrenoreceptors directly.

2. LABORATORY EVALUATION OF AUTONOMIC DISORDERS

Several systemic and neurologic conditions affect the autonomic nervous system. In some cases, involvement of the sympathetic or parasympathetic component predominates, but it is rare to have involvement of only one division of the autonomic nervous system. In this chapter, we will review the standard tests of autonomic function (2–5). The main indications for diagnostic laboratory evaluation are:

1. generalized autonomic failure;
2. distal small fiber neuropathy;

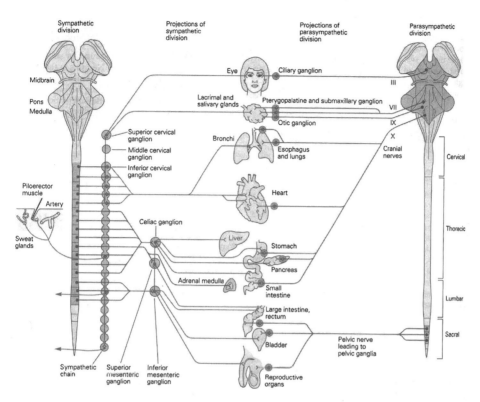

Figure 4.1 Comparison of sympathetic system with parasympathetic system.

3. syncope, orthostatic intolerance, and postural tachycardia;
4. other limited dysautonomias (gastrointestinal, urologic); and
5. sweating disorders (anhidrosis, hyperhidrosis).

Autonomic testing is also used to evaluate the progression and therapeutic responses in dysautonomia. Very specialized dysautonomias, such as pupillary, genitourinary, or gastrointestinal disorders, are beyond the scope of this chapter.

Given the influence of many substances on autonomic function, it is important to withhold these substances, if medically possible, for variable periods before testing. Caffeine and nicotine should be held at least 4 h before testing. Alcohol should be held 8 h. Over-the-counter drugs (decongestants) and anticholinergics (including tricyclic anti-depressants) should be held 48 h. Sympathomimetics should be held 24 h. The patient should be quietly seated indoors for 30 min before the test to allow for adequate rest and thermal equilibration.

2.1. Tests of Sudomotor Function

The three main tests are:

1. quantitative sudomotor axon reflex test (QSART);
2. thermoregulatory sweat test (TST); and
3. sympathetic skin responses (SSR).

2.1.1. Quantitative Sudomotor Axon Reflex Test

In this test, a multi-compartment sweat capsule is attached to the skin. Acetylcholine 10% is iontophoresed through one compartment using a low intensity (up to 2 mA) constant current to activate cutaneous axon terminals. The action potentials propagate antidromically to the next branch-point, then propagate orthodromically to the next nerve terminal. This releases endogenous acetylcholine, which binds to muscarinic receptors on eccrine sweat glands (3). The evoked sweat response is recorded from a second compartment of the sweat capsule using a sudorometer (3). This reflex response is mediated by postganglionic sympathetic sudomotor axons. The test is noninvasive, but subjects often describe a transient local burning or stinging sensation lasting several seconds following the iontophoresis. After the capsule is removed, a small erythematous flare may persist for up to 20 min. QSART is sensitive and reliable in controls and in patients with autonomic neuropathy. Intra-subject reproducibility is high. There is little asymmetry from side to side; in our laboratory, this difference is <40%. Therefore, recording from either side should suffice, except when local factors are present (skin injury or infection, previous trauma, or biopsy). When symptoms are unilateral, it is useful to evaluate both sides. Standard recording sites are the volar mid-forearm, the anterior proximal leg, the anterior distal leg, and the dorsolateral proximal foot. These sites are innervated by the ulnar, peroneal, saphenous, and sural nerves, respectively. Normal data from the Mayo clinic and from our laboratory have been published (3,6).

2.1.2. Thermoregulatory Sweat Test

The TST is a sensitive qualitative test of sudomotor function that provides important information on the pattern and distribution of sweat loss. The original method applied quinizarin indicator to dry skin. Sweating changes the indicator from brown to violet. Because quinizarin is highly allergenic, alizarin-red is currently used, and the color changes from orange to purple (7). Skin reactions are rare, but staining of clothing may occur. The test is conducted in a heated tent or a sweat cabinet. The subject should be well hydrated. Anticholinergic agents, some antihistamine, antidepressant, and some antiparkinsonian drugs, should be held for 24–48 h before the test. A commonly used endpoint is a rise in oral temperature of 1°C provided the resting baseline temperature is >36.5°C. A minimum of 25% ambient humidity is usually necessary to facilitate sweating and slow the evaporation. There are some variations in normal sweat patterns, but all normal subjects should perspire over the forehead, trunk (particularly torso), hands, and feet; and most normal subjects perspire over the legs and forearms. In our experience, some normal subjects, particularly women, may not sweat over the thighs and arms. The test is highly sensitive because it detects pre- or postganglionic sudomotor dysfunction. In a study by Fealey et al. (8) on 51 diabetics, 94% of those with clinical findings of neuropathy had abnormal TST. Anhidrosis occurred distally in 65%, or regionally—including dermatomal distribution—in 50%; 78% of patients had more than one pattern. Global anhidrosis was noted in 16% and all had symptomatic dysautonomia.

In autonomic disorders, TST is a useful adjuvant to autonomic testing. Distal anhidrosis is the most common pattern and is usually indicative of a distal small fiber neuropathy. Most often, it is symmetric. When there is significant asymmetry, a microangiopathic or dysimmune condition should be considered. Global anhidrosis is characteristic of pure autonomic failure (PAF), multisystem atrophy (MSA), and pan-autonomic neuropathy. Regional anhidrosis can be dermatomal or segmental. Hemihidrosis is an extreme example of segmental anhidrosis typically seen in myelopathies or after a cerebral infarction.

2.1.3. Sympathetic Skin Responses

Also known as galvanic skin responses (GSR), SSR is an electrodermal response recorded from sweat glands after stimulation of type II mechanoreceptors in a mixed nerve (9). Standard EMG surface electrodes are placed over the hands and feet. The response is recorded from the active electrodes over the palmar or plantar surface, while the reference electrode is placed over the dorsal surface. An electrical stimulus with duration of 0.2 ms and an intensity of 30–50 mA is delivered to the contralateral wrist or ankle. The response waveform has a slow latency (1–3 s) and a long duration, which requires a low frequency filter of <0.20 Hz. The high frequency filter is usually <2000 Hz. The sweep speed should be 500–1000 ms/cm. Owing to the large variability among normal subjects, and the habituation of the response with repeated stimulation, only an absent SSR is of pathological significance and indicates abnormal sudomotor adrenergic innervation of the affected limb.

2.2. Tests of Cardiovagal Function

The three main tests are:

1. heart rate response to deep breathing (HR)
2. Valsalva ratio (VR)
3. heart rate response to standing "30:15" ratio

In the first test, the variation of heart rate (HR) depends on vagal innervation, and is abolished by the muscarinic antagonist atropine. In the other two tests, the HR is determined by the vagal component of the barorcflex arc, while blood pressure (BP) responses are determined by sympathetic factors. BP changes also depend on the magnitude of forced expiratory pressure during the Valsalva maneuver, the patient's volume and cardiac status, and the patient's position. BP and HR can also be recorded noninvasively using plethysmographic equipment, such as finapres or arterial tonometry (Table 4.1) (10).

2.2.1. HR Response to Deep Breathing

Age, resting HR, rate of breathing, body mass index, cardiac status, and medications affect this test. It is not affected by gender. Heart rate variations (R–R variation) is maximal at a respiratory rate of 6 bpm (Beats or breaths per minute) (11,12). Breathing should be as smooth as possible and a visual guide—such as an oscillating bar—is very helpful. Six to eight cycles are recorded, and the five cycles with the largest R–R differences are averaged to derive a mean HR range. Breathing at higher rates or for longer periods reduces the

Table 4.1 Test Results in Various Types of Autonomic Failure

Condition	TST	QSART	VR/ΔHRDB	HUT
Autonomic NP	↓↓, Distal	↓↓, Distal	Reduced	↓↓ BP
Adrenergic NP	↓, Distal	↓, Distal	Normal	↓↓ BP
Cholinergic NP	↓↓, Diffuse	↓↓, Diffuse	Reduced	NL
Botulism	↓↓, Diffuse	↓↓, Diffuse	Reduced	NL or ↓
Riley–Day	↓ Distal, ↑ proximal	↓↓, Distal	Reduced	↓↓ BP
PAF	↓↓, Diffuse	↓, Distal	Reduced	↓↓ BP
MSA	↓↓, Diffuse	Normal	Reduced	↓↓ BP
Syncope	NL or ↓	NL or ↓	NL or ↓	↓↓ BP
POTS	NL or ↓	NL or ↓	NL or ↓	↑↑ HR

HR change because of hyperventilation and hypocapnia. If the test is repeated, 3–5 min of rest should be allowed. Overweight patients will have reduced HR variation (13). Normal data from the Mayo clinic and from our laboratory have been published (3,6).

2.2.2. Valsalva Ratio

For the Valsalva maneuver, the subject is asked to blow into a tube to maintain a column of mercury at 40 mmHg for 15 s. The patient is usually rested and supine, but sitting does not affect the ratio. The maneuver may be repeated to ensure reproducible BP responses. Blowing for <10 s or at a pressure <20 mm is suboptimal. The VR is derived from the maximum HR divided by the minimum HR. Most centers select the lowest HR within 30 s of maximal HR, but a few centers select the minimal value within 60 s of maneuver onset. The maximal HR is a response to the fall in BP, while the minimal HR is a response to the baroreflex. The VR is a measure of baroreflex sensitivity. The different phases of the valsalva response are discussed in section 2.3.1.

Reflex bradycardia is blunted in cardiovagal dysfunction, while both the BP overshoot and the reflex bradycardia are blunted in generalized dysautonomia. Factors that affect VR are age, gender, position of the subject, expiratory pressure, duration of effort, and medications.

Occasionally, patients may not generate two reproducible BP curves despite identical expiratory pressures; in these cases, the better VR should be taken. The VR is less reliable in patients with pacemakers, or when BP excursions are minimal for iatrogenic or health (pulmonary) reasons. Some subjects, including controls, may not decrease their BP during early phase II; this curve is referred to as a "flat top" response, and VR may be underestimated. Conversely, VR may be normal in mild cardiovagal impairment if sympathetic cardiac responses are compensatory. Normal data from the Mayo clinic and from our laboratory have been published (Table 4.2) (3,6).

2.2.3. HR Response to Standing Up

The earliest HR changes to standing consist of a tachycardia between 5 and 15 s, followed by a bradycardia between 20 and 30 s. Subsequently, there is an increase in HR and BP before returning to baseline after several minutes. The early bradycardia is baroreflex—mediated. The original study found that the largest HR changes occur at 15 and 30 s after standing, hence the term "30:15 ratio." This tachycardia/bradycardia ratio (R–R interval at beat 30)/(R–R interval at beat 15) is a valid index of cardiovagal function.

Table 4.2 Components of Valsalva Maneuver in Types of Autonomic Failure (3)

Condition	Early Phase II	Late Phase II	Phase IV	VR
Normal	SBP drop <21 mm	SBP = baseline	SBP rise >11 mm	Normal
Vagal lesion	SBP drop <21 mm	SBP = baseline	SBP rise >11 mm	Reduced
Sympathetic lesion, mild	SBP drop >21 mm	SBP < baseline	SBP rise >11 mm	Normal
Sympathetic lesion, moderate	SBP drop >21 mm	SBP < baseline	SBP rise >5 mm	Low, normal
Sympathetic lesion, marked	SBP drop >30 mm	SBP < baseline	SBP = baseline	Reduced

2.3. Tests of Adrenergic Function

The main tests are the head-upright tilt (HUT) and the Valsalva maneuver.

2.3.1. BP Responses to the Valsalva Maneuver

As already mentioned, the VR is a reliable parasympathetic test. The dynamic alterations of the BP during the Valsalva maneuver are important measures of adrenergic function. Invasive (arterial line) and noninvasive (Finapres or arterial tonometry) recordings reveal four phases in the Valsalva maneuver. In phase I, there is increased intrathoracic and intra-abdominal pressure causing mechanical compression of the aorta and a brief rise in BP. Phase II begins with a drop of BP secondary to reduced venous return and cardiac output. This produces efferent sympathetic volleys to the muscles, and the cardiovagal withdrawal leads to tachycardia (Table 4.3). The fall in BP is arrested within 4–6 s, and the BP returns to or exceeds the resting values. Following the release of Valsalva in phase III, the fall in intrathoracic pressure causes a decrease in BP lasting 1–3 s. There is another burst of sympathetic activity and the arteriolar bed remains vasoconstricted. The resumption of normal venous return and cardiac output leads to an overshoot of BP above baseline values in phase IV. Normally, systolic blood pressure (SBP) drop should not exceed 21 mm during early phase II, and should return to its baseline value by late phase II or phase III. α-Adrenergic blockers (phentolamine 10 mg) eliminate late phase II but increase phase IV. β-Adrenergic blockers (propranolol 10 mg) eliminate phase IV.

2.3.2. BP Responses to HUT

The assumption of the upright posture results in the pooling of 500–1000 cc of blood in the lower extremities and splanchnic circulation. The reduced venous return decreases ventricular filling, cardiac output, and BP. These changes lead to parasympathetic inhibition and sympathetic activation. There is subsequent constriction of the vessels and an increase in HR (14).

Orthostatic BP recordings to tilt are usually recorded with the patient supine and after upright tilt to 70–80°. An automated tilt-table allows consistent slow tilt over 20 s. Serial recordings are obtained but the most relevant ones are usually at 1 and 5 min after tilt. It is preferable to perform the tilt after 20 min of rest to maximize the orthostatic reduction in BP. If using plethysmography, the arm should remain at the heart level to avoid positional artifacts of BP values. During upright tilt in normal persons, there may be a brief reduction in BP that fully recovers within 1 min. The decrement should not exceed 20 mmHg of systolic blood pressure, 15 mmHg of mean blood pressure or 10 mmHg of diastolic blood pressure. In the presence of adrenergic failure, there is marked and progressive reduction in BP. The HR response depends on cardiac

Table 4.3 Valsalva-Related BP Changes: Results in Various Types of Autonomic Failure

Condition	↓ BP (Phase II)	↑ BP (Phase IV)
Autonomic NP	Excessive	Reduced
Botulism	Normal	Normal or reduced
Riley–Day	Excessive	Reduced
PAF	Excessive	Reduced
MSA	Normal or excessive	Reduced

adrenergic innervation; if spared, there will be compensatory tachycardia. Orthostatic drop of SBP by >30 mmHg without tachycardia indicates definite adrenergic failure. In mild adrenergic impairment, there may be excessive BP oscillations, a significant orthostatic tachycardia (increment in HR exceeding 30 bpm) or both. These changes are often associated with premonitory signs of syncope.

3. CLINICAL APPLICATIONS

3.1. Acute Autonomic Neuropathies (15)

Acute autonomic neuropathies may have only minor accompanying somatic manifestations or may be part of a more generalized acute peripheral neuropathy, such as the Guillain–Barré syndrome (16), in which motor and sensory disturbances dominate the clinical picture. The isolated autonomic form may be paraneoplastic or immunological, and sometimes occurs after viral infections (17). The clinical presentation is dominated by autonomic dysfunction which can be severe. Postural hypotension and anhidrosis are due to sympathetic impairment, and gastrointestinal and sexual disturbances are due to parasympathetic dysfunction. CSF abnormalities with albumino–cytologic dissociation have been described in some cases. The HR is typically fixed, the skin is dry, and the pupils sluggish or non-reactive to light. Minor sensory, motor, or reflex abnormalities may be present distally in the extremities.

Nerve conduction studies are commonly normal. Minor distal neurogenic changes can be seen on needle EMG. All autonomic function studies are markedly abnormal. The disorder follows a monophasic course. The prognosis is variable, and approximately one-third of patients remain severely disabled. Improvement usually occurs 1 year after the onset. Treatment is symptomatic. Anecdotal reports suggest that plasmapheresis or intravenous immunoglobulin (IVIG) therapy may be helpful.

3.1.1. Botulism

Ingestion of food contaminated by *Clostridium botulinum* often leads to cholinergic failure. The manifestations are anhidrosis, xerostomia, xerophthalmia, gastroparesis, ileus, urinary retention, and BP disturbances (6). There are signs of cranial neuropathies, usually extraocular, and subsequent development of generalized weakness and respiratory difficulties. The diagnosis can be confirmed by identification of the toxins in food or serum.

3.1.2. Porphyria

Sympathetic overactivity is the most common abnormality. In acute intermittent porphyria, persistent tachycardia, and hypertension may herald an attack. Both sympathetic and parasympathetic functions are affected. There is often concomitant large fiber involvement that can be detected by nerve conduction studies.

3.1.3. Drug or Toxin-Induced Autonomic Neuropathies

Autonomic neuropathies may occur in patients receiving a variety of medications including cisplatin, vinca alkaloids, amiodarone, perhexiline maleate, and taxol. Postural hypotension often dominates the presentation, but there are usually other sensory and motor signs of polyneuropathy. Organic solvents also cause a sensorimotor and autonomic polyneuropathy, with abnormal valsalva maneuver and HR response to deep breathing (18). Thallium and arsenic intoxication leads to a peripheral neuropathy with hypertension, tachycardia, and disturbances of sweating (19,20).

3.2. Chronic Autonomic Neuropathies (8)

Autonomic dysfunction is present in many chronic axonal neuropathies, particularly those involving the small fibers.

3.2.1. Diabetic Autonomic Neuropathy

Autonomic neuropathy is present in at least 25% of diabetic patients. Parasympathetic tests are usually impaired before sympathetic tests (21–23). Sweating is often abnormal (8). Other neuropathic complications of diabetes are common and include a distal polyneuropathy, diabetic amyotrophy, lumbosacral radiculo–plexopathy, and truncal radiculopathy.

3.2.2. Amyloid Neuropathy

Autonomic dysfunction is prominent in the Portuguese type of familial amyloid polyneuropathy (FAP type 1). The inheritance is autosomal dominant. The onset is usually in young adulthood. There is often superimposed sensory neuropathy involving mainly the small fibers. Motor and reflex abnormalities are infrequent or late (24).

In sporadic systemic amyloidosis, a neuropathy usually develops in mid—to late adulthood. The neuropathy is usually painful. Autonomic failure is often severe and early. Postural hypotension, syncope, and impotence are frequent. Sudomotor function is impaired. Gastrointestinal disturbances are common. Some patients have dysphagia caused by infiltration of the lower esophagus. Peripheral nerve biopsy shows amyloid deposits with loss of thinly myelinated and unmyelinated fibers. The prognosis is worse than in the inherited form.

3.2.3. Familial Dysautonomia (Riley-Day Syndrome)

Familial dysautonomia is also known as hereditary sensory and autonomic neuropathy type III. It begins in childhood with impaired lacrimation, hyperhidrosis, postural hypotension, and poor temperature control (25). Autonomic testing abnormalities are both sympathetic and parasymapthetic.

3.2.4. Pure Autonomic Failure

Pure Autonomic Failure (PAF) is an idiopathic, sporadic, adult-onset, and progressive disorder of the autonomic nervous system. Bradbury and Eggleston first described it in 1925 (26). Patients present with autonomic dysfunction such as urinary retention, erectile dysfunction, constipation, and orthostatic hypotension with syncope (27). The presence of extrapyramidal deficit, cerebellar deficit, or both indicates multiple system atrophy (MSA) rather than PAF.

3.2.5. Multiple System Atrophy

MSA is a progressive neurodegenerative disease that causes parkinsonism and cerebellar, pyramidal, and autonomic dysfunction in any combination (28,29). Wenning et al. (30) detailed the clinical features of 203 published cases of MSA. Men are more commonly affected than women (ratio of 1.3:1). Autonomic failure is present in 74% of patients.

Parkinsonism affects 87%, cerebellar ataxia 54%, and pyramidal signs are present in 49%. Life expectancy in MSA is usually shorter than in PAF. Anal sphincter electromyography and urodynamic studies are often abnormal.

3.2.6. Pure Adrenergic Neuropathy

Occasional patients with PAF and MSA present with pure adrenergic failure. There is postural hypotension but normal tests of cardiovagal function.

3.2.7. Chronic Idiopathic Anhidrosis

Patients present with heat intolerance. Vasomotor function is usually preserved. There is no associated somatic neuropathy. Some patients have Adie's tonic pupil (Ross syndrome). Adie's pupil is often a large pupil that is poorly reactive to light. Unlike the normal pupil, it constricts after topical application of diluted (2.5%) methacholine. The disorder is often asymmetric or unilateral. Some tendon reflexes, especially the ankle jerks, may be lost. Treatment is usually prophylactic with avoidance of heat.

3.2.8. Small-Fiber Sensory Neuropathies

Patients present with painful dysesthetic feet, allodynia, and sympathetic disturbances, with an impairment of vasomotor function and of sweating. Many have distal sensory nociceptive abnormalities. The motor examination is normal, and tendon reflexes are often preserved. Nerve conduction studies are not helpful. Causes are diabetes, monoclonal gammopathies, primary systemic amyloidosis, AIDS, nutritional deficiencies, certain hereditary sensory, and autonomic neuropathies, Tangier disease, and Fabry disease. Many cases are idiopathic (31,32). Quantitative sensory testing reveals abnormal thermal and pain perception modalities (33). Sudomotor function is impaired, particularly distally. Cardiovagal abnormalities are less common than sudomotor disturbances. When technically available, intraepidermal nerve fiber analysis reveals reduced fiber density, especially distally (34). A large component of the treatment is symptomatic.

3.3. Orthostatic Hypotension, Syncope, and Orthostatic Intolerance

As discussed earlier, the assumption of the erect posture reduces cardiac output and BP. There is subsequent constriction of the vessels and an increase in HR. When these mechanisms fail, the patient develops hypotension and syncope. The normal response to standing is a transient fall in systolic BP (<10 mmHg), an increase in diastolic BP (<10 mmHg), and an increase in the pulse rate (<25 bpm). The changes are usually less pronounced than during passive upright tilt, in part because of the compensatory muscular contraction of the lower limbs.

Orthostatic hypotension and syncope are the most incapacitating symptoms of autonomic failure. Patients typically present with lightheadedness after sudden postural changes, meals, exertion, or prolonged standing. Other pre-syncopal complaints include generalized fatigue, leg weakness, blurred vision, and headache. Syncope may be gradual or sudden, and some patients may have brief myoclonus, raising the possibility of a seizure.

Syncope occurs when orthostatic hypotension exceeds the capacity of cerebral autoregulation. This leads to a transient loss of consciousness and postural tone. In addition to all causes of orthostatic hypotension, cardiac disease should be ruled out. The most common types of syncope are noncardiac. Iatrogenic factors particularly in the elderly may precipitate syncope. Among cardiac causes, vascular obstruction (aortic or pulmonary) and arrythmias predominate. Up to 50% of patients may not have a detectable cause.

Orthostatic intolerance, also known as postural orthostatic tachycardia syndrome (POTS), is characterized by the development orthostatic tachycardia that exceeds 30 bpm after assuming the erect position. HR in excess of 120 bpm is also diagnostic. Patients often describe dizziness, blurred vision and epigastric discomfort. There is occasional venous pooling in the lower limbs. Around 50–60% of patients have evidence of autonomic neuropathy, primarily adrenergic (35,36). The condition likely represents a milder form of neurogenic orthostatic hypotension and syncope. The management depends on the underlying etiology, and follows the same guidelines as orthostatic hypotension.

Treatment of neurogenic orthostatic hypotension can be difficult (37). Two approaches are required. Nonpharmacological measures emphasize patient education. Patients should stand up gradually, particularly in the morning. A tailored program of exercise, particularly isotonic, is recommended. Precipitating factors include exercise in warm weather, hot baths, and showers and particularly when sweating is impaired. Medications that cause orthostatic hypotension should be revised and possibly removed or modified. Patients often benefit from increasing sodium intake. Custom fitted elastic stockings to the waist minimize peripheral blood pooling, but tend to be poorly tolerated.

Pharmacological measures begin with fludrocortisone acetate. Sympathomimetic agents can be added to fludrocortisone acetate. Commonly used α-adrenergic agonists include ephedrine, pseudoephedrine, and midodrine. Midodrine produces arterial and venous constriction and is quite effective. For refractory patients, recombinant human erythropoietin and somatostatin analogs such as octreotide can be useful. β-Adrenergic blockers with intrinsic sympathomimetic activity, such as pindolol, may have a limited role, particularly when there is symptomatic tachycardia.

REFERENCES

1. Kandel ER, Schwartz JH, Jessell TM. The autonomic nervous ystem and the hypothalamus. In: Kandel ER, Schwartz JH, Jessell TM, eds. Principles of Neural Science. Amsterdam: Elsevier, 2000:961–981.
2. Anonymous. Clinical autonomic testing report of the Therapeutics and Technology Assessment Subcommittee of the American Academy of Neurology. Neurology 1996; 46:873–880.
3. Low PA. Laboratory evaluation of autonomic function. In: Low PA, ed. Clinical Autonomic Disorders: Evaluation and Management. Philadelphia: Lippincott-Raven, 1997:179–208.
4. Low PA. Pitfalls in autonomic testing. In: Low PA, ed. Clinical Autonomic Disorders: Evaluation and Management. Philadelphia: Lippincott-Raven, 1997:391–401.
5. Low PA, Suarez GA, Benarroch EE. Clinical autonomic disorders: classification and clinical evaluation. In: Low PA, ed. Clinical Autonomic Disorders. Philadelphia: Lippincott-Raven, 1997:3–15.
6. Jaradeh SS, Smith TL, Torrico L et al. Autonomic nervous system evaluation of patients with vasomotor rhinitis. Laryngoscope 2000; 110:1828–1831.
7. Fealey RD. The thermoregulatory sweat test. In: Low PA, ed. Clinical Autonomic Disorders: Evaluation and Management. Philadelphia: Lippincott-Raven, 1997:245–257.
8. Fealey RD, Low PA, Thomas JE. Thermoregulatory sweating abnormalities in diabetes mellitus. Mayo Clin Proc 1989; 64:617–628.
9. Baba M, Watahiki Y, Matsunaga M et al. Sympathetic skin response in healthy man. Electromyogr Clin Neurophysiol 1988; 28:277–283.
10. Benarroch EE, Opfer-Gehrking TL, Low PA. Use of the photoplethysmographic technique to analyze the Valsalva maneuver in normal man. Muscle Nerve 1991; 14:1165–1172.

11. Angelone A, Coulter NA. Respiratory sinus arrhythmia: a frequency dependent phenomenon. J Appl Physiol 1964; 19:479–482.

12. Hirsch JA, Bishop B. Respiratory sinus arrhythmia in humans: how breathing pattern modulates heart rate. Am J Physiol 1981; 241:H620–H629.

13. Hirsch J, Leibel RL, Mackintosh R et al. Heart rate variability as a measure of autonomic function during weight change in humans. Am J Physiol 1991; 261:R1418–R1423.

14. Borst C, Wieling W, van Brederode JF et al. Mechanisms of initial heart rate response to postural change. Am J Physiol 1982; 243:H676–H681.

15. Low PA, McLeod JG. Autonomic neuropathies. In: Low PA, ed. Clinical Autonomic Disorders: Evaluation and Management. Philadelphia: Lippincott-Raven, 1997:463–486.

16. Tuck RR, McLeod JG. Autonomic dysfunction in Guillain-Barre syndrome. J Neurol Neurosurg Psychiatry 1981; 44:983–990.

17. Young RR, Asbury AK, Corbett JL, Adams RD. Pure pan-dysautonomia with recovery. Description and discussion of diagnostic criteria. Brain 1975; 98:613–636.

18. Matikainen E, Juntunen J. Autonomic nervous system dysfunction in workers exposed to organic solvents. J Neurol Neurosurg Psychiatry 1985; 48:1021–1024.

19. Bank WJ, Pleasure DE, Suzuki K et al. Thallium poisoning. Arch Neurol 1972; 26:456–464.

20. LeQuesne PM, McLeod JC. Peripheral neuropathy following a single exposure to arsenic. J Neurol Sci 1977; 32:437–451.

21. Bennett T, Fentem PH, Fitton D et al. Assessment of vagal control of the heart in diabetes. Measures of R-R interval variation under different conditions. Br Heart J 1977; 39:25–28.

22. Low PA, Zimmerman BR, Dyck PJ. Comparison of distal sympathetic with vagal function in diabetic neuropathy. Muscle Nerve 1986; 9:592–596.

23. Wheeler T, Watkins PJ. Cardiac denervation in diabetes. Br Med J 1973; 4:584–586.

24. Bergfeldt BL, Olofsson BO, Edhag KO. Electrophysiologic evaluation of the cardiac conduction system and its autonomic regulation in familial amyloid polyneuropathy. Am J Cardiol 1985; 56:647–652.

25. Axelrod FB. Familial dysautonomia. In: Low PA, ed. Clinical Autonomic Disorders. 2nd ed. Philadelphia: Lippincott-Raven Publishers, 1997:525–535.

26. Bradbury S, Eggleston C. Postural hypotension. Report of 3 cases. Am Heart J 1925; 1:73–86.

27. Bannister R, Sever P, Gross M. Cardiovascular reflexes and biochemical responses in progressive autonomic failure. Brain 1977; 100:327–344.

28. Anonymous. Consensus statement on the definition of orthostatic hypotension, pure autonomic failure, and multiple system atrophy. Neurology 1996; 46:1470.

29. Cohen J, Low PA, Fealey R et al. Somatic and autonomic function in progressive autonomic failure and multiple system atrophy. Ann Neurol 1987; 22:692–699.

30. Wenning GK, Tison F, Ben Shlomo Y et al. Multiple system atrophy: a review of 203 pathologically proven cases. Mov Disord 1997; 12:133–147.

31. Stewart JD, Low PA, Fealey RD. Distal small fiber neuropathy: results of tests of sweating and autonomic cardiovascular reflexes. Muscle Nerve 1992; 15:661–665.

32. Suarez GA et al. Idiopathic autonomic neuropathy: clinical, neurophysiologic, and follow-up studies on 27 patients. Neurology 1994; 44:1675–1682.

33. Jamal GA, Hansen S, Weir AI et al. The neurophysiologic investigation of small fiber neuropathies. Muscle Nerve 1987; 10:537–545.

34. Holland NR, Crawford TO, Hauer P et al. Small-fiber sensory neuropathies: clinical course and neuropathology of idiopathic cases. Ann Neurol 1998; 44:47–59.

35. Jaradeh SS, Maas EF. Postural orthostatic tachycardia syndrome: diagnostic value of thermoregulatory sweat test. Clin Auton Res 1997; 7:258–259.

36. Low PA, Opfer-Gehrking TL, Textor SC et al. Postural tachycardia syndrome (POTS). Neurology 1995; 45(suppl 5):S19–S25.

37. Fealey RD, Robertson D. Management of orthostatic hypotension. In: Low PA, ed. Clinical Autonomic Disorders: Evaluation and Management. Philadelphia: Lippincott-Raven, 1997:763–775.

5

Peripheral Nerve Histology and Pathology

Mark B. Bromberg
University of Utah, Salt Lake City, Utah, USA

ABSTRACT

There are many causes of peripheral neuropathy, but peripheral nerve has a limited repertoire of pathological response to injury. Despite this, microscopic inspection of nerve provides information on the underlying causative process that is not available from other techniques. Basic pathologic changes are described, and findings in selected neuropathies are presented. An understanding of peripheral nerve histology and pathology is also instructive for interpreting clinical and electrodiagnostic aspects of neuropathies.

1. NERVE HISTOLOGY

1.1. Gross Structure

Sensory and motor fibers are, for the most part, intermixed within peripheral nerves. Exceptions suitable for biopsy are cutaneous sensory nerves such as the sural, superficial peroneal, and superficial radial nerves. Within the peripheral nerve, groups of several hundred nerve fibers are surrounded by layers of connective tissue and bundled into fascicles (Fig. 5.1). Nerves contain 4–10 or more fascicles, but individual fascicles are not continuous, and there is merging and branching of fascicles along the length of the peripheral nerve, with fibers moving from one fascicle to another.

1.2. Connective Tissue

Three layers of connective tissue surround nerves to provide structural support and metabolic boundaries (Fig. 5.2). Epineurium is the outer-most layer that is continuous with surrounding connective tissue, and binds fascicles into a nerve trunk. This connective tissue layer tends to be longitudinally arranged and provides strength to nerve stretching. Perineurium is the intermediate layer, consisting of a multilayered sheath of flat cells that invest fascicles. It is continuous from nerve roots to terminal ends. Cells are circumferentially arranged and are surrounded by a basement membrane. The arrangement of cells and their metabolic activity supports their role as a blood–nerve barrier that regulates the

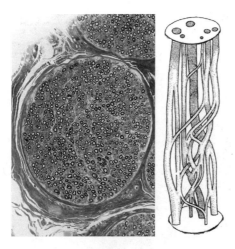

Figure 5.1 Fascicular arrangement of nerves. Photomicrograph of one complete and three neighboring fascicles (left). Drawing of branching and merging fascicles within nerve (right). [Modified from Sunderland (1).]

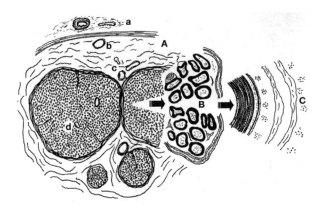

Figure 5.2 Schematic arrangement of connective tissues and blood vessels in nerve. (A) Whole nerve showing epineurium as continuous with connective tissue. (B) Enlarged section showing perineurium with circumferential cells. (C) Further enlargement showing portion of a myelinated fiber with compact myelin and endoneurium with longitudinal cells. a, indicates Nutrient artery; b, Epineurial vessels; c, Perineurial vessels; d, Intrinsic vessels. [Modified from Low (2).]

endoneuronal milieu. Endoneurium, the inner-most layer, is the infrafascicular connective tissue surrounding individual nerve fibers. The infrafascicular compartment also contains fine fibrillary material and fluid.

1.3. Vasculature

The blood supply to nerve can be divided into extrinsic and intrinsic systems. The extrinsic system includes arterioles, capillaries, and venules in the epineurium and perineurium. Vessels pierce through to connect to an intrinsic system that consists of longitudinal microvessels within the fascicular endoneurium (Fig. 5.2). Anastomoses between the external and internal vascular systems constitute a collateralized blood supply that helps maintain blood flow under conditions of ischemia. Nerve fibers are also able to use anerobic metabolism. These factors can account for the relative insensitivity of peripheral nerve to all but extreme degrees of general ischemia. Ischemia at the microvascular level, such as in the vasculidities, can cause localized nerve damage.

2. NERVE FIBER HISTOLOGY

2.1. Numbers and Sizes

Individual nerve axons vary in diameter. Larger diameter axons are individually wrapped by Schwann cells (myelinated fibers), while smaller diameter axons are wrapped in groups by Schwann cells (unmyelinated fibers) (Fig. 5.3). Myelinated fiber diameters range from 2 to 22 μm: sensory fibers have bimodal distributions with peak diameters at 4 and 10 μm, and motor fibers have bimodal distributions with peak diameters at 2 and 6 μm. The number of myelinated fibers, measured in sensory nerves, ranges from 5000 to 9000, with considerable variability between individuals. Unmyelinated fibers are challenging to count and measure, but are 3–6 times more numerous than myelinated fibers. Diameters range from 0.5 to 3.0 μm, with a unimodal peak at $\sim$1.5 μm.

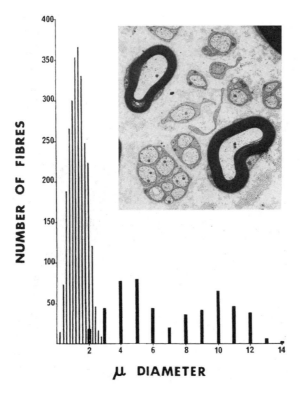

Figure 5.3 Photomicrograph and fiber diameter histogram of myelinated and unmyelinated fibers. [Modified from Ochoa and Mair (3).]

2.2. Myelinated Fibers

Myelinated axons are surrounded by a linear series of Schwann cells. Each Schwann cell is long and flat, and tightly wraps the axon in a spiral fashion (Fig. 5.4). The wrapping results in compacted layers of membranes, with little cytoplasm in between myelin. Schwann cell nuclei lie external to the wrapping. Schwann cells are arranged serially along an axon, with each Schwann cell covering 300–2000 μm of axon length, with longer length associated with larger diameter axons (Fig. 5.5). The thickness of the myelin wrapping increases with the diameter of the axon. Myelin wrappings are of uniform thickness in the internodal region, but taper at the perinodal region of the axon. There is a 1 μm space between two adjacent Schwann cells called the node of Ranvier. The axon is of uniform caliber in the internodal region, but becomes fluted in the paranodal region, and thinned by 50% at the node of Ranvier. A basement membrane covers both Schwann cells and nodes of Ranvier, and provides a guiding tube for regenerating axons.

2.3. Unmyelinated Fibers

Unmyelinated fibers, in groups of one to six, are loosely invested by single Schwann cells, forming a Remake bundle (Fig. 5.3). Schwann cells are arranged serially along axons, with each cell covering 300–500 μm. The ends of Schwann cells interdigitate, leaving no bare axonal segments. Unmyelinated fibers also cross from one Remake bundle to another. Within a fascicle, unmyelinated and small myelinated fibers tend to be clustered.

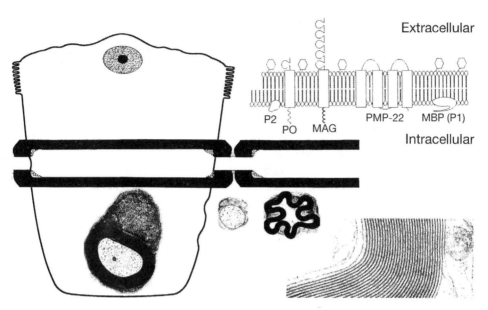

Figure 5.4 Composite figure showing components of myelinated fibers. The middle of the figure shows the outline of two myelinated fibers and a node of Ranvier. At the left is an outline of an unrolled Schwann cell, with the nucleus at the top. Within this outline is a cross-section electron micrograph of compact myelin and Schwann cell nucleus. The electron micrograph below the node of Ranvier shows the reduced diameter of the axon through this region. The micrograph to the right shows the crinkled shape of the axon in the paranodal region. The electron micrograph at lower right shows the lamallar arrangement of compact myelin. Constituent proteins in myelin are shown at the upper right. [Modified from Midroni and Bilbao (4).]

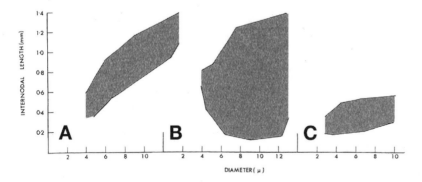

Figure 5.5 Changes in internode length, comparing neuropathies with primary demyelination to those with primary axonal loss and secondary demyelination. The boundary lines enclose the range of internode lengths. (A) Normal range of internode lengths, showing linear relationship between axon diameter and internode length with mild degree of internode variability. (B) General reduction of internode lengths in primary demyelinating neuropathy (animal model of diptheric neuropathy), with a loss of the linear relationship and greater variability. (C) Range of internode lengths in secondary demyelinating neuropathy (Wallerian degeneration) with markedly shorter internode lengths but less variability. [Modified from Fullerton et al. (5).]

3. PATHOLOGIC CHANGES

The repertoire of pathologic changes in peripheral nerve is limited. Findings observed at
the light microscopic level are emphasized. Changes to other structures, such as vessels
and connective tissue, are discussed in detail under individual types of neuropathy.

3.1. Axonal Changes

The cell body is responsible for metabolic maintenance of the long axonal process. It is felt
that many acquired neuropathies primarily affect some aspect of the cell body function or
axonal transport, leading to early changes in distal portions of the nerve. Metabolic
abnormalities and their mechanistic effects vary among diseases that cause peripheral
neuropathies, but specific mechanisms are incompletely understood. Despite this lack of
specific knowledge, many disorders lead to a common set of pathologic observations.
This has given rise to a variety of terms, including dying-back neuropathy or distal
axonopathy. Animal models of toxic neuropathies have been important sources of information on morphologic changes. The pathological changes in dying-back neuropathies
are similar to those seen with distal Wallerian degeneration following an axonal lesion,
except that dying-back changes evolve more slowly and co-exist with regenerative changes.

The most distal, large diameter myelinated fibers are the first to be affected. A
schematic representation of changes is depicted in Fig. 5.6. The initial change is felt
to be in the axon, with an accumulation of abnormal mitochondria, organelles, and
disorganized microtubules and neurofilaments. Changes to myelin occur soon after
acute injury (7). Myelin swells at the paranodal regions, leading to secondary changes
in myelin. The earliest observed changes at the light microscopic level are the formation
of rows of myelin ovoids that are best viewed in teased fiber preparation (Fig. 5.7). Ovoids

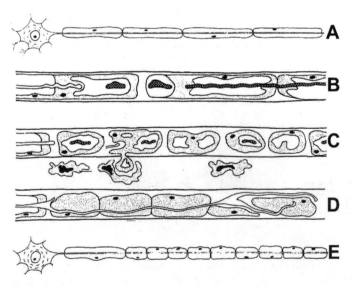

Figure 5.6 Schematic drawing of primary axonal neuropathy with secondary demyelination, and
subsequent remyelination. (A) Normal nerve. (B) Early axonal degeneration with subsequent
demyelination and formation of myelin ovoids. (C) Formation of digestion chambers with macrophages removing myelin debris. (D) Early axonal regeneration and remyelination. (E) Regenerated
axon with shorter internode lengths. [Modified from Bradley (6).]

Figure 5.7 Outline drawings of teased fibers comparing normal to changes in a primary axonal neuropathy. (Top) Normal fiber showing uniform myelin thickness and normal paranodal and node of Ranvier. (Middle) Early secondary changes in myelin consisting of irregularities and retraction of myelin at nodes of Ranvier. (Bottom) More severe changes with myelin ovoids. [Drawn from Dyck et al. (8).]

increase in size, and become larger digestion chambers that are seen on routine longitudinal nerve preparations (Fig. 5.8). Macrophages appear, filled with myelin debris. Schwann cell nuclei divide and cells begin to proliferate.

In acute axonopathy models, axonal regeneration occurs after degeneration. In chronic neuropathies, axonal regeneration frequently takes place in parallel with ongoing degeneration. Multiple growth cones sprout from a single axon and become remyelinated. Regenerating fibers are of small diameter and are thinly myelin (Fig. 5.9). This leads to several small myelinated axons within the space previously occupied by single large axons. Regenerating clusters can be distinguished from unmyelinated fibers by the presence of individual myelin sheaths. Division of Schwann cells leads to shorter internode lengths (Fig. 5.5).

The changes observed on nerve biopsy depend upon the severity and rapidity of the neuropathy. Although most neuropathies have a chronic course, a reduction in the number of axons within a fascicle will be appreciated when loss exceeds 25%. Axonal loss may be diffuse within a fascicle, or involve focal areas. In severe neuropathies there may be no visible fibers. Changes within the fascicle that support a chronic and ongoing process include endoneural fibrosis and hypercellularity (fibroblasts).

3.2. Myelin Changes

Primary segmental demyelination refers to disorders that initially affect myelin, but the pathologic process can secondarily damage axons. The segmental distribution means

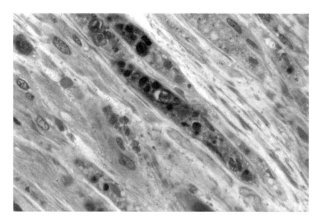

Figure 5.8 Longitudinal section micrograph showing digestion chambers in myelin due to axonal degeneration. (Figure courtesy of J. Townsend.)

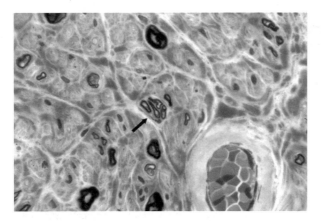

Figure 5.9 Cross-sectional micrograph of diabetic neuropathy showing marked axonal loss and clusters of regenerating fibers (arrow). (Figure courtesy of J. Townsend.)

that adjacent Schwann cells may be affected to different degrees. Elucidation of changes in primary myelinating neuropathies is derived from animal models, using various toxins such as diptheria toxin. A schematic representation of changes is depicted in Fig. 5.10. The earliest change is widening of the nodal gap. Electron-microscopy (EM) studies in acute demyelinating disorders show finger-like projections from macrophages between layers of myelin as the likely mechanism that strips away myelin. With further damage

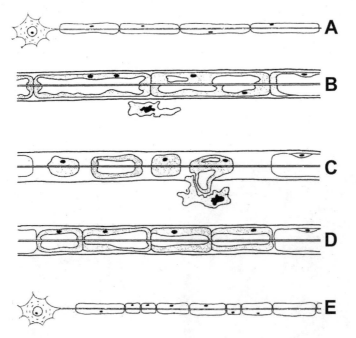

Figure 5.10 Schematic drawing of primary demyelinating neuropathy (dyptheric neuropathy). (A) Normal nerve. (B) Early changes to myelin with duplication of Schwann cell nuclei. (C) Formation of myelin ovoids and removal by macrophages. (D) Remyelinated fiber. (E) Remyelinated fiber with shorter and variable internode lengths. [Modified from Bradley (6).]

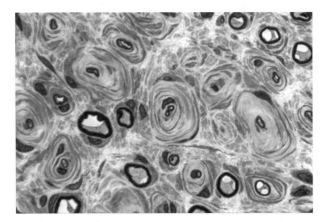

Figure 5.11 Cross-sectional micrograph of onion bulb formation characterized by multiple layers of Schwann cells around myelinated fibers. (Figure courtesy of J. Townsend.)

to myelin, macrophages can be appreciated on light microscopy to phagocytize myelin debris. Schwann cell nuclei divide, and remyelination occurs early on, initially with thin layers. Each Schwann cell contributes to the remyelination process, and internodal lengths are shorter and highly variable (Fig. 5.5).

Onion bulb formation refers to intertwined and attenuated Schwann cell processes surrounding axons (Fig. 5.11). This reflects underlying pathologic processes of repeated demyelination and remyelination. Collagen separates Schwann cell processes. Onion bulb formation is not specific to a particular type of neuropathy, and is encountered in both hereditary and acquired neuropathies that involve repeated myelin breakdown.

Secondary demyelination refers to degeneration of Schwann cells consequent to primary axonal degeneration. There is a degree of initial autophagocytosis by the Schwann cell, and subsequent removal of myelin debris by macrophages. Changes in Schwann cells and myelin subsequent to axonal damage have been discussed (Fig. 5.5–5.9).

3.3. Connective Tissue Changes

Changes in connective tissue are usually of a nonspecific nature. Vessels course through the epineurium. Perivascular cuffing with mononuclear cells is common but nonspecific, and is not synonymous with vasculitis. Epineurial vascular proliferation is indirect evidence for vasculitis. Amyloid deposition may be observed in amyloidosis. Inflammatory cells may be found in the perineurium, but is also a nonspecific finding.

3.4. Vascular Changes

Endoneurial edema may be observed as an increase in interstitial space or as a widening of subperineurial space. The space is filled with an amorphous substance, which may represent different constituents, including mucopolysaccharides, or an osmotic shift of fluid. Fluid accumulations are a nonspecific finding, but do suggest chronicity.

Focal ischemia, as in vasculitic neuropathy, results in incomplete loss of axons within a fascicle. Large axons are not preferentially affected. Changes to vessels include luminal narrowing with thrombosis, vessel sclerosis, disorganization of the vessel wall with change in the media and breakup of the internal elastic layer, focal calcification, hemosiderin indicating old hemorrhage, and recanalization and proliferation of capillaries (4).

Chronic vascular (arterial) insufficiency results in nonspecific changes. There may be reductions in axonal numbers, from mild to severe and without correlation with the degree of vascular insufficiency. Frequently, there is evidence for axonal regeneration.

4. NERVE BIOPSY

4.1. Uses and Limitations

Clinical and electrodiagnostic tests cannot reliably distinguish among underlying mechanisms. Nerve biopsies provide unique information, but the type of information may be limited for several reasons. First, biopsies view a microscopic length of nerve, and multifocal pathologic processes may be missed. Second, the spectrum of pathologic processes is limited. For example, axonal loss is a common consequence of many underlying pathologic processes. Nerve biopsies are most informative when the clinical and electrodiagnostic tests suggest specific diagnoses that require pathologic confirmation (Table 5.1).

4.2. Suitable Nerves

Most nerve biopsies are of sensory nerves because permanent sensory loss from the biopsy is better tolerated than weakness that would result if a mixed nerve was biopsied. The additional sensory loss from the biopsy will be less noticed in the context of the sensory disturbance from the underlying neuropathy. Fortunately, most neuropathies involve both sensory and motor fibers and a sensory nerve will be representative. The nerve chosen should show clinical and electrodiagnostic evidence of pathologic involvement. Nerves most commonly biopsied are the sural and superficial peroneal nerves, and occasionally the superficial radial. Fascicular motor nerve biopsies are feasible in pure motor neuropathies. A simultaneous muscle biopsy may increase the yield of finding pathologic changes, especially for vasculitis (9).

4.3. The Biopsy

Biopsies are performed under local anesthesia with minimal morbidity, although wound healing may be an issue (7). A several centimeter segment of nerve is taken, and cut into a number of pieces for different pathologic processing. A cross-sectional piece and longitudinal piece are imbedded in paraffin, and another cross-sectional piece flash-

Table 5.1 Neuropathies
that can be Diagnosed
by Nerve Biopsy

Vasculitis
Leprosy
Sarcoidosis
Amyloidoisis
Infiltrative neoplasms
Hexacarbon inhalation
HNPP
Charcot–Marie–Tooth
Giant axonal neuropathy
Storage diseases

frozen for immunologic studies. Another piece is fixed in gluteraldehyde for plastic-embedded 1 μm plastic sections. EM may be performed on plastic sections if necessary. A segment can be prepared for fiber teasing. Not all techniques are necessary or available in a given laboratory (especially teased fiber analysis), and plans for specific preparations and staining can be made depending upon diagnostic questions.

4.4. Biopsy Review

Steps in reviewing a nerve biopsy include general fascicular histology for adequacy of the preparation, inspection of connective tissue, and assessment of individual fascicules for changes to axons and myelin. The pathophysiological questions to be answered are: (1) Is the biopsy normal, or is there evidence for a peripheral neuropathy? (2) If abnormal, is there evidence for a primary axonal, a primary demyelinating, or a mixed neuropathy? (3) What is the time course, acute or chronic? (4) Are there pathologic features supporting a specific diagnosis? Finally, the biopsy findings must be placed in the context of the clinical and electrodiagnostic findings to make a final diagnosis that makes sense.

4.5. Biopsy Yield

The question of the diagnostic yield of a nerve biopsy is important but difficult to answer because there is sample bias based on what types of patients are sent for biopsy. A biopsy is most informative if a specific question is asked, and the most common clinical question is whether there is a vasculitis (9). Studies in the elderly suggest that vasculitis is not uncommon, but the clinical and therapeutic significance is not clear (10). Nerve biopsy gives little discriminative information in toxic neuropathies, except for hexacarbon toxicity. Inflammatory neuropathies can be more accurately diagnosed by electrodiagnostic studies than by biopsy (11). Idiopathic peripheral neuropathies represent a common class for which the question of whether to biopsy is difficult to answer. When a peripheral neuropathy has a very slow progressive course with little functional disability, a biopsy is unlikely to identify a specific cause (12,13).

5. CLASSES OF NEUROPATHY

5.1. Inflammatory Neuropathies

Nerve biopsy findings are similar for the Guillain–Barré syndrome, or acute inflammatory demyelinating polyradiculoneuropathy (AIDP), and chronic inflammatory demyelinating polyradiculoneuropathy (CIDP).

Pathologic changes are dependent upon the stage of the neuropathy, and are more specific in the acute phase of AIDP and less specific in CIDP. Endoneurial mononuclear cell infiltration is a prominent feature in AIDP, and less common in CIDP. Cells are mostly lymphocytes and macrophages, with fewer polymorphonuclear leukocytes. The cells are found in association with venules and precapillaries. Macrophages are observed in close association with axons. Endoneurial edema is often present. Segmental demyelination and remyelination is the most important feature (Fig. 5.10). This includes combinations of fibers with normal myelin, thin myelin and bare axons, and macrophages with myelin debris (Fig. 5.12). Schwann cells proliferate and remyelinate with shorter internodal segments (Fig. 5.5). Axonal loss may be marked in severe cases of AIDP, but is more common in CIDP. Onion bulb formations also occur in CIDP.

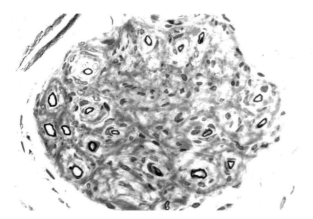

Figure 5.12   Cross-sectional micrograph in CIDP showing axonal loss, hyper cellularity and evidence of remyelination with small diameter fibers and thin myelin. (Figure courtesy of J. Townsend.)

5.2.   Vasculitic Neuropathies

The vasculitidies that affect peripheral nerve are characterized by small vessel occlusion causing axonal loss. Vessel destruction is characterized by the presence of inflammatory infiltrates within the vessel wall, leading to fibrinoid necrosis and thrombosis (Fig. 5.13). Transmural damage is an essential pathologic feature of vasculitis, and perivascular inflammation without fibrinoid necrosis is a nonspecific finding and insufficient for the diagnosis of vasculitis. Acute vessel changes include infiltration of the muscularis and endothelial layers with inflammatory cells, and fragmentation of the internal elastic lamina is characteristic. Old lesions may be recognized as fibrous obliteration of vessels in association with hemosiderin-laden macrophages.

The amount of fiber loss varies from none to severe, presumably depending upon the degree of involvement of the biopsied nerve. The pattern of fiber loss within a fascicle also varies, but characteristically affects discrete areas, and is not randomly scattered

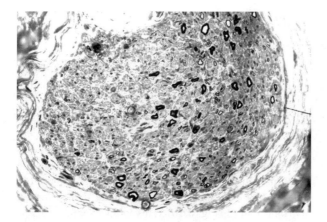

Figure 5.13   Cross-sectional micrographs in vasculitis. (A) Small vessel showing fibrinoid necrosis and partial occlusion of the vessel lumen. (B) Nerve fascicle showing discrete area of axonal loss. (Figure courtesy of J. Townsend.)

throughout the fascicle (Fig. 5.13). Vascular lesions may be focal or patchy in distribution, and multiple sections along the length of the biopsied nerve should be studied if clinical suspicion is high and no involved vessels are found with the initial survey. A combination biopsy of nerve and neighboring muscle may increase the diagnostic yield (9).

5.3. Amyloid Neuropathies

Amyloid is an extra cellular protein composed of beta-pleated sheets that accumulate in the epineurium, perineurium or endoneurium, or in adipose tissue. Neuropathies attributed to excess amyloid occur in both acquired and hereditary forms of amyloidosis. Amyloid deposition can be identified with Congo red stain by its characteristic apple-green yellow birefringence stain. The primary nerve pathology is axonal loss, of varying degrees. The degree of loss may not correlate with the degree of amyloid observed in the biopsied nerve segment, and is attributed to the effects of amyloid at more proximal locations along the nerve. The mechanism of amyloid-induced damage is not clear. One is mechanical pressure on nerves from extraneural depositon within connective tissue. Another is deposition of amyloid within vessel walls (Fig. 5.14). Patients with amyloid neuropathy may not show amyloid deposition in nerve, and if suspected, other tissues should be biopsied, such as rectal tissue and fat aspirates (14).

5.4. Hereditary Neuropathies

Charcot–Marie–Tooth neuropathies represent a heterogeneous group of hereditary nerve disorders. The most common forms have been broadly divided by electrodiagnostic and pathologic criteria into hypertrophic (type 1) and neuronal (type 2) forms. Both types include axonal loss. Further subtyping is based on genotypes, but genetic subtypes cannot be distinguished pathologically.

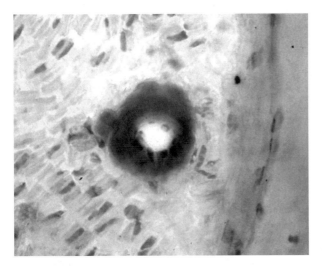

Figure 5.14   Cross-sectional micrograph showing amyloid deposition (Congo red stain) in a small vessel. (Figure courtesy of J. Townsend.)

Hypertrophic type 1 neuropathies are characterized pathologically by enlarged nerves due to increased numbers of Schwann cells with frequent onion bulb formations and a myxoid-appearing interstitium composed largely of collagen. This results in enlarged fascicles, up to several times normal. There is a variable degree of fiber loss, dependant upon the severity of the neuropathy, and there may be no nerve fibers in a distal biopsy. Unmyelinated fibers are less affected.

Neuronal type 2 neuropathies have normal or smaller fascicles, and there is no edema. The number of myelinated fibers is reduced and frequently there are no fibers in a distal biopsy. Clusters of regenerating fibers are common, but there is no evidence for demyelination or onion bulb formation. Unmyelinated fibers are normal.

Hereditary predisposition to pressure palsies (HNPP) has unique pathological features. Myelinated fibers with very thick myelin sheaths (tomaculi) are observed (Fig. 5.15). Some myelin may be thickened circumferentially or eccentrically and may have focal out- or in-foldings of myelin. The number of myelinated fibers is usually normal, with little evidence for axonal degeneration.

5.5. Diabetic Neuropathies

Pathologic changes in diabetic distal symmetric neuropathies are primarily axonal in nature, with secondary changes to myelin. These pathologic findings are not specific for diabetes. There is loss of large and small myelinated fibers, roughly in proportion to clinical severity. Neuropathies classified clinically as affecting predominantly small fiber function may show corresponding predominant loss of unmyelinated fibers. Axonal loss leads to frequent regenerating clusters of axons and fibers with thin myelin, and there is segmental demyelination (Fig. 5.9).

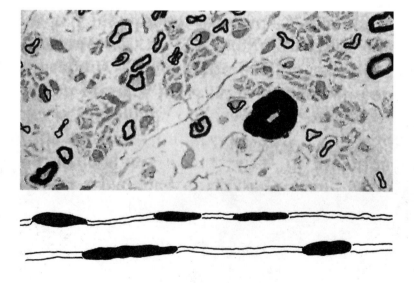

Figure 5.15 HNPP. (Top) Micrograph comparing thick myelin of tomaculi with normal myelin. (Bottom) Teased fiber preparation showing focal enlargement of myelin (tomaculi). [Drawn and modified from Mendell et al. (15).]

Pathologic findings in proximal focal diabetic neuropathies (lumbosacral radiculoplexus neuropathies) are primarily implicated from distal nerve biopsies. Focal nerve fiber loss, reflecting primary axonal damage, is prominent. There is also evidence for perineural thickening and inflammatory cells in perivascular and vascular location. These changes are interpreted as reflecting an inflammatory microvasculitis leading to multifocal nerve ischemia (16). In contrast to the vasculidities described earlier, that involve larger vessels, fibrinoid necrosis is rarely observed in lumbosacral radiculoplexus neuropathies, presumably due to the small size of involved vessels.

5.6. Toxic Neuropathies

Neuropathies may be caused by a diverse group of exogenous toxins such as drugs and industrial solvents. Included in this category are neuropathies associated with altered metabolic states due to vitamin deficiencies and systemic diseases. The primary pathology is axonal loss, in a length-dependent fashion. Large myelinated fibers are affected earlier and more severely than small fibers. The degree of axonal loss depends upon the dose and length of exposure. Early changes are restricted to individual fibers, and late in the course there may be no fibers in distal specimens. In chronic disorders, there will be endoneurial fibrosis and hypercellularity reflecting Schwann cell proliferation. Of note, the length-dependent pathology includes the central processes of dorsal root ganglion neurons resulting in axonal loss in rostral portions of the funiculus gracilis. In severe cases, dorsal root ganglion and anterior horn cell bodies may undergo chromatolytic changes.

Several toxins have unique pathologic features. n Hexane neuropathy from inhaling rubber cement results in characteristic fusiform swelling of distal axonal segments due to accumulation of neurofilaments (Fig. 5.16). Swollen segments are mainly in the internode segment, and the overlying myelin may be thin. Axonal diameters in swollen segments may be several times normal axonal diameters.

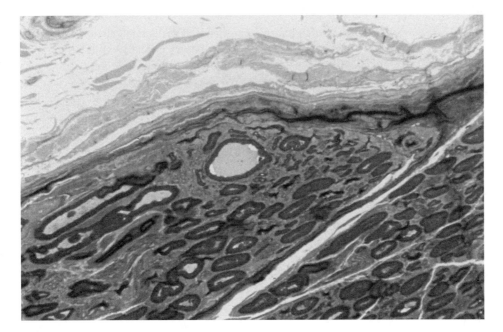

Figure 5.16 Micrograph of n-hexane neuropathy showing enlarged axons. Some fibers are cut in oblique section. (Figure courtesy of A.G. Smith.)

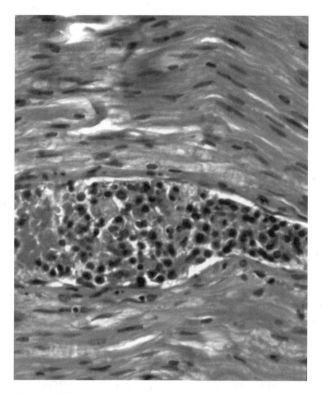

Figure 5.17 Longitudinal section micrograph showing B-cell infiltration. (Figure courtesy of J. Townsend.)

5.7. Neuropathies Associated with Cancer

Neuropathies may be associated with direct infiltration of malignant cells or as a remote effect (paraneoplastic syndrome). Nerve infiltration occurs primarily with hematologic malignancies. In lymphomatous neuropathies, diffuse and massive infiltration may occur, frequently involving all compartments (endoneurium, perineurium, and epineurium) (Fig. 5.17). Collections of cells are noted around vessels. Chronic axonal damage with segmental demyelination and remyelination are observed.

5.8. Other Neuropathies

There are other uncommon conditions with suggestive or characteristic pathologic features on nerve biopsy that will not be covered because of their rarity and the clinical picture is sufficiently distinct to be diagnostic. These include metachromatic leukodystrophies, globoid cell leukodystrophy, Fabry disease, Niemann–Pick, and Tangier disease.

ACKNOWLEDGMENTS

I thank Jeannette Townsend, MD, for her review of the manuscript, and Becky Guertler for her help with the figures.

REFERENCES

1. Sunderland S. Nerves and Nerve Injuries. 2nd ed. Edinburgh: Churchill Livingstone, 1978.
2. Low R. The perineurium and connective tissue of peripheral nerve. In: Landon D, ed. The Peripheral Nerve. London: Chapman and Hall, 1976:159–187.
3. Ochoa J, Mair W. The normal sural nerve. Acta Neuropathologica 1969; 13:197–216.
4. Midroni G, Bilbao J. Biopsy Diagnosis of Peripheral Neuropathy. Boston: Butterworth-Heinemann, 1995.
5. Fullerton P, Gilliatt R, Lancelles R, Morgan-Huges J. Relation between fibre diameter and internodal length in chronic neuropathy. J Physiol 1965; 178:26P–28P.
6. Bradley W. Disorders of Peripheral Nerves. Oxford: Blackwell, 1974.
7. Dyck P, Giannini C, Lais A. Pathologic alternations of nerves. In: Dyck P, Thomas P, Griffin J, Low P, Poduslo J, eds. Peripheral Neuropathy. 3rd ed. Philadelphia: WB Saunders Company, 1993:514–595.
8. Dyck P, Johnson W, Lambert E, O'Brien P. Segmental demyelination secondary to axonal degeneration in uremic neuropathy. Mayo Clin Proc 1971; 46:406–431.
9. Collins M, Periquet M, Mendell J, Sahenk Z, Nagaraja H, Kissel J. Nonsystemic vasculitic neuropathy. Insights from a clinical cohort. Neurology 2003; 61:623–630.
10. Chia L, Fernandez A, Lacroix C, Adams D, Planté V, Said G. Contribution of nerve biopsy findings to the diagnosis of disabling neuropathy in the elderly. A retrospective review of 100 consecutive patients. Brain 1996; 119:1091–1098.
11. Krendel D, Parks H, Anthony D, St Clair M, Graham D. Sural nerve biopsy in chronic inflammatory demyelinating polyradiculoneuropathy. Muscle Nerve 1989; 12:257–264.
12. Wolfe G, Baker N, Amato A, Jackson C, Nations S, Saperstein D et al. Chronic crytogenic sensory polyneuropathy. Clinical and laboratory characteristics. Arch Neurol 1999; 56:540–547.
13. Notermans M, Wokke J, Franssen H, van der Graaf Y, Vermeulin M, van den Berg L et al. Chronic idiopathic polyneuropathy presenting in middle or old age: a clinical and electrophysiological study of 75 patients. J Neurol Neurosurg Psychiatr 1993; 56:1066–1071.
14. Simmons Z, Blaivas M, Aguilera A, Feldman E, Bromberg M, Towfighi J. Low diagnostic yield of sural nerve biopsy in patients with peripheral neuropathy and primary amyloidosis. J Neurol Sci 1993; 120:60–63.
15. Mendell J, Kissel J, Cornblath D. Diagnosis and Management of Peripheral Nerve Disorders. Oxford: Oxford University Press, 2001.
16. Dyck P, Norell J, Dyck P. Microvasculitis and ischemia in diabetic lumbosacral radiculoplexus neuropathy. Neurology 1999; 53:2113–2121.

6
Skin Biopsy

A. Gordon Smith
University of Utah, Salt Lake City, Utah, USA

ABSTRACT

One of the most common clinical situations encountered in general neurologic practice is numb painful feet. Patients often complain of numbness and significant pain, but have minimal objective findings on neurologic examination. Nerve conduction studies are often normal. Skin biopsy stained for peripheral nerve axons is usually abnormal in these patients and is often the only objective evidence of peripheral neuropathy. Other structures including sensory receptors and sweat glands may also be observed. Because the density of epidermal innervation is a quantitative and reproducible measure of small fiber neuropathy severity, skin biopsy is also a useful research tool and may be used to follow neuropathy progression and evaluate potential therapies.

1. INTRODUCTION

Although the routine use of skin biopsy as a means of studying peripheral neuropathy is a recent development, the existence of epidermal nerve fibers was first demonstrated by Langerhans (1) in 1868. Langerhans' initial description was accurate, including a drawing demonstrating several epidermal fibers branching from the dermal plexus, and

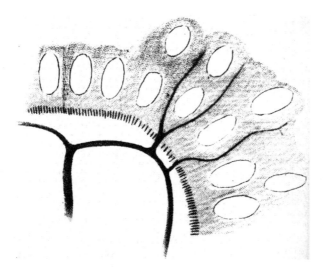

Figure 6.1 A drawing from Langerhans' in 1868 accurately depicts the anatomy of epidermal innervation.

ascending in between keratinocytes toward the epidermal surface (Fig. 6.1). Despite the fact that other investigators in the first-half of the 20th century confirmed his observations (2), the technical difficulties encountered in attempts to stain the fine epidermal fibers led to a belief developed that the epidermis was devoid of significant innervation (3). The development of an antibody against neuropeptide protein gene product 9.5 (PGP 9.5) in the 1980s (4), which effectively stains all axons, allowed Kennedy and Wendelschafer-Crabb (5) to demonstrate numerous nerve fibers in all layers of human epidermis. Since this confirmation of Langerhans' initial observation, several groups have demonstrated the utility of skin biopsy as a means of evaluating patients with small fiber neuropathy.

2. TECHNIQUE

Skin biopsies are performed using a 3 mm punch after injection of a local anesthetic. The biopsy procedure is generally very well tolerated with only minimal risk of infection (1/1000). The biopsy site heals over ~2 weeks, similar to a deep scratch, resulting in a small scar that fades over months. Because the procedure is so well tolerated, it may be repeated over time to measure changes in nerve fiber density. The sites biopsied depend on the clinical question. Most subjects with a diagnostic question of a distal polyneuropathy undergo biopsy of a distal site (ankle) and a proximal site (thigh) in order to evaluate a length dependent pattern of fiber loss. Biopsy of truncal skin may be useful in evaluating thoracic radiculopathy or sensory ganglionopathy (6). Although rarely used clinically, biopsy of glabrous skin (finger or toe pad) may be used to study Meissner's and Pacinian corpuscles, sensory receptors important in touch and vibration sensation (Fig. 6.2).

Biopsy tissue is immediately placed in fixative (paraformaldehyde lysine phosphate). After several hours, fixed skin is placed in a cryoprotectant and cut into 50 μm thick sections using a freezing sliding microtome. The free floating sections are stained with PGP 9.5. Biopsy slides may be analyzed using either standard light microscopy or confocal microscopy. Confocal microscopy facilitates staining with multiple antibodies simultaneously and provides a three-dimensional picture of the skin and is therefore a powerful research technique. However, light microscopy is equally useful for most clinical purposes.

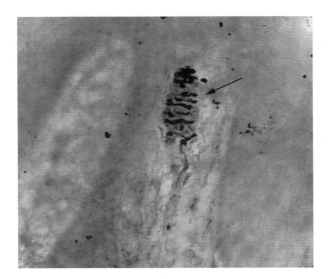

Figure 6.2 A Meissner's corpuscle located at the apex of a dermal papillae.

PGP 9.5, the most commonly used antibody, binds to the C terminus of ubiquitin hydrolase and therefore robustly stains all neurons and axons. PGP 9.5 is the primary antibody used in clinical testing. Other antibodies may be useful in research and rare clinical settings. For example, antibodies against calcitonin gene-related proteins (CGRP), vasoactive intestinal polypeptide (VIP), and substance P may be used to stain sweat glands or blood vessels.

3. NORMAL INNERVATION

Skin is divided into several layers (Fig. 6.3). The epidermis is the most superficial layer of skin. Immediately underlying the epidermis is the dermis. Several different types of nerves supply the dermis and epidermis. There is a rich plexus of myelinated nerve fibers in the dermis that supplies piloerector muscles (Fig. 6.4) and sweat glands (Fig. 6.5), as well as

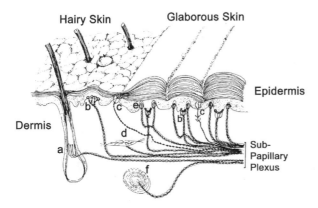

Figure 6.3 Normal skin contains a variety of sensory organs. (A) Palisade sensory endings in a hair follicle (hair movement). (B) Merkel cells (touch). (C) Intraepidermal "free" nerve fibers (pain sensation). (D) Ruffini ending (touch). (E) Meissner's corpuscles (touch). (F) Pacinian corpuscle (vibration).

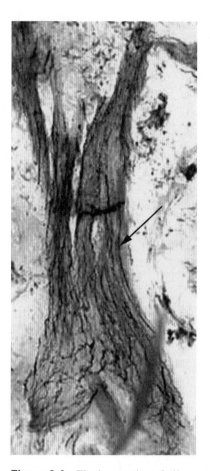

Figure 6.4   The innervation of piloerector muscles (arrow) is easily observed in skin biopsy.

specialized sensory organs including Meissner's and Pacinian corpuscles and Merkel cells that are important in perception of vibration and touch. The dermis normally invaginates the epidermis as papillae. Dermal nerve fibers approach and enter the dermis at the apex of papillae and subsequently branch into several unmyelinated axons which extend to the surface of the skin in a parallel fashion (Fig. 6.6). These fibers terminate immediately beneath the surface of the skin and often have a small terminal enlargement (5).

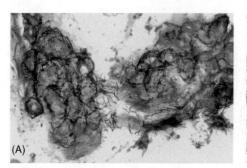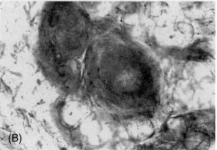

Figure 6.5   (A) Normal innervation of two sweat glands. (B) Absent innervation of sweat glands in a patient with congenital insensitivity to pain due to a mutation of the tyrosine kinase A receptor.

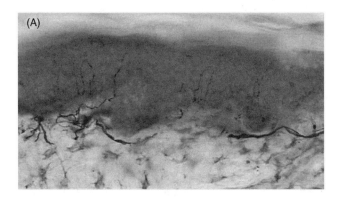

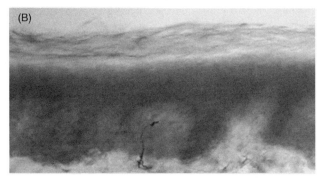

Figure 6.6   (A) Normal innervation with nerve fibers extending through the epidermis, parallel to one another, extending toward the skin surface. (B) A patient with small fiber neuropathy has a total absence of epidermal nerve fibers with a single dermal fiber terminating prematurely beneath the epidermis.

The pattern of skin innervation varies with anatomic location. For example, Meissner's and Pacinian corpuscles are most commonly observed in glabrous skin of the finger and toe pads. Epidermal nerve fibers are distributed throughout the body but density varies with location, with intraepidermal nerve fiber density (IENFD) highest at distal sites (7).

The effects of aging on cutaneous innervation are controversial. Dermal papillae become lower in height and there is denervation of sweat glands with aging (8). There is also a reduction in the density of both myelinated and unmyelinated sensory nerve fibers within the sural nerve with aging (9). In contrast to these observations, the density of epidermal nerve fibers appears to remain constant, although few subjects >75 years old have been studied (7,10). The reason for the discrepancy between sural nerve and IENFD data is unknown. However, the stability of epidermal nerve fiber density facilitates the use of skin biopsy as a sensitive clinical tool in the evaluation of small fiber peripheral neuropathy at advanced ages.

4. CLINICAL APPLICATIONS

Skin biopsy was first used in the study of peripheral neuropathy in the 1960s, when investigators at the Mayo Clinic demonstrated reduced numbers of Meissner's corpuscles from glabrous skin of subjects with a variety of inherited neuropathies, including Charcot–Marie–Tooth disease. The first routine use of skin biopsy for neuropathy came after the development of PGP 9.5, which allowed for the easy identification of epidermal nerve fibers. Several investigators have demonstrated reduced density of epidermal fibers in a length dependent fashion in sensory neuropathies caused by HIV, antiretroviral therapy, diabetes, and in idiopathic neuropathy [Fig. 6.6(B)] (11–14). Surviving fibers often have morphologic abnormalities including axonal swellings or unusual branching patterns [Fig. 6.7(A)]. These morphologic changes are frequently observed at sites well proximal to the area of symptoms. In areas with reduced epidermal fiber density, dermal fibers may approach the dermal–epidermal junction, but either end abruptly or branch beneath the epidermis [Fig. 6.7(B)]. Patients with pain and numbness limited to the feet often have these changes in skin from the proximal thigh. Analysis of other structures, particularly sweat glands, may also be useful, and patients with peripheral neuropathy often have denervated sweat glands [Fig. 6.5(B)].

Fiber density does not correlate with nerve conduction study parameters, an expected observation given that routine electrophysiologic evaluation is limited to large diameter fibers, whereas skin biopsy specifically evaluates small fibers. As anticipated, there is good correlation with the number of small unmyelinated fiber in sural nerve biopsy tissue (15). Fiber density correlates with pain but not sudomotor function (16,17). These findings suggest that epidermal nerve fibers are normally responsible for pain sensation and damage results in abnormal sensations including pain.

Skin biopsy is a very useful tool in the diagnosis of peripheral neuropathy, particularly for patients who have painful feet. Approximately 30–50% of patients presenting with foot pain and numbness have normal nerve conduction studies (17,18). Even when other specialized tests such as quantitative sensory testing and sudomotor testing are used, one-third of patients with this common clinical presentation require skin biopsy to confirm the diagnosis of neuropathy. When a normal skin biopsy is obtained, a careful search for a central nervous system cause for pain is warranted (17). Although processing of skin biopsy tissue requires a specialized laboratory, biopsy tissue may be easily shipped to laboratories offering this test. Therefore, no special equipment or training (aside from performing the skin biopsy itself) is necessary to use this test in routine clinical practice.

5. WHEN TO PERFORM A SKIN BIOPSY?

Skin biopsy is most often used in the evaluation of patients with foot pain and numbness but a normal nerve conduction study. In this setting, an abnormal skin biopsy confirms the

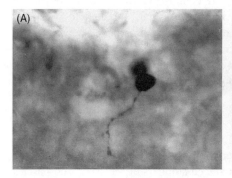
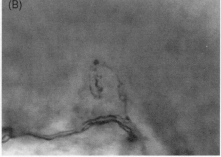

Figure 6.7 Predegenerative structural changes in small fiber neuropathy. (A) Axonal swellings at a proximal site (thigh) in a patient with symptoms limited to the feet. (B) Excessive branching and premature termination of nerve fibers as they approach the epidermal surface.

clinical suspicion of a small fiber predominant neuropathy. Skin biopsy may also be useful in patients with suspected painful neuropathy in whom measurement of distal lower extremity sensory responses is complicated by technical issues (edema and obesity) or advanced age.

A rare syndrome of acute diffuse burning pain, often following a viral illness, has been described. Most patients describe their pain as resembling a sunburn. This syndrome is presumably due to postinfectious injury to small cutaneous nerve fibers in a nonlength dependent fashion or the dorsal root ganglion neurons responsible for small fiber sensory function. Nerve conduction studies are normal, but skin biopsy reveals diffusely reduced IENFD (19).

Broadly speaking, skin biopsy is useful in any situation where the demonstration of peripheral sensory axonal loss, especially if it involves small fibers, is diagnostically important, but impractical using other available means. For example, skin biopsy may occasionally be of use in confirming a diagnosis of thoracic radiculopathy due to Herpes Zoster. Although this diagnosis is usually strait forward, if there is no clear history of vesicles, skin biopsy may be used to confirm the presence of sensory denervation corresponding to a thoracic dermatome. In this instance, a biopsy of the involved area should be compared with another proximal site other than the opposite side, because bilateral denervation is often observed (20).

6. RESEARCH APPLICATIONS

In addition to providing a clinically useful diagnostic test, skin biopsy is also a useful research tool. Skin biopsy tissue stained for peripheral nerve can be used to study the neurobiology of disease. For example, skin biopsy has demonstrated that sensory axonal loss occurs bilaterally in postherpetic neuralgia, even when symptoms are unilateral (20). Because skin biopsy is a very sensitive measure of small fiber sensory integrity, it may be used to study subclinical peripheral nerve changes. For example, many patients with late onset sporadic restless legs syndrome have evidence of a neuropathy using skin biopsy, supporting the role of sensory neuropathy in the development of restless legs syndrome (21). Following a skin biopsy, sensory nerves from adjacent skin reinnervate the biopsy site. Skin biopsy may therefore be used to study cutaneous reinnervation.

Perhaps, the most useful research application is as an endpoint measure for treatment trials for peripheral neuropathy. Many common neuropathies cause prominent small fiber injury, including diabetes and HIV. Traditional surrogate measures of neuropathy progression measure large fiber loss (e.g., nerve conduction studies). In neuropathies with mixed small and large fiber loss, specific therapies may preferentially target small fiber function (e.g., nerve growth factor for diabetic neuropathy). Because skin biopsy provides a reproducible and quantitative means of evaluating cutaneous innervation, it holds promise as an endpoint measure for neuropathy trials and has been used as a secondary progression measure in one study of nerve growth factor in HIV neuropathy (22). By causing focal epidermal denervation by injecting capsaicin and the effect of different agents on the rate or degree of reinnervation may also be studied.

7. CONCLUSION

Skin biopsy is a useful clinical and research tool in the evaluation of patients with painful sensory peripheral neuropathy. Epidermal denervation may be the only laboratory evidence confirming the suspicion of a neuropathy prominently involving small diameter nerve fibers. Skin biopsy may also be used in other clinical settings to confirm and quantitate sensory axonal loss. Because skin biopsy is minimally invasive and well tolerated it may be repeated in order to evaluate neuropathy progression.

REFERENCES

1. Langerhans P. Uber die nerven der menschlichen haut. Virchows Arch Pathol Anat 1868; 44:325–337.
2. Arthur R, Shelley W. The innervation of human epidermis. J Invest Dermatol 1959; 32:397–411.
3. Winkelmann R. Cutaneous sensory nerves. Semin Dermatol 1988; 7:236–268.
4. Thompson R, Doran J, Jackson P, Dhillon A, Rode J. PGP 9.5—a new marker for vertebrate neurons and neuroendocrine cells. Brain Res 1983; 278:224–228.
5. Kennedy W, Wendelschafer-Crabb. The innervation of human epidermis. J Neurol Sci 1993; 115:184–190.
6. Lauria G, McArthur J, Hauer P, Griffin J, Cornblath D. Neuropathological alterations in diabetic truncal neuropathy: evaluation by skin biopsy. J Neurol Neurosurg Psychiatry 1998; 65:762–766.
7. McArthur JC, Stocks EA, Hauer P, Cornblath DR, Griffin JW. Epidermal nerve fiber density: normative reference range and diagnostic efficiency. Arch Neurol 1998; 55:1513–1520.
8. Abdel-Rahman T, Collins K, Cown T, Rustin M. Immunohistochemical morphological and functional changes in the peripheral sudomotor neuro-effector system in elderly people. J Auton Nerv Syst 1992; 37:187–198.
9. Jacobs J, Love S. Qualitative and quantitative morphology of human sural nerve at different ages. Brain 1985; 108:897–924.
10. Lauria G, Holland N, Hauer P, Cornblath DR, Griffin JW, McArthur JC. Epidermal innervation: changes with aging, topographic location, and in sensory neuropathy. J Neurol Sci 1999; 164:172–178.
11. Hirai A, Yasuda H, Joko M, Maeda T, Kikkawa R. Evaluation of diabetic neuropathy through the quantitation of cutaneous nerves. J Neurol Sci 2000; 172:55–62.
12. Holland NR, Stocks A, Hauer P, Cornblath DR, Griffin JW, McArthur JC. Intraepidermal nerve fiber density in patients with painful sensory neuropathy. Neurology 1997; 48:708–711.
13. Kennedy WR, Wendelschafer Crabb G, Johnson T. Quantitation of epidermal nerves in diabetic neuropathy. Neurology 1996; 47:47–59.
14. Smith AG, Tripp C, Singleton JR. Skin biopsy findings in patients with neuropathy associated with diabetes and impaired glucose tolerance. Neurology 2001; 57:1701.
15. Herrmann D, Griffin J, Hauer P, Cornblath D, McArthur J. Epidermal nerve fiber density and sural nerve morphometry in peripheral neuropathies. Neurology 1999; 53:1634–1640.
16. Polydefkis M, Yiannoutsos C, Cohen B et al. Reduced intraepidermal nerve fiber density in HIV associated sensory neuropathy. Neurology 2002; 58:115–119.
17. Periquet MI, Novak V, Collins MP et al. Painful sensory neuropathy prospective evaluation using skin biopsy. Neurology 1999; 53:1641–1647.
18. Wolfe GI, Barohn RJ. Cryptogenic sensory and sensorimotor polyneuropathies. Semin Neurol 1998; 18:105–111.
19. Holland NR, Crawford TO, Hauer P, Cornblath DR, Griffin JW, McArthur JC. Small-fiber sensory neuropathies: clinical course and neuropathology of idiopathic cases. Ann Neurol 1998; 44:47–59.
20. Oaklander AL, Romans K, Horasek S, Stocks A, Hauer P, Meyer RA. Unilateral postherpetic neuralgia is associated with bilateral sensory neuron damage. Ann Neurol 1998; 44:789–795.
21. Polydefkis M, Allen R, Hauer P, Earley C, Griffin J, McArthur J. Subclinical small fiber neuropathy in late-onset restless legs syndrome. Neurology 2000; 55:1115–1121.
22. McArthur J, Yiannoutsos C, Simpson DM et al. A phase II trial of nerve growth factor for sensory neuropathy associated with HIV infection. Neurology 2000; 54:1080–1088.

7
MR Imaging of the Peripheral Nerve

Kevin R. Moore
University of Utah, Salt Lake City, Utah, USA

ABSTRACT

Magnetic resonance imaging (MRI) is the best modality for evaluating the integrity and architecture of peripheral nerve. High quality peripheral nerve imaging can be performed on routine clinical MRI scanners using commercially available MRI coils. Peripheral nerve imaging is a useful adjunct to the clinical examination and electrodiagnostic testing and can anatomically localize a lesion, provide important details about internal nerve architecture integrity, and in some cases, provide a specific diagnosis. Normal nerve on MRI is anatomically continuous and discrete, and well-defined fascicles can be discerned that are isointense to adjacent muscle tissue on T1 weighted sequences and slightly hyperintense to adjacent muscle tissue on fat saturated T2 weighted or short tau inversion recovery sequences. Abnormal nerve may demonstrate segmental nerve enlargement, disruption of nerve anatomic continuity, distortion of normal fascicular architecture, or T2 signal hyperintensity approaching that of regional blood vessels. The effects of motor nerve damage can be assessed in muscle as changes from acute and chronic denervation. MRI of muscle can help confirm a suspected peripheral nerve lesion and may augment incomplete or nonconclusive electrodiagnostic testing results.

1. INTRODUCTION

An expanding variety of techniques applicable to peripheral nerve imaging are available including conventional X-rays, ultrasonography, computed tomography (CT), and MR imaging (MRI). Each has advantages and disadvantages. Conventional X-ray studies lack contrast resolution and the ability to image structures in multiple planes (multiplanar capabilities) and are of limited use in evaluating peripheral nerve abnormalities. X-ray studies are useful in the evaluation of adjacent osseous structures. Ultrasound is inexpensive and useful for real time static and dynamic evaluation of peripheral nerves and adjacent tendons, but is highly operator dependent and has lower contrast resolution than MRI. CT provides better contrast resolution than conventional X-ray and permits multiplanar reconstruction in nonaxial planes, but has lower contrast resolution relative to MRI. Its reliance on ionizing radiation also limits its applicability. Only MRI has sufficient contrast and spatial resolution, multiplanar capabilities, and flexibility for evaluating peripheral nerve and muscle.

All images in this chapter were obtained using currently available clinical (1.5 T) MR scanners and FDA approved and commercially available volume or surface coils. The best quality images are obtained using dedicated phased array surface coils and high performance MR scanner gradients. Insurmountable spatial resolution limits and the inability to perform chemical fat saturation on many low-field scanners seriously limit their utility for examining peripheral nerves. It is not possible to achieve consistently high-quality imaging of peripheral nerve structures using an MR scanner with field strengths <1.5 T.

Both conventional and high-resolution imaging approaches are possible. Conventional MRI protocols use commonly available general-purpose volume or phase array coils, and with careful attention to optimizing imaging parameters, can produce acceptable images. High-resolution MR peripheral nerve imaging (MRPNI), also known as MR neurography (1), is the most sensitive imaging modality for characterizing peripheral nerve and plexus abnormalities (1–4) and for directing treatment planning (4,5). High-resolution MRPNI uses a small field of view (FOV), an optimized signal-to-noise ratio (SNR), and high contrast resolution to depict subtle internal nerve architectural details.

MRI is an invaluable adjunct to the clinical examination and electrodiagnostic evaluation of peripheral nerve disease. It provides anatomic lesion localization and details about internal nerve architecture, and in some cases, may provide a specific diagnosis. MRPNI studies must be interpreted in context with pertinent clinical, laboratory, and electrophysiologic data. Successful high quality peripheral nerve imaging requires an understanding of relevant anatomy and close attention to technical details. MRPNI is typically more sensitive for the presence of disease than specific for a particular disease process. For example, MRPNI is sensitive to nerve anatomical and signal abnormalities due to neoplastic and inflammatory lesions, but often cannot distinguish between them. However, MRPNI frequently permits a specific answer when the primary questions involve assessment of nerve integrity and the presence or absence of edema in causes of nerve trauma.

This chapter describes MRI findings of normal and abnormal nerves including abnormalities of nerve size, T2 signal intensity, and definition of internal architecture (3,6,7). MRI of muscles is included because acute and chronic muscle denervation have distinctive imaging appearances that may help confirm a suspected peripheral nerve lesion. In certain situations, it is possible to confirm the existence of a specific peripheral nerve lesion based on the pattern of abnormal muscle imaging, when identification the affected nerve as a discrete structure is impossible because it is too small or the imaging abnormality too subtle. MRI of muscle may provide useful corollary information when a patient is not able to undergo definitive electrodiagnostic testing.

2. NEURAL STRUCTURES AMENABLE TO MRPNI

In theory, nerves 4–5 mm or larger in diameter that have a known course can be imaged with MRPNI. In practice, however, artifacts caused by adjacent structures may prevent useful imaging. Commonly imaged nerves include the brachial plexus, lumbosacral plexus, sciatic nerve, ulnar nerve, and common peroneal nerve (at the fibular head). Less frequently imaged nerves include the median, radial, tibial, and femoral nerves. In cases where the nerve of interest is too small to be resolved as a discrete structure (e.g., long thoracic nerve, spinal accessory nerve, posterior interosseous nerve in the forearm), it is usually possible to follow the nerve's expected course and indirectly deduce anatomical lesions producing the observed clinical findings.

3. ROLE OF THE ORDERING PHYSICIAN

It is very difficult for the radiologist to perform and accurately interpret peripheral nerve imaging studies without full clinical information. Availability of pertinent clinical data facilitates designing appropriate imaging of the relevant region in a time efficient manner. MRPNI sequences are relatively lengthy and sensitive to patient movement, and it is not generally feasible to screen a whole extremity from root to distal nerve branches in a single sitting. Radiology scheduling constraints and limited patient tolerance for prolonged MRI generally limit scanning time to ~1 h. Accordingly, it is important for the ordering physician to specify the area of interest based on clinical and electrodiagnostic data prior to initiating scanning. It is also important to clearly state on the requisition when a neoplastic on infectious process is suspected to insure that intravenous contrast is appropriately administered.

In situations where clinical data do not allow for precise anatomic localization, a decision must be made about which region to image first. A routine screening MR study of the cervical or lumbar spinal region contributing nerve roots to the clinically abnormal nerve is generally recommended prior to MRPNI in order to exclude common abnormalities such as spinal stenosis or disc disease as the sole or contributing cause. If the clinical symptoms are not explained by the routine study, further imaging with MRPNI can be considered. However, when the lesion can be definitively localized clinically or electrically to a region within the extremity (e.g., ulnar nerve entrapment at the elbow), a focused MRPNI study is more appropriate as the initial imaging study.

4.   TECHNICAL POINTS AND IMAGING PARAMETERS

High quality high-resolution peripheral nerve imaging requires close attention to several technical elements including FOV, spatial resolution, SNR, imaging time, and contrast resolution. Although it is possible to use a "cookie-cutter" approach to nerve imaging, careful attention to the clinical question to be answered will help determine which parameters to emphasize. Readers interested in a more technical discussion are referred to references on general MR physics (8) and high spatial resolution peripheral nerve imaging (2,6,7,9). The appendix outlines effective imaging parameters for common nerves.

4.1.   Hardware

4.1.1.   MR Scanner

High quality peripheral nerve imaging requires a high-field strength MR scanner (1.5 T or higher). Technical limitations of low-field scanners (relatively large minimum FOV, relatively thick minimum slice thickness, and lack of availability or practicality of chemical fat saturation pulse sequences) preclude their routine use for peripheral nerve imaging.

4.1.2.   Coils

A variety of MR coils are available that are satisfactory for peripheral nerve imaging. Coil are either volume coils that provide homogeneous coverage of a structure that fits within the coil, or surface coils that directly contact the body surface and provide best imaging parameters at the surface of the object. Examples of common volume MR coils suitable for peripheral nerve imaging include the body radiofrequency coil built into the MR scanner bore, the birdcage head coil, and the knee coil. Common surface coils suitable for peripheral nerve imaging include the shoulder coil, multipurpose flexible phase array coil, torso wraparound phased array coil, and pelvic coil. It is often possible to use a coil designed for one part of the body to image another. For example, high quality imaging of the wrist may be performed using the head volume coil when a surface coil study is impossible because of patient mobility limitations or body habitus. The coil that maximizes technical quality and patient comfort should be used independent of its designated purpose.

4.2. Patient Comfort

A comfortable patient is more likely to hold still to yield high quality imaging studies. Poor patient satisfaction also limits imaging time and willingness to comply with future imaging requests. Careful attention should be paid to appropriate placement of supporting pillows and padding as well as immobilization of the limb.

4.3. Technical Imaging Parameters and Their Adjustment

Successful identification of fascicular morphology and subtle nerve signal intensity abnormalities requires optimal scan parameters to maximize SNR and produce sufficient spatial and contrast resolution within a reasonable imaging time. A basic introduction to the most clinically pertinent technical parameters and their importance will help achieve better imaging quality. The most important technical parameters to understand are FOV, spatial resolution, SNR, imaging time, and contrast resolution.

4.3.1. Field of View

It is most important to define the study FOV so that the nerve of interest is displayed as a large discrete structure. Choosing a large FOV may make it difficult to resolve the nerve as a discrete structure, much less discern internal architecture. For example, imaging the sciatic nerve within the pelvis and proximal thigh using a single large FOV results in a tiny, poorly visualized nerve structure. To detect subtle differences in nerve size or signal intensity, it is often best to image each side separately or to compare the symptomatic side to normal imaging studies stored in an institutional normative database.

4.3.2. Spatial Resolution

Spatial resolution is maximized by choosing the largest practical matrix size and thinnest reasonable slice thickness to make voxels as small as possible. However, there are trade-offs with an increase in imaging time and decrease in the SNR.

4.3.3. Signal-to-Noise Ratio

SNR may be improved by increasing imaging time (increasing the number of excitations), increasing slice thickness, or decreasing the matrix size. Higher SNR produces a smoother and more pleasing image that facilitates the detection of subtle abnormalities.

4.3.4. Imaging Time

Short imaging time is important for patient comfort and for maintaining reasonable patient throughput. Best quality imaging is usually acquired within the first 20 min of the session, before the patient becomes restless and begins to move. Most patients are intolerant of individual imaging sequences lasting >8–10 min.

4.3.5. Contrast Resolution

Contrast resolution is the ability to distinguish individual structures on the basis of differences in intrinsic tissue contrast. T1 weighted images (T1WI) provide excellent anatomical definition and fat/muscle contrast resolution and are useful for delineating underlying architecture of macroscopic structures, but provide relatively poor contrast resolution for structures of varying water content. Fat saturated T2 weighted image (T2WI) sequences, on the other hand, do not display underlying anatomy as well and have relatively poor muscle and fat contrast resolution, but are excellent for portraying relatively subtle differences in tissue water content. For these reasons both sequences should be obtained, T1WI for anatomical information and T2WI to identify inflammatory or neoplastic changes manifesting as differences in water content.

4.4. Pulse Sequences and Imaging Scan Planes

MRPNI technique exploits differences in water content between endoneurium, perineurium, and surrounding epineurium. MRPNI protocols use high resolution T1 weighted sequences to delineate anatomical detail and fat suppressed T2 weighted or *short tau inversion recovery* (STIR) sequences to detect abnormal nerve water content due to inflammation or neoplasm.

4.4.1. Pulse Sequences

It is not possible to discern subtle abnormalities in nerve water T2 signal without suppressing the fat signal, because increased nerve water secondary to pathology and fat both appear bright on the T2WI. Intrinsic fat signal on the T2WI is negated using chemical fat saturation pulses or STIR technique. STIR is an extremely useful pulse sequence that provides T2 weighting, excellent homogeneous suppression of fat signal, and accentuates nerve water content by removing the intrinsic high signal from fat containing structures. Fat saturated T2WI and STIR sequences each have their merits and limitations. T2WI technique generally provides better SNR and is more time efficient than STIR sequences, but may be compromised by inhomogeneous fat suppression. On the other hand, STIR technique gives very homogeneous fat signal suppression and is effective for demonstrating nerve hyperintensity, but is generally a longer sequence with more background noise and vascular flow artifacts than T2WI. As a general rule, intravenous contrast agents do not confer appreciable additive value to current MRPNI technique. However, the selected use of contrast is helpful in patients with known scarring or neoplasm in the vicinity of the area of interest, or if either of those entities is discovered unexpectedly during the study. Chemical fat saturation technique on post-contrast enhanced T1WI sequences negates fat signal and accentuates abnormal nerve lesion or scar enhancement.

4.4.2. Imaging Scan Planes

Imaging in two orthogonal planes, dependant on the nerve orientation, is preferable. Axial imaging (relative to the short axis of the nerve) is indispensable for studying intrinsic fascicular architecture and the nerve's relationship to adjacent structures. When imaging extremity nerves, such as the sciatic nerve in the thigh or the ulnar nerve at the elbow, the axial plane is usually the only imaging plane necessary. For nerves that travel within two different planes, imaging should be performed in both orthogonal planes. For example, when imaging the lumbosacral plexus within the pelvis, the coronal plane best depicts the proximal nerve roots and the ventral primary rami, whereas an oblique axial plane permits imaging of the lumbosacral plexus in short axis.

5. NORMAL PERIPHERAL NERVE

Perineural fat provides excellent visualization of nerves, and allows clear differentiation from adjacent soft tissues. Normal nerve is a well-defined oval structure containing discrete fascicles that are isointense to adjacent muscle tissue on T1WI (Fig. 7.1). On fat saturated T2WI or STIR images, normal nerve is slightly hyperintense to adjacent

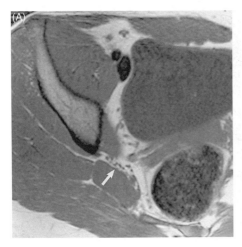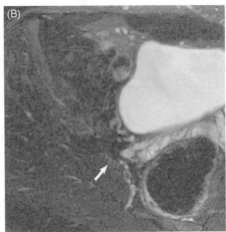

Figure 7.1 Normal sciatic nerve at the level of piriformis muscle. (A) Oblique axial T1WI oriented through the sciatic nerve short axis (arrow) shows normal fascicles that are isointense to muscle, surrounded by bright fatty connective tissue. (B) Oblique axial fat saturated T2WI shows mildly hyperintense fascicles with surrounding dark fatty connective tissue (dark due to the fat saturation pulse).

muscle and hypointense to regional vessels, with clearly defined fascicles separated by interposed lower signal intensity connective tissue. Normal nerve fascicles should be of uniform size and shape, and this distinct fascicular pattern distinguishes peripheral nerves from lesions such as schwannoma or ganglion cyst, which also have high intrinsic T2 signal intensity. Intrafascicular signal intensity is determined by endoneurial fluid and axoplasmic water, whereas the interfascicular signal is dominated by fibro-fatty connective tissue that is amenable to fat suppression.

It is sometimes difficult to distinguish a peripheral nerve from adjacent vascular structures, particularly if the nerve is abnormal and displays high T2 signal intensity. Both nerves and vessels are round or ovoid linear structures, but vessels have characteristics that often permit their distinction from nerves. Vessels demonstrate internal flow voids, branch at large angles, and show intense contrast enhancement. Nerves on the other hand do not show flow voids, branch at relatively acute angles, enhance minimally, and display a discrete distinctive fascicular architecture on transverse imaging.

6. ABNORMAL NERVE IMAGING DIAGNOSTIC CRITERIA

Abnormal MRPNI findings include segmental nerve enlargement, disruption of normal nerve anatomy, T2 signal intensity approaching that of regional blood vessels on fat saturated T2WI or STIR sequences, or disruption or distortion of normal fascicular architecture (Fig. 7.2).

Goals of MRPNI are localization of the site of nerve "injury" or tumor, determination of the pathologic process, formulation of a treatment plan, and prognosis. Nerve injuries result in gross changes in nerve configuration, loss or distortion of the characteristic fascicular pattern, and/or swelling of individual fascicles with abnormally high signal on T2 weighted and STIR sequences. Abnormal nerves are isointense on T1WI, but become increasingly hyperintense to muscle on T2WI. The cause of abnormal high

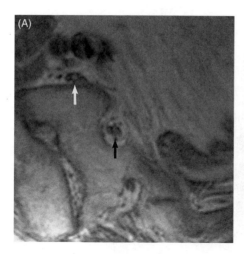 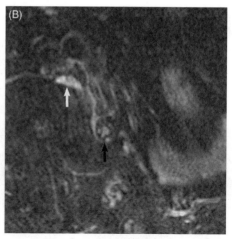

Figure 7.2 Lumbosacral trunk neuropathy. A 62-year-old man presents with pain radiating down the leg and a clinical diagnosis of compression of the sciatic nerve within the piriformis muscle. (A) Oblique axial T1WI shows enlargement of the right lumbosacral trunk (white arrow). The adjacent normal S1 root (black arrow) may be used for comparison. (B) Oblique axial fat saturated T2WI confirms abnormal increased T2 signal intensity, with several enlarged "hot" fascicles that are particularly bright (white arrow). The adjacent normal S1 root (black arrow) for comparison.

signal on T2WI and STIR sequences is not definitively known, but edema from increased endoneurial fluid due to disordered endoneurial fluid flow or local venous obstruction may be factors (6). Alterations in axoplasmic flow may also produce T2 hyperintensity, including impeded flow due to compression (1,4,6).

MRPNI is sensitive for detecting and discriminating among the three types of peripheral nerve injury. Neurapraxia is the least severe type of injury, and is characterized by focal damage to the myelin sheath without axonal disruption. It is identifiable on MRPNI by swollen and hyperintense nerve fascicles. Axonotmesis is an intermediate level of crush or traction injury that produces axonal disruption and subsequent Wallerian degeneration, but leaves Schwann cells and endoneurium intact. Axonotmesis results in homogeneously increased signal intensity with loss of fascicular architecture at the injury site. Neurotmesis is the most severe form of nerve injury, and represents complete interruption of nerve continuity. MRPNI cannot always distinguish axonotmesis from neurotmesis, but the latter may be inferred with there is discontinuity of surrounding connective tissues.

MRPNI should be considered a companion to electrodiagnostic testing. Abnormal high signal in nerve fascicles correlates well with clinical and electrodiagnostic evidence of nerve injury (4). Electromyography does not show denervation until 1–2 weeks following injury, whereas MR neurography can allow assessment of nerve integrity immediately after injury (6).

7. ABNORMAL MUSCLE IMAGING DIAGNOSTIC CRITERIA

MRPNI is sensitive to muscle denervation, and correlates well with denervation changes on electrodiagnostic studies (10). Denervation results in T2 signal hyperintensity on fat saturated T2WI or STIR sequences, and normal or increased muscle volume (Fig. 7.3). Acute denervation changes are not reliably identified earlier than 4 days post nerve

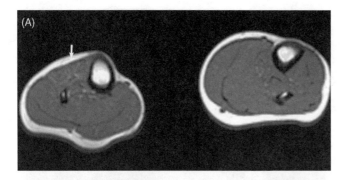

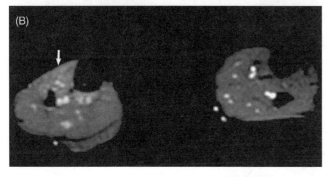

Figure 7.3 Superimposed acute and chronic muscle denervation in a patient with a right peroneal mononeuropathy after femoral osteotomy. (A) Conventional resolution axial T1WI of both legs (for comparison purposes) demonstrating volume loss and fatty replacement (arrow) of the right lower extremity anterior compartment muscles when compared with the normal left leg. (B) Conventional resolution axial STIR image of both legs at the same level as (A) showing T2 hyperintensity characteristic of acute or ongoing denervation (arrow).

injury (10). Chronic denervation is characterized by decreased muscle volume (atrophy) and strands of interspersed high T1 signal intensity representing fatty replacement of muscle tissue. Acute and chronic changes may coexist in diseases with ongoing denervation. Although a preponderance of either type of findings is useful for characterizing the length of denervation, subacute denervation can show both types of findings simultaneously for considerable time periods.

8. IMAGING ATLAS

The following case studies provide illustrative examples of how MRI can be effectively applied to the evaluation of peripheral nerve disease. Examples of normal and abnormal nerve and muscle images are provided. A variety of structural and nonstructural nerve lesions are reviewed. The appendix provides details on the specific imaging techniques for each major peripheral nerve. All images are used with permission Electronic Medical Education Resource Group, Salt Lake City, Utah, USA.

9. CONCLUSIONS

This chapter considers principles necessary to produce and interpret peripheral nerve imaging studies. MRI is the only clinically available imaging technique with suitable contrast and spatial resolution to permit characterization of nerve architecture. Optimizing technical parameters and patient comfort are critical to achieve consistently high quality imaging studies. It is difficult to achieve consistently satisfactory peripheral nerve imaging on MR scanners with <1.5 T field strength. Normal nerve demonstrate well-defined fascicles on transverse imaging, and T2 signal intensity slightly greater than regional muscle structures but not as bright as adjacent vessels. Abnormalities of size, T2 signal hyperintensity, and internal architecture facilitate diagnosis of the abnormal nerve. Attention to muscle volume and signal intensity on T1WI and T2WI may permit detection of acute or chronic denervation that can help confirm a suspected nerve injury, and based on denervation pattern, may assist lesion localization in clinically or electrographically difficult cases.

APPENDIX: GUIDELINES FOR IMAGING SPECIFIC NEURAL STRUCTURES

Technical parameters for imaging nerve structures should be specific to the clinical question to be answered. This appendix provides technical guidelines to assist the clinician and consulting radiologist in imaging specific neural structures, including suggested coils, imaging planes, and sequences.

A.1. Brachial Plexus (Figs. 7.4 and 7.5)

Preferred coil: Multipurpose flexible phase array surface coil

Alternative coil: Neurovascular phase array coil

Imaging planes: Coronal and oblique sagittal planes from C3 (rostral) through T2 (caudal), nerve roots (medial) through axilla (lateral).

Imaging sequences: Coronal T1WI, Coronal STIR, Oblique sagittal T1 SE, and Oblique sagittal STIR.

Optional sequences: Oblique sagittal and coronal contrast enhanced fat saturated T1WI (for cases of known or suspected neoplasm, scar, or infection).

Comments: It is easier for technical reasons to evaluate the supraclavicular plexus than the infraclavicular plexus. STIR provides more reliable fat suppression than chemical fat saturated T2WI.

A.2. Lumbosacral Plexus (Fig. 7.6)

Preferred coils: Torso wrap-around or pelvis phase array coil.

Alternative coil: Spine phase array coil

Imaging planes: Coronal and oblique sagittal planes with scan coverage from L3 (rostral) through the ischial tuberosity (caudal), spinal axis (medial) through greater trochanter (lateral).

Imaging sequences: Coronal T1WI, coronal STIR or fat saturated T2WI, direct axial or oblique axial T1 spin echo, and direct axial or oblique axial fat saturated T2WI or STIR.

Optional sequences: Coronal and oblique axial contrast enhanced fat saturated T1WI (for cases of known or suspected neoplasm, scar, or infection).

Comments: Compared with the torso phase array coil, the spine and pelvis phase array coils provide inferior SNR in the lateral aspects of the pelvis, which may limit evaluation of the proximal sciatic nerve in larger patients.

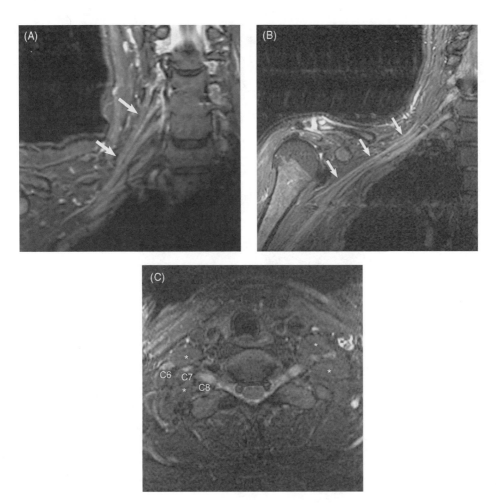

Figure 7.4 Normal brachial plexus. (A and B) Coronal STIR images show normal size and normal mild T2 hyperintensity of the upper and lower plexus elements (arrows). (C) Axial STIR image shows the normal size and signal intensity brachial plexus (annotations) passing through the anterior and middle scalene muscles (asterisks).

Although the body coil will provide adequate coverage, it is severely limited by poor SNR and spatial resolution. The neural foramina, proximal L4 and L5 ventral rami, lumbosacral trunk, S1 contribution to the sciatic nerve, and sciatic nerve continuation into the greater sciatic foramen are best evaluated in direct coronal and axial planes. The oblique axial plane permits optimal visualization of internal architecture of the sacral plexus and proximal sciatic nerve.

A.3. Sciatic Nerve (Figs. 7.7 and 7.8)

Preferred coil: Torso wrap-around phase array coil
Alternative coil: Flexible extremity surface coil
Imaging planes: Coronal and oblique axial or direct axial planes (see subsequently).
Imaging sequences: Coronal T1WI, coronal STIR or fat saturated T2WI, direct axial or oblique axial T1 spin echo, and direct axial or oblique axial fat saturated T2WI or STIR.

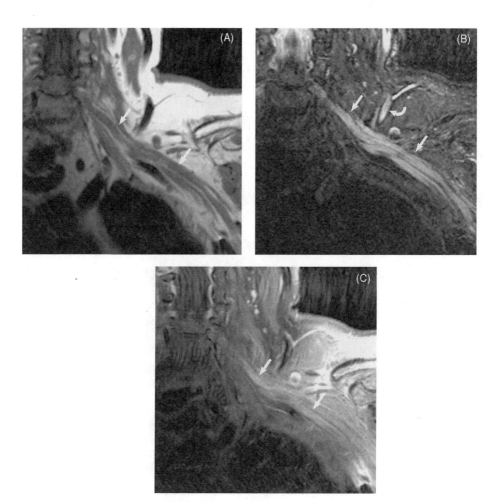

Figure 7.5 Radiation plexitis following breast cancer treatment. A 55-year-old woman with known metastatic breast cancer presents with arm pain and numbness. MRNI was performed in order to differentiate radiation plexitis from metastatic infiltration. (A) Coronal T1WI shows mild enlargement of the brachial plexus (arrows). (B) Coronal STIR image shows diffuse enlargement (straight arrows) and increased T2 signal intensity of the plexus elements that approaches that of regional vessels (curved arrow). (C) T1WI fat saturated image following contrast administration reveals mild patchy enhancement (arrows) without focal mass to suggest malignant infiltration.

Optional sequences: Coronal and direct or oblique axial contrast enhanced fat saturated T1WI (for cases of known or suspected neoplasm, scar, or infection).

Comments: Although the body coil will provide adequate coverage, it is severely limited by poor SNR and spatial resolution. For lesions clinically localized to proximal sciatic nerve, oblique axial T1WI, and fat saturated T2WI on the symptomatic side from the sacral ala (superior) through the ischial tuberosity (inferior) are preferable. For lesions localized to the sciatic nerve within the thigh (below the ischial tuberosity), direct axial T1WI and fat saturated T2WI on the symptomatic side from the ischial tuberosity (superior) to the tibioperoneal bifurcation (inferior) are preferable.

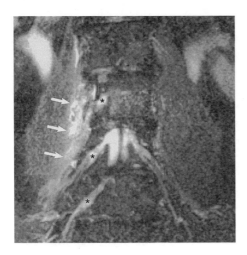

Figure 7.6 Neurolymphomatosis. A 69-year-old man with a history of successfully treated thoracic nonHodgkin's lymphoma presents with progression right leg pain and weakness, clinically and electrodiagnostically localized to the right lumbar plexus. Coronal STIR image shows diffuse enlargement and abnormal increased T2 signal intensity (arrows) of the right lumbosacral plexus that also involves the right L4, L4 and L5 dorsal root ganglia (asterisks), and ventral primary rami.

A.4. Tibial and Peroneal Nerves (Fig. 7.9)

Preferred coils: Torso wrap-around phase array coil or knee coil (produces excellent images but limited to coverage of the common peroneal nerve at the fibular head).

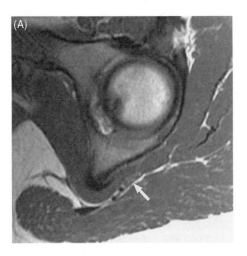
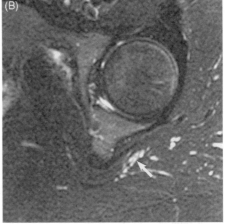

Figure 7.7 Compressive injury of the sciatic nerve at the obturator internus level. A 24-year-old woman presents with a 13 month history of pain in the left buttock radiating to the left calf. The pain was exacerbated by long periods of sitting. (A) Oblique axial T1WI oriented through the sciatic nerve short axis (arrow) shows enlarged, hypointense fascicles. Architectural preservation implies a relatively mild (neuropraxic) injury. (B) Oblique axial fat saturated T2WI confirms abnormal T2 hyperintensity of several fascicles similar to that of regional vessels.

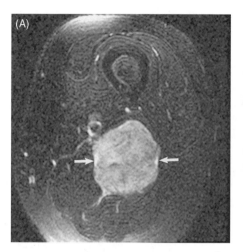 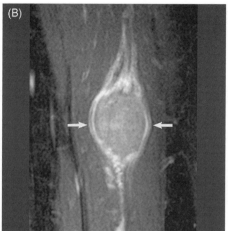

Figure 7.8 Sciatic nerve metastasis (surgically confirmed). A 49-year-old woman with widely metastatic (stage IV) dermatofibrosarcoma protuberans presents with progressive left leg pain and weakness in a sciatic distribution. (A) Axial fat saturated T2WI shows a large hyperintense mass superimposed over the expected location of the sciatic nerve in the thigh (arrows). (B) Coronal T1WI fat saturated image following contrast administration confirms expected extensive enhancement of the mass (arrows) due to absence of blood-neural barrier.

Alternative coil: Flexible extremity surface coil
Imaging plane: Direct axial plane only.
Imaging sequences: Direct axial T1WI and direct axial STIR or fat saturated T2WI.
Optional sequence: Direct axial contrast enhanced fat saturated T1WI (for cases of known or suspected neoplasm, scar, or infection).
Comments: A torso coil is useful for most sciatic and tibial-peroneal nerve imaging indications because of its excellent SNR and large coverage distance. Imaging both legs simultaneously substantially reduces spatial resolution by increasing the FOV, but although the coil is wrapped around both legs, one leg can be imaged at a time to maximize spatial resolution. The knee coil is useful for imaging the common peroneal nerve at the fibular head.

A.5. Femoral Nerve (Fig. 7.10)

Preferred coil: Torso wrap-around phase array coil.
Alternative coil: Flexible extremity surface coil
Imaging planes: Coronal and direct axial planes.
Imaging sequences: Coronal T1WI, coronal STIR or fat saturated T2WI, direct axial T1WI, and direct axial fat saturated T2WI or STIR.
Optional sequences: Coronal and direct axial contrast enhanced fat saturated T1WI (for cases of known or suspected neoplasm, scar, or infection).
Comments: Imaging parameters similar to sciatic nerve imaging in the thigh, except that coronal images must extend from sacrum (posterior) to groin (anterior) in order to image femoral nerve at the inguinal ligament.

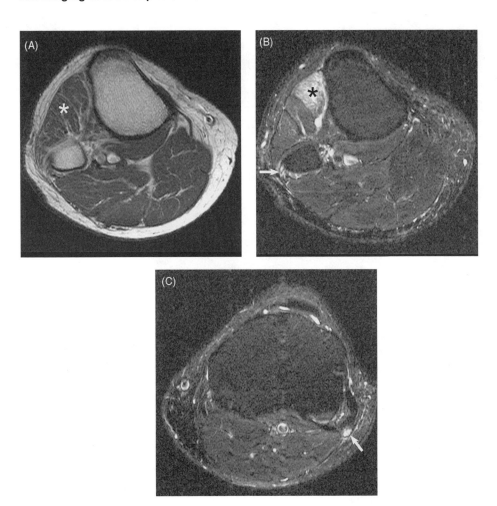

Figure 7.9 Bilateral peroneal nerve palsy with muscle denervation. A 33-year-old man developed sudden left foot drop followed 1 month later by a sudden right foot drop. (A) Axial T1WI shows fatty replacement of the anterior muscle compartment (asterisk) indicating chronic denervation. (B) Axial fat saturated T2WI image of the right lower extremity confirms that there is an acute ongoing component of denervation in the medial portion of the compartment (asterisk), and abnormal T2 signal of the peroneal nerve as it crosses the fibular head (arrow). (C) Axial fat saturated T2WI image of the left lower extremity shows similar imaging characteristics of the peroneal nerve at the fibular head (arrow).

A.6. Ulnar Nerve (Fig. 7.11)

> Preferred coil: Multipurpose flexible phase array surface coil; may need to use in sequential stations to achieve desired coverage.
> Alternative coil: Flexible extremity surface coil
> Imaging plane: Direct axial plane only.
> Imaging sequences: Direct axial T1WI and direct axial STIR or fat saturated T2WI.
> Optional sequence: Direct axial contrast enhanced fat saturated T1WI (for cases of known or suspected neoplasm, scar, or infection).
> Comments: It is important to prospectively localize the lesion to the elbow (cubital tunnel) or wrist (Guyon's tunnel) to correctly place the coil.

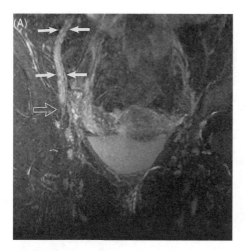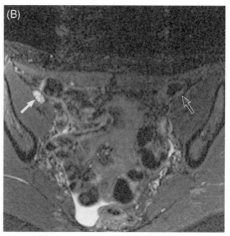

Figure 7.10 Femoral neuropathy following surgical herniorrhaphy. A 27-year-old woman presents with right anterior thigh and inguinal pain following a second herniorrhaphy for a direct inguinal hernia. Electrodiagnostic testing reveals denervation changes in quadriceps muscles, although thigh adductor muscles could not be examined because of pain. (A) Coronal fat saturated T2WI shows a markedly enlarged and hyperintense femoral nerve (arrows) with an abrupt transition to normal signal (open arrow). (B) Axial STIR image shows a markedly enlarged right femoral nerve with swollen hyperintense fascicles (white arrow) as it courses along the ventral iliopsoas muscle. The normal left femoral nerve (open arrow) serves as comparison. A suture ligature was found encircling the femoral nerve (at the level of transition in (A) during surgical exploration.

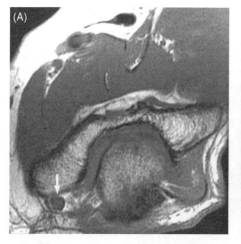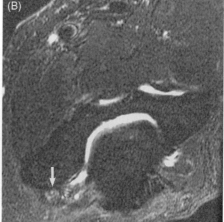

Figure 7.11 Ulnar nerve compressive neuropathy. A 65-year-old man has a 15 year history of intermittent pain in the left elbow and forearm. Examination reveals reduced sensation in the fourth and fifth digits. (A) Axial T1WI shows marked enlargement of the ulnar nerve (arrow) at the cubital tunnel. (B) Axial fat saturated T2WI confirms enlargement and abnormal increased fascicular signal (arrow).

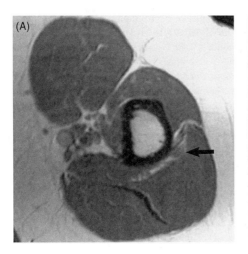 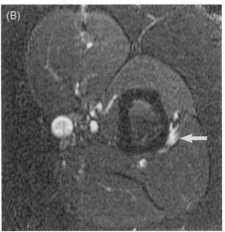

Figure 7.12   Radial neuropathy. A 58-year-old woman with Parkinson's disease awoke in the morning with a complete wrist drop and numbness of the first three fingers. (A) Axial T1WI shows enlargement of the radial nerve along the spiral groove (arrow). (B) Axial STIR image confirms enlargement and abnormal nerve signal intensity (arrow).

A.7.   Median Nerve

Preferred coil: Multipurpose flexible phase array surface coil in sequential stations to achieve desired coverage.

Alternative coil: Flexible extremity surface coil

Imaging plane: Direct axial plane only.

Imaging sequences: Direct axial T1WI and direct axial STIR or fat saturated T2WI.

Optional sequence: Direct axial contrast enhanced fat saturated T1WI (for cases of known or suspected neoplasm, scar, or infection).

Comments: Nerve entrapment by the flexor retinaculum at the wrist is the most common site, but it is important to extend imaging distally into the palm to include distal nerve entrapments.

A.8.   Radial Nerve (Fig. 7.12)

Preferred coil: Multipurpose flexible phase array surface coil

Alternative coil: Flexible extremity surface coil

Imaging planes: Direct axial plane only.

Imaging sequences: Direct axial T1WI and direct axial STIR or fat saturated T2WI.

Optional sequence: Direct axial contrast enhanced fat saturated T1WI (for cases of known or suspected neoplasm, scar, or infection).

Comments: It is difficult to image the distal radial nerve after its bifurcation, but relatively easy within the arm along the spiral groove.

REFERENCES

1. Filler AG, Howe FA, Hayes CE, Kliot M, Winn HR, Bell BA, Griffiths JR, Tsuruda JS. Magnetic resonance neurography. Lancet 1993; 341:659–661.

2. Aagaard BD, Maravilla KR, Kliot M. Magnetic resonance neurography: magnetic resonance imaging of peripheral nerves. Neuroimaging Clin N Am 2001; 11(8):131–146.
3. Filler AG, Kliot M, Howe FA, Hayes CE, Saunders DE, Goodkin R, Bell BA, Winn HR, Griffiths JR, Tsuruda JS. Application of magnetic resonance neurography in the evaluation of patients with peripheral nerve pathology. J Neurosurg 1996; 85:299–309.
4. Kuntz C, Blake L, Britz G, Filler A, Hayes CE, Goodkin R, Tsuruda J, Maravilla K, Kliot M. Magnetic resonance neurography of peripheral nerve lesions in the lower extremity. Neurosurgery 1996; 39:750–756; discussion 756–757.
5. Grant G, Goodkin R, Kliot M. Evaluation and surgical management of peripheral nerve problems. Neurosurgery 1999; 44:825–840.
6. Maravilla K, Aagaard B, Kliot M. MR neurography: MR imaging of peripheral nerves. MRI Clin N Am 1998; 6:179–194.
7. Maravilla K, Bowen B. Imaging of the peripheral nervous system: evaluation of peripheral neuropathy and plexopathy. Am J Neuroradiol 1998; 19:1011–1023.
8. Hashemi R, Bradley W. MRI: the basics. Lippincott, Williams, and Wilkins, 1997:307.
9. Moore KR, Tsuruda JS, Dailey AT. The value of MR neurography for evaluating extraspinal neuropathic leg pain: a pictorial essay. AJNR Am J Neuroradiol 2001; 22:786–794.
10. West G, Haynor D, Goodkin R, Tsuruda J, Bronstein A, Kraft G, Winter T, Kliot M. Magnetic resonance imaging signal changes in denervated muscles after peripheral nerve injury. Neurosurgery 1994; 35:1077–1086.

Inflammatory Demyelinating Neuropathies

8

Acute Inflammatory Demyelinating Polyradiculoneuropathy (Guillain–Barré Syndrome)

Amanda C. Peltier and James W. Russell

University of Michigan and Veterans Affairs Medical Center, Ann Arbor, Michigan, USA

ABSTRACT

Guillain–Barré Syndrome is used to describe several related syndromes, the most common being acute inflammatory demyelinating polyneuropathy (AIDP). AIDP is associated with acute onset of a radiculopolyneuropathy affecting to variable extents motor, sensory, and autonomic function in the peripheral nervous system, and rare involvement of the central nervous system. Approximately two-thirds of affected patients have an antecedent illness 1–4 weeks prior to the onset of symptoms. Demyelinating features predominate in AIDP, but in a more severe variant, acute motor-sensory axonal neuropathy, axonal degeneration predominates. Intensive clinical support coupled with immunomodulators such as intravenous immunoglobulin and plasma exchange significantly reduce the length of illness, and probably reduce morbidity and mortality.

1. INTRODUCTION

Guillain–Barré Syndrome (GBS) was described by Guillain et al. (1) in 1916 as "a syndrome of radiculoneuritis with increased albumin in the cerebrospinal fluid without cellular reaction." Since that time several entities have come under the umbrella of GBS: acute inflammatory demyelinating polyneuropathy (AIDP), acute motor, and sensory axonal neuropathy (AMSAN) (2), acute motor axonal neuropathy (AMAN) (3), acute pandysautonomia, and Fisher syndrome (4). What unifies these as a syndrome are: (i) acute onset, (ii) monophasic course with recovery, (iii) increased protein with cyto-albumin disassociation found in cerebrospinal fluid (CSF), and (iv) overlap among the disorders seen clinically. AIDP is the most common, and will be the focus of this chapter, but the other forms will also be reviewed.

2. SPECTRUM OF GBS

AIDP is the demyelinating variant of GBS. The incidence of AIDP is $1-2/100,000$ per year and it occurs in all geographical regions and in all age groups, but tends to be slightly more common in males (1:2) (5,6). AIDP is usually a sporadic disorder, but occasional epidemiological clusters are observed, such as during the swine flu vaccination program in the United States in 1976. The most prominent symptom of AIDP is weakness, which typically begins distally and ascends to the upper extremities and trunk, and in some cases to bulbar musculature. AIDP may affect both proximal and distal limb nerve roots, as well as the phrenic nerve and cranial nerves. The net effect of the ubiquitous inflammatory response is a neuropathy that can result in quadriplegia in 30% of subjects, restriction to bed in another 30%, and a need for respiratory therapy in one-third of subjects. AIDP may have dysautonomia, bulbar weakness, and axonal damage as part of the syndrome, overlapping with the other syndromes included under the eponym of GBS.

In 1986, Feasby et al. (2) described five patients with clinical features similar to AIDP, but with electrodiagnostic evidence and pathologic evidence of primarily axonal degeneration without significant demyelination. Axonal degeneration was described in 3% of the patients evaluated by Albers et al. in 1985, but Feasby suggested that cases with primarily axonal involvement should be considered as a separate variant, as they had a worse prognosis. Patients with AMSAN characteristically have a severe, progressive paralysis with sensory loss, and incomplete recovery. Griffin et al. (7) subsequently named this variant acute motor-sensory axonal polyneuropathy (AMSAN), and described the pathology in autopsy specimens as primarily wallerian-like degeneration with periaxonal macrophages, and little demyelination present on teased-fiber specimens. They also noted a high correlation with antecedent *Campylobacter jejuni* infection.

In 1991, McKhann et al. (8) described a primary axonal form of pure motor involvement in Shijiazhung, China. They termed this variant acute motor axonal neuropathy (AMAN). In comparison to AMSAN, AMAN typically is associated with acute weakness or paralysis without sensory loss. Like AMSAN, an antecedent *Campylobacter* infection is common (3,9). AMAN occurs more commonly in Japan, China, and developing countries, and is rare in the United States and Europe (9). The pathology of AMAN suggests an antibody-mediated attack, based on immunohistochemistry demonstrating the presence of IgG and complement bound to the axolemma of motor fibers (10). It is associated with a prodrome of diarrhea, followed by a rapid motor syndrome reaching a nadir at 6 days (2,11).

The distribution of weakness in AMAN is distal greater than proximal, and there is involvement of cranial nerves in ~25% of patients (2,9). Reflexes are most often reduced, and the sensory examination is normal both clinically and on electrodiagnostic testing. A subset of patients with AMAN recover over two months, although some forms result in a rapidly progressive severe weakness with poor recovery. Positive *C. jejuni* titers are found in over 65% and the risk of neuropathy is greatest with the O-19 serotype association. Positive GM1 ganglioside antibodies are found in ∼30% of affected subjects and GD1a antibodies in up to 60% of subjects (12). Emperic treatment trials indicate that IVIg may be effective, but plasma exchange or corticosteroids are not.

The triad of ophthalmoplegia, ataxia, and areflexia (4,13) characterize the Fisher syndrome. Facial weakness, ptosis, and pupillary abnormalities are also commonly seen (4,13–15). The incidence of Fisher syndrome is estimated to be 0.09/100,000 (16). Most cases are associated with anti-GQ1b antibodies (17) that cross-react with siali-dase-sensitive epitopes associated with *C. jejuni*. The sensitivity of the anti-GQ1b antibody has been reported to be between 90% and 95% (17–19). These antibodies have been shown to have *ex vivo* and *in vivo* activity at the neuromuscular junction, and may cause terminal axon degeneration at the endplate, diminishing acetylcholine quanta (20,21). The presence of GQ1b ganglioside is higher in human extraocular nerves, which may explain the prevalence of extraocular muscle weakness (22). The level of the anti-GQ1b antibody correlates with the severity of the disease and correlates to the clinical improvement. The Fisher variant has also been associated with systemic lupus erythematosis, Q fever, toxoplasmosis, mycoplasma, and treatment with gold salts.

A sensory variant of AIDP has been proposed, characterized by acute loss of distal sensory function with preservation of strength (23,24).

Acute pandysautonomia has been grouped with GBS primarily because of clinical similarities, for example, acute onset, albuminocytologic dissociation in the spinal fluid, and frequent antecedent infection. AIDP often has significant autonomic involvement as well, further strengthening the association. Autonomic failure includes both sympathetic and parasympathetic functions. Symptoms are orthostatic hypotension, gastrointestinal symptoms of nausea, vomiting, severe constipation or diarrhea, decreased sweating, urinary retention, and impotence. Some patients have been treated with plasmapheresis with success (25).

3. FEATURES OF AIDP

3.1. Clinical Features

The diagnosis of AIDP is based on the clinical history and examination findings, abnormal CSF studies and electrodiagnostic testing. The difficulty lies in that during the first week many patients will have normal CSF results and few or no abnormalities on electro-diagnostic testing. However, patients tend to do better if treatment with IVIg or plasma exchange is initiated early. Treatment may need to be started based on clinical suspicion without confirmatory laboratory testing.

In the most common varieties of GBS, AIDP and AMSAN, weakness is the main initial complaint. In most patients, weakness affects the legs first and ascends. However, 5% of patients present with isolated cranial nerve involvement, followed by descending limb weakness (13). The severity of weakness varies from mild gait difficulty to total limb and respiratory paralysis with death from respiratory failure. Oropharyngeal dysfunc-tion is observed in severe cases and facial diplegia occurs in at least 50% of patients (13) and unilateral in 10% of patients (26). Sensory loss occurs in most patients. Muscle pain or aches occur in up to 50% of cases. Signs of AIDP typically include decreased or absent deep tendon reflexes.

The diagnostic criteria put forth by the National Institute of Neurological Disorders and Stroke (NINDS) in 1978 and evaluated by Asbury and Cornblath (27) require progressive motor weakness of more than one limb and areflexia to make a diagnosis of AIDP. Weakness should be symmetric. Prominent central nervous system findings other than cerebellar ataxia should cast the diagnosis of GBS in doubt. Areflexia may be relative (some reflexes may become hypoactive rather than absent) (27). These criteria do not differentiate among AIDP and AMSAN, which are only differentiated on electrodiagnostic and pathologic grounds.

Autonomic nervous system involvement affecting both sympathetic and parsympathetic function occurs in 65% of patients. Sinus tachycardia is the most common feature, and may be coupled with bradycardia, loss of orthostatic control, and hypohidrosis. Autonomic changes may result in sudden death, and monitoring is critical in affected patients. Occasional patients may have involvement of the urethral sphincter resulting in transient urinary retention or incontinence. Another major complication of AIDP is the development of respiratory insufficiency secondary to diaphragmatic and intercostal muscle weakness. Approximately 10–20% of patients develop respiratory failure requiring mechanical ventilation, and 2–5% die of complications.

In 60% of patients there is a viral or other prodrome occurring within 2 weeks of disease onset (28). The "acute" designation comes from data that on average progression is usually complete after 2 weeks in 50% of cases, after 3 weeks in >80%, and after 4 weeks in >90% (13,29). The disease usually occurs once, and true relapses are very rare.

3.2. Laboratory Evaluation

The classic CSF abnormality found in AIDP is albumin–cytologic dissociation, an elevated protein without associated pleocytosis. An elevated white blood cell count, often lymphocyte predominant, can be seen, but more than 50 white blood count (WBC)/mL suggests another diagnoses, such as human immunodeficiency virus (HIV) or Lyme disease. Oligoclonal bands and elevated myelin basic protein can also be seen. Most patients with an initially normal CSF protein will have elevated levels later in the course of their illness, but in 10% of patients, CSF protein may remain normal throughout their illness (30).

3.3. Electrodiagnostic Evaluation

Electrodiagnostic testing is important because it gives insight into the underlying pathology (Table 8.1). However, it may not be informative in the first week of symptoms and repeat evaluation may be necessary. Early in the course of AIDP, absent or prolonged H-reflexes and F-wave responses may be the only abnormality (31). In sequential studies, multifocal conduction block and slowing, and temporal dispersion become apparent. These lead to slowed conduction velocity, prolonged distal latency, and reduction in the compound muscle action potential (CMAP) wave form in two or more peripheral nerves are seen (32,33). Approximately 50% of patients will fit criteria in the first week, but by 3 weeks, up to 85% will have diagnostic findings on nerve conduction studies. At minimum, sural, peroneal, and median nerves should be examined. Three of the following four criteria are suggestive of demyelination: (i) reduced conduction velocity in two or more nerves to <80% of the lower limit of normal (LLN) if amplitude is >80% of normal, or to <70% of LLN if amplitude <80% of LLN; (ii) partial conduction block or abnormal temporal dispersion in one or more motor nerves; (iii) prolonged distal latencies in two or more nerves to >125% of the upper limit of normal (ULN) if amplitude >80% LLN, or to >150% of ULN if amplitude <80% of LLN; and

(iv) absent F waves or prolonged minimum F-wave latencies in two or more motor nerves to >120% of ULN if amplitude >80% of LLN, or to >150% of ULN if amplitude <80% of LLN. In AMSAN, typically there are no responses after stimulation in several nerves, or there is decreased CMAP below 80%, with sensory nerve involvement, which distinguishes it from AMAN (34). Summed proximal and distal motor amplitudes <20% of normal have been associated with poorer prognosis (35,36). Sensory changes in AIDP may be prominent clinically, but are less severe electrodiagnostically. During the

Table 8.1 Clinical and Electrodiagnostic Criteria for Acute Neuropathies

AIDP (NINDS criteria)	AMSAN	AMAN
Reduction in conduction velocity in two or more motor nerves a. <80% of LLN if amplitude >80% of LLN. b. <70% of LLN if amplitude <80% of LLN.	No evidence of significant reduction in conduction velocity	No evidence of significant reduction in conduction velocity
Conduction block or abnormal temporal dispersion in one or more motor nerves Criteria for conduction block a. <15% change in duration between proximal and distal sites and >20% drop in negative peak-to-peak amplitude between proximal and distal sites. Criteria as for temporal dispersion a. >15% change in duration between proximal and distal sites and >20% drop in negative-peak area or peak-to-peak amplitude between proximal and distal sites.	No evidence of abnormal temporal dispersion	No evidence of abnormal temporal dispersion
Prolonged distal latencies in two or more nerves a. >125% of ULN if amplitude >80% of LLN. b. >150% of ULN if amplitude <80% of LLN. Absent F-waves or prolonged minimum F-wave latencies (10–15 trials) in two or more nerves a. >120% of ULN if amplitude >80% of LLN. b. >150% of ULN if amplitude <80% of LLN.	Prolonged distal latency not considered demyelination if amplitude <10% LLN	
	Decrease in CMAP and SNAP to <80% of LLN or inexcitable (absent evoked response) in two or more nerves	Decrease in CMAP to <80% of LLN or inexcitable (absent evoked response) in two or more motor nerves

Source: The following references were used to create this table: Andersson and Siden (28), McKhann (35), Rees et al. (40), Donofrio et al. (41).

first few weeks, only 25% of patients have sensory nerve abnormalities. After 3 weeks, 80% develop abnormal sensory studies with absent or reduced sensory nerve action potential (SNAP) amplitudes, typically in the median greater than sural nerves (24,33).

Because so few patients fulfill these electrodiagnostic criteria, especially early in the course of illness, other sets of criteria have been suggested. How many abnormalities should be found and in how many nerves has challenged electrodiagnostic testing. Serial electrodiagnostic findings in the Dutch Guillain–Barré trial showed that if patients had three abnormalities in two or more nerves, sensitivity was 85% and specificity 100% (37). Evidence of demyelination was felt to present if at least one finding suggestive of demyelination was seen in two or more nerves (60% in first electrodiagnostic study) (37). Hadden et al. (36) also used the ratio of proximal CMAP to distal CMAP (pCMAP/dCMAP) <0.5 as a sign of conduction block, and allowed motor conduction velocity to be <90% instead of <80%, which increased the sensitivity of their criteria.

Needle EMG is less helpful in initial diagnosis of AIDP, with many patients having only decreased motor unit action potential recruitment (33). Electromyography in AIDP initially demonstrates decreased motor unit action potential recruitment, without change in configuration or spontaneous activity. Myokymic discharges can be seen in the first few weeks. Fibrillation potentials and positive waves appear between 2 and 5 weeks (33). In AMSAN, abundant early fibrillation potentials were seen diffusely by 16 days (34).

MRI may be used in AIDP to exclude other causes (such as transverse myelitis or brainstem stroke) in unusual clinical presentations, but is not necessary in most patients. A small percentage of AIDP patients will also have CNS lesions with abnormal T2 signal, suggesting an overlap with acute demyelinating encephalomyelitis. This is also found in several children with AIDP (38). Enlargement of peripheral nerves or of lumbosacral nerve roots may be observed on MRI. Actively inflamed roots may be demonstrated by gadolinium enhancement.

Serologic evaluation in AIDP for antibodies to specific gangliosides has been the focus of much research. Antibodies to GalNAc–GD1a, GM1, GM2, GM3, GD1a, GD1b, GD3, GT1b, GM1b, and GQ1b have been tested (39), with the greatest specificity in the Fisher syndrome where 89% of patients have elevated titers of GQ1b IgG antibody. GM1 antibodies have also been found to be present in 20–30% of patients, and are associated with previous infection of C. jejuni infection and possibly more axonal involvement (40). Other ganglioside antibodies have been positive in patients with AMAN variants (GD1b, GalNAc–GD1a). However, the usefulness of antibody testing is unclear, and is not recommended.

3.4. Differential Diagnosis

When evaluating a patient with AIDP it is important to consider other causes of rapidly progressive weakness (Table 8.2). Atypical features such as continued fever, loss of pupillary reflexes, retained reflexes or a spinal cord level should alert the physician to other diagnoses. Spinal cord compression, postinfectious transverse myelitis, and brainstem infarcts acutely may have loss of reflexes and sensory findings. Excluding toxin exposure and abnormal electrolytes such as hypokalemia is necessary.

Toxins can cause an acute neuropathy, which can mimic AIDP. These can be environmental or iatrogenic secondary to prescribed medications. Organophosphates, thallium, arsenic, acrylamide, lead, and n-hexane can cause rapidly progressive neuropathies. Arsenic-induced polyneuropathy can present initially with findings of demyelination as in AIDP (41). Tick exposure and shellfish and other toxin exposure (tetrodotoxin, saxitoxin, and ciguaratoxin) can masquerade as AIDP. Tick paralysis occurs over hours to days, and

Table 8.2 Differential Diagnosis of GBS

Localization	Etiology	CSF	NCS/EMG	Clinical features
Spinal cord	Acute cord compression	Normal or pleocytosis	Normal	Acutely: areflexic, flaccidity, sensory level, then ↑ reflexes, no bulbar symptoms
	Transverse myelitis	+/− Pleocytosis ↑ protein Oligoclonal bands	Normal	Acutely: areflexic, flaccidity, sensory level, then ↑ reflexes, no bulbar symptoms
Motor neuron	Poliomyelitis	Inflammatory (pleocytosis), lymphocyte predominant	Denervation, reduced CMAP amplitude, reduced motor unit recruitment	Flaccid weakness with no sensory symptoms, asymmetric
Multiple radiculopathies	Carcinomatous meningitis	Pleocytosis, abnormal cytology, ↑ protein	Denervation in radicular pattern	Asymmetric sensory findings and weakness, suspicion of neoplasm
Neuromuscular junction	Botulism	Normal	Posttetanic amplification, low CMAP amplitudes	Loss of pupil reflex, bulbar findings, rapid onset (24 h), motor only
	Organo-phosphate poisoning	Normal		History of exposure, acute weakness with no sensory symptoms
Muscle (periodic paralysis)	Hypokalemia	Normal		Low serum potassium
Neuropathy	Porphyria	Normal	Axonal neuropathy	GI symptoms, psychiatric symptoms, urine porphyrins
	Thallium	Normal or ↑ protein	Axonal neuropathy	Alopecia, history of exposure
	Arsenic	Normal	Initially demyelinating neuropathy, then axonal	Alopecia, Mees' lines, history of exposure
	Hypophosphatemia	Normal or ↑ protein	Demyelinating neuropathy	Resolves with PO_4
	Uremia	Normal or ↑ protein	Demyelinating neuropathy	Abnormal creatine, history of renal failure
	Viral hepatitis	Normal or ↑ protein	Demyelinating neuropathy	Elevated liver enzymes, jaundice

presents as a rapidly progressing descending paralysis, with decreased CMAP responses. Treatment consists mainly of removing the tick and supportive therapy (42). HIV patients receiving stavudine (d4T) have been reported to develop a rapid neuropathy similar to AIDP (43).

Metabolic disturbances such as severe hypophosphatemia, hypermagnesemia, and hypokalemia may cause acute weakness. Hypermagnesemia and hypokalemia can also cause acute weakness (30). The periodic paralyses (hypokalemic, hyperkalemic, thyrotoxic) can cause rapidly progressive flaccid paralysis. These resolve over hours to days, and the time course should allow discrimination of these disorders from GBS.

Other diseases rarely causing a rapid progression of weakness include viral hepatitis (most often Hepatitis B), uremia, and porphyria. Except for porphyria, these can have demyelination on nerve conduction studies. The other clinical findings such as sore throat, jaundice, renal failure, GI upset, and cognitive changes should enable the clinician to distinguish these entities from AIDP.

Botulism causes a rapidly progressive weakness with predominant bulbar symptoms and may be confused with the Fisher variant. However, botulism often causes loss of pupillary reflexes, a finding not often observed in AIDP. There is no sensory involvement, as is usually present in AIDP. CSF studies are normal. The time course is usually more rapid in botulism, with maximal weakness in 48 h vs. up to 2 weeks in AIDP. Electrodiagnostic study reveals diffusely decreased CMAP amplitudes with significant posttetanic facilitation. Short duration small amplitude motor unit action potentials are typical of botulism, however, rarely there can be neuropathic findings on needle EMG testing (44). Although the presence of a focal skin wound or history of ingestion of home-canned foods should alert the physician to botulism as a possible etiology, this history is rarely present. Botulism is now rare in adults, but is considerably more common in infants who often are exposed by ingesting contaminated dust or, less commonly, contaminated food (e.g., honey).

Other causes of acute weakness with loss of reflexes include poliomyelitis, which is rarely caused by the poliovirus in the United States, but may occur as the result of other coxsackie or echovirus infection. These can be distinguished from AIDP by lack of sensory symptoms, continued fever at the height of weakness, and asymmetric or regional weakness. Poliomyelitis can also cause abnormal signal in the anterior spinal cord on MRI T2-weighted images, unlike AIDP. Electromyographic studies demonstrate a pure motor axonopathy, with significantly reduced CMAP amplitudes and evidence of denervation, without significant demyelination. CSF studies show a pleocytosis, often lymphocytic predominant that is much higher than typical for AIDP (45). West nile virus infection may cause a poliomyelitis like illness. This topic is discussed in Chapter 38.

Another infectious cause of rapidly progressive polyneuropathy is diphtheritic polyneuropathy. This also causes a demyelinating neuropathy with predominant bulbar symptoms and laryngeal weakness; however, there can also be loss of pupil accommodation, and other autonomic features (tachycardia, hypotension, and hyperhidrosis). The latency between the infection and the onset of neurologic symptoms is significantly longer (5–7 weeks) when compared with AIDP. The CSF typically mimics AIDP with an elevation in protein without pleocytosis. Diphtheria typically causes myocardial damage with electrocardiographic changes in over one-half of cases that can distinguish it from AIDP (46).

3.5. Treatment

There are several treatment options that shorten recovery time and may improve prognosis. Plasma exchange was the first treatment found to be beneficial (6,47,48).

The continuous flow plasma exchange technique may be superior to intermittent flow, and albumin is superior to fresh frozen plasma as the exchange fluid. Plasma exchange is most beneficial when started within seven days after disease onset, but may still have a beneficial impact when started later in the course of disease. Intravenous immunoglobulin (IVIg) therapy has been established as equally effective to plasma exchange when given during the first two weeks. A combination of both treatments is not recommended at this time. The major effect of either treatment is to shorten the recovery time (49). Unlike chronic inflammatory demyelinating polyneuropathy, corticosteroids are not beneficial in AIDP (50,51), and are not recommended, although currently trials of steroids and IVIg are being conducted.

Both plasma exchange and IVIg have potentially significant side effects. The typical course of treatment with plasma exchange is five treatments with 40–50 cc/kg exchange, spaced every other day, of at least 200–250 mL/kg total plasma volume exchanged using an IBM-2997 or an aminco-Cell-trifuge. Using a Haemanetics-30 machine, a typical schedule is 40 cc/kg every other day for at least 200 cc/kg total plasma exchange (52,53). Albumin and saline are used as replacement fluid. Treatments closer together can significantly decrease the concentration of clotting factors, increasing the risk of coagulopathy. To ensure a reasonable flow rate, most patients require a central venous catheter placement, which significantly increases the risk of treatment, such as pneumothorax secondary to catheter placement and septicemia from the catheter. Additional complications of plasma exchange include hypotension.

Because of the limited availability of plasma exchange machines and trained technicians, IVIg has become the more common treatment for many patients. The mechanism of action of IVIg is unknown but includes neutralization of anti-idiotypic antibodies, suppression of cytokines, inhibition of complement binding, blockade of Fc receptors, modulation of T-cell function, and selective modulation of circulating proinflammatory cytokines. The half-life of intravenous immune globulin varies from 2 to 4 weeks. A total infusion of 2 g/kg, over 2–5 days has been recommended (54). A regimen of 400 mg/kg per day over 5 days has been used in therapeutic trials of AIDP (53). The rate of infusion is not recommended to exceed 200 mL/h or 0.08 mL/kg per min. Since most AIDP patients requiring IVIg are hospitalized longer than 5 days, using a more conservative approach is reasonable.

Serious adverse reactions with IVIg are relatively uncommon. Patients who receive intravenous immune globulin treatment may have an acute inflammatory reaction manifested by fever, nausea, and vomiting that may lead to hypotension. Patients with IgA deficiency may be at risk for an anaphylaxis, although this side effect is primarily seen in patients being treated for idiopathic thrombocytopenic purpura, and products depleted of IgA are available. IVIg therapy causes an increase in serum viscosity in normal patients, up to 0.5 cP (centipoise). Serum hyperviscosity causing thromboembolism and other complications may be observed in patients with high-normal or slightly elevated serum viscosity such as hypercholesterolemia and cryoglobulinemia (54). IVIg-induced nephropathy has been reported (55), and acute renal tubular necrosis may occur rarely in patients with preexisting renal disease, and probably related to the concentration of hypertonic sucrose in the solution (certain brands of IVIg have lower concentrations than others). Dilution of intravenous immune globulin preparation and a slowing of the rate of infusion lowers the risk. Stroke and encephalopathy may also occur as a result of hyperviscosity or cerebral vasospasm (56–58). In most cases, patients recover after discontinuation of IVIg, and no special treatment is required. Other complications of IVIg include congestive heart failure, serum sickness, and migraine headache—this can be prevented by pretreatment with propranolol (59) or sumatriptan (60). Headaches may also be associated with aseptic meningitis, which is usually subsides 24–48 h after stopping the IVIg infusion. Transmission of viral infections is extremely rare. Hepatitis C infection prior to development of appropriate screening technology has been reported.

Treatment dilemmas may occur in patients with mild AIDP, who are still ambulating. In most of the trials, ability to ambulate was an exclusionary criterion for IVIg and plasma exchange. Because of the significant potential complications of IVIg and plasma exchange and lack of improvement of morbidity, most neurologists do not treat mildly affected AIDP patients or who are stable. However, early presenting ambulatory patients with rapidly progressive weakness should be treated aggressively and monitored very closely for decline in pulmonary function (61).

3.6. Management

A treatment algorithm is outlined in Fig. 8.1. Causes of mortality in AIDP are from respiratory failure and autonomic dysfunction, and secondarily from medical complications. Intubation should be considered for impending respiratory failure and to protect the airway when bulbar function is compromised. Patients should be intubated electively, in a controlled environment to decrease the complications of intubation (aspiration, hypoxia). If possible, depolarizing paralytic medications should not be used, as there is a small risk of hyperkalemia in patients with significant denervation. Features suggestive of increased risk for respiratory failure include bulbar weakness and inability to clear secretions. Respiratory strength should be monitored with bedside spirometry, including forced vital capacity, and maximum negative inspiratory force (NIF). A vital capacity of <20 mL/kg (1 L in a 70 kg patient), an NIF <30 cm H_2O, correlate with progression to respiratory failure and should strongly indicate the need for intubation (49). Patients whose respiratory parameters are falling should be transferred to an ICU for closer monitoring. Patients at risk for aspiration should be fed by alternate means, and those requiring frequent suctioning for secretions need intubation.

Autonomic dysfunction can be a difficult to manage and requires intensive monitoring. Conditions include tachycardia, malignant hypertension, and significant hypotension, fever, and sweating. Myocardial infarctions have occurred from malignant hypertension. Hypertension can be difficult to treat because patients may become hypotensive after small doses of antihypertensive agents, and rapidly reversible medications in small doses are preferable. Fever should prompt an evaluation for underlying infection as nosocomial infection are common, but repeatedly negative cultures and negative chest X-ray may signal a fever caused by dysautonomia.

Complications from immobility are deep venous thromboses and pulmonary emboli. All non-ambulatory patients should receive heparin or heparinoid agents if not contraindicated. Sequential compression devices can also be used. A high suspicion for pulmonary embolus in patients with tachypnea, unexplained alveolar–arterial mismatch, fever or pleuritic chest pain should be employed by all treating physicians, as this is a significant cause of death in AIDP patients.

Nursing care is important to prevent skin breakdown and contractures in immobile AIDP patients. Frequent position changes and turning, and vigilance for skin breakdown are also required in these patients. Range of motion should be performed daily as soon as medically tolerated. Patients frequently complain of deep, aching pain in the back and buttocks, as well as neuropathic pain (tingling, burning or shooting) in the extremities. Pain control can be an issue. Gabapentin and tricyclic antidepressants are helpful for both types of pain, and gabapentin has the advantage of fewer side effects and can be titrated up more rapidly. Opiates may be necessary for some patients.

3.7. Prognosis

The North American GBS Study Group identified several factors that indicated a worse prognosis in AIDP (6). These include: age >60 years, ventilatory failure requiring support, rapid progression, and mean distal CMAP amplitudes 20% of the LLN. These poor prognostic factors were associated with <20% probability of walking independently

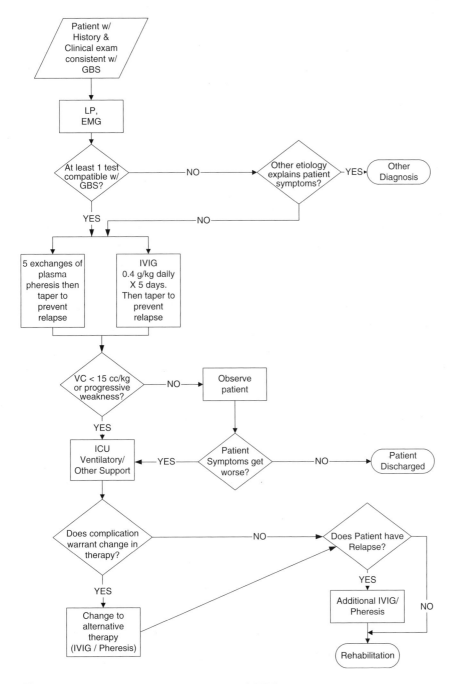

Figure 8.1 Algorithm for the management of AIDP.

at 6 months. Most patients regain a degree of strength, but 20% are left with residual motor weakness 1 year later.

Outcome analysis in the Plasma Exchange/Sandoglobulin GBS Trial Group demonstrated worse outcome (measured as being unable to walk unaided after 1 year) in patients with inexcitable nerves or low mean distal CMAP amplitude (consistent with AMSAN). Patients with an obvious GI illness preceding their symptoms were more likely to develop AMSAN, and had a worse prognosis. Patients with pure motor involvement electrodiagnostically were more likely to have GM1 antibodies, but did not differ in outcome from other patients (36). Patients identified with axonal involvement tend to have a worse prognosis, with prolonged need for ventilation and higher residual weakness (2). Patients described with AMAN usually have good recovery, similar to that of AIDP. The prognosis for AIDP has improved with better treatment, although up to 10% of patients are confined to a wheelchair at six months.

3.8. Pathogenesis

There is evidence in AIDP of segmental demyelination and mononuclear cellular infiltration (11,62). Infiltrates are observed not only in peripheral nerves, but also in cranial nerves, nerve roots, dorsal root ganglia, and autonomic ganglia (11,62). Macrophage infiltration of the nerve is associated with phagocytosis, segmental myelin degeneration, and paranodal sheath retraction. Severe demyelinating neuropathy may be associated with axonal degeneration (63). The etiology for the neuronal inflammatory changes is unknown. Several viral and nonviral infections have been associated with AIDP including CMV (18%), *Mycoplasma pneumonia* (5%), Epstein–Barr virus, HIV, Hepatitis A and B, *Coxiella burnetii*, *Streptococcus pyogenes*, *Staphylococcus aureus*, and Lyme disease (11,30,33,39). Several vaccines have been associated with demyelinating neuropathy including tetanus toxoid, influenza, the oral polio, and the rabies vaccines. Some cases of vaccine mediated AIDP are associated with sensitization to myelin basic protein and occur in clusters. Other evidence of immune reactivity includes increased serum GM2 and GalNAc–GD1a gangliosides, and immunoglobulin or complement activation affecting the Schwann cell or axolemma (10,64). In patients with gastrointestinal symptoms there is an increase in *C. jejuni* titers (28%) (10). These patients are more likely to have pure motor involvement, axonal degeneration, and a poorer prognosis. Other potential associations with acquired demyelinating neuropathy include the postpartum period, the postsurgical period, autoimmune rejection (graft vs. host disease), and Hodgkin's and non-Hodgkin's lymphoma.

The immune response in AIDP is thought to be secondary to activation of autoreactive T-cells and antibodies secondary to molecular mimicry. Certain *C. jejuni* serotypes such as HS:19, which are associated with AIDP, contain sialyated oligosaccharide structures in their outer core identical to peripheral nerve gangliosides GM1, GD1a, GT1a. Other ganglioside antibodies associated with specific pathogens are GM2 with CMV, GQ1b with Haemophilus influenzae, and Gal-C with Mycoplasma pneumoniae (39,65,66).

In the case of *C. jejuni*, there is no evidence that one specific clone or serotype is associated with AIDP (67,68). In addition, sera from healthy blood donors has been found to contain fragments of *C. jejuni* DNA, suggesting that host immune factors are also important in determining whether or not an immune reaction will occur (69). Analysis of IgG Fc-receptors, which are important in linking cellular and humoral immunity shows that homozygosity for certain receptors are associated with better or worse outcomes (70,71). A variety of cytokines, chemokines and proteolytic enzymes have been found to be elevated in the peripheral nerves and CSF of AIDP patients, which may lead to additional therapeutic options or aid in selecting therapy for patients (72–74).

The role of ganglioside antibodies in AIDP is unknown. There is evidence that they may play a pathogenetic role in the disease (21,75). This correlates with evidence of humoral factors involved in the pathology of peripheral nerve myelin in biopsies of patients with AIDP and the response of patients to plasmapheresis. Anti-GM1 or anti-GD1a IgG is present in ~50% of those with AIDP, 35% of those with mixed Fisher syndrome and AIDP, and 16% of subjects with Fisher syndrome. The presence of common antibodies suggests a continuous spectrum in the pathogenesis of acute inflammatory peripheral and central nervous system disorders.

ACKNOWLEDGMENTS

The authors would like to thank Ms. Denice Janus for secretarial assistance. The authors were supported in part by NIH NS42056, NS40458, The Juvenile Diabetes Research Foundation Center for the Study of Complications in Diabetes (JDRF), Office of Research Development (Medical Research Service) and Geriatric Research Educational and Clinical Center (GRECC), Department of Veterans Affairs.

REFERENCES

1. Guillain G, Barre JA, Strohl A. Sur un syndrome de radiculo-nevrite avec hyperalbuminose du liquide cephalorachidien sans reaction cellulaire: remarques sur les caracteres cliniques et graphiques des reflexes tendineux. Bull Soc Med Hop Paris 1916; 40:1462–1470.
2. Feasby TE, Gilbert JJ, Brown WF, Bolton CF, Hahn AF, Koopman WF, Zochodne DW. An acute axonal form of Guillain–Barré polyneuropathy. Brain 1986; 109:1115–1126.
3. McKhann GM, Cornblath DR, Griffin JW, Ho TW, Li CY, Jiang Z, Wu HS, Zhaori G, Liu Y, Jou LP, Liu TC, Gao CY, Mao JY, Blaser MJ, Mishu B, Asbury AK. Acute motor axonal neuropathy: a frequent cause of acute Baccid paralysis in China. Ann Neurol 1993; 33:333–342.
4. Fisher M. An unusual variant of acute idiopathic polyneuritis (syndrome of ophthalmoplegia, ataxia and areflexia). N Engl J Med 1956; 255:57–65.
5. Schonberger LB, Hurwitz ES, Katona P, Holman RC, Bregman DJ. Guillain–Barré syndrome: its epidemiology and associations with influenza vaccination. Ann Neurol 1981; 9(suppl):31–38.
6. Mobley W, Wolinsky J. Scientific overview of inflammatory demyelinating polyneuro-pathy and design of the North American Collaborative Study of plasma exchange in Guillain–Barré syndrome. In: Tindall R, ed. Therapeutic Apheresis and Plasma Perfusion. New York: Alan R. Liss, 1982:159–187.
7. Griffin JW, Li CY, Ho TW, Tian M, Gao CY, Xue P, Mishu B, Cornblath DR, Macko C, McKhann GM, Asbury AK. Pathology of the motor-sensory axonal Guillain–Barré syndrome. Ann Neurol 1996; 39(1):17–28.
8. McKhann GM, Cornblath DR, Ho T, Li CY, Bai AY, Wu HS, Yei QF, Zhang WC, Zhaori Z, Jiang Z et al. Clinical and electrophysiological aspects of acute paralytic disease of children and young adults in northern China. Lancet 1991; 338(8767):593–597.
9. Ho TW, Mishu B, Li CY, Gao CY, Cornblath DR, Griffin JW, Asbury AK, Blaser MJ, McKhann GM. Guillain–Barré syndrome in northern China: relationship to *Campylobacter jejuni* infection and anti-glycolipid antibodies. Brain 1995; 118:597–605.
10. Hafer-Macko C, Hsieh ST, Li CY, Ho TW, Sheikh K, Cornblath DR, McKhann GM, Asbury AK, Griffin JW. Acute motor axonal neuropathy: an antibody-mediated attack on axolemma. Ann Neurol 1996; 40(4):635–644.

11. Arnason B, Soliven B. Acute inflammatory demyelinating neuropathy. In: Dyck P, Thomas P, eds. Peripheral neuropathy. Philadelphia: WB Saunders, 1993:1437–1497.

12. Ho TW, Willison HJ, Nachamkin I, Li CY, Veitch J, Ung H, Wang GR, Liu RC, Cornblath DR, Asbury AK, Griffin JW, McKhann GM. Anti-GD1a antibody is associated with axonal but not demyelinating forms of Guillain–Barré syndrome. Ann Neurol 1999; 45(2):168–173.

13. Ropper A, Wijdicks E, Truax B. Guillain–Barré syndrome. Philadelphia: FA Davis, 1991.

14. Service FJ, O'Brien PC. The relation of glycaemia to the risk of development and progression of retinopathy in the Diabetic Control and Complications Trial. Diabetologia 2001; 44:1215–1220.

15. Mori M, Kuwabara S, Fukutake T, Yuki N, Hattori T. Clinical features and prognosis of Miller Fisher syndrome. Neurology 2001; 56(8):1104–1106.

16. Emilia–Romagna Study Group on Clinical and Epidemiological Problems in Neurology. Guillain–Barré syndrome variants in Emilia–Romagna, Italy, 1992–1993: incidence, clinical features, and prognosis. J Neurol Neurosurg Psychiatry 1998; 65(2):218–224.

17. Yuki N, Sato S, Tsuji S, Ohsawa T, Miyatake T. Frequent presence of anti-GQ1b antibody in Fisher's syndrome. Neurology 1993; 43(2):414–417.

18. Chiba A, Kusunoki S, Obata H, Machinami R, Kanazawa I. Serum anti-GQ$_{1b}$ IgG antibody is associated with ophthalmoplegia in Miller Fisher syndrome and Guillain–Barré syndrome: Clinical and immunohistochemical studies. Neurology 1993; 43:1911–1917.

19. Odaka M, Yuki N, Hirata K. Anti-GQ1b IgG antibody syndrome: clinical and immunological range. J Neurol Neurosurg Psychiatry 2001; 70(1):50–55.

20. O'Hanlon GM, Plomp JJ, Chakrabarti M, Morrison I, Wagner ER, Goodyear CS, Yin X, Trapp BD, Conner J, Molenaar PC, Stewart S, Rowan, EG, Willison HJ. Anti-GQ1b ganglioside antibodies mediate complement-dependent destruction of the motor nerve terminal. Brain 2001; 124(Pt 5):893–906.

21. Buchwald B, Bufler J, Carpo M, Heidenreich F, Pitz R, Dudel J, Nobile-Orzaio E, Toyka KV. Combined pre- and postsynaptic action of IgG antibodies in Miller Fisher syndrome. Neurology 2001; 56(1):67–74.

22. Chiba A, Kusunoki S, Obata H, Machinami R, Kanazawa I. Ganglioside composition of the human cranial nerves, with special reference to pathophysiology of Miller Fisher syndrome. Brain Res 1997; 745(1–2):32–36.

23. Young RR, Asbury AK, Corbett JL, Adams RD. Pure pan-dysautonomia with recovery. Description and discussion of diagnostic criteria. Brain 1975; 98(4):613–636.

24. Oh SJ, LaGanke C, Claussen GC. Sensory Guillain–Barré syndrome. Neurology 2001; 56(1):82–86.

25. Suarez GA, Fealey RD, Camilleri M, Low PA. Idiopathic autonomic neuropathy: clinical, neurophysiologic, and follow-up studies on 27 patients. Neurology 1994; 44(9):1675–1682.

26. Maile LA, Badley-Clarke J, Clemmons DR. Structural analysis of the role of the beta 3 subunit of the alpha V beta 3 integrin in IGF-I signaling. J Cell Sci 2001; 114:1417–1425.

27. Asbury AK, Cornblath DR. Assessment of current diagnostic criteria for Guillain–Barré syndrome. Ann Neurol 1990; 27(supplement):21–29.

28. Andersson T, Siden A. A clinical study of the Guillain–Barré Syndrome. Acta Neurol Scand 1982; 66(3):316–327.

29. Masucci EF, Kurtzke JF. Diagnostic criteria for the Guillain–Barré syndrome. An analysis of 50 cases. J Neurol Sci 1971; 13(4):483–501.

30. Bosch E, Smith B. Disorders of peripheral nerves. In: Bradley W, Daroff R, Fenichel F, Marsden C, eds. Neurology in Clinical Practice. Boston: Butterworth–Heinemann, 2000: 2079–2086.

31. Gordon PH, Wilbourn AJ. Early electrodiagnostic findings in Guillain–Barré syndrome. Arch Neurol 2001; 58(6):913–917.

32. Jacobs BC, Meulstee J, van Doorn PA, van der Meche FG. Electrodiagnostic findings related to anti-GM1 and anti-GQ1b antibodies in Guillain–Barré syndrome. Muscle Nerve 1997; 20(4):446–452.

33. Albers JW, Kelly JJ. Acquired inflammatory demyelinating polyneuropathies: Clinical and electrodiagnostic features. Muscle Nerve 1989; 12:435–451.
34. Brown WF, Feasby TE, Hahn AF. Electrophysiological changes in the acute "axonal" form of Guillain–Barré syndrome. Muscle Nerve 1993; 16(2):200–205.
35. McKhann GM. Guillain–Barré syndrome: clinical and therapeutic observations. Ann Neurol 1990; 27 Suppl:S13–16.
36. Hadden RD, Cornblath DR, Hughes RA, Zielasek J, Hartung HP, Toyka KV, Swan AV. Electrophysiological classification of Guillain–Barré syndrome: clinical associations and outcome. Plasma Exchange/Sandoglobulin Guillain–Barré Syndrome Trial Group. Ann Neurol 1998; 44(5):780–788.
37. Meulstee J, van der Meche FG. Electrodiagnostic criteria for polyneuropathy and demyelination: application in 135 patients with Guillain–Barré syndrome. Dutch Guillain–Barré Study Group. J Neurol Neurosurg Psychiatry 1995; 59(5):482–486.
38. Okumura A, Ushida H, Maruyama K, Itomi K, Ishiguro Y, Takahashi M, Osuga A, Negoro T, Watanabe K. Guillain–Barré syndrome associated with central nervous system lesions. Arch Dis Child 2002; 86(4):304–306.
39. Ang CW, Jacobs BC, Brandenburg AH, Laman JD, van der Meche FG, Osterhaus AD, van Doorn PA. Cross-reactive antibodies against GM2 and CMV-infected fibroblasts in Guillain–Barré syndrome. Neurology 2000; 54(7):1453–1458.
40. Rees JH, Soudain SE, Gregson NA, Hughes RAC. *Campylobacter jejuni* infection and Guillain–Barré Syndrome. N Engl J Med 1995; 333:1374–1379.
41. Donofrio PD, Wilbourn AJ, Albers JW, Rogers L, Salanga V, Greenberg HS. Acute arsenic intoxication presenting as Guillain–Barré-like syndrome. Muscle Nerve 1987; 10(2):114–120.
42. Greenstein P. Tick paralysis. Med Clin North Am 2002; 86(2):441–446.
43. Wollerton E. HIV drug stavudine and symptons mimicking Guillain–Barré syndrome. Can Med Assoc J 2002; 166(8):1067.
44. Chang VH, Robinson LR. Serum positive botulism with neuropathic features. Arch Phys Med Rehabil 2000; 81(1):122–126.
45. Gorson KC, Ropper AH. Nonpoliovirus poliomyelitis simulating Guillain–Barré syndrome. Arch Neurol 2001; 58(9):1460–1464.
46. Piradov MA, Pirogov VN, Popova LM, Avdunina IA. Diphtheritic polyneuropathy: clinical analysis of severe forms. Arch Neurol 2001; 58(9):1438–1442.
47. The French Cooperative Group on Plasma Exchange in Guillain–Barré Syndrome. Appropriate number of plasma exchanges in Guillain–Barré syndrome. Ann Neurol 1997; 41(3):298–306.
48. French Cooperative Group on Plasma Exchange in Guillain–Barré syndrome. Efficiency of plasma exchange in Guillain–Barré syndrome: role of replacement fluids. Ann Neurol 1987; 22(6):753–761.
49. Fletcher DD, Lawn ND, Wolter TD, Wijdicks EF. Long-term outcome in patients with Guillain–Barré syndrome requiring mechanical ventilation. Neurology 2000; 54(12):2311–2315.
50. Hughes RAC, Newsom-Davis JM, Perkin GD, Pierce JM. Controlled trial of prednisolone in acute polyneuropathy. Lancet 1978; 2:750–753.
51. Guillain–Barré Syndrome Steroid Trial Group. Double-blind trial of intravenous methylprednisolone in Guillain–Barré syndrome. Lancet 1993; 341(8845):586–590.
52. Guillain–Barré Syndrome Study Group. Plasmapheresis and acute Guillain–Barré syndrome. Neurology 1985; 35:1096–1104.
53. van der Meche FG, Schmitz PI. A randomized trial comparing intravenous immune globulin and plasma exchange in Guillain–Barré syndrome. Dutch Guillain–Barré Study Group. N Engl J Med 1992; 326(17):1123–1129.
54. Dalakas MC. Intravenous immunoglobulin in the treatment of autoimmune neuromuscular diseases: present status and practical therapeutic guidelines. Muscle Nerve 1999; 22(11): 1479–1497.
55. Gabarra-Niecko V, Keely PJ, Schaller MD. Characterization of an Activated Mutant of Focal Adhesion Kinase: SuperFAK. Biochem J 2002; 365(Pt 3):591–603.

56. Tsiouris J, Tsiouris N. Hemiplegia as a complication of treatment of childhood immune thrombocytopenic purpura with intravenously administered immunoglobulin. J Pediatr 1998; 133(5):717.

57. Steg RE, Lefkowitz DM. Cerebral infarction following intravenous immunoglobulin therapy for myasthenia gravis. Neurology 1994; 44(6):1180–1181.

58. Harkness K, Howell SJ, Davies-Jones GA. Encephalopathy associated with intravenous immunoglobulin treatment for Guillain–Barré syndrome. J Neurol Neurosurg Psychiatry 1996; 60(5):586.

59. Constantinescu CS, Chang AP, McCluskey LF. Recurrent migraine and intravenous immune globulin therapy. N Engl J Med 1993; 329(8):583–584.

60. Finkel AG, Howard JF Jr. Mann JD. Successful treatment of headache related to intravenous immunoglobulin with antimigraine medications. Headache 1998; 38(4):317–321.

61. Green DM, Ropper AH. Mild Guillain–Barré syndrome. Arch Neurol 2001; 58(7):1098–1101.

62. Asbury AK, Arnason BG, Adams RD. The inflammatory lesion in idiopathic polyneuritis: its role in pathogenesis. Medicine 1969; 48:173–215.

63. Prineas JW. Acute idiopathic polyneuritis. An electron microscope study. Lab Invest 1972; 26(2):133–147.

64. Hafer-Macko CE, Sheikh KA, Li CY, Ho TW, Cornblath DR, McKhann GM, Asbury AK, Griffin JW. Immune attack on the Schwann cell surface in acute inflammatory demyelinating polyneuropathy. Ann Neurol 1996; 39(5):625–635.

65. Koga M, Yuki N, Tai T, Hirata K. Miller Fisher syndrome and Haemophilus influenzae infection. Neurology 2001; 57(4):686–691.

66. Kusunoki S, Shiina M, Kanazawa I. Anti-Gal-C antibodies in GBS subsequent to mycoplasma infection: evidence of molecular mimicry. Neurology 2001; 57(4):736–738.

67. Engberg J, Nachamkin I, Fussing V, McKhann GM, Griffin JW, Piffaretti JC, Nielsen EM, Gerner–Smidt P. Absence of clonality of Campylobacter jejuni in serotypes other than HS:19 associated with Guillain–Barré syndrome and gastroenteritis. J Infect Dis 2001; 184(2):215–220.

68. Nachamkin I, Engberg J, Gutacker M, Meinersman RJ, Li CY, Arzate P, Teeple E, Fussing V, Ho TW, Asbury AK, Griffin JW, McKhann GM, Piffaretti JC. Molecular population genetic analysis of Campylobacter jejuni HS:19 associated with Guillain–Barré syndrome and gastroenteritis. J Infect Dis 2001; 184(2):221–226.

69. Van Rhijn I, Bleumink-Pluym NM, Van Putten JP, Van den Berg LH. Campylobacter DNA is present in circulating myelomonocytic cells of healthy persons and in persons with Guillain–Barré syndrome. J Infect Dis 2002; 185(2):262–265.

70. van der Pol WL, Van den Berg LH, Scheepers RH, van der Bom JG, van Doorn PA, Van Koningsveld R, van den Broek MC, Wokke JH, van de Winkel JG. IgG receptor IIa alleles determine susceptibility and severity of Guillain–Barré syndrome. Neurology 2000; 54(8): 1661–1665.

71. Vedeler CA, Raknes G, Myhr KM, Nyland H. IgG Fc-receptor polymorphisms in Guillain–Barré syndrome. Neurology 2000; 55(5):705–707.

72. Kieseier BC, Tani M, Mahad D, Oka N, Ho T, Woodroofe N, Griffin JW, Toyka KV, Ransohoff RM, Hartung HP. Chemokines and chemokine receptors in inflammatory demyelinating neuropathies: a central role for IP-10. Brain 2002; 125(Pt 4):823–834.

73. Nagai A, Murakawa Y, Terashima M, Shimode K, Umegae N, Takeuchi H, Kobayashi S. Cystatin C and cathepsin B in CSF from patients with inflammatory neurologic diseases. Neurology 2000; 55(12):1828–1832.

74. Press R, Ozenci V, Kouwenhoven M, Link H. Non-T(H)1 cytokines are augmented systematically early in Guillain–Barré syndrome. Neurology 2002; 58(3):476–478.

75. Kanda T, Yamawaki M, Iwasaki T, Mizusawa H. Glycosphingolipid antibodies and blood-nerve barrier in autoimmune demyelinative neuropathy. Neurology 2000; 54(7):1459–1464.

9
Chronic Inflammatory Demyelinating Polyradiculoneuropathy

Zachary Simmons
Penn State College of Medicine, Hershey, Pennsylvania, USA

ABSTRACT

Chronic inflammatory demyelinating polyradiculoneuropathy (CIDP) is usually idiopathic
and presents with relatively symmetric, progressive or relapsing weakness, sensory loss,
and hypo- or areflexia. The key to diagnosis is the presence of a sensorimotor polyneuropathy with multifocal demyelination on electrodiagnostic examination. Most patients
respond well to immunotherapy. Intravenous immunoglobulin is usually considered the
treatment of first choice, although a variety of other immunotherapies including plasma
exchange and corticosteroids are also effective. CIDP occurs less commonly in children
than in adults, but is treated similarly, and usually has an excellent prognosis. CIDP
may be associated with a monoclonal gammopathy of undetermined significance. When
associated with IgM, deficits are primarily sensory and response to treatment is unreliable
and often poor. In contrast, when associated with IgG or IgA, deficits and treatment are
similarly to those with idiopathic CIDP. An asymmetric pattern of deficits occurs and
treatment is similar to idiopathic CIDP.

1. INTRODUCTION

Chronic inflammatory demyelinating polyradiculoneuropathy (CIDP) is an acquired
demyelinating disorder affecting nerve roots and peripheral nerves. The pattern of nerve
involvement is usually symmetric, although asymmetric variants occur. Adults are
more commonly affected than children. Most cases are idiopathic, and respond well to

immunotherapy. CIDP can be associated with a monoclonal gammopathy of undetermined significance (MGUS). Under these circumstances, the response to treatment varies with the associated monoclonal subtype.

2. IDIOPATHIC CHRONIC INFLAMMATORY DEMYELINATING POLYRADICULONEUROPATHY IN ADULTS

CIDP is a chronic sensorimotor disorder most commonly affecting sensory and motor functions. It may follow monophasic, relapsing, or progressive courses, which distinguish it from acute inflammatory demyelinating polyradiculopathy (AIDP) or the Guillain–Barré Syndrome (GBS). A variety of names have been used, including chronic relapsing polyneuropathy, chronic relapsing Guillain–Barré polyneuritis, relapsing corticosteroid-dependent polyneuritis, steroid-responsive recurrent polyneuropathy, chronic relapsing polyneuritis, and chronic inflammatory polyradiculoneuropathy (1–6). The disorder was formally defined in 1975, and formal research criteria established in 1991 (7). A number of patient series have described the spectrum of clinical and electrodiagnostic findings, course, and prognosis (8–13).

2.1. Clinical Features

CIDP may affect individuals at any age, including into the ninth decade (14). The mean age in adults varies from 31.6 to 51 years in different patient series. It is slightly more common in men than in women. Antecedent events occur in ~30% of patients, most commonly upper respiratory infections, gastroenteritis, other infections, vaccinations, surgery, and trauma (9,11–13,15). This is in contrast to a much higher incidence (~60–70%) of antecedent events in AIDP/GBS (16,17).

In general, CIDP develops rather slowly, and the mean time from symptom onset to initial presentation from different series is 11.7 months (13) to 24 months (15). Research clinical criteria for CIDP (7) and many clinical series require a minimum period of 2 months of symptom progression, but others accept a shorter period of progression (8,12). However, the range is broad, and some patients present acutely, resembling AIDP/GBS, before going on to develop a relapsing course typical of CIDP. Most patient series include up to 20% of patients reaching a nadir of symptoms within 4 weeks, but they are distinguished from AIDP/GBS by developing a relapsing or a progressive course that responds to immunotherapy (9,11,13,18). However, a subacute time course (subacute idiopathic demyelinating polyradiculoneuropathy—SIDP) has been recognized and proposed as a separate clinical entity for patients who have a monophasic course and progression for 4–8 weeks (19). As awareness of CIDP grows and the diagnosis is made more rapidly, it is increasingly likely that decisions regarding diagnosis and treatment will be made prior to the development of a 2 month period of symptoms.

CIDP is a strikingly heterogeneous disease (20). Most patients present with both sensory and motor symptoms, although small percentages present with predominantly motor (10–22%) or sensory involvement (6%). Weakness may be severe, and in our series we found that 13 of 77 patients (17%) were severely disabled (unable to carry our activities of daily living) at our evaluation. Numbness and paresthesias, most commonly in feet and hands, occurred in 64–82% at onset. Pain was a less common presenting feature (14–20%) (13). Cranial nerve symptoms, which occur in a minority, include dysarthria, dysphagia, facial numbness, facial weakness, blurred or double vision, and ptosis (8,11–13). Symptoms of dysautonomia are uncommon, although urinary dysfunction and impotence have been reported (8,21).

Examination findings include both proximal and distal weakness, usually in a symmetric manner, with distal weakness more common and severe than proximal weakness. Tendon reflexes are decreased or absent in most patients, with areflexia in 70% and absent Achilles reflexes in most patients. Sensory deficits are present in >80% of patients, with vibratory impairment more common than deficits to pinprick. Cranial nerve dysfunction can be found in up to 16%, including ophthalmoplegia, facial weakness, and bulbar weakness. Papilledema may also occur (8,11–13).

Among CIDP variant patients who present clinically with only a sensory syndrome and normal strength, electrodiagnostic evidence for demyelination in motor nerves may be found in some (22–26). Patients with acquired demyelinating neuropathies localized to the upper limbs have been described and included as a variant of CIDP (27,28). These patients likely represent examples of the Lewis–Sumner syndrome or multifocal motor neuropathy, and are discussed elsewhere. Nerve root hypertrophy can result in cervical myelopathy (29) or in findings of lumbar radiculopathy (30–32) superimposed upon CIDP.

2.2. Laboratory Evaluation

Establishing a set of diagnostic criteria for CIDP has been challenging. A set of research criteria have been proposed that categorize patients as definite, probable, or possible CIDP-I based upon clinical, electrodiagnostic, pathologic, and cerebrospinal fluid (CSF) findings (Table 9.1) (7). Such criteria are very useful but strict, and many patients who do not meet criteria for definite CIDP are (and should be) diagnosed with and treated for CIDP. If CIDP is suspected from the history and examination findings, the following laboratory evaluation should be undertaken.

2.2.1. Serum Laboratory Studies

Few routine metabolic studies are informative in diagnosing CIDP, and largely represent an exclusion of other causes or concurrent medical conditions. Erythrocyte sedimentation rate is commonly normal in CIDP. Anti-DNA titer and other tests for collagen vascular disease are also usually normal. A 2 h glucose tolerance test may be helpful if a diabetic neuropathy is included as a diagnostic possibility. HIV titers should be drawn in those patients suspected to be at risk for HIV infection because CIDP can appear in this setting. Tests for other causes of polyneuropathy, including thyroid function tests, vitamin B12 level, VDRL, and (in some geographic regions) Lyme titer, may be helpful if nerve conduction findings are equivocal. Serum and urine immunofixation or immunoelectrophoresis should be performed looking for a monoclonal gammopathy in the serum and Bence–Jones proteins in the urine. If the IgM level is elevated, antibody titers to myelin-associated glycoprotein (anti-MAG) should be assessed (discussed subsequently). If a monoclonal antibody is detected a skeletal X-ray survey should be performed and an evaluation by a hematology/oncology specialist is warranted.

2.2.2. Electrodiagnostic Studies

Motor nerve conduction abnormalities are similar to those seen in AIDP/GBS, and include multifocal demyelination characterized by prolonged distal latencies, slowed conduction velocities, prolonged F-wave latencies, and evidence of partial conduction block or abnormal temporal dispersion (8–13,33) (Fig. 9.1). Several sets of formal

Table 9.1   Research Criteria for Diagnosis of CIDP

CIDP is a diagnosis of pattern recognition, based on clinical symptoms and signs, electrodiagnostic studies, cerebrospinal fluid examination, laboratory tests appropriate to the specific clinical situation, and, on occasions, results from nerve biopsy.

Four features are used as the basis of diagnosis: clinical, electrodiagnostic, pathologic, and cerebrospinal fluid studies. These are further divided into (A) mandatory, (B) supportive, and, where appropriate (C) exclusion. Mandatory features are those required for diagnosis and should be present in all Definite cases. Supportive features are helpful in clinical diagnosis but by themselves do not make a diagnosis, and are not part of the diagnostic categories. Exclusion features strongly suggest alternative diagnoses.

I.   Clinical
    A.   Mandatory
        1.   Progressive or relapsing motor and sensory, rarely, only motor or sensory, dysfunction of more than one limb of a peripheral nerve nature, developing over at least 2 months.
        2.   Hypo- or areflexia. This usually involves all four limbs.
    B.   Supportive
        1.   Large-fiber sensory loss predominates over small-fiber sensory loss.
    C.   Exclusion
        1.   Mutilation of hands or feet, retinitis pigmentosa, ichthyosis, appropriate history of drug or toxic exposure known to cause a similar peripheral neuropathy, or family history of an inherited peripheral neuropathy.
        2.   Sensory level.
        3.   Unequivocal sphincter disturbance.

II.   Electrodiagnostic studies
    A.   Mandatory
    Nerve conduction studies including studies of proximal nerve segments in which the predominant process is demyelination. Must have three of following four:
        1.   Reduction in conduction velocity (CV) in two or more motor nerves:
           a.   <80% of lower limit of normal (LLN) if amplitude >80% of LLN.
           b.   <70% of LLN if amplitude <80% of LLN.
        2.   Partial conduction block[a] or abnormal temporal dispersion[b] in one or more motor nerves: either peroneal nerve between ankle and below fibular head, median nerve between wrist and elbow or ulnar nerve between wrist and below elbow.
        3.   Prolonged distal latencies in two or more nerves:
           a.   >125% of upper limit of normal (ULN) if amplitude >80% of LLN.
           b.   >150% of ULN if amplitude <80% of LLN.
        4.   Absent F-waves or prolonged minimum F-wave latencies (10–15 trials) in two or more motor nerves:
           a.   >120% of ULN if amplitude >80% of LLN.
           b.   >150% of ULN if amplitude <80% of LLN.
    B.   Supportive
        1.   Reduction in sensory CV <80% of LLN.
        2.   Absent H reflexes.

III. CSF studies
    A.   Mandatory
        1.   Cell count <10/mm^3 if HIV-seronegative or <50/mm^3 if HIV-seropositive.
        2.   Negative VDRL.
    B.   Supportive
        1.   Elevated protein.

(continued)

Table 9.1 *Continued*

IV. Pathologic features
    A. Mandatory
        Nerve biopsy showing unequivocal evidence of demyelination and remyelination.[c]
    B. Supportive
        1. Subperineurial or endoneurial edema.
        2. Mononuclear cell infiltration.
        3. "Onion-bulb" formation.
        4. Prominent variation in the degree of demyelination between fascicles.
    C. Exclusion
        Vasculitis, neurofilamentous swollen axons, amyloid deposits, or intracytoplasmic inclusions in Schwann cells or macrophages indicating adrenoleukodystrophy, metachromatic leukodystrophy, globoid cell leukodystrophy, or other evidence of specific pathology.

Diagnostic categories for research purposes

DEFINITE: Clinical A and C, Electrodiagnostic A, CSF A, and Pathology A and C.
PROBABLE: Clinical A and C, Electrodiagnostic A, and CSF A.
POSSIBLE: Clinical A and C and Electrodiagnostic A.

Laboratory studies

Depending on the results of the laboratory tests, those patients meeting the criteria above will be classified into the groups listed below. The following studies are suggested: CBC, ESR, SMA6/12, CK, ANA, thyroid functions, serum and urine immunoglobulin studies (to include either immunofixation electrophoresis or immunoelectrophoresis), and HIV and hepatitis serology. The list of laboratory studies is not comprehensive. For instance, in certain clinical circumstances other studies may be indicated, such as phytanic acid, long-chain fatty acids, porphyrins, urine heavy metals, α-lipoprotein, β-lipoprotein, glucose tolerance test, imaging studies of the central nervous system, and lymph node or bone marrow biopsy.

A. Idiopathic CIDP: no concurrent disease.
B. Concurrent disease with CIDP (depending on laboratory studies or other clinical features):
    1. Systemic lupus erythematosus.
    2. HIV infection.
    3. Monoclonal or biclonal gammopathy (macroglobulinemia, POEMS syndrome, osteosclerotic myeloma).
    4. Castleman disease.
    5. Monoclonal gammopathies of undetermined significance.
    6. Diabetes.
    7. Central nervous system demyelinating disease.

---

[a]Criteria suggestive of partial conduction block: >20% drop in area or amplitude with <15% change in duration between proximal and distal sites.

[b]Criteria for abnormal temporal dispersion and possible conduction block: >20% drop in area or amplitude between proximal and distal sites with >15% change in duration between proximal and distal sites. These criteria are only suggestive of partial conduction block as they are derived from studies of normal individuals. Additional studies, such as stimulation across short segments or recording of individual motor unit potentials, are required for confirmation.

[c]Demyelination by either electron microscopy (>5 fibers) or teased fiber studies (>12% of 50 teased fibers, minimum of four internodes each, demonstrating demyelination/remyelination).

Source: Adapted from *Ad hoc* subcommittee of the American Academy of Neurology AIDS task force (7).

electrodiagnostic criteria have been proposed based on these abnormalities to distinguish between primary demyelinating and primary axonal neuropathies (7,33). However, these abnormalities may not be found in all motor nerves, likely reflecting different degrees of nerve involvement and different distributions of involvement (e.g., changes in nerve

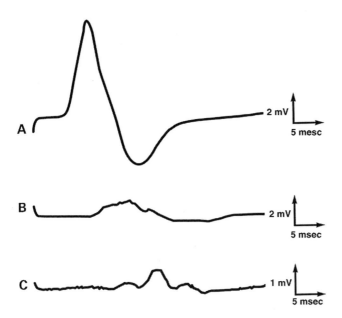

Figure 9.1 Ulnar motor nerve conduction study performed on a patient with CIDP, recording with surface electrodes over the abductor digiti quinti muscle and stimulating at the wrist (A), below elbow (B), and above elbow (C). There is partial conduction block and abnormal temporal dispersion with proximal stimulation. [Adapted from Simmons and Albers (209).]

conduction along segments not routinely tested). A review of 70 CIDP patients found that only 48–64% fulfilled any one of the sets of electrodiagnostic criteria for CIDP (34). Attempts to make the criteria less stringent to include CIDP of lesser severity result in the inclusion of patients with Charcot–Marie–Tooth (CMT) type I neuropathies (35). These criteria, therefore, best serve as guidelines and should be considered in conjunction with clinical, pathological, and CSF studies.

Electrodiagnostic studies are helpful in distinguishing between CIDP and CMT type I, the most common form of hereditary neuropathy (36). Motor nerve conduction in CIDP is characterized by abnormal temporal dispersion and conduction block on proximal stimulation, whereas conduction in CMT type I is characterized by uniform slowing (Fig. 9.2).

Sensory responses may vary from normal to absent (9–11,13). A unique pattern of sensory nerve findings observed more commonly in CIDP than in distal-predominant neuropathies is the combination of an abnormal median response and a normal sural response (37).

Needle EMG findings reflect the degree of secondary axonal degeneration. Abnormalities from acute and chronic partial denervation include fibrillation potentials and positive sharp waves. Recruitment will be decreased and motor unit potentials will show varying degrees of increased amplitude, long-duration, and increased polyphasia (12,33,38,39).

2.2.3. Cerebrospinal Fluid

CSF protein is frequently elevated without a pleocytosis (albuminocytologic dissociation), with mean values ~140 mg/dL (range 20–1200 mg/dL) (8,11–13). Cell counts are rarely greater than five.

2.2.4. Nerve Biopsy

The findings on nerve biopsy are not sensitive or specific for CIDP, and a nerve biopsy is not necessary to make the diagnosis in most patients with suspected CIDP. When the

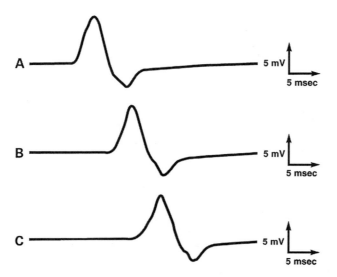

Figure 9.2   Ulnar motor nerve conduction study performed on a patient with Type I Charcot–Marie–Tooth disease, recording with surface electrodes over the abductor digiti quinti muscle and stimulating at the wrist (A), below elbow (B), and above elbow (C). The distal latency is prolonged at 6.8 ms (normal ≤3.5 ms). The conduction velocities in the forearm and across the elbow are 30 m/s and 38 m/s, respectively (normal ≥49 m/s). Slowing is uniform, and partial conduction block and temporal dispersion are absent, in contrast to CIDP. [Adapted from Simmons and Albers (209).]

diagnosis is unclear, a biopsy may be helpful if the differential diagnosis includes vasculitis, amyloidosis, sarcoidosis, or neoplastic infiltration of the nerve. In CIDP, the degree of demyelination varies widely between patients, being predominant in only about half of patients (8,9,12,40). Predominant axonal degeneration and mixed axonal and demyelinating patterns also occur (12). A comparison of sural nerve biopsies from patients with CIDP or chronic idiopathic axonal neuropathies found no difference in demyelinating features between the two (41). Endoneurial perivascular mononuclear inflammatory infiltrates and endoneurial edema are not specific for CIDP (41,42).

2.2.5.   Radiologic Studies

A skeletal X-ray survey of bone should be performed in patients with a monoclonal gammopathy. Occasional patients have a combined central and peripheral demyelinating disorder manifest clinically by a myelopathy superimposed upon clinical and electrodiagnostic evidence of CIDP, and a magnetic resonance image (MRI) of the brain and spinal cord may be useful. Cervical and lumbosacral MRI scans in CIDP patients may show hypertrophy of roots caused by demyelination and remyelination with onion-bulb formation (29–32,43–45). These findings do not appear to correlate with disease severity (46). MRI scanning of the cord should be performed when a combined central and peripheral disturbance of myelin is suspected with evidence of a myelopathy.

2.3.   Differential Diagnosis

The differential diagnosis includes hereditary and acquired neuropathies, disorders of neuromuscular transmission, and primary diseases of muscle. Patients with an insidious onset and very slow progression may resemble CMT, but will lack characteristic orthopedic abnormalities (high arched feet and hammer toes), and will demonstrate distinct electro-diagnostic findings (see section on "Laboratory Evaluation"). Patients who have an acute onset may initially resemble AIDP/GBS, but will progress to a chronic or relapsing course. The Lewis–Sumner syndrome and multifocal motor neuropathy are similar to each other with asymmetric limb involvement, which is distinct from CIDP. Axonal neuropathies may resemble CIDP, although clinically they have a distal predominance of sensory loss and weakness, and electrodiagnostically they lack conduction block, temporal dispersion, and severely slow conduction velocities. Axonal neuropathies are-frequently painful, whereas CIDP is not. The proximal weakness in CIDP may resemble disorders of neuromuscular junction transmission, but myasthenia gravis and Lambert–Eaton myasthenic syndrome frequently include bulbar and ocular involvement, and lack features of acquired demyelination on nerve conduction testing. Primary disorders of muscle such as inflammatory myopathies, toxic myopathies, and muscular dystrophies include proximal weakness but lack the sensory loss and nerve conduction abnormalities characteristic of CIDP.

CIDP may coexist with other diseases including systemic lupus erythematosus, HIV infection, and central nervous system demyelination (47–57). CIDP has rarely been reported in association with malignancies, including pancreatic adenocarcinoma, rectosig-moid adenocarcinoma, cholangiocarcinoma, hepatocellular carcinoma, seminoma, and malignant melanoma (58–63), but it is not necessary to evaluate every CIDP patient for all these disorders, but only when clinically indicated. CIDP with atypical clinical findings or a poor response to standard therapies should lead to a broader search for associated diseases.

CIDP has been described in association with diabetic neuropathy. It can be challenging to diagnose and manage CIDP in diabetic patients, but important because it is treatable. Clinical clues to a superimposed primary inflammatory neuropathy are a rapid change in clinical symptoms that include proximal weakness. Electrodiagnostic findings will include features of primary demyelination (64–66). Nerve biopsy does not distinguish between diabetic neuropathy and CIDP. The inflammatory neuropathy does respond to immunotherapy, and a treatment trial should be considered for diabetic patients who meet two of four electrophysiologic criteria for CIDP (66). Overall, patients with CIDP and diabetes have more axonal loss and respond more poorly to treatment than those with idiopathic CIDP (67).

2.4. Management

2.4.1. Overview of Treatment

A variety of immunosuppressive agents have been demonstrated effective in a large number of controlled and uncontrolled studies and retrospective reviews (3–6,8–13). They include corticosteroids, plasma exchange, intravenous immunoglobulin (IVIg), azathioprine, and cyclophosphamide. In most series, the overall response rate has been good, with 65–95% of patients responding to these therapies, either alone or in combination (11–13,15). However, the response to any single therapy is not predictable, and failure to respond to one modality should lead to treatment with another (8,11–13,15). A summary of the major treatment modalities, followed by a recommended approach is provided.

2.4.2. Corticosteroids

Corticosteroids represent the earliest effective treatment for CIDP (3–6). A prospective, randomized, placebo-controlled trial of prednisone demonstrated a small but significant improvement in patients with CIDP (68). The effects of prednisone are not immediate, and the mean time for initial improvement is $\sim$2 months, and the mean time to reach a clinical plateau is $\sim$6 months (12).

2.4.3. Azathioprine

The combination of azathioprine and prednisone has been assessed in a controlled trial and was found to be no better than prednisone alone, at least over a 9 month period (69). However, clinicians commonly add azathioprine as a "steroid-sparing" agent when treating patients with CIDP, particularly those with relative contraindications to steroids, such as diabetics or those with severe osteoporosis.

2.4.4. Plasma Exchange

Randomized sham-controlled studies have confirmed the efficacy of plasma exchange in some patients with CIDP (70,71) supplemented by uncontrolled studies (72–79), but not all patients respond. The time to improvement is generally short, 2 days to 3 weeks after beginning plasma exchange (79). Plasma exchange is often given 2–3 times per week until clear improvement is obtained, then tapered to a lower frequency. The duration of efficacy varies. Some patients have a monophasic course and do not relapse after plasma exchange treatment, but most relapse after 7–14 days (70,71). Thus, concomitant immunosuppressive therapy is frequently required.

2.4.5. Intravenous Immunoglobulin

There are a number of reports and studies which are retrospective, uncontrolled, or nonrandomized, and which appear to demonstrate the efficacy of IVIg in some, but not all, patients with CIDP. Randomized controlled studies, supplemented by uncontrolled studies, confirm that IVIg is efficacious, being equal to plasma exchange (80–82) or corticosteroids (83). Traditional dosing is 1–2 g/kg divided over 3–5 consecutive days (84–90). The response rate is >60% (81,89), and improvement is rapid, but often transient. The time to onset of improvement is 3–8 days, with maximal improvement within 2–16 weeks (mean 5 weeks) (86,89). Although some patients have a monophasic course characterized by a sustained response, the duration of efficacy ranges from 3 to 22 weeks (mean 6.4 weeks) (81,87).

IVIg can be effective as long-term treatment for relapsing CIDP, with responds to intermittent infusions of IVIg for 4 years or longer (81,89,91). For patients who require regular IVIg infusions, dosages, and intervals vary greatly, ranging from 0.025 g/kg every 10 days to 0.4 g/kg once every 2–4 days (80).

For patients who do not improve with IVIg, improvement with prednisone, azathioprine, plasma exchange, or cyclosporine A has been described (81,89).

2.4.6. Pulse Cyclophosphamide

An uncontrolled trial of pulse cyclophosphamide (1 g/m^2) at monthly intervals for 6 months led to improved strength in two-thirds of 15 patients (92). Most received concomitant prednisone, with no demonstrable added effect from the prednisone.

2.4.7. Cyclosporine A

Cyclosporine A is usually reserved patients who are refractory to standard treatment (corticosteroids, azathioprine, and plasma exchange). Uncontrolled trials of cyclosporine A in patients with idiopathic CIDP and CIDP associated with a MGUS yielded mixed results, with some responding excellently, whereas others have been able to reduce the amount of other immunosuppressive agents (93–95).

2.4.8. *Interferon*

Case reports suggest that interferon-α 2a might be effective for some patients with CIDP poorly responsive or unresponsive to standard therapy (96–101). Strikingly, interferon-α 2a has also been associated with the development of CIDP in patients with hepatitis C, and the role of interferon-α in the treatment of patients with CIDP remains uncertain (102,103).

2.4.9. *Tacrolimus*

Benefits have been reported in one patient with CIDP (104).

2.4.10. *Autologous Stem Cell Transplantation*

Autologous stem cell transplantation resulted in marked clinical and electrodiagnostic improvement in one patient with chronic CIDP refractory to standard therapy, and allowed for a daily prednisone dose of 5 mg/day for maintenance (105).

2.4.11. *Immunoadsorption*

A single patient responded less well to immunoadsorption than to plasma exchange in a crossover study (106).

2.5. An Approach to Treatment of the Patient with CIDP

The goal should be to induce and maintain remission with the minimum dosage of immunosuppressive medication or procedures to reduce medication side effects. Periodic attempts should be made to taper the patient off immunosuppressive medication. It may be challenging when patients do not respond to initial medications among immunosuppressive medications. A treatment algorithm is provided in Fig. 9.3.

Patients with mild sensory deficits and no weakness can be observed without treatment for days to weeks, because spontaneous improvement may occur. If a patient does not improve or worsens, or has weakness, treatment should be initiated. IVIg, plasma exchange, and prednisone are beneficial in most CIDP patients, and the choice of initial therapy should be based on other factors such as speed of onset action, side effect profile, concurrent diseases, availability, convenience, and cost (80). IVIg or plasma exchange is reasonable as the initial treatment because some patients experience sustained improvement with these treatments, and the adverse effects of long-term corticosteroid treatment can be avoided in these responders. The widespread availability of IVIg has made this the initial treatment of choice for most neurologists. However, both are very expensive.

The standard dose of IVIg is 2 g/kg infused over 2–3 consecutive days. The onset of action is rapid, and the side effect profile in most patients is rather benign. A single dose of IVIg may bring about a sustained remission. If relapses occur, IVIg at 1 g/kg can be given again, and at monthly intervals. Maintenance doses should be tapered, and efficacy is often maintained for years. An alternative if several doses of IVIg are not fully effective is the addition of prednisone 60–80 mg/day for 2–3 months. The prednisone dose is then gradually tapered over another 6–9 months, aiming for an alternate-day regimen at the

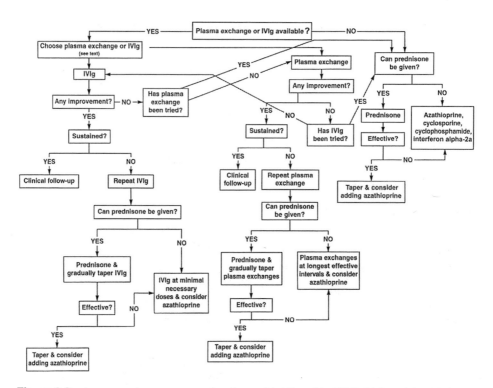

Figure 9.3 An approach to treatment of patients with idiopathic CIDP. [Adapted from Simmons and Albers (209).]

lowest dose that maintains the patient in remission. Supplemental calcium and vitamin D, and monitoring of glucose and electrolytes are prudent, and for those maintained on long-term prednisone, bone density studies should be included and aggressive treatment of osteoporosis may be necessary. Azathioprine 3, 5 mg/kg (with dose escalation starting at 50 mg), can be added in an attempt to minimize the prednisone dose. Long-term IVIg is appropriate for patients in whom prednisone is contraindicated, such as those with brittle diabetes mellitus, or for those who do not tolerate prednisone. In some patients, immunosuppressive therapy can be eventually discontinued, but most patients require maintenance therapy.

Plasma exchange is usually given as one plasma volume per exchange, five times over 2 weeks. As with IVIg, the onset of action generally is rapid. If the effect is sustained, no further treatment is required. If relapse occurs, plasma exchange may be repeated, but prednisone should be started according to the earlier guidelines. For patients who cannot tolerate prednisone, plasma exchange can be used alone and tapered to maintain remission.

Prednisone can be given without IVIg or plasma exchange for patients with mild to moderate chronic deficits, or for those patients for whom IVIg and plasma exchange are not available. Although the onset of action is typically slower than that with IVIg or plasma exchange, it is easy to administer and inexpensive. Azathioprine can be added as a steroid-sparing agent.

Cyclophosphamide should be considered for patients who fail to respond to these therapies, or who do not tolerate them. Cyclophosphamide dosages are 1–2 mg/kg orally on a daily basis or 1 g/m^2 of body surface area by monthly intravenous infusion. Monitoring of hematologic and renal parameters and urine are essential to manage transient immunosuppresssion and minimize long-term risk for developing malignancies.

Cyclosporine can be given at 3–5 mg/kg orally in twice daily doses, with close monitoring of renal function. Interferon α-2a may represent an alternative, as described earlier. For cases of refractory CIDP, autologous stem cell transplantation holds promise.

2.6. Prognosis

CIDP may follow monophasic, relapsing or progressive courses. A monophasic illness includes a single episode of deterioration followed by sustained improvement. A relapsing course includes at least two discrete episodes of deterioration, separated by at least one episode of improvement. A progressive course is characterized by gradually increasing deficits with no episodes of improvement. A relapsing course has been noted in 34–65% of patients, although most series have found that less than half the patients have such a course. The proportions identified as having monophasic, relapsing, and progressive courses vary widely among patient series (8,11,12,107,108). Differences are not surprising, because they include a wide variety of treatment regimens and length of follow-up times. In our series, 45% of patients demonstrated a monophasic course, whereas 13% had progressive disease (107).

Although CIDP may demonstrate a relapsing course even in the absence of treatment, relapses often occur in conjunction with attempts to taper immunosuppressive medication (3,8–11), or after a course of plasma exchange or IVIg. In the modern treatment era, it is increasingly difficult to determine whether the natural course of the disease in a particular individual is relapsing or not.

Relapses may occur abruptly or progress gradually (average time to peak impairment 5 months, range weeks to years), and the number of relapses varies widely (average number of relapses 4, range 2–7) (107). Respiratory failure requiring ventilatory support is rare (12%) (13).

Prognosis has improved. In the older literature, 10% of patients died from CIDP, 30% were nonambulatory, and only 65% were able to work (8). Subsequent reports include a satisfactory outcome in over three-quarters of patients (11,107). Good outcomes are still not universal, and the death rate from CIDP remains 3–6% and 2–4% are unable to live independently (4%) (11,12,107,108).

Continued long-term immunosuppressive treatment will be required to treat or prevent relapses in 60–70% of CIDP patients (12,107). A major factor influencing long-term outcome in CIDP is the degree of axon loss, with greater axon loss associated with a poorer prognosis (109).

2.7. Pathogenesis

CIDP is an autoimmune disorder, supported by the clinical improvement with immunosuppressive therapy. Experimental evidence is provided by the similarity between CIDP and chronic experimental allergic neuritis (EAN) (108) and by the development of conduction block and demyelination in rats receiving intraneural or systemic injections of IgG or serum from patients with CIDP (110). Both humoral and cell-mediated responses against a variety of myelin-derived antigens have been detected in CIDP patients (111–117). It is unclear whether CIDP is due to a single pathogenic cause or it represents a syndrome with more than one pathogenetic mechanism. No one specific antigen has been identified as the common target in all patients with CIDP, however antibodies to P0 glycoprotein have been found in the serum of some patients with CIDP, and these antibodies have the ability to produce conduction block and demyelination when injected into rat sciatic nerve (118). Most likely, there are other autoantibodies involved as well, and the mechanism of CIDP is probably mediated by both T and B cells (119).

3. IDIOPATHIC CIDP IN CHILDREN

CIDP is an uncommon cause of childhood polyneuropathy, making up 9–12% in several series (90,114,120–126).

3.1. Clinical Features

Antecedent events, usually an upper respiratory infection, have been reported in 30–56% of pediatric CIDP patients (127–131). CIDP in children generally presents more precipitously than in adults, mimicking AIDP/GBS one-third of the time (128), and this feature has been recognized in recently-published clinical criteria (132). Symptoms are diffuse and symmetric, with early leg weakness (gait disturbance) common, and overall greater impairment of function than in adults (Table 9.2) (128–131).

Table 9.2   Presenting Symptoms and Signs: Pediatric vs. Adult CIDP Patients

Clinical feature	Pediatric CIDP (15 patients)	Adult CIDP (69 patients)	p-value[a]
Initial symptoms[b]			
Weakness	100.0	95.7	0.41
Numbness/paresthesias	53.3	85.5	0.005
Numbness/paresthesias (age ≥8 years old)	66.7	85.5	0.11
Gait abnormality	40	13	0.01
Gait abnormality (age <10 years only)	100	13	0.0001
Pain	0	15.9	0.1
Cranial nerve dysfunction	13.3	5.8	0.3
Dysarthria	6.7	0	
Blurred or double vision	13.3	4.4	
Ptosis	0	1.5	
Strength[c]			
Composite MRC score	3.5 (1.5–4.1)	3.5 (0–5)	0.49
Sensation[b]			
Vibratory impairment	64.3	88.4	0.02
Pinprick impairment	35.7	66.7	0.03
Reflexes[b]			
Absent biceps reflex	85.7	73.9	0.35
Absent brachioradialis reflex	92.9	82.6	0.34
Absent quadriceps reflex	92.9	79.7	0.24
Absent achilles reflex	100.0	92.8	0.30
Total areflexia	85.7	69.6	0.22
Functional level[c]			
Rankin score	3.5 (3–5)	3.3 (1–5)	0.3

[a]Mann–Whitney U-test for ordinal measures and scaled responses; chi-square analysis for categorical responses.
[b]Percent of patients.
[c]Mean (range).
Source: Adapted from Simmons et al. (128).

3.2. Laboratory Evaluation

As with adult CIDP, the research criteria for pediatric CIDP include "confirmed" or "poss-ible" diagnoses based on clinical, electrodiagnostic, CSF, and nerve biopsy findings (Table 9.3) (132). For clinical use, the criteria should be used as a guideline so as not to exclude from treatment patients who do not fulfill all items in the list.

Blood tests for pediatric CIDP are similar to those for adults, although the probability of finding an MGUS or a lymphoproliferative disorder is much lower. Electrodiagnostic findings in children do not differ in most measures from those in adults (11,12,120,121,126–131). Slowed conduction velocity, prolonged distal latency, and partial conduction block or temporal dispersion are the major findings. As with adult CIDP, not all children satisfy electrodiagnostic criteria, and an extensive evaluation should be attempted despite the normal lack of cooperation demonstrated by some children.

CSF protein level is usually but not invariably elevated, and mean values do not differ from those found in adult CIDP (8,9,11,12,120,121,126,128,130,132). Guidelines for performing a nerve biopsy are similar to those for adults. Nerve biopsies demonstrate myelinated fiber loss, segmental demyelination and remyelination, and inflammatory changes consisting of mononuclear cell infiltration (129–131).

3.3. Differential Diagnosis

Differential diagnosis is similar to adult CIDP. The primary challenges in children are the differentiation of CIDP from AIDP/GBS when the onset is rapid onset, and hereditary neuropathies when the onset is gradual. Differentiation from AIDP/GBS is often possible only after a period of observation to determine whether a relapsing or progressive course ensues. Differentiation from hereditary neuropathies may be particularly challenging in very young children because nerve conduction velocity values gradually increase with the process of myelination. Genetic testing for CMT type I can be helpful making this dis-tinction. In some such patients, a therapeutic trial of immunotherapy is warranted.

3.4. Management

Treatment of pediatric CIDP is similar to that in adults. IVIg, plasma exchange, and predisone have been used, but there are no controlled trials of these therapies in children. Children with CIDP respond at least as well, and probably better, to initial treatment than adults because all children in our series and most of the children in other series improved with initial therapy (120,121,126–130).

IVIg usually is very effective (90,129,130). Some patients have a sustained response and a monophasic course, whereas for other patients the effect of IVIg is transient and the course relapsing. As in adults, IVIg can be given repeatedly with continued effectiveness for years (120,129,130). Plasma exchange appears to have efficacy similar to that seen in adults, and may have to be repeated periodically (129,130,133). Prednisone is usually effective in high dose (1 mg/kg for small children, 60–80 mg for adult-sized children), but some chil-dren relapse when the dose is lowered or the prednisone is discontinued. Other treatments used in few children include cyclophosphamide, azathioprine, and methotrexate (130).

3.5. An Approach to Treatment of Pediatric CIDP

The principles of treatment are the same as those for adults. IVIg, plasma exchange, and prednisone are reasonable first choices. The relative paucity of side effects, general

Table 9.3   Diagnostic Criteria for Childhood CIDP

Mandatory clinical criteria
A.   Progression of muscle weakness in proximal and distal muscles of upper and lower extremities over at least 4 weeks, or alternatively when rapid progression (GBS-like presentation) is followed by relapsing or protracted course ($>$1 year).
B.   Areflexia or hyporeflexia

Major laboratory features
A.   Electrophysiological criteria
Must demonstrate at least three of the following four major abnormalities in motor nerves (or two of the major and two of the supportive criteria):
   1.   Major electrophysiological criteria
      a.   Conduction block or abnormal temporal dispersion in one or more major nerves at sites not prone to compression.
         i.   Conduction block: at least 50% drop in negative peak area or peak-to-peak amplitude of proximal compound muscle action potential (CMAP) if duration of negative peak of proximal CMAP is $<$130% of distal CMAP duration.
        ii.   Temporal dispersion: abnormal if duration of negative peak of proximal CMAP is $>$130% of distal CMAP duration.
        Recommendations: (i) Conduction block and temporal dispersion can be assessed only in nerves where amplitude of distal CMAP is $>$1 mV. (ii) Supramaximal stimulation should always be used.
      b.   Reduction in conduction velocity (CV) in two or more nerves: $<$75% of the mean minus standard deviations (SD) CV value for age.
      c.   Prolonged distal latency (DL) in two or more nerves: $>$130% of the mean $+2$ SD DL value for age.
      d.   Absent F waves or prolonged F-wave minimal latency (ML) in two or more nerves: $>$130% of the mean $+$ 2SD F-wave ML for age.
      Recommendation: F-wave study should include a minimum of 10 trials.
   2.   Supportive electrophysiological criteria
     When conduction block is absent, the following abnormal electrophysiological parameters are indicative of nonuniform slowing and thus of an acquired neuropathy:
      a.   Abnormal median sensory nerve action potential (SNAP) while the sural nerve SNAP is normal.
      b.   Abnormal terminal latency index (TLI)
      c.   Difference of $>$10 m/s in motor CVs between nerves of upper or lower limbs (either different nerves from the same limb or the same nerve from different sides)
B.   Cerebrospinal fluid (CSF)
      a.   CSF protein $>$35 mg/dL
      b.   Cell count $<$10 cells/mm^3
C.   Nerve biopsy features
      a.   Nerve biopsy with predominant features of demyelination.

Exclusion criteria
A.   Clinical features or history of a hereditary neuropathy, other diseases or exposure to drugs or toxins that are known to cause peripheral neuropathy.
B.   Laboratory findings (including nerve biopsy or DNA studies) that show evidence for a different etiology other than CIDP.
C.   Electrodiagnostic features of abnormal neuromuscular transmission, myopathy, or anterior horn cell disease.

(*continued*)

Table 9.3 *Continued*

Diagnostic criteria (must have no exclusion criteria)
A. Confirmed CIDP
    1. Mandatory clinical features.
    2. Electrodiagnostic and CSF features.
B. Possible CIDP
    1. Mandatory clinical features.
    2. One of the three laboratory findings.

Source: Adapted from Nevo and Topaloglu (132).

availability, and lack of need for large-bore needles as required for plasma exchange have led many clinicians to use IVIg as initial therapy. Subsequent courses of IVIg may be given as required. Plasma exchange can be given for severe weakness. Prednisone 1–2 mg/kg per day can be given alone or in conjunction with IVIg, and taper guidelines outlined for adults can be followed. Failure to respond to one modality of treatment should lead to treatment with another. One goal is to avoid long-term immunosuppression if possible, and the generally favorable response in children aids this goal.

3.6. Prognosis

Improvement after initial therapy in children is very rapid (mean 1 week, range 0.3–3 weeks) (128). Relapse rates have been found to vary, from 30% to 80% (120,127,128, 133), Relapse episodes develop more rapidly, but improve more rapidly and completely than in adults (133). Ventilatory failure and support is rare (129,130,133).

Long-term prognosis for children with CIDP is excellent, and deaths have not been reported (120,126,129–131,133). Overall, residual deficits, if present, are minor, and few children have significant residual disability (127–129,133). Data from one series found that children who experienced acute onset weakness (peak disability in <3 months) were more likely to have a monophasic course and complete recovery. In contrast, children with slower progression were more likely to have severe long-term disability, corticosteroid dependence, and require other immunosuppressive agents (127).

3.7. Pathogenesis

The pathogenesis for CIDP in children is felt to be similar to that in adults.

4. CIDP ASSOCIATED WITH MONOCLONAL GAMMOPATHY OF UNDETERMINED SIGNIFICANCE

MGUS is characterized by low levels of serum monoclonal (M) protein (<3 g/dL), low levels or absent Bence–Jones proteins in the urine, bone marrow plasma cell counts of <5%, and no bone lesions, anemia, hypercalcemia, or renal insufficiency (134). The association of CIDP with MGUS is of interest because of the possible causal pathologic relationship between the neuropathy and the MGUS, particularly IgM.

4.1. Clinical Features

Patients with CIDP and MGUS (CIDP-MGUS) have been compared with those who have idiopathic CIDP (CIDP-I) (12). (Table 9.4). CIDP-MGUS patients generally present with more slowly progressing disease. Other features of CIDP-MGUS compared with CIDP-I are less severe weakness and more sensory impairment (13,135). Comparisons are problematic because patients with CIDP-MGUS are a heterogeneous group with IgM, IgG, and IgA monoclonal gammopathies, and IgM when associated with high levels of anti-MAG activity may play a unique role (see Pathogenesis). Patients with IgM CIDP-MGUS and high titers of anti-MAG activity likely constitute a relatively homogeneous group of predominantly male, middle aged to elderly patients with chronic, slowly progressive polyneuropathies characterized by distal sensory loss, gait ataxia, normal strength or mild distal weakness, and some distinguishing features on their nerve conduction studies (see section on "Laboratory Evaluation"). In contrast, IgM CIDP-MGUS patients who lack reactivity to MAG form a more heterogeneous group (136–143). Further, IgM CIDP-MGUS patients may differ clinically from those with IgG or IgA CIDP-MGUS patients

Table 9.4 Presenting Symptoms and Signs: CIDP-I vs. CIDP-MGUS Patients

Clinical feature	CIDP-I (77 patients)	CIDP-MGUS (26 patients)	p-value[a]
Initial symptoms[b]			
Weakness	94.8	76.9	0.008
Numbness/paresthesias	81.8	96.2	0.07
Pain	14.3	7.7	0.38
Gait ataxia	13.0	19.2	0.44
Cranial nerve dysfunction	7.8	3.9	0.49
Dysarthria	1.3	3.8	
Blurred or double vision	6.4	0.0	
Ptosis	1.3	0.0	
Strength (MRC score)[c]			
Proximal upper extremity	3.9 (0–5)	4.8 (3–5)	0.0001
Distal upper extremity	3.6 (0–5)	4.5 (2–5)	0.0001
Proximal lower extremity	3.6 (0–5)	4.4 (2–5)	0.003
Distal lower extremity	2.9 (0–5)	3.9 (0–5)	0.001
Average MRC	3.5 (0–5)	4.4 (2–5)	0.0001
Sensation[b]			
Vibratory impairment	87.0	100.0	0.05
Pinprick impairment	63.6	92.3	0.005
Reflexes[b]			
Absent biceps reflex	75.3	53.9	0.04
Absent brachioradialis reflex	84.4	61.5	0.01
Absent quadriceps reflex	81.8	65.4	0.08
Absent achilles reflex	93.5	88.5	0.41
Total areflexia	71.4	50.0	0.05
Functional level[c]			
Rankin score	3.3 (1–5)	2.4 (1–5)	0.0006

[a]Mann–Whitney U-test for ordinal measure and scaled responses; chi-square analysis for categorical responses.
[b]Percent of patients.
[c]Mean (range).
Source: Adapted from Simmons et al. (13).

as the former have frequent sensory loss, more frequent ataxia, greater symptom progression, and a higher frequency of nerve conduction abnormalities (13,15,144–147).

CIDP is characterized by multifocal demyelination affecting both distal and proximal segments of nerve. A distal acquired demyelinating symmetric neuropathy (DADS) has been identified in patients with distal, symmetric, sensory or sensorimotor involvement, sparing proximal limb, neck, and facial muscles. Most such patients have an IgM kappa monoclonal gammopathy and elevated titers of anti-MAG antibodies (148,149).

4.2. Laboratory Evaluation

The evaluation is similar to that CIDP-I. Diagnostic criteria have been proposed for CIDP-MGUS (135) (Table 9.5). The presence of a monoclonal protein should be further evaluated to determine if it represents a plasma cell dyscrasia by a skeletal X-ray survey and evaluation by a hematology/oncology specialist. For CIDP-MGUS patients as a group, electrodiagnostic findings in motor nerves are similar to those of patients with CIDP-I, whereas sensory nerve conduction studies are more abnormal (13,15). However, patients with IgM-MGUS and high titers of anti-MAG antibodies have several unique features, including disproportionately prolonged motor distal latencies, as measured by the terminal latency index, compared to those patients with CIDP-I and to those with CIDP-MGUS but without elevated anti-MAG titers and less conduction block (136–143,150).

Table 9.5 Proposal for Criteria for Demyelinating Polyneuropathy Associated with MGUS

A causal relation between demyelinating polyneuropathy and MGUS should be considered in a patient with:
1. Demyelinating polyneuropathy according to the electrodiagnostic AAN criteria for idiopathic CIDP
2. Presence of an M protein (IgM, IgG, or IgA), without evidence of malignant plasma cell dyscrasias like multiple myeloma, lymphoma, Waldenstrom's macroglobulinemia, or amyloidosis
3. Family history negative for neuropathy
4. Age >30 years

The relationship is *definite* when the following is present:
1. IgM M protein with anti-MAG antibodies

The relationship is *probable* when at least three of the following are present in a patient without anti-MAG antibodies:
1. Time to peak of the neuropathy >2 years
2. Chronic slowly progressive course without relapsing or remitting periods
3. Symmetrical distal polyneuropathy
4. Sensory symptoms and signs predominate over motor features

A causal relation is *unlikely* when at least three of the following are present in a patient without anti-MAG antibodies:
1. Median time to peak of the neuropathy is within 1 year
2. Clinical course is relapsing and remitting or monophasic
3. Cranial nerves are involved
4. Neuropathy is asymmetrical
5. Motor symptoms and signs predominate
6. History of preceding infection
7. Presence of abnormal median SNAP in combination with normal sural SNAP

Source: Adapted from Notermans et al. (135).

Further, the combination of an abnormal median sensory nerve action potential with a normal sural nerve action potential is more likely to be present in patients with CIDP-I than in those with CIDP-MGUS (135). CSF findings are similar to those in CIDP-I (107). Nerve biopsy is rarely needed, but patients with anti-MAG activity may demonstrate unique findings discussed under Pathogenesis. Increased sural nerve T-cells are seen in patients with a more progressive disease course and more pronounced weakness (151). MRI scanning of the brachial plexus, when performed, reveals increased signal intensity on T2-weighted imaging in most patients with CIDP-MGUS, and may demonstrate swelling of the brachial plexus (152).

4.3. Differential Diagnosis

The differential diagnosis of other peripheral nerve disorders is similar to CIDP-I. However, the clinical and electrodiagnostic features of CIDP-MGUS may be similar or identical to those seen in the presence of osteosclerotic myeloma and POEMS syndrome (polyneuropathy, organomegaly, endocrinopathy, M-protein, and skin changes) (153–156). Amyloidosis may present with neuropathy and a monoclonal protein in serum or urine, but symptoms usually include marked pain and the neuropathy is usually axonal (157–161). This pattern warrants a nerve biopsy, which generally demonstrates amyloid deposition (157,159,162).

4.4. Management

Treatment of CIDP-MGUS follows that for CIDP-I. In general, the response is better in patients with IgG and IgA than with IgM (139,163,164). Although lowering IgM levels by 50% for several months with immunosuppressive therapy may be beneficial (141), the overall response to treatment is not reliable, and is often limited and transient, without a consistent relationship between the lowering of antibody titers and improvement in the neuropathy (138,165–169). Experience with IVIg in patients with IgM-MGUS is varied, but generally poor (165,170–172). Case reports treating with cyclosporine A were favorable patients with various monoclonal gammopathies (93,94,173,174). Chlorambucil has been reported to produce improvement in up to one-third of patients with IgM monoclonal gammopathy (175).

Several recent treatment modalities show promise. Fludarabine has been efficacious in a small series (176). Interferon-α was more beneficial than IVIg, primarily due to an improvement in the sensory component of the neuropathy (168). This is encouraging, because the poor response of CIDP-MGUS patients to standard immunomodulating therapy is largely due to persistence of sensory deficits (13,107). Rituximab has been reported effective in patients with IgM and anti-MAG antibodies (177,178). Autologous bone marrow transplantation has been described to induce an improvement in the demyelinating polyneuropathy of a patient with Waldenstrom's macroglobulinemia and elevated titers of anti-MAG antibodies who failed to respond to standard immunosuppressive therapies (169).

4.5. An Approach to Treatment of Monoclonal Gammopathy of Undetermined Significance

Patients with IgG or IgA MGUS should be treated using the same approach as those with CIDP-I. A protocol for patients with CIDP-IgM might start with IVIg; with three monthly treatments before assessment for response. Rituximab could be considered for nonresponders to IVIg. If there is no response to Rituximab, a series of plasma exchanges over several weeks attempting to lower the serum IgM level to ≤50% of baseline. The other agents discussed earlier can then be tried, but the probability of a response to any one of them cannot be predicted. Corticosteroids are less likely to be beneficial.

4.6. Prognosis

The course of CIDP-MGUS is more likely to be progressive than that of CIDP-I (107,135). CIDP-MGUS also evolves more slowly, with a longer time from onset of deterioration to peak impairment for each episode, and at their worst, patients with CIDP-MGUS demonstrate a lesser degree of measured weakness than those with CIDP-I. Much of the functional impairment in CIDP-MGUS patients is due sensory impairment. The overall prognosis varies among patient series, from a course similar to CIDP-I (15) to a less favorable one (107). Patients with IgM-MGUS have a more problematic course. Most patients require continued immunosuppressive treatment to maintain remission (107).

Laboratory follow-up is necessary in patients with CIDP-I or CIDP-MGUS. Those with CIDP-I may go on to develop CIDP-MGUS or a lymphoproliferative disorder months or years after the onset of the neuropathy (107,179–184). Immunological re-evaluation should be considered in those patients who have major relapses. Particular attention should be paid to the skeletal survey, since a plasmacytoma may vary greatly in radiographic appearance, and may be mistaken for a more common benign bone lesion such as a nonossifying fibroma, fibrous dysplasia, or an aneurysmal bone cyst (155,185–188). When in doubt, biopsy of such a lesion is indicated.

4.7. Pathogenesis

There is a strong suspicion that IgM monoclonal proteins play a unique role in the pathogenesis of some demyelinating polyneuropathies. Antibodies directed against MAG have been found in over half of patients with polyneuropathy and IgM monoclonal gammopathy (136). Several lines of evidence point to a role for IgM, particularly anti-MAG IgM, in the pathogenesis of polyneuropathy. (i) Monoclonal IgM and complement have been shown to bind to peripheral nerve myelin (136,189–193), and IgM antibody deposits are associated with sites of MAG localization (194). (ii) Widening of myelin lamellae has been observed in virtually all patients with peripheral neuropathy, IgM monoclonal gammopathy, and anti-MAG antibodies (165,195). There is a good correlation between widening of myelin sheaths and IgM penetration level into myelinated fibers (196). (iii) Anti-MAG antibodies alter neurofilament spacing, producing smaller distances between neurofilaments in nerves of patients with anti-MAG antibodies than in those with idiopathic CIDP or normal control subjects (197). (iv) A demyelinating neuropathy can be produced in experimental animals by transfer of serum from patients with IgM monoclonal gammopathy and anti-MAG antibodies either intraneurally or systemically (198–201). (v) IgM monoclonal gammopathies are more common compared with IgG among patients with peripheral neuropathy and MGUS than among the general population of patients with MGUS (144,145). Conversely, the prevalence of peripheral neuropathy is higher in patients with IgM-MGUS than in patients with IgA-MGUS or IgG-MGUS (202). (vi) A much higher proportion of patients with IgM monoclonal gammopathy and clinical neuropathy had high levels of anti-MAG IgM antibodies than patients with IgM monoclonal gammopathy and no clinical neuropathy (56% vs. 11.5%) (136). (vii) More patients with high anti-MAG reactivity have a subclinical neuropathy compared with those with low or no MAG reactivity. At follow-up of patients with a subclinical neuropathy or no neuropathy, more patients with high anti-MAG reactivity went on to develop a clinical neuropathy than patients with low or no MAG reactivity (203).

Despite these strong points, there are observations that confound a simple pathogenic relationship. Patients may have anti-MAG IgM without neuropathy (136). A patient with CIDP has been observed to develop anti-MAG IgM after the onset of the neuropathy (180).

5. LEWIS–SUMNER SYNDROME

The Lewis–Sumner syndrome is chronic, acquired, asymmetric sensorimotor demyelinating polyneuropathy which clinically resembles a mononeuritis multiplex (204–208). Electrodiagnostic studies demonstrate multifocal conduction block in motor nerves. CSF protein is normal to mildly elevated. In contrast to multifocal motor neuropathy, patients may improve with prednisone. This clinical pattern has been given various names, including Lewis–Sumner syndrome, motor and sensory demyelinating mononeuropathy multiplex, multifocal motor and sensory demyelinating neuropathy, multifocal inflammatory demyelinating neuropathy, and multifocal acquired demyelinating sensory and motor (MADSAM) neuropathy.

5.1. Clinical Features

This appears to be a disease of adults, with a mean age of symptom onset in the sixth decade (range of 18–77 years). Progression is slow, commonly over many years. Upper extremities are usually involved before lower extremities. Both weakness and numbness may be present, in an asymmetric pattern, usually in the distribution of discrete nerves. Pain is present in a minority. Cranial neuropathies may occur, but are rare. Reflexes are usually decreased in an asymmetric multifocal manner, but rarely are completely absent (206–208).

5.2. Laboratory Evaluation

Blood and urine tests are the same as those for CIDP. In contrast to multifocal motor neuropathy, anti-GM1 antibodies are rarely present (205–208). Electrodiagnostic studies demonstrate features of multifocal demyelination in motor nerves, including prolonged distal latencies, slowed conduction velocities, temporal dispersion, conduction block, and prolonged F-wave latencies in an asymmetric manner. Sensory studies are also abnormal. Needle EMG demonstrates active and chronic denervation. CSF protein is usually normal to mildly elevated, but one patient has been reported with a protein level of 459 mg/dL. Sural nerve biopsy usually is not necessary, but shows primary demyelination. MRI of the brachial plexus may reveal swollen nerves and increased signal intensity on T2-weighted imaging (208).

5.3. Differential Diagnosis

The Lewis–Sumner syndrome is to be differentiated from multifocal motor neuropathy because of differences in response to treatment. The clinical and electrodiagnostic sensory involvement usually are sufficient to make this distinction. The asymmetric presentation may mimic motor neuron disease or a mononeuritis multiplex, but electrodiagnostic findings of multifocal demyelination are not seen in these other disorders (except possibly in the acute stage of a mononeuritis multiplex). The presence of sensory involvement and decreased to absent reflexes distinguishes this syndrome from motor neuron disease.

5.4. Management and Prognosis

Corticosteroids are effective in greater than half of patients (206,207). IVIg has also been effective (206–208).

5.5. Pathogenesis

This syndrome is considered to be a variant of CIDP, in view of the sensory and motor involvement, the electrodiagnostic finding of multifocal primary demyelination, and the response of some patients to steroids.

6. SUMMARY

CIDP represents a heterogeneous autoimmune disorder of the peripheral nervous system producing weakness and sensory loss as a result of multifocal demyelination in children as well as in adults. There is no single test diagnostic for CIDP, and the diagnosis rests on a considered evaluation starting with a thorough history and neurologic examination, an electrodiagnostic evaluation, an analysis of CSF, and serum studies for a monoclonal protein. Other studies are indicated, such as skeletal X-ray survey and consultation with a hematologist/oncologist in selected cases. Immunotherapy is effective, including IVIg, plasma exchange, corticosteroids, and other immunomodulating therapies, resulting in a good prognosis for most adults and virtually all children with CIDP. A treatment algorithm is provided in Fig. 9.3. CIDP associated with an IgM monoclonal gammopathy, particularly in the presence of anti-MAG antibodies, appears to be distinct clinically, pathologically, and with regard to treatment response, producing a neuropathy with sensory predominance and a poor response to many immunotherapies. Rituximab may play a role in treating such neuropathies, as described earlier in this chapter. An asymmetric CIDP variant, usually termed Lewis–Sumner syndrome, has been described, and resembles idiopathic CIDP electrodiagnostically and with regard to its response to immunotherapy.

REFERENCES

1. Hoestermann E. On recurring polyneuritis. Dtsche Z Nervenheikd 1914; 51:116–123.
2. Roussy G, Cornil L. Progressive hypertrophic non-familial neuritis in adults. Ann Med 1919; 6:206–305.
3. Austin JH. Recurrent polyneuropathies and their corticosteroid treatment. Brain 1958; 81:157–192.
4. Thomas PK, Lascelles RG, Hallpike JF, Hewer RL. Recurrent and chronic relapsing Guillain–Barré polyneuritis. Brain 1969; 92:589–606.
5. DeVivo DC, Engel WK. Remarkable recovery of a steroid-responsive recurrent polyneuropathy. J Neurol Neurosurg Psychiatry 1970; 33:62–69.
6. Matthews WB, Howell DA, Hughes RC. Relapsing corticosteroid-dependent polyneuritis. J Neurol Neurosurg Psychiatry 1970; 33:330–337.
7. *Ad hoc* subcommittee of the American Academy of Neurology AIDS task force. Criteria for diagnosis of chronic inflammatory demyelinating polyneuropathy (CIDP). Neurology 1991; 41:617–618.

8. Dyck PJ, Lais AC, Ohta M, Bastron JA, Okazaki H, Groover RV. Chronic inflammatory polyradiculoneuropathy. Mayo Clin Proc 1975; 50:621–637.

9. Prineas JW, McLeod JG. Chronic relapsing polyneuritis. J Neurol Sci 1976; 27:427–458.

10. Dalakas MC, Engel WK. Chronic relapsing (dysimmune) polyneuropathy: pathogenesis and treatment. Ann Neurol 1981; 9(suppl):134–145.

11. McCombe PA, Pollard JD, McLeod JG. Chronic inflammatory demyelinating poly-radiculoneuropathy: a clinical and electrophysiological study of 92 cases. Brain 1987; 110:1617–1630.

12. Barohn RJ, Kissel JT, Warmolts JR, Mendell JR. Chronic inflammatory demyelinating polyradiculoneuropathy: clinical characteristics, course, and recommendations for diagnostic criteria. Arch Neurol 1989; 46:878–884.

13. Simmons Z, Albers JW, Bromberg MB, Feldman EL. Presentation and initial clinical course in patients with chronic inflammatory demyelinating polyradiculoneuropathy: comparison of patients without and with monoclonal gammopathy. Neurology 1993; 43:2202–2209.

14. McLeod JG, Pollard JD, Macaskill P et al. Prevalence of chronic inflammatory demyelinating polyneuropathy in New South Wales, Australia. Ann Neurol 1999; 46:910–913.

15. Gorson KC, Allam G, Ropper AH. Chronic inflammatory demyelinating polyneuropathy: clinical features and response to treatment in 67 consecutive patients with and without a monoclonal gammopathy. Neurology 1997; 48:321–328.

16. Andersonn T, Siden A. A clinical study of the Guillain–Barré syndrome. Acta Neurol Scand 1982; 66:316–317.

17. Ropper AH, Wijdicks EFM, Truax BT. Guillain–Barré Syndrome. Philadelphia: FA Davis, 1991:57.

18. Mori K, Hattori N, Sugiura M, Koike H, Misu K, Ichimura M, Hirayama M, Sobue G. Chronic inflammatory demyelinating polyneuropathy presenting with features of GBS. Neurology 2002; 58:979–982.

19. Hughes R, Sanders E, Hall S, Atkinson P, Colchester A, Payan P. Subacute idiopathic demye-linating polyradiculoneuropathy. Arch Neurol 1992; 49:612–616.

20. Rotta FT, Sussman AT, Bradley WG, Ayyar DR, Sharma KR, Shebert RT. The spectrum of chronic inflammatory demyelinating polyneuropathy. J Neurol Sci 2000; 173:129–139; Dyck PJ, Dyck PJB. Atypical varieties of chronic inflammatory demyelinating neuropathies. Lancet 2000; 355:1293–1294.

21. Sakakibara R, Hattori T, Kuwabara S, Yamanishi T, Yasuda K. Micturitional disturbance in patients with chronic inflammatory demyelinating polyneuropathy. Neurology 1998; 50:1179–1182.

22. Oh SJ, Joy JL, Sunwoo I, Kuruoglu R. A case of chronic sensory demyelinating neuropathy responding to immunotherapies. Muscle Nerve 1992; 15:255–256.

23. Oh SJ, Joy JL, Kuruoglu R. Chronic sensory demyelinating neuropathy: chronic inflammatory demyelinating polyneuropathy presenting as a pure sensory neuropathy. J Neurol Neurosurg Psychiatry 1992; 55:677–680.

24. Simmons Z, Tivakaran S. Acquired demyelinating polyneuropathy presenting as a pure clinical sensory syndrome. Muscle Nerve 1996; 19:1174–1176.

25. Uncini A, DiMuzio A, De Angelis MV, Gioia S, Lugaresi A. Minimal and asymp-tomatic chronic inflammatory demyelinating polyneuropathy. Clin Neurophysiol 1999; 110:694–698.

26. Rubin M, Mackenzie CR. Clinically and electrodiagnostically pure sensory demyelinating polyneuropathy. Electromyogr Clin Neurophysiol 1996; 36:145–149.

27. Thomas PK, Claus D, Jaspert A, Workman JM, King RHM, Larner AJ, Anderson M, Emerson JA, Ferguson IT. Focal upper limb demyelinating neuropathy. Brain 1996; 119:765–774.

28. Gorson KC, Ropper AH, Weinberg DH. Upper limb predominant, multifocal chronic inflam-matory demyelinating polyneuropathy. Muscle Nerve 1999; 22:758–765.

29. Midroni G, Dyck PJ. Chronic inflammatory demyelinating polyradiculoneuropathy: unusual clinical features and therapeutic responses. Neurology 1996; 46:1206–1212.

30. Ginsburg L, Platts AD, Thomas PK. Chronic inflammatory demyelinating polyneuropathy mimicking a lumbar spinal stenosis syndrome. J Neurol Neurosurg Psychiatry 1995; 59:189–191.

31. Goldstein JM, Parks BJ, Mayer PL, Kim JH, Sze G, Miller RG. Nerve root hypertrophy as the cause of lumbar stenosis in chronic inflammatory demyelinating polyradiculoneuropathy. Muscle Nerve 1996; 19:892–896.

32. Schady W, Goulding PJ, Lecky BRF, King RHM, Smith CML. Massive nerve root enlargement in chronic inflammatory demyelinating polyneuropathy. J Neurol Neurosurg Psychiatry 1996; 61:636–640.

33. Albers JW, Kelly JJ. Acquired inflammatory demyelinating polyneuropathies: clinical and electrodiagnostic features. Muscle Nerve 1989; 12:435–451.

34. Bromberg MB. Comparison of electrodiagnostic criteria for primary demyelination in chronic polyneuropathy. Muscle Nerve 1991; 14:968–976.

35. Nicolas G, Maisonobe T, Le Forestier N, Leger J-M, Bouche P. Proposed revised electrophysiological criteria for chronic inflammatory demyelinating polyradiculoneuropathy. Muscle Nerve 2002; 25:26–30.

36. Lewis RA, Sumner AJ. The electrodiagnostic distinctions between chronic familial and acquired demyelinative neuropathies. Neurology 1982; 32:592–596.

37. Bromberg MB, Albers JW. Patterns of sensory nerve conduction abnormalities in demyelinating and axonal peripheral nerve disorders. Muscle Nerve 1993; 16:262–266.

38. Dumitru D. Electrodiagnostic Medicine. Philadelphia: Hanley and Belfus, 1995: 763–767.

39. Preston DC, Shapiro BE. Electromyography and Neuromuscular Disorders: Clinical-Electrophysiologic Correlations. Boston: Butterworth-Heinemann, 1998: 366–367.

40. Krendel DA, Parks HP, Anthony DC, St Clair MB, Graham DG. Sural nerve biopsy in chronic inflammatory demyelinating polyradiculoneuropathy. Muscle Nerve 1989; 12:257–264.

41. Bosboom WMJ, van den Berg LH, Franssen H, Giesbergen PCLM, Flach HZ, van Putten AM, Veldman H, Wokke JHJ. Diagnostic value of sural nerve demyelination in chronic inflammatory demyelinating polyneuropathy. Brain 2001; 124:2427–2438.

42. Bosboom WMJ, Van den Berg LH, De Boer L, Van Son MJ, Veldman H, Franssen H, Logtenberg T, Wokke JHJ. The diagnostic value of sural nerve T cells in chronic inflammatory demyelinating polyneuropathy. Neurology 1999; 53:837–845.

43. De Silva RN, Willison HJ, Doyle D, Weir AI, Hadley DM, Thomas AM. Nerve root hypertrophy in chronic inflammatory demyelinating polyneuropathy. Muscle Nerve 1994; 17:168–170.

44. Mizuno K, Nagamatsu M, Hattori N, Yamamoto M, Goto H, Kuniyoshi K, Sobue G. Chronic inflammatory demyelinating polyradiculoneuropathy with diffuse and massive peripheral nerve hypertrophy: distinctive clinical and magnetic resonance imaging features. Muscle Nerve 1998; 21:805–808.

45. Duggins AJ, McLeod JG, Pollard JD, Davies L, Yang F, Thompson EO, Soper JR. Spinal root and plexus hypertrophy in chronic inflammatory demyelinating polyneuropathy. Brain 1999; 122:1383–1390.

46. Midroni G, de Tilly LN, Gray B, Vajsar J. MRI of the cauda equina in CIDP: clinical correlations. J Neurol Sci 1999; 170:36–44.

47. Dalakas MC, Culper EJ. Neuropathies in HIV infection. Baillieres Clin Neurol 1996; 5:199–218.

48. Mendell JR, Kolkin S, Kissel JT, Weiss KL, Chakeres DW, Rammohan KW. Evidence for central nervous system demyelination in chronic inflammatory demyelinating polyradiculoneuropathy. Neurology 1987; 37:1291–1294.

49. Rubin M, Karpati G, Carpenter S. Combined central and peripheral myelinopathy. Neurology 1987; 37:1287–1290.

50. Thomas PK, Walker RWH, Rudge P, Morgan-Hughes JA, King RHM, Jacobs JM, Mills KR, Ormerod IEC, Murray NMF, McDonald WI. Chronic demyelinating peripheral neuropathy associated with multifocal central nervous system demyelination. Brain 1987; 110:53–76.

51. Thomas PK, Valentine A, Youl BD. Chronic inflammatory demyelinating polyneuropathy with multifocal CNS demyelination in an Afrid. J Neurol Neurosurg Psychiatry 1996; 61:529–530.

52. Liguori R, Rizzi R, Vetrugno R, Salvi F, Lugaresi A, Cevoli S, Montagna P. Steroid-responsive multifocal demyelinating neuropathy with central involvement. Muscle Nerve 1999; 22:262–265.

53. Waddy HM, Misra VP, King RHM et al. Focal cranial nerve involvement in chronic inflammatory demyelinating polyneuropathy: clinical and MRI evidence of peripheral and central lesions. J Neurol 1989; 236:400–410.

54. Feasby TE, Hahn AF, Koopman WJ, Lee DH. Central lesions in chronic inflammatory polyneuropathy: an MRI study. Neurology 1990; 40:476–478.

55. Hawke SHB, Hallinan JM, McLeod JG. Cranial magnetic resonance imaging in chronic demyelinating polyneuropathy J Neurol Neurosurg Psychiatry 1990; 53:794–796.

56. Ormerod IEC, Waddy HM, Kermode AG, Murray NMF, Thomas PK. Involvement of the central nervous system in chronic inflammatory demyelinating polyneuropathy: a clinical, electrophysiological and magnetic resonance imaging study. J Neurol Neurosurg Psychiatry 1990; 53:789–793.

57. Holtkamp M, Zschenderlein R, Bruck W, Weber JR. Acta Neuropathol 2001; 101: 529–531.

58. Antoine JC, Mosnier JF, Lapras J, Convers P, Absi L, Laurent B, Michel D. Chronic inflammatory demyelinating polyneuropathy associated with carcinoma. J Neurol Neurosurg Psychiatry 1996; 60:188–190.

59. Sugai F, Abe K, Fujimoto T, Nagano S, Fujimura H, Kayanoki Y, Oshikawa O, Yamasaki E, Kawata S, Matsuzawa Y, Yanagihara T. Chronic inflammatory demyelinating polyneuropathy accompanied by hepatocellular carcinoma. Inter Med 1997; 36:53–55.

60. Abe K, Sugai F. Chronic inflammatory demyelinating polyneuropathy accompanied by carcinoma. J Neurol Neurosurg Psychiatry 1998; 65:403–404.

61. Greenspan BN, Felice KJ. Chronic inflammatory demyelinating polyneuropathy (CIDP) associated with seminoma. Eur Neurol 1998; 39:57–58.

62. Bird SJ, Brown MJ, Shy ME, Scherer SS. Chronic inflammatory demyelinating polyneuropathy associated with malignant melanoma. Neurology 1996; 46:822–824.

63. Weiss MD, Luciano CA, Semino-Mora C, Dalakas MC, Quarles RH. Molecular mimicry in chronic inflammatory demyelinating polyneuropathy and melanoma. Neurology 1998; 51:1738–1741.

64. Krendel DA, Costigan DA, Hopkins LC. Successful treatment of neuropathies in patients with diabetes mellitus. Arch Neurol 1995; 52:1053–1061.

65. Stewart JD, McKelvey R, Durcan L, Carpenter S, Karpati G. Chronic inflammatory demyelinating polyneuropathy (CIDP) in diabetics. J Neurol Sci 1996; 142:59–64.

66. Uncini A, De Angelis MV, Di Muzio A et al. Chronic inflammatory demyelinating polyneuropathy in diabetics: motor conductions are important in the differential diagnosis with diabetic polyneuropathy. Clin Neurophysiol 1999; 110:705–711.

67. Gorson KC, Roopper AH, Adelman LS, Weinberg DH. Influence of diabetes mellitus on chronic inflammatory demyelinating polyneuropathy. Muscle Nerve 2000; 23:37–43.

68. Dyck PJ, O'Brien PC, Oviatt KF, Dinapoli RP, Daube JR, Bartleson JD, Mokri B, Swift T, Low PA, Windebank AJ. Prednisone improves chronic inflammatory demyelinating polyradiculoneuropathy more than no treatment. Ann Neurol 1982; 11:136–144.

69. Dyck PJ, O'Brien P, Swanson C, Low P, Daube J. Combined azathioprine and prednisone in chronic inflammatory demyelinating polyneuropathy. Neurology 1985; 35:1173–1176.

70. Dyck PJ, Daube J, O'Brien P, Pineda A, Low PA, Windebank AJ, Swanson C. Plasma exchange in chronic inflammatory demyelinating polyradiculoneuropathy. N Engl J Med 1986; 314:461–465.

71. Hahn AF, Bolton CF, Pillay N, Chalk C, Benstead T, Bril V, Shumak K, Vandervoort MK, Feasby TE. Plasma-exchange therapy in chronic inflammatory demyelinating polyneuropathy: a double-blind, sham-controlled, cross-over study. Brain 1996; 119:1055–1066.

72. Levy RL, Newkirk R, Ochoa J. Treating chronic relapsing Guillain–Barré syndrome by plasma exchange. Lancet 1979; 2:259–260.

73. Gross MLP, Thomas PK. The treatment of chronic relapsing and chronic progressive idiopathic inflammatory polyneuropathy by plasma exchange. J Neurol Sci 1981; 52:69–78.

74. Conner RK, Ziter FA, Anstall HB. Childhood chronic relapsing polyneuropathy: dramatic improvement following plasmapheresis. J Clin Apheresis 1982; 1:46–49.

75. Gross MLP, Legg NJ, Lockwood MC, Pallis C. The treatment of inflammatory polyneuropathy by plasma exchange. J Neurol Neurosurg Psychiatry 1982; 45:675–679.

76. Toyka KV, Augspach R, Wietholter H et al. Plasma exchange in chronic inflammatory polyneuropathy: evidence suggestive of a pathogenic humoral factor. Muscle Nerve 1982; 5:479–484.

77. Van Nunen SA, Gatenby PA, Pollard JD, Deacon M, Clancy RL. Specificity of plasmapheresis in the treatment of chronic relapsing polyneuropathy. Aust NZ J Med 1982; 12:81–84.

78. Pollard JD, McLeod JG, Gatenby P, Kronenberg H. Prediction of response to plasma exchange in chronic relapsing polyneuropathy. J Neurol Sci 1983; 58:269–287.

79. Donofrio PD, Tandan R, Albers JW. Plasma exchange in chronic inflammatory demyelinating polyradiculoneuropathy. Muscle Nerve 1985; 8:321–327.

80. Dyck PJ, Litchy WJ, Kratz KM, Suarez GA, Low PA, Pineda AA, Windebank AJ, Karnes JL, O'Brien PC. A plasma exchange versus immune globulin infusion trial in chronic inflammatory demyelinating polyradiculoneuropathy. Ann Neurol 1994; 36:838–845.

81. Hahn AF, Bolton CF, Zochodne D, Feasby TE. Intravenous immunoglobulin treatment in chronic inflammatory demyelinating polyneuropathy: a double-blind, placebo-controlled, cross-over study. Brain 1996; 119:1067–1077.

82. Mendell JR, Barohn RJ, Freimer ML et al. Randomized controlled trial of IVIg in untreated chronic inflammatory demyelinating polyradiculoneuropathy. Neurology 2001; 56:445–449.

83. Hughes R, Bensa S, Willison H, Van den Bergh P, Comi G, Illa I, Nobile-Orazio E, van Doorn P, Dalakas M, Bojar M, Swan A. Randomized controlled trial of intravenous immunoglobulin versus oral prednisolone in chronic inflammatory demyelinating polyradiculoneuropathy. Ann Neurol 2001; 50:195–201.

84. Vermeulen M, van der Meche FDA, Speelman JD, Weber A, Busch JFM. Plasma and gamma-globulin infusion in chronic inflammatory polyneuropathy. J Neurol Sci 1985; 70:317–326.

85. Curro Dossi B, Tezzon F. High-dose intravenous gammaglobulin for chronic inflammatory demyelinating polyneuropathy. Ital J Neurol Sci 1987; 8:321–326.

86. Faed JM, Day B, Pollock M, Taylor PK, Nukada H, Hammond-Tooke GD. High-dose intravenous human immunoglobulin in chronic inflammatory demyelinating polyneuropathy. Neurology 1989; 39:422–425.

87. Van Doorn PA, Brand A, Strengers PFW, Meulstee J, Vermeulen M. High-dose intravenous immunoglobulin treatment in chronic inflammatory demyelinating polyneuropathy: a double-blind, placebo-controlled, crossover study. Neurology 1990; 40:209–212.

88. Cornblath DR, Chaudhry V, Griffin JW. Treatment of chronic inflammatory demyelinating polyneuropathy with intravenous immunoglobulin. Ann Neurol 1991; 30:104–106.

89. Van Doorn PA, Vermeulen M, Brand A, Mulder PGH, Busch HFM. Intravenous immunoglobulin treatment in patients with chronic inflammatory demyelinating polyneuropathy. Arch Neurol 1991; 48:217–220.

90. Vedanarayanan VV, Kandt RS, Lewis DV, DeLong GR. Chronic inflammatory demyelinating polyradiculoneuropathy of childhood: treatment with high-dose intravenous immunoglobulin. Neurology 1991; 41:828–830.

91. Choudhary PP, Hughes RAC. Long-term treatment of chronic inflammatory demyelinating polyradiculoneuropathy with plasma exchange or intravenous immunoglobulin. Q J Med 1995; 88:493–502.

92. Good JL, Chehrenama M, Mayer RF, Koski CL. Pulse cyclophosphamide therapy in chronic inflammatory demyelinating polyneuropathy. Neurology 1998; 51:1735–1738.

93. Hodgkinson SJ, Pollard JD, McLeod JG. Cyclosporin A in the treatment of chronic demyelinating polyradiculoneuropathy. J Neurol Neurosurg Psychiatry 1990; 53:327–330.

94. Mahattankul W, Crawford TO, Griffin JW, Cornblath DR, Goldstein JM. Treatment of chronic inflammatory demyelinating polyneuropathy with cyclosporin-A. J Neurol Neurosurg Psychiatry 1996; 60:185–187.

95. Barnett MH, Pollard JD, Davies L, McLeod JG. Cyclosporin A in resistant chronic inflammatory demyelinating polyradiculoneuropathy. Muscle Nerve 1998; 21:454–460.

96. Sabatelli M, Mignogna T, Lippi G, Milone M, Di Lazzaro V, Tonali P, Bertini E. Interferon-alpha may benefit steroid unresponsive chronic inflammatory demyelinating polyneuropathy. J Neurol Neurosurg Psychiatry 1995; 58:638–639.

97. Gorson KC, Allam G, Simovic D, Ropper AH. Improvement following interferon-alpha 2a in chronic inflammatory demyelinating polyneuropathy. Neurology 1997; 48:777–780.

98. Mancuso A, Ardita FV, Leonardi J, Scuderi M. Interferon alpha-2a therapy and pregnancy. Report of a case of chronic inflammatory demyelinating polyneuropathy. Acta Obstet Gynecol Scand 1998; 77:869–872.

99. Gorson KC, Ropper AH, Clark BD, Dew RB, Simovic D, Allam G. Treatment of chronic inflammatory demyelinating polyneuropathy with interferon-alpha 2a. Neurology 1998; 50:84–87.

100. Hadden RDM, Sharrack B, Bensa S, Soudain SE, Hughes RAC. Randomized trial of interferon beta-1a in chronic inflammatory demyelinating polyradiculoneuropathy. Neurology 1999; 53:57–61.

101. Kuntzer T, Radziwill AJ, Lettry-Trouillat R et al. Interferon-β1a in chronic inflammatory demyelinating polyneuropathy. Neurology 1999; 53:1364–1365.

102. Marzo E, Tintore M, Fabregues O, Montalban X, Codina A. Chronic inflammatory demyelinating polyneuropathy during treatment with interferon-alpha. J Neurol Neurosurg Psychiatry 1998;65:604.

103. Meriggioli MN, Rowin J. Chronic inflammatory demyelinating polyneuropathy after treatment with interferon-alpha. Muscle Nerve 2000; 23:433–435.

104. Ahlmen J, Andersen O, Hallgren G, Peilot B. Positive effects of tacrolimus in a case of CIDP. Transplantation Proceedings 1998; 30:4194.

105. Vermeulen M, Van Oers MH. Successful autologous stem cell transplantation in a patient with chronic inflammatory demyelinating polyneuropathy. J Neurol Neurosurg Psychiatry 2002; 72:127–128.

106. Hadden RDM, Bensa S, Lunn MPT, Hughes RAC. Immunoadsorption inferior to plasma exchange in a patient with chronic inflammatory demyelinating polyradiculoneuropathy. J Neurol Neurosurg Psychiatry 2002; 72:644–646.

107. Simmons Z, Albers JW, Bromberg MB, Feldman EL. Long-term follow-up of patients with chronic inflammatory demyelinating polyradiculoneuropathy, without and with monoclonal gammopathy. Brain 1995; 118:359–368.

108. Harvey GK, Pollard JD, Schindhelm K, Antony J. Chronic experimental allergic neuritis: an electrophysiological and histological study in the rabbit. J Neurol Sci 1987; 81:215–225.

109. Bouchard C, Lacroix C, Planté V, Adams D, Chedru F, Guglielmi J-M, Said G. Clinico-pathologic findings and prognosis of chronic inflammatory demyelinating polyneuropathy. Neurology 1999; 52:498–503.

110. Yan WX, Taylor J, Andrias-Kauba S, Pollard JD. Passive transfer of demyelination by serum of IgG from chronic inflammatory demyelinating polyneuropathy patients. Ann Neurol 2000; 47:765–775.

111. Koski CL, Humphrey R, Shin ML. Anti-peripheral myelin antibody in patients with demyelinating neuropathy: quantitative and kinetic determination of serum antibody by complement component 1 fixation. Proc Natl Acad Sci USA 1985; 82:905–909.

112. Van Doorn PA, Brand A, Vermeulen M. Clinical significance of antibodies against peripheral nerve tissue in inflammatory polyneuropathy. Neurology 1987; 37:1798–1802.

113. Fredman P, Bedeler CA, Nyland H, Aarli JA, Svennerholm L. Antibodies in sera from patients with inflammatory demyelinating polyradiculoneuropathy react with ganglioside LM1 and sulphatide of peripheral nerve myelin. J Neurol 1991; 238:75–79.

114. Ilyas AA, Mithen FA, Dalakas MC, Chen ZW, Cook SD. Antibodies to acidic glycolipids in Guillain–Barré syndrome and chronic inflammatory demyelinating polyneuropathy. J Neurol Sci 1992; 107:111–121.

115. Connolly AM, Pestronk A, Trotter JL, Feldman EL, Cornblath DR, Olney RK. High-titer selective serum anti-β-tubulin antibodies in chronic inflammatory demyelinating polyneuropathy. Neurology 1993; 43:557–562.

116. Khalili-Shirazi A, Atkinson P, Gregson N, Hughes RAC. Antibody responses to P0 and P2 myelin proteins in Guillain–Barré syndrome and chronic idiopathic demyelinating polyradiculoneuropathy. J Neuroimmunol 1993; 46:245–251.

117. Simone IL, Annunziata P, Maimone D, Liguori M, Leante R, Livrea P. Serum and CSF anti-GM1 antibodies in patients with Guillain–Barré syndrome and chronic inflammatory demyelinating polyneuropathy. J Neurol Sci 1993; 114:49–55

118. Yan WX, Archelos JJ, Hartung H-P, Pollard JD. P0 protein is a target antigen in chronic inflammatory demyelinating polyradiculoneuropathy. Ann Neurol 2001; 50:286–292.

119. Hughes RAC. Chronic inflammatory demyelinating polyradiculoneuropathy. Ann Neurol 2001; 50:281–282.

120. Colan RV, Snead OC, Oh SJ, Benton JW. Steroid-responsive polyneuropathy with subacute onset in childhood. J Pediatr 1980; 97:374–377.

121. Sladky JT, Brown MJ, Berman PH. Chronic inflammatory demyelinating polyneuropathy of infancy: a corticosteroid-responsive disorder. Ann Neurol 1986; 20:76–81.

122. Ouvrier RA, Mc Leod JG. Chronic peripheral neuropathy in childhood: an overview. Aust Paediatr J 1988; (suppl):80–82.

123. Faleck H, Cruse RP, Levin KH, Estes M. Response of CSF IgG to steroids in an 18-month-old with chronic inflammatory polyradiculoneuropathy: Clev Clin J Med 1989; 56:539–541.

124. Beydoun SR, Engel WK, Karofsky P, Schwartz MU. Long-term plasmapheresis therapy is effective and safe in children with chronic relapsing dysimmune polyneuropathy. Rev Neurol (Paris) 1990; 146:123–127.

125. Taku K, Tamura T, Miike T. Gammaglobulin therapy in a case of chronic relapsing dysimmune polyneuropathy. Brain Dev 1990; 12:247–249.

126. Uncini A, Parano E, Lange DJ, DeVivo DC, Lovelace RE. Chronic inflammatory demyelinating polyneuropathy in childhood: clinical and electrophysiological features. Child's Nerv Syst 1991; 7:191–196.

127. Nevo Y, Pestronk A, Kornberg AJ, Connolly AM, Yee W-C, Iqbal I, Shield LK. Childhood chronic inflammatory demyelinating neuropathies: clinical course and long-term follow-up. Neurology 1996; 47:98–102.

128. Simmons Z, Wald JJ, Albers JW. Chronic inflammatory demyelinating polyradiculoneuropathy in children: I. Presentation, electrodiagnostic studies, and initial clinical course, with comparison to adults. Muscle Nerve 1997; 20:1008–1015.

129. Korinthenberg R. Chronic inflammatory demyelinating polyradiculoneuropathy in children and their response to treatment. Neuropediatrics 1999; 30:190–196.

130. Ryan MM, Grattan-Smith PJ, Procopis PG, Morgan G, Ouvrier RA. Childhood chronic inflammatory demyelinating polyneuropathy: clinical course and long-term outcome. Neuromusc Disord 2000; 10:398–406.

131. Hattori N, Ichimura M, Aoki S-I et al. Clinicopathological features of chronic inflammatory demyelinating polyradiculoneuropathy in childhood. J Neuro Sci 1998; 154:66–71.

132. Nevo Y, Topaloglu H. 88th ENMC international workshop: childhood chronic inflammatory demyelinating polyneuropathy (including revised diagnostic criteria), Naarden, The Netherlands, December 8–10, 2000. Neuromusc Disord 2002; 12:195–200.

133. Simmons Z, Wald JJ, Albers JW. Chronic inflammatory demyelinating polyradiculoneuropathy in children: II. Long-term follow-up, with comparison to adults. Muscle Nerve 1997; 20:1569–1575.

134. Kyle RA. Diagnostic criteria of multiple myeloma. Hem Onc Clin North Am 1992; 6:347–369.

135. Notermans NC, Franssen H, Eurelings M, Van der Graaf Y, Wokke JHJ. Diagnostic criteria for demyelinating polyneuropathy associated with monoclonal gammopathy. Muscle Nerve 2000; 23:73–79.

136. Nobile-Orazio E, Manfredini E, Carpo M, Meucci N, Monaco S, Ferrari S et al. Frequency and clinical correlates of anti-neural IgM antibodies in neuropathy associated with IgM monoclonal gammopathy. Ann Neurol 1994; 36:416–424.

137. Kelly JJ. The electrodiagnostic findings in peripheral neuropathy associated with monoclonal gammopathy. Muscle Nerve 1983; 6:504–509.

138. Melmed C, Frail D, Duncan I, Braun P, Danoff D, Finlayson M, Stewart J. Peripheral neuropathy with IgM kappa monoclonal immunoglobulin directed against myelin-associated glycoprotein. Neurology 1983; 33:1397–1405.

139. Hafler DA, Johnson D, Kelly JJ, Panitch H, Kyle R, Weiner HL. Monoclonal gammopathy and neuropathy: myelin-associated glycoprotein reactivity and clinical characteristics. Neurology 1986; 36:75–78.

140. Nobile-Orazio E, Marmiroli P, Baldini L, Spagnol G, Barbieri S, Moggio M et al. Peripheral neuropathy in macroglobulinemia: incidence and antigen-specificity of M proteins. Neurology 1987; 37:1506–1514.

141. Kelly JJ, Adelman LS, Berkman E, Bhan I. Polyneuropathies associated with IgM monoclonal gammopathies. Arch Neurol 1988; 45:1355–1359.

142. Kaku DA, England JD, Sumner AJ. Distal accentuation of conduction slowing in polyneuropathy associated with antibodies to myelin-associated glycoprotein and sulphated glucuronyl paragloboside. Brain 1994; 117:941–947.

143. Chassande B, Leger J-M, Younes-Chennoufi AB, Bengoufa D, Maisonobe T, Bouche P, Baumann N. Peripheral neuropathy associated with IgM monoclonal gammopathy: correlations between M-protein antibody activity and clinical/electrophysiological features in 40 cases. Muscle Nerve 1998; 21:55–62.

144. Gosselin S, Kyle RA, Dyck PJ. Neuropathy associated with monoclonal gammopathies of undetermined significance. Ann Neurol 1991; 30:54–61.

145. Suarez GA, Kelly JJ Jr. Polyneuropathy associated with monoclonal gammopathy of undetermined significance: further evidence that IgM-MGUS neuropathies are different than IgG-MGUS. Neurology 1993; 43:1304–1308.

146. Notermans NC, Wokke JHJ, Lokhorst HM, Franssen H, van der Graaf Y, Jennekens FGI. Polyneuropathy associated with monoclonal gammopathy of undetermined significance: a prospective study of the prognostic value of clinical and laboratory abnormalities. Brain 1994; 117:1385–1393.

147. Simovic D, Gorson KC, Ropper AH. Comparison of IgM-MGUS and IgG-MGUS polyneuropathy. Acta Neurol Scand 1998; 97:194–200.

148. Katz JS, Saperstein DS, Gronseth G, Amato AA, Barohn RJ. Distal acquired demyelinating symmetric neuropathy. Neurology 2000; 54:615–620.

149. Saperstein DS, Katz JS, Amato AA, Barohn RJ. Clinical spectrum of chronic acquired demyelinating polyneuropathies. Muscle Nerve 2001; 24:311–324.

150. Cocito D, Isoardo G, Ciaramitaro P et al. Terminal latency index in polyneuropathy with IgM paraproteinemia and anti-MAG antibody. Muscle Nerve 2001; 24:1278–1282.

151. Eurelings M, Notermans NC, Wokke JH, Bosboom WM, Van den Berg LH. Sural nerve T cells in demyelinating polyneuropathy associated with monoclonal gammopathy. Acta Neuropathol 2002; 103:107–114.

152. Eurelings M, Notermans NC, Franssen H, Van Es HW et al. MRI of the brachial plexus in polyneuropathy associated with monoclonal gammopathy. Muscle Nerve 2001; 24:1312–1318.

153. Bardwick PA, Zvaifler NJ, Gill GN, Newman D, Greenway GD, Resnick DL. Plasma cell dyscrasia with polyneuropathy, organomegaly, endocrinopathy, M protein, and skin changes: the POEMS syndrome. Medicine 1980; 59:311–322.

154. Kelly JJ, Kyle RA, Miles JM, Dyck PJ. Osteosclerotic myeloma and peripheral neuropathy. Neurology 1983; 33:202–210.

155. Miralles GD, O'Fallon JR, Talley NJ. Plasma-cell dyscrasia with polyneuropathy: the spectrum of POEMS syndrome. N Engl J Med 1992; 327: 1919–1923.

156. Kyle RA, Dyck PJ. Osteosclerotic myeloma (POEMS syndrome). In: Dyck PJ, Thomas PK, Griffin JW, Low PA, Poduslo JF, eds. Peripheral Neuropathy. 3rd ed. Philadelphia: WB Saunders, 1993: 288–1293.

157. Kyle RA, Greipp PR. Amyloidosis (AL): clinical and laboratory features in 229 cases. Mayo Clin Proc 1983; 58:665–683.

158. Duston MA, Skinner M, Anderson J, Cohen AS. Peripheral neuropathy as an early marker of AL amyloidosis. Arch Intern Med 1989; 149:358–360.

159. Kyle RA, Dyck PJ. Amyloidosis and Neuropathy. In: Dyck PJ, Thomas PK, Griffin JW, Low PA, Poduslo JF, eds. Peripheral Neuropathy. 3rd ed. Philadelphia: WB Saunders, 1993:1294–1309.

160. Kyle RA, Gertz MA. Primary systemic amyloidosis: clinical and laboratory features in 474 cases. Sem Hematol 1995; 32:45–59.

161. Rajkumar SV, Gertz MA, Kyle RA. Prognosis of patients with primary systemic amyloidosis who present with dominant neuropathy. Am J Med 1998; 104:232–237.

162. Janssen S, Van Rijswijk MH, Meijer S, Ruinen L, Van Der Hem GK. Systemic amyloidosis: a clinical survey of 144 cases. Neth J Med 1986; 29:376–385.

163. Sherman WH, Olarte MR, McKiernan G, Sweeney K, Latov N, Hays AP. Plasma exchange treatment of peripheral neuropathy associated with plasma cell dyscrasia. J Neurol Neurosurg Psychiatry 1984; 47:813–819.

164. Dyck PJ, Low PA, Windebank AJ, Jaradeh SS, Gosselin S, Bourque P et al. Plasma exchange in polyneuropathy associated with monoclonal gammopathy of undetermined significance. N Engl J Med 1991; 325:1482–1486.

165. Ellie E, Vital A, Steck A, Boiron J-M, Vital C, Julien J. Neuropathy associated with "benign" anti-myelin-associated glycoprotein IgM gammopathy: clinical, immunological, neurophysiological, pathological findings and response to treatment in 33 cases. J Neurol 1996; 243:34–43.

166. Haas DC, Tatum AH. Plasmapheresis alleviates neuropathy accompanying IgM anti-myelin-associated glycoprotein paraproteinemia. Ann Neurol 1988; 23:394–396.

167. Nobile-Orazio E, Baldini L, Barbieri S, Marmiroli P, Spagnol G, Francomano E, Scarlato G. Treatment of patients with neuropathy and anti-MAG IgM M-proteins. Ann Neurol 1988; 24:93–97.

168. Mariette X, Chastang C, Clavelou P, Louboutin J-P, Leger J-M, Brouet J-C, for the IgM-associated polyneuropathy study group. A randomised clinical trial comparing interferon-α and intravenous immunoglobulin in polyneuropathy associated with monoclonal IgM. J Neurol Neurosurg Psychiatry 1997; 63:28–34.

169. Rudnicki SA, Harik SI, Dhodapkar M, Barlogie B, Eidelberg D. Nervous system dysfunction in Waldenström's macroglobulinemia: response to treatment. Neurology 1998; 51:1210–1213.

170. Cook D, Dalakas M, Galdi A, Biondi D, Porter H. High-dose intravenous immunoglobulin in the treatment of demyelinating neuropathy associated with monoclonal gammopathy. Neurology 1990; 40:212–214.

171. Leger JM, Younes-Chennoufi AB, Chassande B, Davila G, Bouche P, Baumann N, Brunet P. Human immunoglobulin treatment of multifocal motor neuropathy and polyneuropathy associated with monoclonal gammopathy. J Neurol Neurosurg Psychiatry 1994; 57(suppl):46–49.

172. Dalakas MC, Quarles RH, Farrer RG, Dambrosia J, Soueidan S, Stein DP, Cupler E, Sekul EA, Otero C. A controlled study of intravenous immonoglobulin in demyelinating neuropathy with IgM gammopathy. Ann Neurol 1996; 40:792–795.

173. Waterston JA, Brown MM, Ingram DA, Swash M. Cyclosporine A therapy in paraprotein-associated neuropathy. Muscle Nerve 1992; 15:445–448.

174. Barnett MH, Pollard JD, Davies L, McLeod JG. Cyclosporin A in resistant chronic inflammatory demyelinating polyradiculoneuropathy. Muscle Nerve 1998; 21:454–460.

175. Oksenhendler E, Chevret S, Leger J-M, Louboutin L-P, Bussel A, Brouet J-C for the IgM-associated polyneuropathy study group. Plasma exchange and chlorambucil in polyneuropathy associated with monoclonal IgM gammopathy. J Neurol Neurosurg Psychiatry 1995; 59:243–247.

176. Wilson H, Lunn MPT, Schey S, Hughes RAC. Successful treatment of IgM paraproteinaemic neuropathy with fludarabine. J Neurol Neurosurg Psychiatry 1999; 66:575–580.

177. Latov N, Sherman WH. Therapy of neuropathy associated with anti-MAG IgM monoclonal gammopathy with Rituxan. Neurology 1999; 52(suppl 2):A551.

178. Levine TD, Pestronk A. IgM antibody-related polyneuropathies: B-cell depletion chemotherapy using Rituximab. Neurology 1999; 52:1701–1704.

179. Julien J, Bital C, Vallat JM et al. Chronic demyelinating neuropathy with IgM producing lymphocytes in peripheral nerve and delayed appearance of "benign" monoclonal gammopathy. Neurology 1984; 34:1387–1389.

180. Valldeoriola F, Graus F, Steck AJ, Munoz E, de la Fuente M, Gallart T, Ribalta T, Bombi JA, Tolosa E. Delayed appearance of anti-myelin-associated glycoprotein antibodies in a patient with chronic inflammatory demyelinating polyneuropathy. Ann Neurol 1993; 34:394–396.

181. Ponsford S, Willison H, Veitch J, Morris R, Thomas PK. Long-term clinical and neurophysiological follow-up of patients with peripheral neuropathy associated with benign monoclonal gammopathy. Muscle Nerve 2000; 23:164–174.

182. Kyle RA. "Benign" monoclonal gammopathy: a misnomer? J Am Med Assoc 1984; 251:1849–1854.

183. Kyle RA, Garton JP. The spectrum of IgM monoclonal gammopathy in 430 cases. Mayo Clin Proc 1987; 62:719–731.

184. Kyle RA. "Benign" monoclonal gammopathy—after 20–35 years of follow-up. Mayo Clin Proc 1993; 68:26–36.

185. Read D, Warlow C. Peripheral neuropathy and solitary plasmacytoma. J Neurol Neurosurg Psychiatry 1978; 41:177–184.

186. Takatsuki K, Sanada I. Plasma cell dyscrasia with polyneuropathy and endocrine disorder: clinical and laboratory features of 109 reported cases. Jpn J Clin Oncol 1983; 13:543–556.

187. Nakanishi T, Sobue I, Toyokura Y, Nishitani H, Kuroiwa Y, Satoyoshi E et al. The Crow-Fukase syndrome: a study of 102 cases in Japan. Neurology 1984; 34:712–720.

188. Simmons Z. Wald J, Albers JW, Feldman EL. The natural history of a "benign" rib lesion in a patient with a demyelinating polyneuropathy and an unusual variant of POEMS syndrome. Muscle Nerve 1994; 17:1055–1059.

189. Latov N, Sherman WH, Nemni R, Galassi G, Shyong JS, Penn AS et al. Plasma-cell dyscrasia and peripheral neuropathy with a monoclonal antibody to peripheral-nerve myelin. N Engl J Med 1980; 303:618–621.

190. Mendell JR, Sahenk Z, Whitaker JN, Trapp BD, Yates AJ, Griggs RC, Quarles RH. Polyneuropathy and IgM monoclonal gammopathy: studies on the pathogenetic role of anti-myelin-associated glycoprotein antibody. Ann Neurol 1985; 17:243–254.

191. Takatsu M, Hays AP, Latov N, Abrams GM, Nemni R, Sherman WH et al. Immunofluorescence study of patients with neuropathy and IgM M proteins. Ann Neurol 1985; 81:173–181.

192. Hays AP, Lee SSL, Latov N. Immune reactive C3d on the surface of myelin sheaths in neuropathy. J Neuroimmunol 1988; 18:231–244.

193. Monaco S, Bonetti B, Ferrari S, Moretto G, Nardelli E, Tedesco F et al. Complement dependent demyelination in patients with IgM monoclonal gammopathy and polyneuropathy. N Engl J Med 1990; 322:844–852.

194. Gabriel JM, Erne B, Bernasconi L, Tosi C, Probst A, Landmann L, Steck AJ. Confocal microscopic localization of anti-MAG autoantibodies in a patient with peripheral neuropathy initially lacking a detectable IgM gammopathy. Acta Neuropathol 1998; 95:540–546.

195. Vital A, Vital C, Julien J, Baquey A, Steck AJ. Polyneuropathy associated with IgM monoclonal gammopathy: immunological and pathological study in 31 patients. Acta Neuropathol 1989; 79:160–167.

196. Ritz M-F, Erne B, Ferracin F, Vital A, Vital C, Steck AJ. Anti-MAG IgM penetration into myelinated fibers correlates with the extent of myelin widening. Muscle Nerve 1999; 22:1030–1037.

197. Lunn MPT, Crawford TO, Highes RAC, Griffin JW, Sheikh KA. Anti-myelin-associated glycoprotein antibodies alter neurofilament spacing. Brain 2002; 125:904–911.

198. Hays AP, Latov N, Takatsu M, Sherman WH. Experimental demyelination of nerve induced by serum of patients with neuropathy and an anti-MAG IgM M-protein. Neurology 1987; 37:242–256.

199. Willison HJ, Trapp BD, Bacher JD, Dalakas MC, Griffin JW, Quarles RH. Demyelination induced by intraneural injection of human antimyelin-associated glycoprotein antibodies. Muscle Nerve 1988; 11:1169–1176.

200. Trojaborg W, Galassi G, Hays AP, Lovelace RE, Alkaitis M, Latov N. Electrophysiological study of experimental demyelination induced by serum of patients with IgM M proteins and neuropathy. Neurology 1989; 39:1581–1586.

201. Tatum AH. Experimental paraprotein neuropathy, demyelination by passive transfer of human IgM anti-myelin-asociated glycoprotein. Ann Neurol 1993; 33:502–506.

202. Nobile-Orazio E, Barbieri S, Baldini L, Marmiroli P, Carpo M, Premoselli S et al. Peripheral neuropathy in monoclonal gammopathy of undetermined significance: prevalence and immunopathogenetic studies. Acta Neurol Scand 1992; 85:383–390.

203. Meucci N, Baldini L, Cappellari A, Di Troia A, Allaria S, Scarlato G, Nobile-Orazio E. Anti-myelin-associated glycoprotein antibodies predict the development of neuropathy in asymptomatic patients with IgM monoclonal gammopathy. Ann Neurol 1999; 46:119–122.

204. Lewis RA, Sumner AJ, Brown MJ, Asbury AK. Multifocal demyelinating neuropathy with persistent conduction block. Neurology 1982; 32:958–964.

205. Gibbels E, Behse F, Kentenich M, Haupt WF. Chronic multifocal neuropathy with persistent conduction block (Lewis–Sumner syndrome). Clin Neuropathol 1993; 12:343–352.

206. Oh SJ, Claussen GC, Kim DS. Motor and sensory demyelinating mononeuropathy multiplex (multifocal motor and sensory demyelinating neuropathy): a separate entity or a variant of chronic inflammatory demyelinating polyneuropathy? J Periph Nerv Syst 1997; 2:362–369.

207. Saperstein DS, Amato AA, Wolfe GI, Katz JS, Nations SP, Jackson CE, Bryan WW, Burns DK, Barohn RJ. Multifocal acquired demyelinating sensory and motor neuropathy: the Lewis–Sumner syndrome. Muscle Nerve 1999; 22:560–566.

208. Van den Berg-Vos RM, Van den Berg LH, Franssen H et al. Multifocal inflammatory demyelinating neuropathy: a distinct clinical entity? Neurology 2000; 54:26–32.

209. Simmons Z, Albers JW. Chronic inflammatory demyelinating polyradiculoneuropathy and related disorders. In: Katirji B, Kaminski HJ, Preston DC, Ruff RL, Shapiro BE, eds. Neuromuscular Disorders in Clinical Practice. Boston: Butterworth-Heinemann, 2002:567–588.

10
Multifocal Demyelinating Neuropathies

Richard A. Lewis
Wayne State University School of Medicine, Detroit, Michigan, USA

ABSTRACT

Chronic immune-mediated demyelinating neuropathies have a spectrum of clinical presentations, electrodiagnostic findings, laboratory findings, and responses to treatment. Over the past 25 years, a number of different forms have been recognized on the basis of specific features, and these include chronic inflammatory demyelinating polyradiculoneuropathy, multifocal motor neuropathy with conduction block, and the Lewis–Sumner Syndrome (multifocal sensorimotor demyelinating polyneuropathy with persistent conduction block or multifocal acquired demyelination sensory and motor neuropathy). Distinctions between these entities can be challenging, and it is not clear that they represent truly distinct entities. This chapter reviews the recognition of these disorders from a historical perspective, clarifying and contrasting the clinical, diagnostic, and treatment response features.

1. INTRODUCTION

Our understanding of the spectrum of neuropathies that can be considered to be "chronic immune-mediated demyelinating neuropathies" has increased over the past 25 years. Prior to 1980, the only disorders under this heading were chronic inflammatory demyelinating polyradiculoneuropathy (CIDP) and the neuropathy associated with multiple myeloma. Currently, there are over 10 different disorders that fit this classification (Table 10.1). CIDP remains the prototypic immune-mediated neuropathy. It is characterized by greater weakness than sensory loss involving symmetric proximal and distal regions. Many of the other disorders also are symmetric. However, some have a strikingly asymmetric pattern that involves multiple individual nerves, termed *mononeuropathy (or mononeuritis) multiplex*. The term *confluent mononeuropathy multiplex* is used when many nerves have become involved, and it is not possible to identify specific nerves.

Prior to 1980, the cause of mononeuritis multiplex was attributed to collagen vascular disorders and vasculitides, but since then other disorders have been recognized (Table 10.2). Vasculitis is known to cause an ischemic insult leading to Wallerian degeneration as the pathologic consequence of the nerve infarct. Demyelinating mononeuropathy multiplex is seen in only a few conditions. Hereditary neuropathy with liability to pressure palsies (HNPP) is one such disorder. This inherited disorder due to a deletion of the gene for PMP-22 on chromosome 17 presents with multifocal sensorimotor symptoms related to repetitive activity, minor trauma, or moderate compression that would not normally affect peripheral nerve function. An immune mechanism has not been identified. However, two disorders that appear to be immune-mediated have now been recognized as causing a multifocal demyelinating neuropathy. This chapter will describe and contrast these disorders: multifocal motor neuropathy and the Lewis–Sumner Syndrome (LSS) [multifocal sensorimotor demyelinating polyneuropathy with persistent conduction block (MSMDN)].

Table 10.1 Chronic Immune-Mediated Polyneuropathies

CIDP
CIDP variants
  Sensory predominant
  Associated with multiple myeloma
  Associated with MGUS
    POEMS
    Distal acquired demyelinating neuropathy
      Associated with IgM MGUS
      Anti-MAG antibodies in 50%
    CANOMAD
  Associated with CNS demyelination
  Associated with systemic disorders
    ?Associated with Diabetes mellitus
MMN
MSMDN

Note: CIDP, chronic inflammatory demyelinating polyradiculoneuropathy; MGUS, monoclonal gammopathy of undermined significance; POEMS, polyneuropathy, organomegaly, endocrinopathy, M-protein, and skin changes; Anti-MAG, antibody titers to myelin-associated glycoprotein; CANOMAD, chronic ataxic neuropathy ophthalmoplegia M-protein agglutination disialosyl antibodies; CNS, central nervous system; MMN, multifocal motor neuropathy; MSMDN, multifocal sensorimotor demyelinating polyneuropathy with persistent conduction block.

Table 10.2 Mononeuropathy Multiplex

Demyelinating neuropathies
   MMN
   MSMDN
   Block (LSS)
   HNPP
Vasculitic and ischemic neuropathies
   Systemic lupus erythematosis
   Rheumatoid vasculitis
   Systemic sclerosis (Scleroderma)
   Periarteritis nodosa
   Churg–Strauss
   Wegener's granulomatosis
   Paraneoplastic vasculitic neuropathy
   Nonsystemic vasculitic neuropathy
   Behçet Syndrome
   Giant cell arteritis
Diabetes mellitus
   Lumbosacral radiculoplexopathy
   Truncal radiculopathy
   Cranial mononeuropathies
   Sensory perineuritis
Infectious neuropathies
   Leprosy
   Herpes zoster
   Lyme disease
   HIV associated cytomegalovirus
   Hepatitis C and cryoglobulinemia
Other causes
   Sarcoid
   Brachial neuritis (Parsonage–Turner Syndrome)
   Monomelic amyotrophy
   Malignant infiltration of peripheral nerve
   Neurofibromatosis

In 1982 (1), five patients were described who had a sensorimotor mononeuropathy multiplex, but rather than finding prominent Wallerian degeneration, the expected finding in vasculitic mononeuritis multiplex, these patients had striking and persistent multifocal conduction block (CB) and segmental demyelination. The two patients who were treated with prednisone responded in a time frame consistent with recovery from CB rather than the slower time course of recovery from Wallerian degeneration. These patients were described as having MSMDN and were considered to have a variant of CIDP that had previously been described as a symmetric disorder.

In 1988, Parry and Clarke (2), and in a separate report, Pestronk et al. (3), reported patients, who were initially considered to have lower motor neuron forms of amyotrophic lateral sclerosis (ALS), but were found to have a motor mononeuropathy multiplex related to persistent CB. Since then, there have been a number of studies describing patients with multifocal motor neuropathy with persistent conduction block (MMN). Whether patients with MMN and patients with MSMDN have the same disorder with varying degrees of sensory involvement has been debated, and the LSS has been used interchangeably by different authors to describe both entities. Recent reports suggest significant differences between these two disorders which may have therapeutic and pathophysiologic significance. For this reason, the two disorders will be considered separately and the term LSS will be used to describe only the sensorimotor disorder.

The naming of MSMDN has been a topic of discussion. The title of the original paper does not lend itself to a short, easily articulated, name. Saperstein et al. (4) have suggested the term MADSAM, for multifocal acquired demyelinating sensory and motor neuropathy. Although this chapter's author may be somewhat biased, the term MADSAM seems less than ideal. It may be confused with Mad Cow Disease and also seems somewhat prejudicial as the term connotes psychiatric pathology (not a feature of this disorder). Van den Berg-Vos et al. (5) have suggested "multifocal inflammatory demyelinating neuropathy." This is only minimally less awkward than the original title and does not truly separate MSMDN from MMN. As such, for this chapter, the author has taken the liberty of using the term LSS as the preferred name for MSMDN.

2. MULTIFOCAL MOTOR NEUROPATHY WITH PERSISTENT CB

2.1. Background

Most reviews point to the two reports in 1988 of Parry and Clarke (2) and Pestronk et al. (3) for identifying MMN. However, there were other reports that preceded these in which the various aspects of the disorder were described (6–9). The two reports in 1988 described patients who were initially considered to have lower motor neuron forms of ALS but were found to have a multifocal demyelinating neuropathy. Parry's five cases and Pestronk's two cases all presented with multifocal weakness, atrophy, cramps, and fasciculations without significant sensory complaints. Parry and Clarke emphasized that the symptoms began in the arms, that reflexes were usually normal or lost focally, that cerebrospinal fluid (CSF) protein was normal, and that the course was slowly progressive. Treatment responses were variable. One patient did not respond to plasmapheresis, one stabilized when azathioprine was added to prednisone, and one did not respond to plasmapheresis, prednisone, or cyclophosphamide. The cardinal feature of the disorder was multifocal CB and conduction slowing which appeared to be confined to motor nerve fibers. Distal sensory responses were normal and somatosensory evoked responses and compound nerve action potentials were normal across the regions of motor block.

Pestronk also emphasized early involvement of the upper limbs, presence of fasciculations, lack of upper motor neuron (UMN) signs or bulbar involvement, and the normal sensory exam. CSF protein was elevated to 69 mg/dL in one patient and normal in the other. They found similar findings of motor CB as well as conduction slowing with normal distal sensory conduction. Sural nerve biopsy was normal from one patient, but revealed occasional Wallerian-like degeneration from the other. A motor point biopsy showed axonal loss and demyelination of the remaining axons. There was no significant response to treatment with prednisone or plasmapheresis, but both patients responded to intravenous and/or oral cyclophosphamide. Both patients had IgM antibodies that reacted with GM1 ganglioside. The titers of the anti-GM1 antibodies fell after cyclophosphamide treatment.

Both reports mention that some of the patients had mild and vague sensory symptoms but no significant abnormality on clinical examination, and sensory conduction studies were normal. Since these reports, there have been a number of case reports and small series that have defined the clinical syndrome and the electrophysiologic features. They have addressed the controversial issue of the significance of elevated titers of anti-GM1 antibody and response to various treatments. In particular, many authors have emphasized intravenous immunoglobulin (IVIg) and/or cyclophosphamide in the treatment of MMN.

2.2. Clinical Features

MMN is a rare motor disorder that is more common in men than women (2:1 ratio) (4,10–12). The age of onset is between 20 and 70 years, with most patients between 25 and 55 years of age. The disease usually progresses slowly, with some reports indicating a course of over 20 years (10,12), but some patients will have a more rapid decline in function (3,9,11).

Patients may be misdiagnosed with a lower motor neuron form of ALS. Presenting features are usually painless, asymmetric weakness, atrophy, and fasciculations of the upper extremities in a distribution that may be isolated to one or two nerves. Legs may become involved, but rarely as the first limb, and the severity is usually less in legs than in arms, and patients may remain ambulatory despite severe upper extremity weakness. Although some patients describe vague sensory phenomena or intermittent mild sensory symptoms, sensory symptoms are never prominent despite marked lower motor neuron changes. Discrete sensory symptoms in the distribution of the motor abnormalities are not present. Sensory examination is almost always normal, even in patients with sensory symptoms. However, some reports mention distal vibration sense reduction (3) or sensory symptoms later in the course (2). Atrophy, fasciculations, myokymia, and cramps are seen in various combinations (9,12). Tinel's signs at the sites of the CB have not been mentioned. Focal hemiatrophy of the tongue has been described (13), but bulbar and pseudobulbar dysfunction have not been reported. Deep tendon reflexes tend to be preserved despite significant weakness. They can be lost focally, particularly in the arms, but it is unusual to have complete areflexia unless the weakness has become generalized and profound.

Some reports mention relative hyper-reflexia (3) but unequivocal UMN involvement in the form of Babinski responses or sustained clonus are not seen. Whether UMN signs can clinically distinguish ALS from MMN has been addressed (14). In this study of 169 patients with motor neuron disease, 17 were found to have either motor CB (10 patients) or focal temporal dispersion (seven patients). One out of the 10 patients with CB had Babinski signs or sustained clonus, whereas five others had incongruously brisk reflexes. Three of the seven patients with no block but abnormal temporal dispersion had definite UMN signs, and two had brisk reflexes. The implications of this study are that CB, as opposed to abnormal temporal dispersion, appears to best define the syndrome of MMN, and that true UMN signs are rare in patients with MMN, but brisk reflexes may be seen. The diagnosis of MMN should be questioned in patients with otherwise unexplained UMN signs.

2.3. Electrodiagnostic Features: Conduction Block

The defining feature of MMN is motor CB. CB occurs when saltatory transmission is lost over a focal segment of nerve due to structural or physiologic changes at the nodes of Ranvier. This is usually associated with segmental demyelination. The pathophysiologic features of CB have been shown in studies of CB induced by tourniquet (15) and intraneural injection of anti-galactocerebroside serum (16,17). Although CB can occur without segmental demyelination, in most conditions in which CB causes weakness, segmental demyelination will eventually occur (17). Exceptions to this would include the CB due to local anesthetics and acute motor axonal neuropathy (AMAN). AMAN is a form of Guillain–Barré Syndrome associated with IgG antibodies against certain gangliosides including GM1.

The demonstration of CB requires that the amplitude of the motor response on stimulation proximal to the lesion must be substantially less than the amplitude upon stimulation distal to the lesion (Fig. 10.1). The criterion for determining CB remains controversial. In case series of MMN, amplitude reductions ranging from 20% to 60% have been used as indicative of CB (18,19). The issue is that the amplitude reduction cannot be attributed to abnormal temporal dispersion and, in an attempt to exclude abnormal temporal dispersion, many investigators will assess the negative peak area for a confirmatory reduction. If the reduction in negative peak area on proximal stimulation compared with distal stimulation is less than the degree of reduction in amplitude, this would imply that at least some of the amplitude reduction is due to abnormal temporal dispersion (Fig. 10.2), resulting in phase cancellation that reduces the amplitude on prox-imal stimulation (20). Although it is theoretically possible for amplitude reductions as small as 20% to be due to CB, in reality there are too many other causes of reduced amplitude to utilize this value for long nerve segments. The degree of amplitude reduction and temporal dispersion that occurs depends on the length of nerve studied. A 20% drop in amplitude is likely due to CB if the length of nerve between stimulating sites is short (<10 cm) but may be normal if the length of nerve is long (>20 cm). For instance, the long length of the tibial nerve between the ankle and the popliteal fossa may result in a normal amplitude reductions of 20–30% on proximal stimulation. The electrodiagnostic examination must take this and other technical factors into account before deciding that pathophysiologic CB is present. Most authors recommend criteria of ~50% reduction in both amplitude and area to determine CB with <20% increase in duration (21).

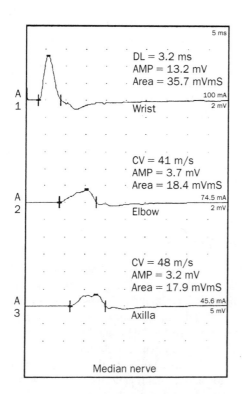

Figure 10.1 Motor CB. DL, distal latency; AMP, amplitude; CV, conduction velocity. The duration of the response on elbow stimulation is increased by 50% when compared with wrist stimulation suggesting that there is some temporal dispersion but the amplitude and area decrease cannot be accounted for by temporal dispersion.

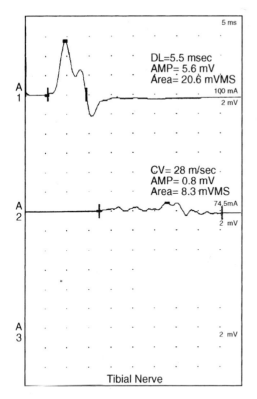

Figure 10.2 Temporal dispersion. The dispersion on proximal stimulation is 300%. The area is also reduced but CB, if present, is not the predominant pathophysiologic process. Abbreviations as in Fig. 10.1.

Consensus criteria have been established which attempt to be more specific for different nerves (22).

Although CB is the defining electrophysiologic feature of MMN, other electrodiagnostic features of segmental demyelination have been noted (11,21,23–25). These include prolonged distal motor latencies, prolonged F-wave latencies, multifocal slow motor conduction velocities, and abnormal temporal dispersion. In most instances, CB is detected in at least one nerve, along with the other features of demyelination that may be observed in nerves without CB.

Whether the diagnosis of MMN can be made without evidence of CB remains controversial. The inability to detect CB may be due to difficulties stimulating above and below very proximal or very distal lesions, or may be due to secondary Wallerian degeneration masking the primary CB lesion. It is reasonable to strongly consider MMN in patients with an appropriate clinical picture and electrodiagnostic evidence of segmental demyelination but without CB. However, response to treatment does not appear to be as good in these patients as with those with CB (26–28). The consensus criteria for the diagnosis of MMN require at least one nerve with CB for definite or probable MMN (29).

Sensory conduction studies are normal in MMN. Those investigators that have attempted to look for sensory conduction changes in the regions of motor block have been unable to detect any abnormality utilizing sensory conduction, compound nerve action potentials, and somatosensory evoked responses (2,13,21,30).

2.4. Laboratory Features

The CSF protein is normal or mildly elevated (4), reflecting the minimal involvement of nerve roots. There are no other significant abnormalities on routine spinal fluid or serum testing.

The most significant, albeit controversial, laboratory finding in MMN is elevated titers of antibody against GM1 ganglioside. GM1 is one of a number of gangliosides that are constituents of cell membranes and have been implicated in neuroimmunologic disorders. GM1, GD1a, GD1b, GT1a, and GT1b constitute >80% of the total gangliosides in most mammalian brains (31), and GM1 is the most abundant ganglioside in human CNS myelin (32). The GM1 epitope is present in motor neurons and their axons and to a lesser extent in dorsal root ganglion cells and sensory axons (33), but there may be differences in the ceramide composition of GM1 in motor and sensory axons (34). Although the total amount of GM1 in peripheral nerve is minimal when compared with other constituents, it is a major peripheral nerve antigen at nodes of Ranvier and on the axolemma (35). The mechanism by which anti-GM1 antibodies might cause conduction block remains unclear. The possibility that the antibodies cause blockade of sodium channels (36,37) has been challenged (33), and an alternate explanation of nerve fiber membrane hyper-polarization mediated by potassium channels has been suggested as a mechanism of increasing nodal threshold to the point of producing CB.

The incidence of anti-GM1 antibodies in MMN varies from 20% to 80% (38). The discrepancy is attributed to multiple factors. It is unclear how high titers must be in order to be considered significant, but the specificity increases if only very high titers are considered significant. Analytic techniques vary among laboratories, and not all laboratories use the same disease controls, making it difficult to compare the results. Pestronk and Choksi (38) report 85% of patients with MMN have elevated titers to GM1 combined with other lipids including galactocerebroside and cholesterol, whereas no patient with ALS had elevated titers. This combination appears to increase sensitivity and maintain specificity of antibody testing. However, Carpo et al. (39), utilizing what they understood to be the same technique, noted elevated titers in only 35% of patients with MMN, which was only an increase from 31% utilizing standard ELISA technique. Thus, the sensitivity of IgM anti-GM1 antibodies remains variable among patients, and possibly dependent upon laboratory techniques. Specificity has also been variable, but most recent studies have found high titers primarily in MMN and rarely in ALS, CIDP, or other neurologic disorders. In a meta-analysis, van Schaik et al. (40) noted that different methodologies, particularly the use of detergent and the duration and temperature of incubation, significantly affect results. ELISA methods utilizing no detergent and longer incubation periods resulted in a specificity of 90% and sensitivity of 38% in a comparison of MMN with other lower motor neuron disorders. The probability of having MMN was between 50% and 85% if titers were highly raised and considered to be clinically significant.

Although there is evidence that anti-GM1 antibodies have the potential for causing CB and demyelination (41), there is still no clear evidence that the antibodies are the specific cause of MMN. Thus, the current state of knowledge points to a correlation between high titer anti-GM1 antibodies and MMN. High titers are rarely seen in ALS or other neurologic disorders. However, the specificity and sensitivity of high titers is probably not strong enough to make detection of high titer antibodies in and of themselves diagnostic. At best, they may be confirmatory of the diagnosis of MMN when the clinical and electrophysiologic findings are unclear. High titer antibodies in patients with other diagnoses might encourage re-evaluation consideration of MMN. On occasion, the detection of high titer antibody may suggest an empiric trial of immunotherapy in a patient with an otherwise untreatable condition. It may be very difficult for a treating physician not to consider IVIg in a patient with possible or probable ALS but who also has high titers of anti-GM1 antibodies. Van den Berg et al. (26) treated five patients with lower motor neuron disorders (LMND) who had high titers of anti-GM1 antibodies but who did not have CB. Only one patient responded to IVIg, but the benefit did not persist despite chronic treatment. The conclusion was that the presence of high titers of anti-GM1 antibodies did not identify a subgroup of patients with lower motor neuron syndromes, but atypical of MMN, who respond to IVIg. Similarly, Azulay et al. (27) in a placebo-controlled, cross-over trial in 12 patients with LMND and high titers of anti-GM1 antibodies showed that only the five patients with CB responded. Tsai et al. (28) reported that 12 patients with LMND and elevated anti-GM1 antibody titers without CB did not improve clinically with intravenous cyclophosphamide despite reductions in antibody titers. Pestronk et al. (42), on the other hand, noted improvement in four patients with LMND and high titer anti-GM1 antibodies without CB when plasmapheresis and cyclophosphamide were combined. Although it is enticing to consider immunomodulating or immunosuppressant treatment in atypical cases of LMND, the experience to date is not supportive.

It would appear that the routine use of anti-GM1 antibodies as a diagnostic tool has limited utility. In those patients who have the typical clinical presentation and electrophysiologic abnormalities, the presence or absence of anti-GM1 antibodies does not add to diagnostic specificity, nor does it help predict who will respond to therapy. The one situation in which it might be helpful, and this requires further study, is when one encounters a patient with a lower motor neuron syndrome but without CB. In this rare clinical situation, the presence of IgM anti-GM1 antibodies may suggest that the patient has MMN and might respond to therapy.

In summary, the diagnosis of MMN depends on the combination of clinical findings including weakness without sensory loss or UMN signs and electrodiagnostic abnormalities of motor CB but normal sensory conduction studies. Currently, there is no role for the use of antibody testing as part of the diagnostic criteria for MMN (29).

2.5. Treatment

2.5.1. *Intravenous Immunoglobulin*

IVIg has been reported to be effective in uncontrolled studies and its efficacy has been confirmed in randomized, double-blind, placebo-controlled trials (27,45–47). More than 50% of patients show improvement after the initial treatment of 2 g/kg, usually administered in divided doses over 2–5 days (10). However, <10% maintain benefit over a year after one treatment, and the majority of patients require intermittent dosing to sustain functional recovery (43,48–50). Patients with definite or probable CB who have disease of shorter duration and less axonal degeneration are more likely to respond to IVIg (51–53). There is no consensus on whether the presence of anti-GM1 antibodies predicts response to treatment.

The dosage and interval between treatments varies from a low dose given weekly to a high dose given every 4 weeks. The treatment must be individualized and the dosing titrated slowly to determine the lowest possible dose at the longest interval that maximizes function. This approach minimizes the cost and inconvenience to the patient without compromising the clinical status of the patient.

The expectations of the physician and patient need to be realistic. A muscle with significant denervation on EMG pointing to secondary Wallerian degeneration will not improve quickly, and is less likely to have complete recovery. It is also known that demyelinating CB lesions may take over 4 weeks to recover (15,16). Therefore, lack of improvement after an initial treatment does not necessarily mean treatment failure. Most clinicians would treat for 2–3 months before considering alternative treatments. However, if a patient develops a new CB lesion during IVIg treatment, alternative therapies should be considered.

It may not be necessary to treat every patient with MMN. With greater recognition of this disorder, patients are being diagnosed earlier, and some may have very few lesions and minimal functional deficit. In addition, the disorder may be very slow and intermittent with long periods of inactivity. In these instances, it may be prudent to withhold treatment until active CB lesions develop or functional disability occurs.

It is important to monitor treatment carefully. Quantitative muscle testing and functional assessments may be helpful. Repeat electrodiagnostic studies frequently show at least partial reversal of the CB. There has been some discrepancy between clinical improvement and electrophysiologic improvement, although it is difficult to understand how strength could improve without the CB improving.

Unfortunately, not all patients benefit from IVIg and new regions of CB or progressive of axonal loss during treatment have been documented (43,54). Alternative treatments of documented benefit are relatively few. Both oral (4,48,49,55) and high dose intravenous (57) corticosteroid treatment have been remarkably ineffective. The few reports utilizing plasmapheresis without other medications have also not been encouraging (2).

Cyclophosphamide is the only immunosuppressive that has been reported to be effective (42,56,58,59). Although the drug is most commonly administered intravenously, there is no consensus on the optimal treatment program. Nobile-Orazio (59) used relatively low dose (1.5–3 mg/kg per day) oral cyclophosphamide in two patients and felt that the frequency of IVIg treatments could be reduced. Pestronk (58), in a review article without published data, recommends six treatments in a monthly basis at 1 g/m^2 preceded by two plasma exchanges. In his experience, this reduces the serum anti-GM1 titer in 60–80% of patients with functional benefit in some of these. Pestronk states that the remission can last for 1–3 years but relapse frequently occurs and retreatment may be necessary. The risks of cyclophosphamide include bone marrow suppression, opportunistic infection, and an increased frequency of neoplasias. It is important to determine whether possible benefits warrant the risks of cyclophosphamide treatment.

There has been recent interest in rituximab, a monoclonal antibody directed against the CD20 epitope on the surface of B-cells. Treatment reduces peripheral B lymphocyte counts by >90% within 3 days of administration. It has therefore been considered for neuropathies associated with IgM monoclonal gammopathies, including MMN. Several reports have been encouraging in IgM related neuropathies (60,61) as well as in MMN (62). In MMN, antibody titers are reduced significantly associated with clinical improvement, but improvement has been delayed by as much as 1 year and the improvement in strength was modest.

3. MULTIFOCAL SENSORIMOTOR DEMYELINATING NEUROPATHY: LEWIS–SUMNER SYNDROME

In 1982, Lewis et al. (1) reported five patients who had a sensorimotor mononeuropathy multiplex. All had symptoms that included pain and numbness as well as weakness in multiple nerve distributions. Motor neuron disease was not considered in the differential diagnosis. Two patients had episodes of optic neuritis with central scotomas, afferent pupillary defects, and prolonged visual evoked responses. CSF protein was normal or mildly increased. Sural nerve biopsy revealed segmental demyelination and a small amount of inflammatory cell infiltrate. Two patients treated with corticosteroids improved. The unique finding in these patients, which distinguished them from patients with vasculitic mononeuritis multiplex, was the presence of CB, which in some cases was demonstrated to persist for many years.

Prior to 1995, the disorder, which has been frequently called the LSS was mostly either ignored or lumped with MMN. However, recent series of patients with sensorimotor symptoms (4,5,63,68), consistent with the original LSS patients, suggest differences between patients with pure motor symptoms and those with sensory and motor symptoms (Table 10.3).

3.1. Clinical Description

The report of Viala et al. (68) summarize the clinical aspects of LSS. It can present at any age (mean age 40–50 years) and is more common in men than women (M/F = 2.8:1). Initial symptoms are sensorimotor in the majority and purely sensory in one-thirds. The upper extremities are more commonly involved first but lower limb onset can occur. Cranial nerve involvement is noted in >25% and optic neuritis has been seen in a few patients. Pain may be significant, and Tinel's sign may be present at the site of the CB. Significant sensory findings are noted, typically in the distribution of specific nerves. Reduction in deep tendon reflexes can be in a multifocal pattern consistent with the clinical symptoms but can occasionally be generalized.

CSF protein levels are elevated in many, but the elevation is usually mild to moderate, rarely >100 mg%. No specific laboratory abnormalities are noted and there are no reported cases of high anti-GM1 antibodies titers.

The disorder can evolve in different patterns over time, including a relapsing–remitting pattern in one-thirds, but a progressive course is seen in the majority. Progression can remain asymmetrical and multifocal, but some will develop a more generalized and symmetric disorder. Spontaneous remission has been noted. However, the majority progress to have new symptoms and require treatment.

3.2. Electrophysiologic Findings

Similar to MMN, the hallmark of LSS is CB, which is more common in the upper extremities and may only be seen in proximal segments. This emphasizes the importance of stimulating at very proximal sites. Conduction slowing, prolonged distal motor latencies, and abnormal F-wave latencies are typically recorded in nerves with CB, but are noted in only a minority of nerves in regions unaffected by CB. Thus, the electrophysiology

Table 10.3 Differences Between MMN and LSS

	MMN	LSS
Sensory symptoms	No	Yes
Pain and Tinel's	No	Yes
Sensory conduction	Normal	Abnormal
Anti-GM1 Abs	High titers in 35–80%	Normal in all patients
CSF protein	Minimal increase	Mild to moderate increase
Prednisone	Poor response	Good response in some

is strikingly multifocal, consistent with the clinical symptoms and signs. Distal sensory amplitudes are reduced in >85%, and if proximal stimulation is performed in nerves with sensory symptoms and motor CB, abnormalities of sensory conduction are usually detected.

3.3. Treatment Response

It appears that 50% of patients have a good response to IVIg (68). However, most require repeated monthly infusions. Prednisone as primary and initial therapy has been associated with remission and improvement. In a small patient series, when prednisone was added to IVIg, IVIg could be discontinued in 33–79% of patients (4,63,68). Plasmapheresis, azathioprine, and cyclophosphamide have all been reported to be beneficial in individual patients.

4. COMPARISON OF MMN AND LSS

Both MMN and LSS are multifocal disorders with CB as the hallmark physiologic finding. Both have a male predominance. However, pain, paresthesias, and Tinel's signs are only seen in patients with sensory symptoms. Sural nerve biopsies of patients with LSS reveal significantly more abnormalities consistent with demyelinating pathology than do biopsies of patients with MMN (4,63,64). High titers of GM1 antibodies have not been reported in LSS although Oh et al. (63) noted one patient out of 16 with mildly elevated titers. CSF protein, while not markedly elevated, tends to be higher in LSS than in MMN, suggesting that nerve roots may be more involved in LSS.

A significant number of patients with LSS respond to corticosteroids whereas patients with MMN either have no response or have accelerated progression (55,57,59). Most cases of MMN that responded to corticosteroids had, at closer view, sensory signs or symptoms, and more likely had LSS (65,66).

The findings on motor conduction studies in LSS are indistinguishable from those found in MMN. However, sensory abnormalities are usually seen, particularly if proximal stimulation is utilized. In contrast to MMN, in which multiple reports have shown normal sensory conduction through areas of motor block, there is now at least one case of LSS demonstrating sensory CB that improved with treatment (67).

There does appear to be a "gray zone" in which occasional patients cannot easily be labeled as MMN or LSS. A few patients who presented with a pure motor syndrome go on to develop sensory symptoms years later. It is also apparent that some patients have few sensory symptoms or minor changes on sensory conduction studies, and it becomes difficult to decide whether these changes are significant enough to warrant a diagnosis of LSS. These are reasons why some investigators suggest "lumping" MMN and MSMDN together as a single entity. Although it will be necessary to identify more patients with MMN and LSS before it can determined if the clinical and electrodiagnostic distinctions are significant, for now it appears prudent to separate the two disorders. First, lumping confuses the issue of GM1 antibodies. The true incidence of these antibodies in MMN will not be known if patients with LSS are included. Second and most important, there appears to be a real difference in response to corticosteroid therapy between the two entities. The potential benefits of long-term prednisone in LSS may outweigh the risks. However, there is currently no evidence in MMN for the use of corticosteroids, and some believe that they are contra-indicated.

Many authors suggest that LSS is a form of CIDP (1,4,63,68), and the response to treatment is similar to that of CIDP, but some favor considering it separately from CIDP. One could make a similar argument about MMN as well. It is increasingly clear that CIDP is not a single disorder, but like its cousin, Guillain–Barrè Syndrome, CIDP should also be considered a syndrome, with subgroups including MMN, LSS, POEMS, the neuropathies associated with monoclonal gammopathies with or without specific antibodies, and sensory predominant CIDP. Clinical recognition of these different disorders will hopefully provide clues that will unravel the immunopathologic causes of these disorders.

REFERENCES

1. Lewis RA, Sumner AJ, Brown MJ, Asbury AK. Multifocal demyelinating neuropathy with persistent conduction block. Neurology 1982; 32:958–962.
2. Parry GJ, Clarke S. Multifocal acquired demyelinating neuropathy masquerading as motor neuron disease. Muscle Nerve 1988; 11:103–107.
3. Pestronk A, Cornblath DR, Ilyas AA, Baba H et al. A treatable multifocal neuropathy with antibodies to GM1 ganglioside. Ann Neurol 1988; 24:73–78.
4. Saperstein DS, Amato AA, Wolfe GI, Katz JS, Nations SP, Jackson CE, Bryan WW, Burns DK, Barohn RJ. Multifocal acquired demyelinating sensory and motor neuropathy: the Lewis–Sumner Syndrome. Muscle Nerve 1999; 22:560–566.
5. Van den Berg-Vos RM, Van den berg LH, Franssen H, Vermeulen M, Witkamp TD, Jansen GH, Van Es HW, Kerkhoff H, Wokke JH. Multifocal inflammatory demyelinating neuropathy: a distinct clinical entity? Neurology 2000; 54:26–32.
6. Chad DA, Hammer K, Sargent J. Slow resolution of multifocal weakness and fasciculation: a reversible motor neuron syndrome. Neurology 1982; 32:958–964.
7. Engel WK, Hopkins LC, Rosenberg BJ. Fasciculating progressive muscular atrophy (F-PMA) remarkably responsive to antidysimmune treatment (ADIT)—a possible clue to more ordinary ALS? Neurology 1985; 335(suppl 1b):72.
8. Freddo L, Yu RK, Latov N, Donofrio PD, Hays AP, Greenberg HS, Albers JW, Allessi AG, Keren D. Gangliosides GM1 and GD1b are antigens for IgM M-protein in a patient with motor neuron disease. Neurology 1986; 36:454–458.
9. Roth G, Rohr J, Magistris MR, Oschner F. Motor neuropathy with proximal multifocal persistent block, fasciculations and myokymia. Evolution to tetraplegia. Eur Neurol 1986; 25:416–423.
10. Bouche P, Moulonguet A, Ben Younes-Chennnoufi A, Adams D, Baumann N, Meninger V, Lèger J-M, Said G. Multifocal motor neuropathy with conduction block: a study of 24 patients. J Neurol Neurosurg Psych 1995; 59:38–44.
11. Comi G, Amadio S, Galardi G, Fazio R, Nemni R. Clinical and neurophysiological assessment of immunoglobulin therapy in five patients with multifocal motor neuropathy. J Neurol Neurosurg Psych 1994; 57(suppl):35–37.
12. Leger J-M, Younes-Chennoufi AB, Chassande B, Davila G, Bouche P, Baumannn N, Brunet P. Human immunoglobulin treatment of multifocal motor neuropathy and polyneuropathy associated with monoclonal gammopathy. J Neurol Neurosurg Psych 1994; 57(suppl):46–49.
13. Kaji R, Shibasaki H, Kimura J. Multifocal demyelinating motor neuropathy: cranial nerve involvement and immunoglobulin therapy. Neurology 1992; 42:506–509.
14. Lange DJ, Trojaberg W, Latov N, Hays AP et al. Multifocal motor neuropathy with conduction block: is it a distinct clinical entity? Neurology 1992; 42:497–505.
15. Rudge P, Ochoa J, Gilliatt RW. Acute peripheral nerve compression in the baboon. J Neurol Sci 1974; 23:403–420.
16. Saida K, Sumner AJ, Saida T, Brown MJ, Silberberg DH. Antiserum-mediated demyelination: relationship between remyelination and functional recovery. Ann Neurol 1980; 8:12–24.

17. LaFontaine S, Rasminsky M, Saida T, Sumner AJ. Conduction block in rat myelinated fibres following acute exposure to anti-galactocerebroside serum. J Physiol 1982; 323:287–306.

18. Brown WF, Feasby TE. Conduction block and denervation in Guillain–Barre polyneuropathy. Brain 1984; 107:219–239.

19. Oh SJ, Kim DE, Kuruguolu HR. What is the best diagnostic index of conduction block and temporal dispersion? Muscle Nerve 1994; 17:489–493.

20. Rhee RK, England JD, Sumner AJ. Computer simulation of conduction block: effects produced by actual block verse interphase cancellation. Ann Neurol 1990; 28:146–159.

21. Chaudhry V, Cornblath DR, Griffin JW, Corse AM, Kuncl RW, Freimer ML, Griffin JW. Multifocal motor neuropathy: electrodiagnostic features. Muscle Nerve 1994; 17:198–205.

22. American Association of Electrodiagnostic Medicine. Consensus criteria for the diagnosis of partial conduction block. Muscle Nerve 1999; 22:S225–S229.

23. Katz JS, Wolfe GI, Bryan WW, Jackson CE, Amato AA, Barohn RJ. Electrophysiologic findings in multifocal motor neuropathy. Neurology 1997; 48:700–707.

24. Pakiam AS, Parry GJ. Multifocal motor neuropathy without overt conduction block. Muscle Nerve 1998; 21:243–245.

25. Weimer LH, Grewal RP, Lange DJ. Electrophysiologic abnormalities other than conduction block in multifocal motor neuropathy. Muscle Nerve 1994; 9:A1089.

26. Van den Berg LH, Franssen H, Van Doorn PA, Wokke JH. Intravenous immunoglobulin treatment in lower motor neuron disease associated with highly raised anti-GM1 antibodies. J Neurol Neurosurg Psych 1997; 63:674–677.

27. Azulay JP, Blin O, Pouget J, Boucrat J, Bille-Turc F, Carles G, Serratrice G. Intravenous immunoglobulin treatment in patients with motor neuron syndromes associated with anti-GM1 antibodies: a double-blind, placebo controlled study. Neurology 1994; 44:429–432.

28. Tsai CP, Lin KP, Liao KK, Wang SJ, Wang V, Kao KP, Wu ZA. Immunosuppressive treatment in lower motor neuron syndrome with autoantibodies against GM1. European Neurology 1993; 33:446–449.

29. Olney RK, Lewis RA, Putnam TD, Campellone JV Jr. Consensus criteria for the diagnosis of multifocal motor neuropathy. Muscle Nerve 2003; 27:117–121.

30. Kaji R, Oka N, Tsuji T, Mezaki T, Nishio T, Akiguchi I, Kimura J. Pathological findings at the site of conduction block in multifocal motor neuropathy. Ann Neurol 1993; 33:152–158.

31. Rapport MM, Donnenfield H, Brunner W, Hungund B, Bartfield H. Ganglioside patterns in amyotrophic lateral sclerosis brain regions. Ann Neurol 1985; 18:60–67.

32. Ledeen R. Gangliosides of the neuron. Trends Neurosci 1985; 8:12–24.

33. Kaji R, Kimura J. Facts and fallacies on anti-GM1 antibodies: physiology of motor neuropathies. Brain 1999; 122:797–798.

34. Ogawa-Goto K, Funamoto N, Abe T et al. Different ceramide compositions of gangliosides between human motor and sensory nerves. J Neurochem 1990; 55:1486–1493.

35. Sheikh KA, Deerinck TJ, Ellisman MH, Griffin JW. The distribution of ganglioside-like moieties in peripheral nerves. Brain 1999; 122:449–460.

36. Takigawa T, Yasuda H, Kikkawa R, Shigeta Y, Saida T, Kitasato H. Antibodies against GM1 ganglioside affect K^+ and Na^+ currents in isolated rat myelinated nerve fibers. Ann Neurol 1995; 37:436–442.

37. Waxman SG. Sodium channel blockade by antibodies: a new mechanism of neurological disease? Ann Neurol 1995; 37:421–423.

38. Pestronk A, Choksi R. Multifocal motor neuropathy. Serum IgM anti-GM1 ganglioside antibodies in most patients detected using covalent linkage of GM1 to ELISA plates. Neurology 1997; 49:1289–1292.

39. Carpo M, Allaria S, Scarlato G, Nobile-Orazio E. Anti-GM1 IgM antibodies in multifocal motor neuropathy: slightly improved detection with covalink ELISA technique. Neurology 1999; 53:2206–2207.

40. van Schaik IN, Bossuyt PM, Brand A, Vermeulen M. Diagnostic value of GM1 antibodies in motor neuron disorders and neuropathies: a meta-analysis. Neurology 1995; 45:1570–1577.

41. Santoro M, Uncini A, Corbo M, Staugaitis SM, Thomas FP, Hays AP, Latov N. Experimental conduction block induced by serum from a patient with anti-GM1 antibodies. Ann Neurol 1992; 31:385–390.

42. Pestronk A, Lopate G, Kornberg AJ, Elliott JL, Blume G, Yee WC, Goodnough LT. Distal lower motor neuron syndrome with high-titer serum IgM anti-GM1 antibodies: improvement following immunotherapy with monthly plasma exchange and intravenous cyclophosphamide. Neurology 1994; 44:2027–2031.

43. Van den Berg LH, Franssen H, Wokke JHJ. The long term effect of intravenous immuno-globulin treatment in multifocal motor neuropathy. Brain 1998; 121:421–428.

44. Van den Berg LH, Franssen H, Wokke JHJ. Improvement of multifocal motor neuropathy during long-term weekly treatment with human immunoglobulin. Neurology 1995; 45:987–988.

45. Van den Berg LH, Kerkhoff H, Oey PL, Franssen H, Mollee I, Vermeulen M, Jennekens FG, Wokke JH. Treatment of multifocal motor neuropathy with high dose intravenous immunoglo-bulin:a double blind, placebo controlled study. J Neurol Neurosurg Psych 1995; 59:248–252.

46. Federico P, Zochodne DW, Hahn AF, Brown WF, Feasby TE. Multifocal motor neuropathy improved by IVIg. Randomized, double-blind, pacebo-controlled, study. Neurology 2000; 55:1257–1262.

47. Léger J-M, Chassande B, Musset L, Meininger V, Bouche P, Bauman N. Intravenous immu-noglobulin therapy in multifocal motor neuropathy: a double-blind placebo-controlled study. Brain 2001; 124:145–153.

48. Azulay J-Ph, Rihet P, Pouget J, Cador F, Blin O, Boucraut J, Serratrice G. Long term follow up of multifocal motor neuropathy with conduction block under treatment. J Neurol Neurosurg Psych 1997; 62:391–394.

49. Meucci N, Cappellari A, Barbieri S, Scarlato G, Nobile-Orazio E. Long term effect of intrave-nous immunoglobulins and oral cyclophosphamide in multifocal motor neruopathy. J Neurol Neurosurg Psych 1997; 63:765–769.

50. Van den Berg-Vos RM, Franssen H, Wokke JHJ, Van den Berg LH. Multifocal motor neuro-pathy: long-term clinical and elctrophysiological assessment of intravenous immunoglobulin maintenance treatment. Brain 2002; 125:1875–1886.

51. Nobile-Orazio E, Meucci N, Carpo M et al. Multifocal motor neuropathy: clinical and immunological features and response to IVIg in relation to the presence and degree of motor conduction block. J Neurol Neurosurg Psych 2002; 72:761–766.

52. Van den Bergh P, Franssen H, Wokke JHJ, Van Es HV, Van den Berg LH. Multifocal motor neuropathy: diagnostic criteria that predict the response to immunoglobulin. Neurology 2000; 48:919–926.

53. Van den Berg-Vos RM, Franssen H, Visser J et al. Disease severity in multifocal motor neuropathy and its association with the response to immunoglobulin treatment. J Neurol 2002; 249–336.

54. Elliott JL, Pestronk A. Progression of multifocal motor neuropathy during apparently success-ful treatment with human immunoglobulin. Neurology 1994; 44:967–968.

55. Donaghy M, Mills KR, Boniface SJ, Simmons J, Wright I, Gregson N, Jacobs J. Pure motor demyelinating neuropathy: deterioration after steroid treatment and improvement with intra-venous immunoglobulin. J Neurol Neurosurg Psych 1994; 57:778–783.

56. Feldman EL, Bromberg MB, Albers JW, Pestronk A. Immunosuppressive treatment in multi-focal motor neuropathy. Ann Neurol 1991; 30:397–401.

57. Van den Berg LH, Lokhorst H, Wokke JHJ. Pulsed high-dose dexamethasone is not effective in patients with multifocal motor neuropathy. Neurology 1997; 48:1135.

58. Pestronk A. Multifocal motor neuropathy: diagnosis and treatment. Neurology 1998; 51(suppl 5)S22–S24.

59. Nobile-Orazio E, Meucci N, Barbieri S, Carpo M, Scarlato G. High-dose intravenous immu-noglobulin therapy in multifocal motor neuropathy. Neurology 1993; 43:537–544.

60. Levine TD, Pestronk A. IgM antibody-related polyneuropathies: B-cell depletion using Rituximab. Neurology 1999; 52:1701–1704.

61. Renaud S, Gregor M, Fuhr P, Lorenz D, Deuschl G, Gratwohl A, Steck AJ. Rituximab in the treatment of polyneuropathy associated with anti-MAG antibodies. Muscle Nerve 2003; 27(5):611–615.

62. Pestronk A, Florence J, Miller T, Choksi R, Al-Lozi MT, Levine TD. Treatment of IgM antibody associated polyneuropathies using rituximab. J Neurol Neurosurg Psychiatry 2003; 74:485–489.

63. Oh SJ, Claussen GC, Kim DS. Motor and sensory demyelinating mononeuropathy multiplex (Multifocal motor and sensory demyelinating neuropathy): a separate entity or a variant of chronic inflammatory demyelinating polyneuropathy. J Periph Nervous System 1997; 2:362–369.

64. Corse AM, Chaudhry V, Crawford TO, Cornblath DR, Kuncl RW, Griffin JW. Sensory nerve pathology in multifocal motor neuropathy. Ann Neurol 1996; 39:319–325.

65. Parry GJ. Are multifocal motor neuropathy and Lewis–Sumner Syndrome distinct nosologic entities? Muscle Nerve 1999; 22:557–559.

66. Lewis RA. Multifocal motor neuropathy and Lewis–Sumner Syndrome: two distinct entitles. Muscle Nerve 1999; 22:1738–1739.

67. Nikhar NJ, Lewis RA. Multifocal sensorimotor demyelinating neuropathy with persistent conduction block is distinct from multifocal motor neuropathy. Neurology 1998; 50(suppl):A206.

68. Viala K, Renié L, Maisonobe T, Béhin A et al. Follow-up study and response to treatment in 23 patients with Lewis–Sumner Syndrome. Brain 2004; 127:2010–2017.

Neuropathies Associated with
Systemic Disease

11
Diabetic Neuropathy

A. Gordon Smith and J. Robinson Singleton
University of Utah, Salt Lake City, Utah, USA

ABSTRACT

Diabetic neuropathy is the most common neuropathy worldwide and is a leading cause of disability. A distal peripheral neuropathy eventually develops in approximately half of diabetic patients and patients with impaired glucose tolerance (prediabetes) may develop end-organ complications of diabetes, including neuropathy. Autonomic neuropathy is also common, resulting in gastroparesis, constipation, diarrhea, and erectile dysfunction, and may be associated with early mortality from cardiac involvement. The role of hyperglycemia is not fully understood, but involves a variety of metabolic consequences leading to direct injury to peripheral nerve and to microvascular endothelium resulting in nerve ischemia. The only effective approach is glycemic control. Other neuropathies occur, including lumbosacral radiculoplexopathies, diabetic truncal, and cranial neuropathies, which likely inflammatory etiology and a favorable prognosis.

1. INTRODUCTION

Diabetes is the most common cause of peripheral neuropathy in the world. In the United States, an estimated 17 million Americans have diabetes, but this is an underestimate as the disease is undiagnosed in approximately half (1). Overall, half of diabetics will develop a neuropathy (2,3). Viewed another way, population studies suggest that up to 7% of the population suffers from peripheral neuropathy and half have diabetes (4). The traditional view holds that neuropathy only develops after years of sustained hyperglycemia, but there is compelling evidence that neuropathy may occur early in the course of glucose dysregulation, including during the stage of impaired glucose tolerance (IGT) (prediabetes) (5–8). Neuropathy is a common cause of disability among diabetic patients because of pain, and a leading risk factor for foot ulceration and amputation.

1.1. Definition of Diabetes

Diabetes mellitus is a group of disorders characterized by high blood sugar (hyperglycemia) related to either a defect in the production of insulin or resistance to the action of insulin, and both often coexist. Hyperglycemia and hyperinsulinemia result in injury to large and small blood vessels, retina, kidney, and peripheral nerve.

In 1997, the American Diabetes Association (ADA) revised criteria for the diagnosis and classification of diabetes mellitus (Table 11.1) (1). Type 1 diabetes is related to destruction of pancreatic β cells, often via an autoimmune mechanism, resulting in insulin deficiency and hyperglycemia. Patients with type 1 diabetes require insulin therapy for survival. Type 2 diabetes is due to peripheral resistance to the action of insulin with resultant hyperinsulinemia and hyperglycemia, and is the most common form of diabetes. Type 2 diabetes is usually managed with diet and exercise therapy and oral hypoglycemic agents, but may eventually require insulin therapy. However,

Table 11.1   Revised Classification of Diabetes Mellitus

Type 1	Cell destruction (usually autoimmune)
Type 2	Insulin resistance
Type 3	Other types
	Genetic defects
	Pancreatic disease
	Drug induced
	Associated with other endocrine disease
Type 4	Gestational diabetes mellitus

the use of insulin does not imply type 1 diabetes. For this reason, the terms insulin dependent and noninsulin dependent diabetes are discouraged. Likewise, the term "adult onset" diabetes is inappropriate because of the growing epidemic of type 2 diabetes among the young obese. Type 3 diabetes is due to other less common mechanisms including genetic defects in β-cell function, drug toxicity, or other endocrinopathies. Gestational diabetes is classified as type 4.

The ADA defined diagnostic criteria for different stages of glucose dysregulation (Table 11.2) based on a standard 2-h oral glucose tolerance test (OGTT) consisting of plasma glucose determinations in the early morning fasting state and 2 h after an oral 75 g anhydrous dextrose load. The OGTT must be performed in the early morning, with the first blood drawn prior to 9 a.m. Impaired fasting glucose (IFG) and IGT represent intermediate levels of glucose dysregulation between the normal state and frank diabetes. IFG and IGT are associated with other features of insulin resistance including obesity, hyperlipidemia, and hypertension as well as an increased risk of large vessel atherosclerotic disease (9). Data suggest that IFG and IGT are also associated with microvascular injury and peripheral neuropathy, traditionally associated with frank diabetes (5–7).

The ADA endorses the use of fasting plasma glucose for screening asymptomatic individuals (1). For patients with peripheral neuropathy, however, the OGTT is preferred (Fig. 11.1) because fasting plasma glucose is often normal in neuropathy patients found to have IGT or diabetes after OGTT. Hemoglobin A1c (HbA1c) provides a valuable tool in estimating overall glucose control over a several month period, but is insensitive to IGT or early diabetes and is therefore a poor diagnostic test (5).

1.2. Spectrum of Diabetic Neuropathy

Neuropathic complications of diabetes may be classified into chronic and acute neuropathies (Table 11.3). The most common chronic neuropathies are distal symmetric polyneuropathy (DSP) and autonomic neuropathy. Acute neuropathies include diabetic lumbosacral radicloplexus neuropathy (DLRPN), truncal radiculopathy, acute painful sensory neuropathy (diabetic neuropathic cachexia (DNC), "insulin neuritis"), and cranial neuropathy. Compressive mononeuropathies are an additional group.

2. CHRONIC NEUROPATHIES

2.1. Distal Symmetric Polyneuropathy

Sensory or combined sensorimotor DSP is the most common form, although autonomic neuropathy is probably at least as common. The diagnosis of DSP requires the presence

Table 11.2 Revised Criteria for Interpretation of OGTT

Diagnosis	Fasting glucose (mg/dL)	2 h glucose (mg/dL)
Normal	<110	<140
IFG	110–125	<140
IGT	<126	140–199
Diabetes (may meet either fasting or 2 h criterion)	>125	>199

Note: Fasting early morning plasma glucose followed by 75 g oral anhydrous dextrose load and a repeat glucose measurement 2 h later.

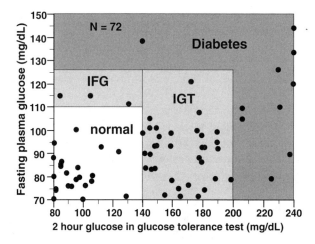

Figure 11.1 Oral glucose tolerance testing is more sensitive than either fasting plasma glucose or glycosylated hemoglobin in the diagnosis of IGT or diabetes. Patients with abnormal OGTT often have normal fasting glucose or glycosylated hemoglobing, while the converse is rare.

of symptoms of sensory loss, paresthesias or neuropathic pain, examination evidence of distal sensory loss, and electrodiagnostic confirmation of distal axonal injury. There is debate regarding how long diabetes must be present to assure that this is the cause. The presence of retinopathy or nephropathy in proportion to the neuropathy is a conservative requirement, which assures a high degree of specificity, but excludes most patients with neuropathy associated with early diabetes or prediabetic hyperglycemia (10).

There is evidence that peripheral nerve injury can occur early in diabetes, as a presenting symptom, and even during a prediabetic state (IGT) (11). Routine nerve conduction studies/electromyography (NCS/EMG) demonstrate diffuse peripheral axonal injury in 10–18% of patients at the time of their diabetes diagnosis (12,13). Further, patients with otherwise idiopathic neuropathy and normal fasting plasma glucose are significantly more likely than age-matched controls to have prolonged postprandial hyperglycemia (5), suggesting that IGT may result in nerve injury even before hyperglycemia crosses the threshold into diabetes.

A reasonable diagnosis of diabetic neuropathy may be made when there are typical symptoms of distal polyneuropathy supported by neurological exam, and electrodiagnostic or histologic data in the setting of diabetes of any duration. With these criteria, a cross-sectional survey of type 2 diabetic patients found 13% that had mild DSP and 1% a

Table 11.3 Spectrum of Diabetic Neuropathies

Chronic neuropathies
  DSP
  Autonomic neuropathy
Acute neuropathies
  DLRPN
  Truncal radiculopathy
  Cranial neuropathy (e.g., Diabetic 3rd nerve palsy)
  DNC
  Insulin neuritis
Compression mononeuropathies

more severe neuropathy (3). A prospective, longitudinal study found 8% that had DSP by clinical examination at the time of diabetes diagnosis, and >50% after 25 years of disease (2). These prevalence figures have been confirmed using a variety of clinical and electrophysiologic diagnostic criteria (14,15).

Patients with retinopathy or overt albuminuria are 2.5× as likely to have neuropathy, confirming the strong co-association of DSP with other complications thought due to microvascular ischemia. Other risk factors are advancing age, duration of known diabetes, poor glycemic control, and surrogates of insulin resistance, including insulin use, increased weight and hypertension, and all are associated with significantly increased risk for DSP. Race and gender are not predictive of DSP (13).

2.1.1. Clinical Features

The dominant symptoms of DSP are sensory, and patients typically describe the insidious onset of distal, symmetric sensory loss, often affecting both small fiber (pain and cold) and large fiber (vibration and joint position sense) sensory modalities. Sensory loss may go unrecognized until postural instability and falls or foot injuries occur. More commonly, patients describe positive symptoms of tingling, lancinating or burning paresthesias or frank pain in their feet or legs, often worse as the patient tries to fall asleep at night. Acute, severe painful neuropathy associated with rapid, profound weight loss may occur as the first sign of diabetes (16). Patients with established diabetes may experience acute worsening of pain with poor glycemic control, or conversely with rapid pharmacologic re-establishment of euglycemic state (insulin neuritis) (17).

These clinical findings suggest prominent early involvement of small unmyelinated nerve fibers. Experiments in animal models and humans indicate that transient hyperglycemia increases spontaneous discharge from small diameter nociceptive afferent C fibers, and is clinically associated with increased neuropathic pain (18,19). Cold sensation (mediated by small fibers) is frequently affected before vibration sense (mediated by large myelinated sensory fibers) in diabetic neuropathy, whereas the reverse scenario is rare, bolstering the concept that diabetic neuropathy disproportionately affects small, unmyelinated fibers early in its course (20). The positive sensory symptoms of pain and paresthesias often bring patients to medical attention before other signs of diabetic end organ injury (retinopathy, nephropathy, and cardiovascular complications) are apparent (21).

Distal lower extremity weakness is rare as a first complaint, and strength is usually normal or minimally affected, even after years of sensory symptoms. However, examination often demonstrates loss of foot intrinsic muscle bulk, and NCS/EMG frequently demonstrate a measure of motor involvement in patients who have no motor symptoms or signs (22). Ankle reflexes are typically diminished or absent. Robust reflexes in the face of diabetic neuropathy should suggest the possibility of a superimposed myelopathy. Erectile dysfunction caused by peripheral autonomic nerve injury occurs in 20–50% of diabetic men (23). Other autonomic complaints are less common (discussed succeedingly). This pattern of clinical involvement is supported by epidemiological studies (21).

2.1.2. Electrodiagnostic Features and Diagnostic Testing

Electrodiagnostic testing may not be necessary to establish a diagnosis of DSP. NCS typically show low amplitude sensory responses with prolonged distal latency. Compound muscle action potential (CMAP) amplitudes are initially normal, but decline with disease progression. Motor conduction velocities are mildly slowed and F-responses are prolonged early in the disease course, suggesting a mild degree of demyelination.

Motor conduction slowing is typical of DSP and represents an important diagnostic clue. However, prior to demyelination out of proportion to axonal loss is rare and should suggest a superimposed inflammatory neuropathy.

EMG in distal muscles may show abnormal spontaneous activity, decreased motor unit recruitment, and increased motor unit amplitude indicating axonal loss with compensatory partial re-innervation.

Small fiber injury leading to prominent neuropathic pain and autonomic dysfunction is often the principle manifestation of neuropathy, especially in IGT or early diabetes. In this setting, NCS/EMG are often normal, but neuropathy can be confirmed by several other methods. Quantitative sensory testing (QST) for cold detection threshold reproducibly measures small fiber function (large fiber function by measuring vibratory perception thresholds). QST is abnormal in 57–72% of patients with small fiber neuropathy (24,25). However, QST is nonspecific in that other causes of sensory loss, including conversion disorder or deliberate deception may result in increased perception thresholds (26). Quantitative sudomotor axon reflex testing (QSART), or demonstration of small diameter, unmyelinated nerve fiber loss by skin biopsy provide more sensitive and specific measures of small fiber function (27).

2.1.3. Pathology

Nerve pathology in moderate diabetic neuropathy typically reflects the combination of axonal injury and segmental demyelination suggested by electrodiagnostic testing. Sural nerve biopsy shows atrophy of nerve fascicles with loss of both myelinated and small unmyelinated axons (28). Wallerian degeneration with formation of digestion chambers is common. Collections of monocytes and macrophages indicate remodeling, but there is rarely evidence of primary inflammatory or autoimmune injury. Relative sparing of individual fascicles suggests an ischemic component to the fascicular injury in some cases. Microvascular injury as a primary pathological mechanism is reinforced by findings of endothelial cell hyperplasia, capillary closure, endothelial and pericyte degeneration, thrombosis, and basement membrane thickening (29,30).

Pathologic and electrodiagnostic evidence of associated demyelination sets diabetic neuropathy apart from other common metabolic neuropathies. The presence of axons with inappropriately thin myelin for axonal diameter and paranodal and segmental internodal demyelination are both common, and onion bulb formation suggest repeated demyelination and demyelination. However, axonal degeneration and regeneration are more common than segmental demyelination and remyelination (28). Overall, the pathologic data support primary axonal injury.

Nerve biopsies are not necessary to diagnose diabetic distal polyneuropathy. In patients with painful neuropathy and normal electrodiagnostic testing, skin biopsy is more sensitive than sural nerve biopsy and less invasive (31).

2.2. Autonomic Neuropathy

Autonomic nerve involvement is common in diabetes, although prevalence figures of diabetic autonomic neuropathy (DAN) depend upon how it is defined. Overt clinical autonomic failure, characterized by variable combination of anhidrosis, gustatory sweating, orthostatic hypotension, supine blood pressure instability, gastroparesis or diarrhea, bladder paresis, and cardiac dysrythmias, develops in <5% of patients with diabetes, typically with prolonged disease (32). However, erectile dysfunction, as well as more subtle evidence for cardiac dysautonomia, gastroparesis, and dysregulation of hormonal response to hypoglycemia, is much more common (33).

Impotence is reported by 20–60% of diabetic men, making it among the most prevalent complications of mild to moderate diabetes (23). Previously undiagnosed diabetes is found in ~10% of patients referred for evaluation of impotence (34–36). Other factors contribute, including microangiopathy and psychiatric disease (37–39). Retrograde ejaculation occurs in up to 40% of men with diabetes as a consequence of autonomic denervation (23). Erectile dysfunction has also been associated with a greater risk for myocardial infarct and peripheral vascular disease.

Heart rate variability with respiration is a sensitive measure of parasympathetic function. Reduced heart rate during deep breathing (HRdb) correlates with development of diabetic peripheral neuropathy and typically precedes the appearance of other autonomic symptoms (40). Depressed HRdb variability is found in 13% of asymptomatic diabetic patients, 50% with clinically recognizable neuropathy, and in every diabetic patient with overt autonomic symptoms (15).

Altered HRdb is associated with a 2.14 fold risk of all causes of mortality (33). Coronary artery disease accounts for 60% of mortality among diabetic patients (41), attributed to accelerated atherosclerosis, hypertension and cardiomyopathy, and autonomic (parasympathetic) denervation predisposing to lethal arrhythmias (42–45).

Gastrointestinal manifestations of autonomic neuropathy include esophageal enteropathy due to lower esophageal sphincter dysfunction, disordered peristalsis leading to gastroparesis or constipation, diarrhea, fecal incontinence, and gallbladder atony and enlargement (33). Vagus nerve dysfunction contributes to both esophageal atony and gastroparesis, causing complaints of early satiety, nausea, vomiting, and epigastric bloating, often in cycles. Diarrhea, often cycling with constipation, occurs in up to 20% of patients, and more frequently in patients with other DAN. Bowel stasis leads to poor motility and bacterial overgrowth, causing diarrhea. Poor sphincter tone can also contribute to diarrhea, or frank incontinence (46).

Blunting of autonomic responses and symptoms (sweating, nausea, and hunger) that accompany hypoglycemia is an important complication of diabetes. Up to one-quarter of patients with type 1 diabetes are unaware of hypoglycemic episodes (43). This autonomic injury may accelerate diabetes by blunting pancreatic α-cell secretion of glucagon in response to hypoglycemia (47–49).

2.2.1. *Pathogenesis of Diabetic Polyneuropathy*

The pathogenesis of diabetic neuropathy has not been fully elucidated, but an appreciation of important mechanisms facilitates an understanding of potential therapies. The pathogenesis of DSP involves an interaction between metabolic and microvascular injury to nerve (50,51). Nerve injury, in some cases, may be accelerated by reactive autoimmune attack and exacerbated by failure of injured nerve axons to undergo efficient regeneration.

Vascular Endothelial Dysfunction and Ischemia. Vascular injury is a feature of all diabetic complications and plays a central role in the development and progression of neuropathy. Severity of neuropathy is correlated with the degree of endoneurial capillary occlusion (52–54), and with the degree of hypoxia within the nerve (55,56). Vascular injury affects vasoregulatory signaling in the endothelial lining of small and large blood vessels. Nerve ischemia occurs initially as a result of decreased capacity for vasodilation. With time, structural injury to microarterial vessels occurs and ultimately leads to permanent neurovascular ischemia. Vasodilatory agents, which have been shown to increase nerve conduction velocity, improve nerve blood flow and slow progression of clinical neuropathic symptoms (57–59).

Vasoregulation is controlled largely through nitric oxide (NO), which is a pivotal link between metabolic and ischemic nerve injury. NO is synthesized by nitric oxide synthase in vascular endothelial cells in response to insulin and other stimuli, and has a half-life of 3–20 s (60,61). Local NO leads to vasodilitation, but also serves to detoxify reactive oxygen species (ROS) that contribute to tissue injury. In situations of excess ROS, less NO is available for vasodilation.

Hyperglycemia depletes NO through several pathways, as outlined in Fig. 11.2. (i) Hyperglycemia leads to activation of the enzyme aldose reductase, which converts excess glucose to sorbitol and fructose (the polyol pathway) (62). Polyol reactions deplete NADPH, which is an obligate cofactor for synthesis of glutathione and NO, resulting in lowered NO. (ii) Excess glucose, and especially sorbitol and fructose, react nonenzymatically with proteins, lipids, and nucleic acids to produce advanced glycation endproducts (AGEs), which induce ROS generation (63). (iii) Endothelial ROS formation is also increased by peroxidation of the more abundant glucose and low density lipoproteins, and by dysregulation of transition metals that serve as catalysts for auto-oxidation (64). (iv) Finally, ischemia itself accelerates ROS formation by decreasing mitochondrial efficiency and by reperfusion injury. The end result is local endothelial damage by ROS and impaired vasodilation from depleted NO. Small arteries are more vulnerable and leading to tissue ischemia.

Endoneurial ischemia occurs by several mechanisms. (i) Vasodilatory signaling pathways, including prostacyclins and endothelium-derived hyperpolarizing factor, are

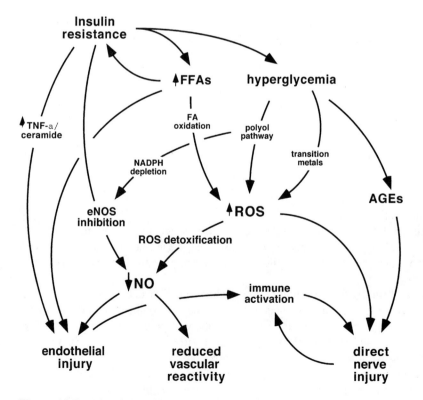

Figure 11.2 DSP nitric oxide pathophysiology.

inhibited (65,66). Increased production of prostanoid endothelium-derived constricting factors and angiotensin II promote vasoconstriction (64,67). (ii) Inapropriate arteriovenous shunting in epineurial arterioles, due to loss of autonomic fibers innervating them, diverts blood flow from endoneurial capillary beds (32,68,69). (iii) Direct occlusion of vessels due to thickening of endothelial basal lamina and fibrin and platelet deposition is a consequence of altered endothelial mitogenic signaling associated with insulin resistance (70,71).

Direct Metabolic Injury. Direct toxic and metabolic damage also has a role. Long axons may be particularly susceptible to direct metabolic consequences of hyperglycemia (72). Alternate processing of excess glucose down the hexosamine pathway serves as a signal to reduce cellular insulin sensitivity, thus reducing neuronal glucose uptake (73). Increased polyol production by overexpression of aldose reductase induces neuropathy in animal models (74), and aldose reductase inhibitor drugs, which reduce shunting of glucose into the polyol pathway, improve neuropathy in animals (75). AGEs are directly neurotoxic by promoting inappropriate covalent cross-links among proteins (62), which is accelerated in response to hyperglycemia and greater polyol pathway flux (63). AGEs cause neuronal-specific injury by inhibiting axonal transport (72,76,77). ROS damage proteins, and inhibit mitochondrial electron transport, and mitochondrial dysfunction may serve as a common final pathway for neuronal damage mediated by polyol, AGE, and hexosamine pathways (78). Mitochondrial dysfunction might account for persistent injury that occurs during periods of relative normoglycemia and contributes to genetic differences in susceptibility to hyperglycemic complications (78).

Nerve repair processes are inhibited in diabetes by a number of factors. Mitochondrial dysfunction decreases ATP generation and increases ROS. Slow and fast axonal transport is inhibited by inappropriate protein glycosylation and ROS damage. Vascular insufficiency limits distal axonal perfusion. Schwann cells in diabetic animal models are slow to synthesize trophic proteins and hormones that prevent neuronal cell death (79).

Growth Factor Depletion. Growth factors and neurotrophic factors act to promote neuronal development during embryogenesis, but also promote axonal sprouting and neuronal function in adults. Nerve growth factor (NGF) supports the growth of small unmyelinated nerve fibers, and is reduced in the serum of diabetic patients and in dorsal root ganglia of diabetic rats (80). NGF is transported in a retrograde direction to the cell body where it exerts its effect, and transport may be disrupted by AGE formation and other consequences of diabetes (63,81). Insulin-like growth factors (IGF-I) is also reduced in the serum of diabetic patients with neuropathy (82). Experimental depletion of IGF-I or blockade of its receptor-specific signaling results in apoptotic death or dorsal root ganglia neurons, and limits new axonal sprouting and Schwann cell repair following injury (83,84). Therapeutic trials of neurotrophic agents have been promising in animal models, but disappointing in humans (85,86).

Immune and Inflammatory Neuronal Injury. Some forms of diabetic neuropathy may include immune activation as a primary or accelerating factor. In type 1 diabetes, atrophy of cervical sympathetic ganglia, with infiltration by lymphocytes, plasma cells and macrophages, indicating vigorous immune response has been demonstrated (87). Circulating antibodies in sera react with sympathetic ganglia and vagus nerve. Autonomic nervous tissue and pancreatic islet cells share cell surface epitopes that could serve as common immune targets (87,88). By analogy, several "factors," thought to be autoantibodies, have been found in sera of patients with type 2 diabetes that are capable of killing neuronal cells in culture through apoptosis (89,90).

An autoimmune cause has been linked to diabetic lumbosacral radiculoplexus neuropathy. Patients with diabetes may also be more likely to develop chronic inflammatory demyelinating polyradiculoneuropathy (CIDP) (91).

2.2.2. Management

Currently, no medication or course of treatment has been shown to reverse neuropathy. Pancreas transplants in type I diabetes results only in stabilization of neuropathy with minimal improvement over many years despite a cure of diabetes (92). Management involves three principal aspects: (i) disease-modifying therapy with glucose control, (ii) surveillance and adaptive changes to prevent secondary tissue injury, and (iii) adequate treatment of neuropathic pain. Recognition of neuropathy as a complication of diabetes should also prompt screening for other micro- and macrovascular complications.

Control of Blood Glucose.   Aggressive control of blood glucose is central to treatment of diabetes and remains the only treatment shown to delay onset and slow progression neuropathy (93). The Diabetes Control and Complications Trial followed 1,441 insulin dependent type I diabetic patients prospectively for 3.5–9 years to assess the effect of intensive glucose control on the development of diabetic complications, including neuropathy. Those who received intensive insulin therapy and glucose monitoring aimed at achieving normoglycemia (with a sustained mean HbA1c of 7.2%) were one-third as likely to develop clinically confirmed neuropathy over a five-year follow-up when compared with diabetic patients receiving routine care (mean HbA1c 9.1%) (93–95).

There is no HbA1c threshold below which patients avoid risk for neuropathy (96), indicating glucose altering therapy should be undertaken in all patients with diabetic neuropathy. For patients with very early or mild diabetes, this treatment may take the form of individualized diet and exercise modification, similar to that used in the Diabetes Prevention Program (97).

Aldose Reductase Inhibitors and Other Rational Therapies.   Because even strict glucose control does not prevent neuropathy progression, there is a need for therapies which address the neuropathy. Agents tested in preclinical studies and human trials for diabetic neuropathy have been based on altering pathways leading to NO inhibition (51). Agents that have been tested and shown to slow or reverse nerve injury in animal models include aldose reductase inhibitors that reduce shunting of glucose into the polyol pathway (75), drugs that decrease ROS (αLipoic acid, glutathione, dimethylthiourea (51), and vitamin E), lipid lowering agents, and transition metal chelators (desferoxamine and αLipoic acid).

Unfortunately, none of these agents have been effective in human clinical trials. Although aldose reductase inhibitors improve nerve conduction velocity and the density of small diameter nerve fibers on sural nerve biopsy, and αLipoic acid improved in pain following short term intravenous administration, no agent has resulted in clinically meaningful improvement in neuropathy (98–101). Differences between animal and human trials may have been influenced by selection of subjects with relatively advanced neuropathy, or low sensitivity of endpoint measures (75,98,101).

Foot Care.   Foot ulcers occur in 15% of patients with diabetes and are responsible for 20% of hospitalizations among diabetic patients with an average cost of approximately $25,000 per episode (102,103). Peripheral neuropathy causes loss of protective sensation. Loss of the ability to detect pressure of a 10 g monofilament has been closely correlated with the degree of sensory loss necessary to permit painless foot injury (104). Intrinsic foot weakness and atrophy associated with moderate and advanced neuropathy alter the anatomy of the foot and potentiate friction injury. Autonomic injury reduces foot sweating and increases foot edema, increasing friction. Limited joint mobility and increased arch associated with foot weakness increase force transmission to the heel, and to a lesser degree, the ball of the foot. Small and large vessel stenosis and loss of vasodilatory regulation result in distal limb ischemia promoting tissue fragility and impairing wound healing (102).

Surveillance for foot skin breakdown requires daily visual inspection by the patient. Routine evaluation by health professionals (Fig. 11.3) significantly reduces the incidence of foot ulcers. The use of a 10 g monofilament greatly increases the sensitivity of this screening protocol, while the use of plantar foot pressure testing increases specificity (105).

Exercise is an important part of diabetes management. However, many patients have difficulty exercising due to exacerbation of foot pain. Aggressive pain management facilitates weight loss and glucose control. Patients may worry that physical stress on the feet will make their neuropathy worse, but need to be reassured that this will not happen, but that they attend to proper footwear and visual inspection. Appropriate footwear, including high-top shoes for improved ankle fixation, a custom orthotic insole, a rocker at the ball of the foot, and a well-cushioned heel should be considered. Properly fit footwear can reduce foot pain, prevent traumatic foot injury and encourage exercise (102). Patients with significant weakness, or with gait ataxia due to joint position sense loss should be encouraged to exercise in a setting position with a recumbent stationary bicycling or engage in water walking.

Treatment of Neuropathic Pain.   Neuropathic pain rarely responds to glycemic control alone, and the mainstays of therapy are anticonvulsant agents, tricyclic antidepressants, and opiates. Each of these classes of medications has drug interactions and side effects that may be more profound in the elderly. Most have been extensively evaluated in clinical patients with diabetes. Individual agents are discussed elsewhere in this volume.

2.2.3. Neuropathy Associated with Impaired Glucose Tolerance

Traditional view held that prolonged exposure to severe hyperglycemia is necessary for development of neuropathy (10). However, the concept that peripheral neuropathy may be the first clinical sign of prolonged hyperglycemia was proposed over 40 years ago (11). Routine NCS/EMG demonstrate diffuse peripheral nerve axonal injury in 10–18% of patients at the time of diabetes diagnosis (12,13), suggesting that nerve injury can predate development of other diabetic symptoms.

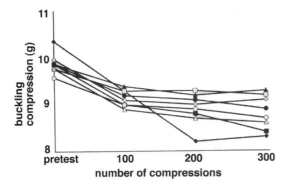

Figure 11.3   Prevention of diabetic foot ulcers should include an algorithmic approach to risk stratification. The reflex and sensory examination and 10 g monofilament testing are highly sensitive. When abnormalities are found, plantar foot pressure testing specifically identifies patients who should be referred for custom shoe and sock fitting.

The ADA recognizes IGT and IFG as part of the spectrum of hyperglycemia (Table 11.2). Accumulating evidence supports the concept of IGT as a disease entity in its own right (106). IGT is associated with the syndrome of insulin resistance, hyper-insulinemia, hyperlipidemia, and hypertension, and is a potent risk factor for cardio-vascular and peripheral vascular occlusive disease, independent of IGT risk for diabetes (107–109).

Recent studies show that axonal neuropathy may also be associated with IGT. Neuropathy is three times more frequent in patients with IGT than in age matched normal controls (14). Conversely, patients with otherwise idiopathic neuropathy are three times more likely to have IGT than are age matched controls (Fig. 11.4) (5–8). Neuropathy patients in whom IGT is discovered have a sensory or painful sensory neuropathy, similar to that seen in early diabetes.

Recent large prospective trials demonstrate that lifestyle modification programs aimed at reducing weight by 7% and increasing exercise to 150 min weekly are more effective than glucose lowering agents in preventing progression from IGT to diabetes (97,110). An ongoing 3-year prospective, longitudinal study in patients with IGT and neuropathy will more clearly test a causative association between IGT and neuropathy, suggesting mechanisms other than chronic hyperglycemia are important.

3. ACUTE NEUROPATHIES

3.1. Diabetic Lumbosacral Radiculoplexus Neuropathy

3.1.1. Historical Perspective and Nomenclature

Diabetes is associated with an acute neuropathy resulting in asymmetric lower extremity pain and weakness. A variety of descriptive terms and eponyms have been given (Table 11.4) (111,112), but only recently has the exact localization of the causative lesion and underlying pathophysiology been elucidated, supporting the preferred term diabetic lumbosacral radicoloplexus neuropathy (DLRPN). Early and accurate diagnosis of DLRPN may prevent unnecessary surgical procedures and facilitate early appropriate therapy. Patients are often initially misdiagnosed as having either lumbar spinal stenosis or other unusual compressive neuropathies (femoral and obturator).

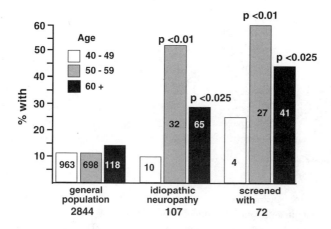

Figure 11.4 An IGT is significantly more common among neuropathy patients than in age matched normal subjects.

Table 11.4 Terms Used for the
Syndrome of DLRPN

Diabetic amyotrophy
Bruns garland syndrome
Diabetic lumbosacral radiculopathy
Diabetic plexopathy
Diabetic myelopathy
Proximal diabetic neuropathy
Ischemic mononeuritis multiplex
Femoral neuropathy
Femoral sciatic neuropathy
DLRPN

3.1.2. Clinical Features

DLRPN occurs most frequently in older patients with type 2 diabetes, although it may occur in type 1 diabetes. Although most patients have long established diabetes, DLRPN may be the first sign of diabetes (113). When compared with patients having DSP, those with DLRPN have better glycemic control, fewer other end-organ complications and a lower body mass index (114). This observation has important pathogenetic implications.

DLRPN most often presents with sudden-onset of asymmetric lower extremity pain typically involving the thigh more than the lower leg. Pain may be deep and aching or sharp and lancinating. The pain is soon followed by progressive weakness and atrophy of involved muscles, and is often associated with significant weight loss. Progression to the contralateral limb occurs in most patients, and many have associated truncal radiculopathies. Autonomic symptoms including sexual, bowel and bladder dysfunction, and orthostatic hypotension occur in half (114,115).

Upper extremities are clinically affected in ~10–15%, predominantly with distal numbness and weakness, although proximal involvement also occurs (114,116). Pain is frequent, although usually not the dominant symptom. Upper extremity involvement usually immediately follows lower extremity onset, but may occur weeks or months later. Regardless, the onset and electrophysiologic features are similar in upper and lower extremities suggesting axonal injury to roots and plexus. Patients who develop upper extremity symptoms are more likely to have associated truncal radiculopathies, an observation that links these findings to classical DLRPN (116).

The natural history of DLRPN is progression over several months, with nadir within 6 months, although occasional patients achieve their peak disability as rapidly as weeks or as slowly as a year or more (114,117,118). Most patients are disabled due to both severe pain and weakness. Pain control usually necessitates opiate therapy. Weakness may be significant, with half of patients using a wheelchair for ambulation. After the nadir, symptoms typically remain stable for several months and then improve spontaneous over the following year (Fig. 11.5) (118). Because of spontaneous recovery, the true severity of DLRPN is often underemphasized. Although most patients recover substantially, most have significant residual symptoms with half requiring long term assistance with ambulation (114).

3.1.3. Laboratory and Electrodiagnostic Evaluation

DLRPN is usually associated with spinal fluid cyto-albuminemic dissociation, with protein 200 mg/dL and above. Oligoclonal bands may be observed in one-third of patients

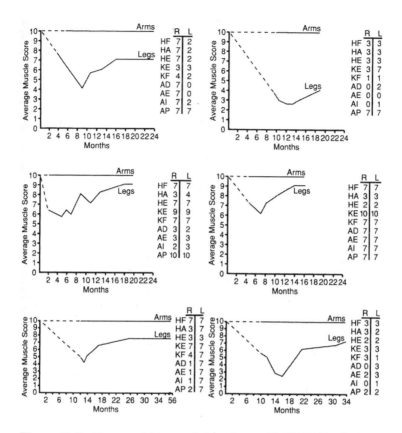

Figure 11.5 The natural history of six patients with DLRPN is displayed. The average muscle strength measured using an expanded Medical Research Council scale initially declines and then improves over the following years. Despite significant improvement, no patient achieves normal strength.

(115). DLRPN with an elevated serum erythrocyte sedimentation rate has been thought to represent a distinct disorder (119), but current consensus is that these patients fall within the spectrum of a single disorder (113).

NCS/EMG studies reveal a distal diabetic peripheral polyneuropathy, with reduced sensory and motor responses, slowed conduction velocity and prolonged F-wave latencies in the legs, in 75% of patients (118). Demyelinating features are not of sufficient severity to fulfill formal electrodiagnostic criteria for an acquired demyelinating neuropathy (e.g., CIDP) (115). EMG reveals fibrillations and positive sharp waves with reduced recruitment and increased motor unit amplitude in weak limb and paraspinal muscles, with findings more widespread than clinical symptoms. Thoracic paraspinal muscles may also have evidence for ongoing denervation. This constellation of findings is consistent with involvement of both nerve root and plexus in addition to peripheral neuropathy and forms the basis of the term DLRPN.

3.1.4. Differential Diagnosis

The differential diagnosis of DLRPN is limited. Lumbosacral disc disease is the most common cause for diagnostic confusion, especially among non-neurologists. CIDP may be considered because both have proximal and distal weakness associated with lower extremity areflexia and cyto-albuminemic dissociation, however asymmetry and severe pain are atypical for CIDP, and evidence for primary demyelination is lacking in DLRPN (114,115). In occasional patients, differentiation may be difficult, and empiric treatment with corticosteroids or intravenous immunoglobulin may be appropriate, especially given evidence that DLRPN may respond to treatments typically used for CIDP.

A syndrome otherwise identical to DLRPN may occur in nondiabetic subjects, lumbosacral radiculoplexus neuropathy (LRPN), but these patients should undergo a careful evaluation for diabetes, including a OGTT (120).

3.1.5. Pathology and Pathogenesis

DLRPN causes multifocal fiber loss with perivascular inflammation in nerve biopsy tissue (117,119,121,122). It had been suggested that metabolic factors are primarily involved in milder disease and that a superimposed inflammatory process with nerve ischemia are also involved in more severe disease (123,124). However, a vasculitis involving vessels in the epineurial and perineurial with transmural inflammation is observed in half of patients, and significant perivascular lymphocytic infiltrates in most others, but frank vasculitis not observed (114,125,126). Other findings supporting a vasculitis are hemosiderin in macrophages, neovascularization, and multifocal fiber loss. Immunoglobulin and complement deposition may also occur (Fig. 11.6) (125).

Supportive evidence for inflammatory vs. metabolic-induced microvascular injury includes better glycemic control in patients with DLRPN than those with DSP and the observation that DLRPN may herald the diagnosis of diabetes (113). Further, spontaneous improvement in nearly all patients would be unexpected in a metabolic or degenerative process. The observation of occasional oligoclonal bands also supports an inflammatory process. Lastly, the apparent response of some patients to immunomodulatory therapy is consistent with an autoimmune etiology.

3.1.6. Treatment

Immune-suppressing therapy has been used in DLRPN based on evidence that it may have an autoimmune basis. Therapies tried include intravenous corticosteroids, IVIG, and plasma exchange (115,120,127,128). It is challenging to assess treatment efficacy in a disorder whose natural history is spontaneous improvement (124). Two double-blind placebo controlled studies are ongoing, one with intravenous corticosteroids and the other with IVIG (113), and routine use of IVIG or corticosteroids to treat patients with

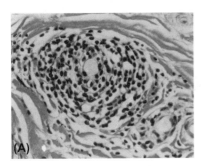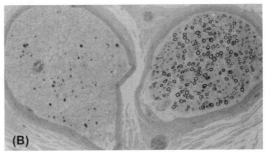

Figure 11.6   Pathologic data support an inflammatory etiology for DLRPN. Sensory nerve biopsy reveals inflammation involving small blood vessels (A) and fascicle-to-fascicle variation in fiber loss, supporting an ischemic process (B).

DLRPN should await the results of these studies. Aggressive therapy for pain is important. Agents specifically directed at neuropathic pain (e.g., tricyclic antidepressants and anticonvulsants) are appropriate, but most patients require the use of oral opiates.

3.2.   Truncal Radiculopathy

Patients present with the acute onset of pain and numbness involving the trunk (129–131). Abdominal wall muscles may become weak, mimicking a hernia (132). The distribution of sensory loss is variable, ranging from a discrete area within one dermatome, to bilateral involvement spanning several dermatomes. Low thoracic dermatomes are most commonly involved, although high thoracic dermatomes may be affected, including the axilla (Fig. 11.7) (129). Truncal radiculopathy shares many features with DLRPN, and the two often coexist. Elderly subjects with type 2 diabetes are most commonly affected and the syndrome spontaneously resolves over a period of months.

There are no data on peripheral nerve or root pathology. Skin biopsy reveals epidermal denervation, indicating that the lesion involves the dorsal root ganglion or its distal process. Repeat skin biopsy after clinical improvement reveals re-innervation of skin (133). EMG studies reveal denervation of paraspinal and abdominal muscles at the affected level (130). The acute nature, spontaneous recovery, and association with DLRPN support an inflammatory etiology.

There are no controlled trials to guide treatment. When truncal radiculopathy occurs with DLRPN, immune therapy may be appropriate in the acute phase. However, immune

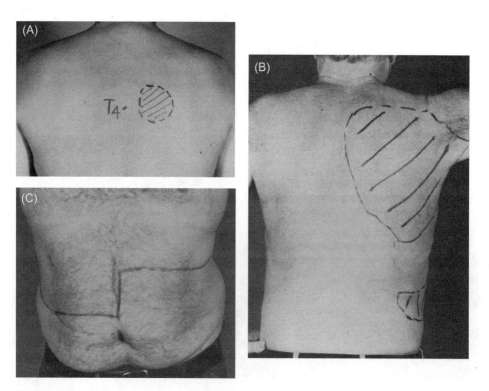

Figure 11.7   Diabetic truncal radiculopathy may cause sensory loss and pain in a small region within a single dermatome (A) or may involve multiple dermatomes on one side (B) or bilaterally (C).

treatment of isolated truncal radiculopathy is unwarranted given the disorder is self limited and causes no disability beyond pain. Treatment should therefore focus on pain control. Effective strategies include those useful for treatment of pain associated with DSP and DLRPN. Because pain usually involves a focal discrete area, topical lidocaine via a patch is a therapeutic option (134,135).

3.3. Cranial Neuropathy

Cranial mononeuropathies are a complication of diabetes. Nerves supplying extraocular muscles, especially the oculomotor nerve, are most commonly involved (Fig. 11.8). Involvement of the trochlear and abducens nerves is much less common (136). The typical clinical presentation of a third nerve palsy is rapid onset of double vision and ptosis, often associated with periorbital pain, although a wider distribution occurs. Classically, the pupil is spared, although minor degrees of internal ophthalmoplegia may be observed, especially with pupilometry (137–139). Because occasional patients with aneurysmal third nerve palsies may spare the pupil, diabetic patients with headache and a painful oculomotor palsy with pupillary involvement should be evaluated for an aneurysm (140).

The etiology of the third nerve palsy is unknown, but a vascular event within the watershed zone within the third nerve itself is likely (Fig. 11.9) (141). A mesencephalic lesion site has also been described with MRI lesions in the ipsilateral midbrain (142). Prognosis is excellent, with most patients recovering within several months, although occasional patients have a recurrent episode (136,138).

Facial nerve palsy (Bell's palsy) may be more common in diabetic patients, with prevalence rates varying between 6–66% (143–145). Perhaps more compelling data

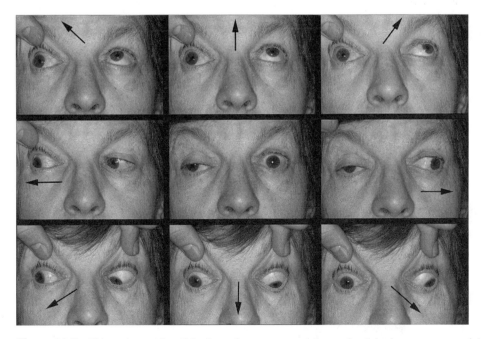

Figure 11.8 This patient with a diabetic oculomotor neuropathy on the right demonstrates partial ptosis and nearly complete paresis of III nerve innervated muscles, without papillary asymmetry. The central panel is in primary gaze and arrows indicate the direction of gaze. (Image provided courtesy of Dr. Kathleen Digre.)

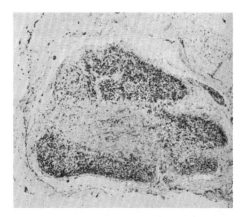

Figure 11.9   The only pathologic data from a patient with diabetic oculumotor neuropathy demonstrates a central region of focal demyelination.

are the observations that 83% of nondiabetic subjects with Bell's palsy have abnormal taste, compared with only 14% of those with diabetes, suggesting more distal involvement in the later group (144).

3.4.   Diabetic Neuropathic Cachexia

The term diabetic neuropathic cachexia (DNC) is used for the rare condition of acute and profound weight loss associated with severe neuropathic pain involving the distal limbs and trunk (Fig. 11.10) (146). There is associated depression and impotence. The original description included older men with type 2 diabetes, but other reports include women and patients with type 1 diabetes (147–150). There is spontaneous recovery over months without specific therapy (146).

The etiology of DNC is unknown. Nerve biopsy reveals axonal degeneration of both large myelinated and small unmyelinated fibers with axonal regeneration (16,148). No inflammatory changes have been observed. Unlike DSP, DNC does not appear to be

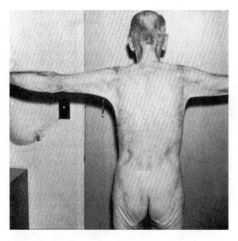

Figure 11.10   This image from Ellenberg's initial description of DNC highlights the severity of cachexia that may be observed.

related to the severity and length of hyperglycemia and is not correlated with retinopathy or nephropathy. The cachexia may be associated with malabsorption due to pancreatic dysfunction and treatment with pancreatic supplements and a high calorie diet may be of benefit (147).

An identical syndrome has been described after initiation of insulin or oral hypogly-cemic therapy following a period of significant hyperglycemia (151). This entity, which has been termed "insulin neuritis," may be part of the spectrum of DNC (152). The pathogenetic mechanism may be distinct. Intravenous insulin impairs tissue oxygenation in rats when hyperglycemia is corrected. In this setting, nerve injury may be secondary to epineurial arteriovenous shunting (150). Acute retinopathy following rapid glycemic control has also been described and attributed to hypoxic injury (153).

4. MONONEUROPATHIES

Compressive neuropathies are more common among patients with diabetes, particularly those with peripheral neuropathy (154). Mononeuropathies, particularly bilateral mono-neuropathies, can be challenging to recognize in the setting of diabetic neuropathy severe enough to involve hands. The most common compressive neuropathy in diabetes is carpal tunnel syndrome (CTS). There are different clinical and electrodiagnostic criteria, but electrodiagnostic evidence for median nerve slowing across the wrist is more common than symptoms of intermittent hand numbness involving median innervated digits. Up to one-third of unselected diabetic patients have electrophysiologic evidence of median nerve slowing. This figure rises to 60% among older diabetic patients who have an associ-ated peripheral neuropathy (3,155). However, only 5.7% have symptomatic CTS (154).

The pathophysiologic relationship between CTS and diabetes is not clear. The risk of CTS correlates with the duration of diabetes, supporting a direct relationship (3,156). The risk of CTS also correlates with obesity and body mass index (156,157). When body mass index is controlled for, the relationship between diabetes and CTS risk is much less robust, suggesting a more complex relationship with obesity playing an inde-pendent role in the development of each problem (157). The obesity associated with dia-betes may lead to fat accumulation in the carpal tunnel. Diabetic nerve may be more sensitive to compressive injury caused by metabolic injury, microvascular dysfunction, or impaired axonal transport or growth factor physiology. Treatment options are the same as for patients without diabetes, but response to therapy may not be as good.

Other compressive mononeuropathies more common in diabetes include peroneal mononeuropathy at the fibular head and ulnar mononeuropathy at the elbow. Lateral femoral cutaneous mononeuropathies (meralgia paresthetica) may also be more common (154).

5. CONCLUSIONS

Type 2 diabetes prevalence is increasing rapidly in the United States, particularly in children and young adults. These trends assure that diabetic complications will also increase, as more patients live longer with their diabetes. Peripheral neuropathy is one of the most common complications of diabetes, and often occurs early in the spectrum of glycemic dysregulation, during the prediabetic period of IGT. In both, diabetes and IGT, neuropathy is most often sensory predominant and frequently painful. Autonomic neuropathy manifesting as impotence in men, altered cardiac reactivity, gastroparesis or diarrhea, or unawareness of hypoglycemia is probably at least as prevalent as polyneuropathy. Acute complications including DLRPN and truncal radiculopathy likely have an inflammatory basis and may respond to immunomodulatory therapy. Acute oculomotor neuropathies are likely due to an ischemic lesion within the brainstem or nerve fascicle and improve spontaneously. Compressive mononeuropathies, particularly CTS, are common among diabetic patients and may represent a source of diagnostic confusion. Management of diabetic neuropathy requires a multimodal approach, incorporating aggressive glucose regulation, surveillance for and prevention of foot injury and ulcers in the sensation-compromised foot, assistance to prevent falls, and appropriate symptomatic treatment of neuropathic pain. Careful glucose control remains the only proven treatment to alter the course of diabetic neuropathy. In patients with IGT or early diabetes, aggressive, tailored diet, and exercise modification may be the most effective treatment to lower glucose and prevent progression of hyperglycemia.

REFERENCES

1. The Expert Committee on the Diagnosis and Classification of Diabetes Mellitus. Report of the expert committee on the diagnosis and classification of diabetes mellitus. Diabetes Care 1997; 20:1183–1199.
2. Pirart J. Diabetes mellitus and its degenerative complications: a prospective study of 4,400 patients observed between 1947 and 1973. Diabetes Care 1978; 1:168.
3. Dyck PJ, Kratz JM, Karnes JL, Litchy WJ, Klein R, Pach JM, Wilson DM, O'Brien PC, Melton LJ. The prevalence by staged severity of various types of diabetic neuropathy, retinopathy and nephropathy in a population-based cohort: The Rochester Diabetic Neuropathy Study. Neurology 1993; 43:817–824.
4. The Italian General Practitioner Study Group. Chronic symmetric symptomatic polyneuropathy in the elderly: a field screening investigation in two italian regions. I. Prevalence and general characteristics of the sample. Neurology 1995; 45:1832–1836.
5. Singleton JR, Smith AG, Bromberg MB. Increased prevalence of impaired glucose tolerance in patients with painful sensory neuropathy. Diabetes Care 2001; 24:1448–1453.
6. Singleton JR, Smith AG, Bromberg MB. Painful sensory polyneuropathy associated with impaired glucose tolerance. Muscle Nerve 2001; 24:1225–1228.
7. Novella SP, Inzucchi SE, Goldstein JM. The frequency of undiagnosed diabetes and impaired glucose tolerance in patients with idiopathic sensory neuropathy. Muscle Nerve 2001; 24:1229–1231.
8. Sumner C, Seth S, Griffin J, Cornblath D, Polydefkis M. The spectrum of neuropathy in diabetes and impaired glucose tolerance. Neurology 2003; 60:108–111.
9. Alberti KG. Impaired glucose tolerance: what are the clinical implications? Diabetes Res Clin Pract 1998; 40:S3–S8.
10. Dyck JB, Dyck PJ. Diabetic Polyneuropathy. In: Dyck PJ, Thomas PK, eds. Diabetic Neuropathy. Philadelphia: WB Saunders, 1999:255–278.
11. Ellenberg M. Diabetic neuropathy presenting as the initial clinical manifestation of diabetes. Ann Intern Med 1958; 49:620–631.
12. Lehtinen JM, Uuistupa M, Siitonen O, Pyorala K. Prevalence of neuropathy in newly diagnosed NIDDM and nondiabetic control subjects. Diabetes 1989; 38:1308–1313.
13. Cohen JA, Jeffers BW, Faldut D, Marcoux M, Schrier RW. Risks for sensorimotor peripheral neuropathy and autonomic neuropathy in non-insulin dependent diabetes mellitus (NIDDM). Muscle Nerve 1998; 21:72–80.
14. Franklin GM, Kahn LB, Marshall JA, Hamman RF. Sensory neuropathy in non-insulin-dependent diabetes mellitus. The San Luis Valley Diabetes Study. Am J Epidemiol 1990; 131:633–643.

15. Ziegler D, Gries FA, Spuler M, Lessmann F. The epidemiology of diabetic neuropathy. J Diab Comp 1992; 6:49–57.

16. Archer A, Watkins PJ, Thomas PK. The natural history of acute painful neuropathy in diabetes mellitus. J Neurol Neurosurg Psych 1983; 46:491–497.

17. Tesfaye S, Malik R, Harris N, Jakubowski JJ, Mody C, Rennie IG, Ward JD. Arterio-venous shunting and proliferating new vessels in acute painful neuropathy of rapid glycaemic control (insulin neuritis). Diabetologia 1996; 39:329–335.

18. Burchiel KJ, Russell LC, Lee RP, Sima AAF. Spontaneous activity of primary afferent neurons in diabetic BB/wistar rats: a possible mechanism of chronic diabetic neuropathic pain. Diabetes 1985; 36:1210–1213.

19. Boulton A. What causes neuropathic pain? J Diab Comp 1992; 6:58–63.

20. Guy RJ, Clark CA, Malcolm PN, Watkins PJ. Evaluation of thermal and vibration sensation in diabetic neuropathy. Diabetologia 1985; 28:131–137.

21. Thomas PK. Classification, differential diagnosis, and staging of diabetic peripheral neuropathy. Diabetes 1997; (suppl 2):S54–S57.

22. Brown MJ, Asbury AK. Diabetic neuropathy. Ann Neurol 1984; 15:2–12.

23. Dunsmuir WD, Holmes SA. The aetiology and management of erectile, ejaculatory, and fertility problems in men with diabetes mellitus. Diab Med 1996; 13:700–708.

24. Periquet MI, Novak V, Collins MP, Nagaraja HN, Erdem S, Nash SM, Freimer ML, Sahenk Z, Kissel JT, Mendel JR. Painful sensory neuropathy: prospective evaluation using skin biopsy. Neurology 1999; 53:1641–1647.

25. Holland NR, Crawford TO, Hauer P, Cornblath DR, Griffin JW, McArthur JC. Small-fiber sensory neuropathies: clinical course and neuropathology of idiopathic cases. Ann Neurol 1998; 44:47–59.

26. Freeman R, Chase K, Risk M. Quantitative sensory testing cannot differentiate simulated sensory loss from sensory neuropathy. Neurology 2003; 60:465–470.

27. Smith AG, Tripp C, Singleton JR. Skin biopsy findings in patients with neuropathy associated with diabetes and impaired glucose tolerance. Neurology 2001; 57:1701.

28. Dyck PJ, Lais A, Karnes JL, O'Brien P, Rizza R. Fiber loss is primary and multifocal in sural nerves in diabetic polyneuropathy. Ann Neurol 1986; 19:425–439.

29. Timperley WR, Boulton AJ, Davies-Jones GA, Jarrett JA, Ward JD. Small vessel disease in progressive diabetic neuropathy associated with good metabolic control. J Clin Pathol 1985; 38:1030–1038.

30. Gianni C, Dyck PJ. Basement membrane thickening and pericyte degeneration precede development of diabetes polyneuropathy and are associated with its severity. Ann Neurol 1995; 37:498–504.

31. Herrmann D, Griffin J, Hauer P, Cornblath DR, McArthur JC. Epidermal nerve fiber density: association with sural nerve morphometry and electrophysiology in peripheral neuropathies. Neurology 1999; 52:A309–A310.

32. Low PA. Diabetic autonomic neuropathy. Sem Neurol 1996; 16:143–151.

33. Vinik AI, Maser RE, Mitchell BD, Freeman R. Diabetic autonomic neuropathy. Diabetes Care 2003; 26:1553–1579.

34. Deutsch S, Sherman L. Previously unrecognized diabetes mellitus in sexually impotent men. J Am Med Assoc 1980; 244:2430–2432.

35. Sairam K, Kulinskaya E, Boustead GB, Hanbury DC, McNicholas TA. Prevalence of undiagnosed diabetes mellitus in male erectile dysfunction. BJU Int 2001; 88:68–71.

36. Maatman TJ, Montague DK, Martin LM. Erectile dysfunction in men with diabetes mellitus. Urology 1987; 29:589–592.

37. Bemelmans BL, Meuleman EJ, Doesburg WH, Notermans SL, Debruyne FM. Erectile dysfunction in diabetic men: the neurological factor revisited. J Urol 1994; 151:884–889.

38. Benvenuti F, Boncinelli L, Vignoli GC. Male sexual impotence in diabetes mellitus: vasculogenic versus neurogenic factors. Neurourol Urodyn 1993; 12:145–151.

39. Lustman PJ, Clouse RE. Relationship of psychiatric illness to impotence in men with diabetes. Diabetes Care 1990; 13:893–895.

40. Low PA. Autonomic nervous system function. J Clin Neurophys 1993; 10:14–27.

41. American Diabetes Association. Consensus statement: role of cardiovascular risk factors in prevention and treatment of macrovascular disease in diabetes. Diabetes Care 1993; 16:72–78.

42. Stevens MJ, Feldman EL, Thomas T, Greene DA. Pathogenesis of diabetic neuropathy. In: Veves A, ed. Clinical Management of Diabetic Neuropathy. Totowa: Humana Press, 1998.

43. Maser RE, Pfeifer MA, Dorman JS, Kuller LH, Becker DJ, Orchard TJ. Diabetic autonomic neuropathy and cardiovascular risk. Pittsburgh Epidemiology of Diabetes Complications Study III. Arch Intern Med 1990; 150:1218–1222.

44. Orchard T, CE L, Maser R, Kuller L. Why does diabetic autonomic neuropathy predict IDDM mortality? An analysis from the Pittsburgh Epidemiology of Diabetes Complications Study. Diabetes Res Clin Pract 1996; 34(suppl):S165–S171.

45. Fava S, Azzopardi J, Muscatt HA, Fenech FF. Factors that influence outcome in diabetic subjects with myocardial infarction. Diabetes Care 1993; 16:1615–1618.

46. Schiller LR, Santa Ana CA, Schmulen AC, Hendler RS, Harford WV, Fordtran JS. Pathogenesis of fecal incontinence in diabetes mellitus: evidence for internal-anal-sphincter dysfunction. N Eng J Med 1982; 307:1666–1671.

47. Taborsky GJ, Ahren B, Havel PJ. Autonomic mediation of glucagon secretion during hypoglycemia: implications for impaired alpha-cell responses in type I diabetes. Diabetes 1998; 47:995–1007.

48. Powell AM, Sherwin RS, Shulman GI. Impaired hormonal responses to hypoglycemia in spontaneously diabetic and recurrently hypoglycemic rats. J Clin Invest 1993; 92:2667–2674.

49. Bolli GB, De Feo P, Compagnucci P, Cartechini MG, Angeletti G, Santeusanio F, Brunetti P, Gerich JE. Abnormal glucose counterregulation in insulin-dependent diabetes mellitus: interaction of anti-insulin antibodies and impaired glucagon and epinephrine secretion. Diabetes 1983; 32:134–141.

50. Feldman EL, Stevens MJ, Russell JW, Greene DA. Diabetic neuropathy. In: Taylor S, ed. Current Review of Diabetes. New York, 1999.

51. Cameron N, Eaton S, Cotter M, Tesfaye S. Vascular factors and metabolic interactions in the pathogenesis of diabetic neuropathy. Diabetologia 2001; 44:1973–1988.

52. Dyck P, Hansen S, Karnes J, O'Brien P, Yasuda H, Windebank A. Capillary number and percentage closed in human diabetic sural nerve. Proc Natl Acad Sci 1985; 82:2513–2517.

53. Britland S, Young R, Sharma A, Clarke B. Relationship of endoneurial capillary abnormalities to type and severity of diabetic neuropathy. Diabetes 1990; 39:909–913.

54. Malik R, Newrick PG, Sarma AK, Jennings A, Ah-See AK, Mayhew TM, Jakubowski J, Boulton AJ, Ward JD. Microangiopathy in human diabetic neuropathy: relationship between capillary abnormalities and the severity of neuropathy. Diabetologia 1989; 32:92–102.

55. Ibrahim S, Harris N, Radatz M, Selmi F, Rajbhandari S, Brady L, Jakubowski J, Ward JD. A new minimally invasive technique to show nerve ischaemia in diabetic neuropathy. Diabetologia 1999; 36:737–742.

56. Newrick P, Wilson A, Jakubowski J, Boulton A, Ward J. Sural nerve oxygen tension in diabetes. Brit Med J 1986; 293:1053–1054.

57. Reja A, Tesfaye S, Harris N, Ward J. Is ACE inhibition with lisiopril helpful in diabetic neuropathy? Diabetic Med 1995; 12:307–309.

58. Obrosova I, Van Huysen C, Fathallah L, Cao X, Stevens M, Greene D. Evaluation of a1-adrenoceptor antagonist on diabetes-induced changes in peripheral nerve function, metabolism, and antioidative defense. FASEB J 2000; 14:1548–1558.

59. Malik R, Williamson S, Abbott C, Carrington A, Iqbal J, Schady W, Boulton A. Effect of the angiotensin converting enzyme inhibitor trandalopril on human diabetic neuropathy: a randomised controlled trial. Lancet 1998; 352:1978–1981.

60. Steinberg HO, Brechtel G, Johnson A, Fineberg N, Baron AD. Insulin mediated skeletal muscle vasodilation is nitric oxide dependent: a novel action of insulin to increase nitric oxide release. J Clin Invest 1994; 94:1172–1179.

61. Shankar RR, Wu Y, Shen HQ, Zhu JS, Baron AD. Mice with gene disruption of both endothelial and neuronal nitric oxide synthase exhibit insulin resistance. Diabetes 2000; 49:684–687.

62. Windebank A, Feldman E. Diabetes and the nervous system. In: Aminoff M, ed. Neurology and General Medicine. Philadelphia, PA: Churchill Livingstone, 2001:341–364.

63. Singh R, Barden A, Mori T, Beilin L. Advanced glycation end-products: a review. Diabetologia 2001; 44:129–146.

64. Cameron N, Cotter M, Achibald V, Dines K, Maxfield E. Anti-oxidant and pro-oxidant effects on nerve conduction velocity, endoneurial blood flow and oxygen tension in non-diabetic and streptozotocin diabetic rats. Diabetologia 1994; 37:449–459.

65. Ward K, Low P, Schmelzer J, Zochodne D. Prostacyclin and moradrenaline in peripheral nerve of chronic experimental diabetes in rats. Brain 1989; 112:197–208.

66. Maxfield EK, Cameron NE, Cotter MA. Effects of diabetes on reactivity of sciatic vasa nervorum in rats. J Diabet Complications 1997; 11:47–55.

67. Takahashi K, Ghatei M, Lam H, O'Halloran D, Bloom S. Elevated plasma endothelin levels in patients with diabetes mellitus. Diabetologia 1990; 33:306–310.

68. Suzuki K. Neurological disorders associated with impaired glucose tolerance. Nippon Rinsho 1996; 54:2704–2708.

69. Rezende KF, Melo A, Pousada J, Rezende ZF, Santos NL, Gomes I. Autonomic neuropathy in patients with impaired glucose tolerance. Arq Neuropsiquiatr 1997; 55:703–711.

70. Way KJ, Katai N, King GL. Protein kinase C and the development of diabetic vascular complications. Diabet Med 2001; 18:945–959.

71. Jiang ZY, Lin YW, Clemont A, Feener EP, Hein KD, Igarashi M, Yamauchi T, White MF, King GL. Characterization of selective resistance to insulin signaling in the vasculature of obese Zucker (fa/fa) rats. J Clin Invest 1999; 104:447–457.

72. King RHM. The role of glycation in the pathogenesis of diabetic polyneuropathy. J Clin Pathol Mol Pathol 2001; 54:400–408.

73. McClain DA, Crook ED. Hexosamines and insulin resistance. Diabetes 1996; 45:1003–1009.

74. Yagihashi S, Yamagishi S, Wada R, Baba M, Hohman T, Yabe-Nishimura C, Kokai Y. Neuropathy in diabetic mice overesxpressing human aldose reductase and effects of aldose reductase inhibitor. Brain 2001; 124:2448–2458.

75. Pfeifer MA, Schumer MP, Gelber DA. Aldose reductase inhibitors: the end of an era or the need for different trial designs? Diabetes 1997; 46:82–89.

76. Sugimoto K, Nishizawa Y, Horiuchi S, Yagihashi S. Localization in human diabetic peripheral nerve of N(epsilon)-carboxymethyllysine-protein adducts, an advanced glycation endproduct. Diabetologia 1997; 40:1380–1387.

77. Sima AA, Sugimoto K. Experimental diabetic neuropathy: an update. Diabetologia 1999; 42:773–778.

78. Brownlee M. Biochemistry and molecular cell biology of diabetic complications. Nature 2001; 414:813–820.

79. Pierson CR, Zhang W, Murakawa Y, Sima AA. Early gene responses of trophic factors in nerve regeneration differ in experimental type 1 and type 2 diabetic polyneuropathies. J Neuropathol Exp Neurol 2002; 61:857–871.

80. Faradji V, Sotelo J. Low serum levels of nerve growth factor in diabetic neuropathy. Acta Neurol Scand 1990; 81:402–409.

81. Tomlinson DT, Mayer JH. Defects of axonal transport in diabetes mellitus: a possible contribution to the aetiology of diabetic neuropathy. J Auton Pharmacol 1984; 4:59–68.

82. Migdalis IN, Kalogeropoulou K, Kalantzis L, Nounopoulos C, Bouloukos A, Samartzis M. Insulin-like growth factor-I and IGF-I receptors in diabetic patients with neuropathy. Diabet Med 1995; 12:823–827.

83. Delaney CL, Russell JW, Cheng HL, Feldman EL. Insulin-like growth factor-I and overexpression of Bcl-xL prevent glucose-mediated apoptosis in Schwann cells. J Neuropathol Exp Neurol 2001; 60:147–160.

84. Russell JW, Feldman EL. Insulin-like growth factor-I prevents apoptosis in sympathetic neurons exposed to high glucose. Horm Metab Res 1999; 31:90–96.

85. Christianson J, Riekhof J, Wright D. Restorative effects of neurotrophin treatment on diabetes induced cutaneous axon loss in mice. Exp Neurol 2003; 179:188–199.

86. Apfel S, Schwartz S, Adornato B, Freeman J, Biton V, Rendell M, Ninik A, Giuliani M, Stevens J, Barbano R, Dyck P. Efficacy and safety of recombinant human nerve growth factor in patients with diabetic polyneuropathy a randomized controlled trial. J Am Med Assoc 2000; 284:2215–2221.

87. Ejskjaer NT, Zanone MM, Peakman M. Autoimmunity in diabetic autonomic neuropathy: does the immune system get on your nerves? Diab Med 1998; 15:723–729.

88. Pittenger GL, Liu D, Vinik AI. The neuronal toxic factor in serum of type 1 diabetic patients is a complement-fixing autoantibody. Diab Med 1995; 12:380–386.

89. Srinivasan S, Stevens MJ, Sheng H, Hall KE, Wiley JW. Serum from patients with type 2 diabetes with neuropathy induces complement-independent, calcium-dependent apoptosis in cultured neuronal cells. J Clin Invest 1998; 102:1454–1462.

90. Ristic H, Srinivasan S, Hall KE, Sima AA, Wiley JW. Serum from diabetic BB/W rats enhances calcium currents in primary sensory neurons. J Neurophys 1998; 80:1236–1244.

91. Stewart JD, McKelvey R, Durcan L, Carpenter S, Karpati G. Chronic inflammatory demyelinating polyneuropathy (CIDP) in diabetics. J Neurol Sci 1996; 142:59–64.

92. Navaro X, Sutherland DE, Kennedy WR. Long-term effects of pancreatic transplantation on diabetic neuropathy. Ann Neurol 1997; 42:727–736.

93. Diabetes Control and Complications Trial Research Group. Effect of intensive diabetes treatment on nerve conduction in the diabetes control and complications trial. Ann Neurol 1995; 38:869–880.

94. Diabetes Control and Complications Research Group. The effect of intensive treatment of diabetes on the development and progression of long-term complications in insulin-dependent diabetes mellitus. New Engl J Med 1993; 329:977–986.

95. Diabetes Control and Complications Research Group. Hypoglycemia in the diabetes control and complications trial. Diabetes 1997; 46:271–286.

96. Diabetes Control and Complications Trial Research Group. The absence of a glycemic threshold for the development of long-term complications: the perspective of the diabetes control and complications trial. Diabetes 1996; 45:1289–1298.

97. Diabetes Prevention Program Research Group. Reduction in the incidence of type 2 diabetes with lifestyle intervention or metformin. NEJM 2002; 346:393–403.

98. Krentz A, Honigsberger L, Ellis S, Hardman M, Nattrass M. A 12-month randomized controlled study of the aldose reductase inhibitor ponalrestat in patients with chronic symptomatic diabetic neuropathy. Diabet Med 1992; 9:463–468.

99. Dyck P, O'Brien P. Meaningful degrees of prevention or improvement of nerve conduction in controlled clnical trials of diabetic neuropathy. Diabetes Care 1989; 12:649–652.

100. Greene D, Arezzo J, Brown M, the Zenarestat Study Group. Effect of aldose reductase inhibition on nerve conduction and morphometry in diabetic neuropathy. Neurology 1999; 53:580–591.

101. Pfeifer MA, Schumer MP. Clinical trials of diabetic neuropathy: past, present, and future. Diabetes 1995; 44:1355–1361.

102. Dahmen R, Haspels R, Koomen B, Hoeksma AF. Therapeutic footwear for the neuropathic foot: an algorithm. Diabetes Care 2001; 24:705–709.

103. American Diabetes Association. Preventive foot care in people with diabetes. Diab Care 2002; 25(suppl 1):S69–S70.

104. Abbott C, Carrington A, Ashe H, Bath S, Every L, Griffiths J, Hann A, Hussein A, Jackson N, Johnson K, Ryder C, Torkington R, Van Ross E, Whalley A, Widdows P, Williamson S, Boulton A. The North-West Diabetes Foot Care Study: incidence of, and risk factors for, new diabetic foot ulceration in a community-based patient cohort. Diabet Med 2002; 19:377–384.

105. Pham H, Armstrong DG, Harvey C, Harkless LB, Giurini JM, Veves A. Screening techniques to identify people at high risk for diabetic foot ulceration: a prospective multicenter trial. Diabetes Care 2000; 23:606–611.

106. Perry RC, Baron AD. Impaired glucose tolerance: why is it not a disease? Diabetes Care 1999; 22:883–885.

107. Bonora E, Keichl S, Oberhollenzer, Egger G, Bonadonna RC, Muggeo M, Willeit J. Impaired glucose tolerance, type II diabetes mellitus and carotid atherosclerosis: prospective results from the Bruneck Study. Diabetologia 2000; 42:156–164.

108. Dormandy J, Heeck L, Vig S. Predictors of early disease in the lower limbs. Seminars in Vascular Surgery 1999; 12:109–117.

109. Tominga M, Eguchi H, Igarashi K, Kato T, Sekikawa A. Impaired glucose tolerance is a risk factor for cardiovascular disease but not impaired fasting glucose. The Funagata Diabetes Study. Diabetes Care 1999; 22:920–924.

110. Tuomilehto J, Del Prato S. Mealtime glucose regulation in type 2 diabetes. Int J Clin Pract 2001; 55:380–383.

111. Garland H. Diabetic myelopathy. Br Med J 1955; 2:1405–1408.

112. Bruns L. Ueber neuritsche Lahmungen beim diabetes mellitus. Berlin Klin Wochenschr 1890; 27:509.

113. Dyck PJ, Windebank AJ. Diabetic and nondiabetic lumbosacral radiculoplexus neuropathies: new insights into pathophysiology and treatment. Muscle Nerve 2002; 25:477–491.

114. Dyck P, Norell J, Dyck PJ. Microvasculitis and ischemia in diabetic lumbosacral radiculoplexus neuropathy. Neurology 1999; 53:2113–2121.

115. Jaradeh S, Prieto T, Lobeck L. Progressive polyradiculoneuropathy in diabetes: correlation of variables and clinical outcome after immunotherapy. J Neurol Neurosurg Psychiatry 1999; 67:607–612.

116. Katz J, Saperstein D, Wolfe G, Nations S, Alkhersam H, Amato A, Barohn R. Cervicobrachail involvement in diabetic radiculoplexopathy. Muscle Nerve 2001; 24:794–798.

117. Barohn RJ, Sahenk Z, Warmolts J, Mendell J. The Bruns–Garland syndrome (diabetic amyotrophy) revisited 100 years later. Arch Neurol 1991; 48:1130–1135.

118. Bastron J, Thomas J. Diabetic polyradiculopathy clinical and electromyographic findings in 105 patients. Mayo Clin Proc 1981; 56:725–732.

119. Bradley W, Chad D, Verghese J, Liu H, Good P, Gabbai A, Adelman L. Painful lumbosacral plexopathy with elevated erythrocyte sedimentation rate: a treatable inflammatory syndrome. Ann Neurol 1984; 15:725–732.

120. Dyck P, Norell J, Dyck P. Non-diabetic lumbosacral radiculoplexus neuropathy natural history outcome and comparison with the diabetic variety. Brain 2001; 124:1197–1207.

121. Raff M, Asbury A. Ischemic mononeuropathy and mononeuropathy multiplex in diabetes mellitus. N Engl J Med 1968; 279:17–22.

122. Raff M, Sangalang V, Asbury A. Ischemic mononeuropathy multiplex associated with diabetes mellitus. Arch Neurol 1968; 18:487–499.

123. Said G, Goulon-Goeau C, Lacroix C, Moulonguet A. Nerve biopsy findings in different patterns of proximal diabetic neuropathy. Ann Neurol 1994; 35:559–569.

124. Said G, Elgrably F, Lacroix C, Plante V, Talamon C, Adams D, Tager M, Slama G. Painful proximal diabetic neuropathy: inflammatory nerve lesions and spontaneous favorable outcome. Ann Neurol 1997; 41:762–770.

125. Kelkar P, Masood M, Parry G. Distinctive pathologic findings in proximal diabetic neuropathy (diabetic amyotrophy). Neurology 2000; 55:83–88.

126. Llewelyn J, Thomas P, King R. Epineurial microvasculitis in proximal diabetic neuropathy. J Neurol 1998; 245:159–165.

127. Krendel DA, Costigan DA, Hopkins LC. Successful treatment of neuropathies in patients with diabetes mellitus. Arch Neurol 1995; 52:1053–1061.

128. Pascoe MK, Low PA, Windebank AJ, Litchy WJ. Subacute diabetic proximal neuropathy. Mayo Clin Proc 1997; 72:1123–1132.

129. Stewart J. Diabetic truncal neuropathy: topography of the sensory deficit. Ann Neurol 1989; 25:233–238.

130. Sun S, Streib E. Diabetic thoracoabdominal neuropathy: clinical and electrodiagnostic features. Ann Neurol 1981; 9:75–79.

131. Waxman S, Sabin T. Diabetic truncal polyneuropathy. Arch Neurol 1981; 38:46–47.

132. Parry G, Floberg J. Diabetic truncal neuropathy presenting as abdominal hernia. Neurology 1989; 39:1488–1490.

133. Lauria G, McArthur J, Hauer P, Griffin J, Cornblath D. Neuropathological alterations in diabetic truncal neuropathy: evaluation by skin biopsy. J Neurol Neurosurg Psychiatry 1998; 65:762–766.

134. Rowbotham MC, Davies PS, Verkempinck C, Galer BS. Lidocaine patch: double-blind controlled study of a new treatment method for post-herpetic neuralgia. Pain 1996; 65:39–44.

135. Galer BS, Rowbotham MC, Perander J, Friedman E. Topical lidocaine patch relieves postherpetic neuralgia more effectively than a vehicle topical patch: results of an enriched enrollment study. Pain 1999; 80:533–538.

136. Richards B, Jones F, Younge B. Causes and prognosis in 4,278 cases of paralysis of the oculomotor, trochlear, and abducens cranial nerves. Am J Ophthalmol 1992; 113:489–496.

137. Jacobson D. Pupil involvement in patients with diabetes-associated oculomotor palsy. Arch Ophthalmol 1998; 116:723–727.

138. Goldstein J, Cogan D. Diabetic ophthalmoplegia with special reference to the pupil. Arch Ophthalmol 1960; 64:592–600.

139. Rucker C. The causes of paralysis of the third, fourth and sixth cranial nerves. Am J Ophthalmol 1966; 61:1293–1298.

140. Kissel J, Burde R, Klingele T, Zeiger H. Pupil-sparing oculomotor palsies with internal carotid-posterior communicating artery aneurysms. Ann Neurol 1983; 13:149–154.

141. Asbury A, Aldredge H, Hershberg R, Fisher C. Oculomotor palsy in diabetes mellitus: a clinico-pathological study. Brain 1970; 93:555–566.

142. Hopf H, Gutmann L. Diabetic 3rd nerve palsy: evidence for a mesencephalic lesion. Neurology 1990; 40:1041–1045.

143. Aminoff M, Miller A. The prevalence of diabetes in patients with Bell's palsy. Acta Neurol Scandinav 1972; 48:381–384.

144. Pecket P, Schattner A. Concurrent Bell's palsy and diabetes mellitus: a diabetic mononeuropathy. J Neurol Neurosurg Psychiatry 1982; 45:652–655.

145. Korczyn A. Bell's palsy and diabetes mellitus. The Lancet 1971; 1:108–109.

146. Ellenberg M. Diabetic neuropathic cachexia. Diabetes 1974; 23:418–423.

147. D'Costa D, Price D, Burden A. Diabetic neuropathic cachexia associated with malabsorption. Diabet Med 1992; 9:203–205.

148. Jackson CE, Barohn RJ. Diabetic neuropathic cachexia: report of a recurrent case. J Neurol Neurosurg Psychiatry 1998; 64:785–787.

149. Weintrob N, Josefsberg Z, Galazer A, Vardi P, Karp M. Acute painful neuropathic cachexia in a young type 1 diabetic woman. Diabetes Care 1997; 20:290–291.

150. Yuen K, Day J, Flannagan D, Rayman G. Diabetic neuropathic cachexia and acute bilateral cataract formation following rapid glycaemic control in a newly diagnosed type 1 diabetic patient. Diabet Med 2001; 18:854–857.

151. Llewelyn J, Thomas PK, Fonseca V, King RH, Dandona P. Acute painful diabetic neuropathy precipitated by strict glycaemic control. Acta Neuropathol 1986; 72:157–163.

152. Caravati C. Insulin neuritis: a case report. VA Med Mon 1933; 59:745–746.

153. Patel V, Rassam S, Newsom R, Wiek J, Kohner E. Retinal blood flow in diabetic retinopathy. Br Med J 1992; 305:678–683.

154. Wilbourn AJ. Diabetic entrapment and compression neuropathies. In: Dyck PJ, Thomas PK, eds. Diabetic Neuropathy. Philadelphia: WB Saunders, 1999:481–508.

155. Wilbourn A. Diabetic neuropathies. In: Brown W, Bolton C, eds. Clinical Electromyography. Boston: Butterworth-Heinemann, 1993:477–515.

156. Albers J, Brown M, AA S, Greene D. Frequency of median neuropathy in patients with mild diabetic neuropathy in the early diabetes intervention trial. Tolrestat Study Group for EDIT (early diabetes intervention trial). Muscle Nerve 1996; 19:140–146.

157. Becker J, Nora D, Gomes I, Stringari F, Seitensus F, Panosso J, Ehlers J. An evaluation of gender, obesity, age and diabetes mellitus as risk factors for carpal tunnel syndrome. Clin Neurophys 2002; 113:1429–1434.

12

Endocrine Neuropathies

Patrick M. Grogan and Jonathan S. Katz
Stanford University School of Medicine, Stanford, California, USA

ABSTRACT

Peripheral neuropathies may occur in the setting of various endocrine disorders, but are rare with improvements in the laboratory detection and treatment of the endocrine disorders. The neuropathies generally develop in the setting of general symptoms of the underlying endocrine disorder. Most present with distal extremity sensory loss and paresthesias. Exceptions include predominant motor involvement of upper limbs with

205

insulinoma and generalized weakness in addition to sensory loss with POEMS disease. Focal neuropathies, particularly carpal tunnel syndrome, are also commonly observed. Electrodiagnostic abnormalities vary depending on the type of neuropathy. The diagnosis is confirmed by laboratory identification of the endocrinopathy, and treatment involves reversal of the endocrine imbalance. The neuropathic abnormalities usually resolve once this is achieved.

1. INTRODUCTION

Peripheral neuropathies may occur in association with several endocrine diseases other than diabetes mellitus. However, severe endocrinopathies and associated neuropathies are relatively rare today, as modern testing allows for earlier detection and intervention. Much of the literature is from an earlier era, but knowledge of these disorders is important, as endocrine disorders can be overlooked and are readily treatable. Moreover, earlier associations have influenced modern practice, and thyroid function studies remain in the battery of studies commonly ordered for patients presenting with newly diagnosed peripheral neuropathies. The evidence to determine whether this practice is justified can only be gleaned from this earlier work, although objective support is scant. This chapter considers the clinical features, evaluation, pathophysiology, and treatment of endocrine-related neuropathies.

2. HYPOTHYROIDISM

2.1. Clinical Features

Peripheral neuropathy has been reported in up to 40% of patients with hypothyroidism (1,2). Using a less stringent definition of neuropathy, subjective sensory complaints occur in 40–100% of hypothyroid patients (3–6) and objective sensory loss occurs in 10–60% (5,6). Distal extremity sensory loss associated with pain and paresthesias is the most common neuropathic complaint (3). These symptoms may occur at any time while the patient is hypothyroid, but increase in severity with the degree and duration of hormone deficiency (7). Women report neuropathic complaints more commonly than men, attributed to the increased incidence of hypothyroidism in women rather than a gender-related predilection to develop hypothyroid neuropathy (1,4). Reduced deep tendon reflexes are common in hypothyroidism, but this may result from other neuromuscular conditions, including myopathy. "Hung up" reflexes are distinct diagnostic findings in hypothyroidism that may or may not be associated with a neuropathy (4,5). Myoedema, an electrically silent, focal muscle contraction produced by tapping the muscle, may also be seen but is generally not considered part of the neuropathy. The neuropathy characteristically occurs along with other systemic features of hypothyroidism, including generalized fatigue, cold intolerance, dry skin and hair, weight gain, and constipation. However, in rare instances, the neuropathy may precede the development of generalized hypothyroidism, and this serves as a justification to check thyroid function tests in routine screening for patients presenting with distal neuropathies (3,8). It should be noted that mild hypothyroidism and distal neuropathy are relatively common entities, and there is likely to be a degree of coincidental overlap between idiopathic distal neuropathy and hypothyroidism. Thus, abnormal thyroid studies in a patient without other features of hypothyroidism may be coincidental, and it is questionable whether there is sufficient evidence to justify thyroid studies in chronic axonal polyneuropathies.

Entrapment neuropathies also commonly occur in hypothyroidism. Phalen (9) noted hypothyroidism in only 0.7% of his large series of carpal tunnel syndrome (CTS), but whether this represents an increase over the expected number of cases in the general population is unclear. Smaller studies suggest direct causation, because as many as 75% of patients diagnosed with hypothyroidism report CTS symptoms (10,11). Another review reports that hypothyroid patients are 70% more likely to be referred for carpal tunnel release than the general population (12). Symptoms of median neuropathy at the wrist are identical to patients without hypothyroidism (13). Bilateral symptoms are seen in at least 50% of patients (10,11,14). Tarsal tunnel syndrome has also been reported in hypothyroidism, although nonspecific clinical and electrophysiologic criteria were used (15). Hypothyroidism has also been associated with focal neuropathy of cranial nerve VIII, manifest by hearing loss without vestibular dysfunction. A causal association was assumed based on improvements in subjective hearing and routine audiometric testing with thyroid hormone replacement (16). However, other studies were unable to corroborate these findings and also noted no improvement in brainstem auditory evoked response testing with thyroid replacement (17,18).

2.2. Laboratory

By definition in hypothyroid neuropathy, thyroid stimulating hormone levels are elevated and thyroxine levels are depressed, whereas routine laboratory tests are normal. Elevated serum creatine kinase levels that are seen in the myopathy are not associated with thyroid neuropathy (2,19,20). Cerebral spinal fluid (CSF) protein levels are typically mild-to-moderately elevated in hypothyroidism. Older studies suggest that the elevation is related to disruptions in the blood–brain barrier, alterations in CSF drainage, or even antibody-mediated nerve damage (6,21). CSF protein normalizes with therapy for the hypothyroidism (21).

Nerve conduction studies in hypothyroid neuropathy typically show features of demyelination with reduced motor and sensory velocities in both upper and lower extremities, sometimes with superimposed conduction blocks or abnormal temporal dispersion (8,22–26). Reduced amplitudes are less common (22,25). Nerve conduction abnormalities can be detected in hypothyroid patients even in the absence of neuropathic symptoms (23,26). Needle electromyography (EMG) may show overlapping myopathic changes (2,27), acute denervation (28,29), or myotonic discharges (30), owing to the mixture of myopathic and neuropathic disorders related to hypothyroidism.

Electrodiagnostic abnormalities in CTS related to hypothyroidism are similar to findings in patients with normal thyroid function. Clinical and electrodiagnostic abnormalities improve with treatment and return to the euthyroid state (10,14).

2.3. Pathology/Pathophysiology

The pathophysiology of hypothyroid neuropathy has not been clearly elucidated. Early studies reported changes consistent with primary axonal degeneration and a "mucinous substance" infiltrating the endoneurium and perineurium in many patients (6). Later studies challenged the findings of a primary axonopathy, reporting instead primarily demyelinating changes, including decreased myelin fiber density and segmental demyelination (22,31). Glycogen accumulations within nerve fibers on EM, a feature also seen on muscle biopsy in hypothyroid myopathy, have been reported (22). The pendulum has swung back and recent studies to report axonal changes including disintegrated neurofilaments, altered axoplasmic organelles, and increased numbers of regenerative clusters (24,32,33).

It has been theorized that median nerve compression (CTS) occurs as a result of swollen, myxoedematous tissues under the flexor retinaculum (10,14). However, no biopsy studies of hypothyroid-related median neuropathy have been performed to further clarify this hypothesis. Edematous muscle tissue, the primary diagnostic feature of a subtype of hypothyroid myopathy known as Hoffman's syndrome (28), may cause CTS by similar physiologic mechanisms.

2.4. Treatment

Neuropathic symptoms and clinical examination abnormalities resolve with correction of the hypothyroid state (2,3,24,32,33). Prolonged recovery, up to several years may be noted, although slow and steady improvement is typical (2,7). Nerve conduction study abnormalities (8,22,31), needle EMG changes (30,31), and CSF protein (21) normalize with management of the hypothyroidism.

3. HYPERTHYROIDISM

3.1. Clinical Features

The association between hyperthyroidism and polyneuropathy is unclear. In a small series, electrodiagnostic abnormalities resolved with hyperthyroid management in a quarter of cases (34). The electrodiagnostic findings necessary for inclusion in this unblinded study were decreased motor unit recruitment and increased motor unit action potential amplitude on needle EMG in intrinsic hand and foot muscles, but neither nerve conduction nor clinical histories were reported (34). Other efforts to establish an association between hyperthyroidism and peripheral neuropathy have not lead to a firm conclusion. One report addressing peripheral nervous system dysfunction focused on myopathy, and the small number of patients with neuropathic complaints were not studied in detail (35). It has also been suggested that hyperthyroidism predisposes to Guillain–Barré syndrome, but no clear association is apparent from a small case series (36). Basedow's paraplegia, a rare progressive sensorimotor loss restricted to the legs, has been linked to hyperthyroidism, but responses to hyperthyroid management have been questionable and incomplete (37,38).

A relationship between thyrotoxicosis and a motor neuron disease-like presentation has also been proposed based on a single case report of a patient with limb and bulbar weakness, diffuse hyperreflexia, and acute denervation on EMG that responded to hyperthyroid management (39).

A slightly better argument has been made for focal compressive neuropathies with hyperthyroidism. Two case series associate various entrapment neuropathies, including CTS, peroneal neuropathy at the fibular head, and lateral femoral cutaneous neuropathy (meralgia paresthetica), with thyrotoxicosis, many of which display symptomatic improvement to hyperthyroid therapy (40,41). A recent prospective study reported that 5% of hyperthyroid patients develop clinical and electrophysiologic evidence of CTS, and the majority of these patients respond to hyperthyroid management alone (42).

4. ACROMEGALY

4.1. Clinical Features

Acromegaly is caused by elevated levels of growth hormone (GH), usually due to a pituitary adenoma. Neuropathic complaints, suggestive of a generalized polyneuropathy, occur in 30–40% of patients and commonly include paresthesias, numbness, and pain involving the distal extremities (43–45). Distal extremity weakness may also occur (46). Peripheral nerves may be palpably enlarged (44,47). A myopathy, manifested by proximal limb weakness of insidious onset, may develop late in the disease course, and may confound the clinical picture if the two occur concurrently (48).

Compression neuropathies, in particular CTS, have been reported to occur with increased frequency in acromegaly, with incidences in 35–65% of patients, and include bilateral symptoms in many patients (46,49,50).

4.2. Laboratory

Nerve conduction studies in acromegalic polyneuropathy reveal mild-to-moderate conduction velocity slowing in both motor and sensory nerves. Sural sensory amplitudes are reduced (44,45). Needle EMG typically shows mild chronic denervation (51), but shows nonspecific myopathic abnormalities if the myopathy occurs concurrently (48). Nerve conduction studies in CTS show prolonged median motor and sensory latencies in only 50% of cases. This raises questions about the accuracy of the clinical assessment and the reported incidence of CTS in acromegaly (50,52). A magnetic resonance imaging (MRI) study of the median nerve in symptomatic acromegalic patients noted hyperintense signals on T2-weighted images within the nerve suggesting intraneural edema (53). However, this finding is also seen in typical CTS and is again not specific for acromegaly. The features of a polyneuropathy due to acromegaly are not specific, the diagnosis of the underlying condition rests on recognizing the presence of other features of the condition and demonstrating elevated GH levels. It should be noted that diabetes is commonly associated with acromegaly and may affect the interpretation of electrodiagnostic features of the neuropathy (44,45,47,52).

4.3. Pathology/Pathophysiology

Nerve biopsies in acromegalic patients reveal demyelinating changes, including paranodal and internodal loss of myelin, decrease in myelin fiber density, and frequent "onion bulb" formations (44,46). The severity of the demyelinating abnormalities has been directly correlated with the duration of excess GH levels (46). Massive collagen deposits in the epineurium and perineurium, and axons packed with membranous debris have been observed on electron microscopy, which may explain the clinically enlarged nerves occasionally seen on examination (51).

The pathophysiology of the polyneuropathy in acromegaly is unknown. GH alters energy metabolism toward an anabolic state. Elevated GH levels may induce the conversion from carbohydrate to lipid utilization for energy, increase fatty acid oxidation, impair glycolysis, increase protein synthesis, and reduce protein breakdown. In CTS, the observation that patients who symptomatically improve if GH levels normalize, whereas those with ongoing elevations do not also suggests direct causation (49). Edematous, hypertrophied synovial tissue, with or without intraneural edema of the median nerve, is considered the most likely pathophysiologic mechanism (44,53–57). GH is suspected to trigger the pronounced soft tissue enlargement and edema, given its known anabolic properties. GH also produces electrolyte abnormalities, including sodium retention, which may cause soft tissue edema (54). A reduction in the size of the carpal tunnel from bony overgrowth is unlikely given the rapid symptomatic improvement that is often seen following treatment (52).

4.4. Treatment

Clinical (44,54,55) and electrophysiologic (50,53) improvement with treatment and resolution of elevated GH levels is well documented. The most significant benefits have been obtained with pituitary surgery to remove a GH-producing adenoma, but radiotherapy of the pituitary gland has also produced clinical improvement (49). The improvement mainly occurs within a few weeks of the procedure (49,54–56). Bromocriptine, which can block excess GH levels, has also produced rapid symptomatic improvement (56). Routine carpal tunnel release is a procedure of last resort (49).

5. HYPOPARATHYROIDISM

Hypoparathyroidism and pseudohypoparathyroidism are not known to cause a polyneuropathy. The most common neuromuscular problem associated with hypoparathyroidism is tetany, which is the result of hyperexcitable peripheral nerves. Tetany is elicited by hyperventilation, tapping the face (Chvostek's sign) or impeding venous return in a limb to induce carpopedal spasm (Trousseau's sign). Other neurologic complaints that may be confused with peripheral neuropathy include paresthesias, carpopedal spasms, fatigue, and cramps, all of which are related to nerve hyperexcitability associated with low levels of calcium and magnesium (48,58). The tetany and paresthesias resolve with calcium and vitamin D replacements (58,59). Magnesium supplements are also recommended, if levels are reduced.

6. INSULINOMA

6.1. Clinical Features

A rare neuropathy with distinct features occurs in patients with recurrent hypoglycemic episodes due to an insulinoma of the pancreas (60). Men are affected more than women, and the mean age at presentation is 40 years. Episodic confusion and disorientation are the hallmarks of insulinoma, and the neuropathy develops after variable time periods following the onset of a relatively severe episodic disturbance in mental status (61). The unique features are a symmetric predominantly motor neuropathy marked by weakness and atrophy affecting the upper extremities more than the lower with burning pain and paresthesias (61). There may be an objective sensory loss, and deep tendon reflexes are reduced or absent on examination.

6.2. Laboratory

Diagnosis is based on demonstrating low glucose levels after overnight fasting and inappropriately elevated insulin levels (60). Nerve conduction studies typically reveal a sensorimotor polyneuropathy marked by reduced motor and sensory nerve amplitudes with normal or mildly reduced conduction velocities (60). Computed tomography imaging of the abdomen is used to identify single or multiple pancreatic lesions. Tumors associated with neuropathy are most commonly islet-cell adenomas, although islet-cell carcinomas are described (61). There are two reports of patients with multiple endocrine neoplasia (MEN-1), with insulinoma and parathyroid adenomas who developed a similar polyneuropathy (61,62). Nerve biopsies display evidence of primarily axonal neuropathy (61).

6.3. Pathology/Pathophysiology

The underlying pathophysiology is not known. Historically, mild distal sensory polyneuropathies were described in psychiatric patients receiving insulin shock therapy.

However, the phenotype of this neuropathy differs from that seen in insulinoma, and hypoglycemic episodes were induced much less frequently and over longer periods of time, suggesting an alternative underlying cause (61). Prolonged hypoglycemia is not likely a direct cause as peripheral nerves are less dependent on glucose and may utilize alternate nutrient sources compared with central nervous system neurons (60). Other theories include toxic effects of elevated insulin, unknown factors released by the tumor, or a paraneoplastic syndrome (60,61).

6.4. Treatment

Surgical removal of the insulinoma reliably results in resolution in sensory abnormalities. Resolution of motor abnormalities is less common, although dramatic improvements in strength are reported (61).

7. POEMS SYNDROME

POEMS syndrome [polyneuropathy, organomegaly (hepatosplenomegaly or lymphadenopathy), endocrinopathy, M protein, and skin changes] is an uncommon plasma cell dyscrasia with diverse manifestations. It is also known as Crow–Fukase syndrome. The multisystem dysfunction occurs frequently in association with osteosclerotic myeloma. Castleman's syndrome (multicentric angiofollicular lymph node hyperplasia) may have some features POEMS such as polyneuropathy, Addison's disease, and sclerotic bone lesions. In contrast to the other polyneuropathies in this chapter, the endocrine disorder is not thought to be the direct cause of the neuropathic abnormalities, but instead, an underlying plasma-cell dyscrasia causes both the neuropathy and the endocrinopathy. However, POEMS should be kept in the differential diagnosis of patients with both endocrine dysfunction and polyneuropathy. Of the endocrinopathies associated with POEMS syndrome, diabetes mellitus is the most common, occurring in 30–50% (63,64). Thyroid dysfunction has been reported in 40–60% in nonAsian populations (63). Other endocrine abnormalities are less common and include impotence, gynecomastia, amenorrhea, hypogonadism, hyperestrogenemia, and hyperprolactenemia (63,64).

The onset of the neuropathy is subacute affecting both proximal and distal strength in a symmetric distribution involving all extremities (63). Sensory loss is distal in distribution and may affect the hands and the feet. Examination shows generalized areflexia or hyporeflexia. Electrodiagnostic testing reveals sensory and motor axonal changes, with varying degrees of superimposed conduction slowing. The latter finding may be near the range of that seen in chronic demyelinating polyneuropathy.

The combination of a recent-onset endocrine disorder and a generalized, subacute polyneuropathy may be an initial clue for POEMS syndrome. Overlooking the significance of the endocrinopathy has frequently led to the misdiagnosis of chronic inflammatory demyelinating polyradiculoneuropathy (CIDP) and to endocrine-related neuropathies in this clinical setting. Many patients with POEMS have been diagnosed with diabetes and a diabetic neuropathy, but most neuropathies in POEMS have a relatively more rapid onset than a diabetic neuropathy. Similar time courses apply to patients who have a recent onset of hypothyroidism and a neuropathy. The finding of a monoclonal gammopathy, most commonly IgG or IgA λ, is an important clue to the diagnosis. The quantity of monoclonal immunoglobulin is commonly small, and may be missed on protein electrophoresis, and immunofixation testing is recommended. Nonneurologic abnormalities, including endocrine-related symptoms, should also be sought, as patients may not volunteer them. Dermatologic abnormalities include hyperpigmentation, thickened skin, hypertrichosis, and papular angiomas (63,65). Enlargement of the spleen, liver, or lymph nodes is rarely obvious on examination, but easily diagnosed on imaging of the chest and abdomen. Thrombocytosis, papilledema, and peripheral edema also occur commonly (63,64).

REFERENCES

1. Watanakunakorn C, Hodges RE, Evans TC. Myxedema: a study of 400 cases. Arch Intern Med 1965; 116:183–190.
2. Duyff RF, Van den Bosch J, Laman DM, Potter van Loon BJ, Linssen WHJP. Neuromuscular findings in thyroid dysfunction: a prospective clinical and electrodiagnostic study. J Neurol Neurosurg Psychiatry 2000; 68(6):750–755.
3. Crevasse LE, Logue RB. Peripheral neuropathy in myxedema. Ann Intern Med 1959; 50:1433–1437.
4. Bloomer HA, Kyle LH. Myxedema: a reevaluation of clinical diagnosis based on 80 cases. Arch Intern Med 1959; 104:234–242.
5. Nickel SN, Frame B. Neurologic manifestations of myxedema. Neurology 1958; 8:511–517.
6. Nickel SN, Frame B, Bebin J, Tourtellotte WW, Parker JA, Hughes BR. Myxedema neuropathy and myopathy: a clinical and pathological study. Neurology 1961; 11:125–137.
7. Torres CF, Moxley RT. Hypothyroid neuropathy and myopathy: clinical and electrodiagnostic longitudinal findings. J Neurol 1990; 237:271–274.
8. Dick DJ, Nogues MA, Lane RJM, Fawcett PRW. Polyneuropathy in occult hypothyroidism. Postgrad Med J 1983; 59:518–519.
9. Phalen GS. The carpal tunnel syndrome: 17 years' experience in diagnosis and treatment of 654 hands. J Bone Joint Surg 1966; 48A(2):211–228.
10. Murray IP, Simpson JA. Acroparaesthesia in myxoedema: a clinical and electromyographic study. Lancet 1958; 1:1360–1363.
11. Palumbo CF, Szabo RM, Olmsted SL. The effects of hypothyroidism and thyroid replacement on the development of carpal tunnel syndrome. J Hand Surg [Am] 2000; 25(4):734–739.
12. Solomon DH, Katz JN, Bohn R. Nonoccupational risk factors for carpal tunnel syndrome. J Gen Intern Med 1999; 14:310–314.
13. Amato AA, Kissel JT, Mendell JR. Neuropathies associated with organ system failure, organ transplantation, metabolic disturbances and cancer. In: Mendell JR, Kissel JT, Cornblath JT, eds. Diagnosis and Management of Peripheral Nerve Disorders. Oxford: Oxford University Press, 2001:575–577.
14. Purnell DC, Daly PD, Lipscomb PR. Carpal tunnel syndrome associated with myxedema. Arch Intern Med 1961; 108:751–756.
15. Schwartz MS, Mackworth-Young CG, McKeran RO. The tarsal tunnel syndrome in hypothyroidism. J Neurol Neurosurg Psychiatry 1983; 46(5):440–442.
16. Anand VT, Mann SB, Dash RJ, Mehra YN. Auditory investigations in hypothyroidism. Acta Otolaryngol 1989; 108(1–2):83–87.
17. Parving A. Hearing problems and hormonal disturbances in the elderly. Acta Otolaryngol 1990; 476(suppl):44–53.
18. Vanasse M, Fischer C, Berthezene F, Roux Y, Volman G, Mornex R. Normal brainstem auditory evoked potentials in adult hypothyroidism. Laryngoscope 1989; 99(3):302–306.
19. Graig F, Smith J. Serum creatine phosphokinase activity in altered thyroid states. J Clin Endocrinol 1965; 25:723–731.
20. Scott KR, Simmons Z, Boyer PJ. Hypothyroid myopathy with a strikingly elevated serum creatine kinase level. Muscle Nerve 2002; 26(1):141–144.
21. Bloomer HA, Papadopoulos NM, Mclane JE. Cerebrospinal fluid gamma globulin concentration in myxedema. J Clin Endocrinol Metab 1960; 20:869–875.

22. Dyck PF, Lambert EH. Polyneuropathy associated with hypothyroidism. J Neuropathol Exp Neurol 1970; 29:631–658.
23. Yamamoto K, Saito K, Takai T. Unusual manifestations in primary hypothyroidism. Prog Clin Biol Res 1983; 116:169–187.
24. Nemni R, Bottacchi E, Fazio R. Polyneuropathy in hypothyroidism: electrophysiologic and morphologic findings in 4 cases. J Neurol Neurosurg Psychiatry 1987; 50:1454–1460.
25. Fincham RW, Cape CA. Neuropathy in myxedema: a study of sensory nerve conduction in the upper extremities. Arch Neurol 1968; 19:464–466.
26. Bastron JA. Neuropathy in diseases of the thyroid and pituitary glands. In: Dyck PJ, Thomas PK, Lambert EH et al., eds. Peripheral Neuropathy. 2nd ed. Philadelphia: WB Saunders, 1986:1833–1846.
27. Khaleeli AA, Griffith DG, Edwards RHT. The clinical presentation of hypothyroid myopathy and its relationship to abnormalities in structure and function of skeletal muscle. Clin Endocrinol 1983; 19:365–376.
28. Klein I, Parker M, Shebert R, Ayyar DR, Levey GS. Hypothyroidism presenting as muscle stiffness and psudohypertrophy: Hoffman's syndrome. Am J Med 1981; 70:891–894.
29. Frank B, Schonle P, Klingelhofer J. Autoimmune thyroiditis and myopathy: reversibility of myopathic alterations under thyroxine therapy. Clin Neurol Neurosurg 1989; 91(3):251–255.
30. Venables GS, Bates D, Shaw A. Hypothyroidism with true myotonia. J Neurol Neurosurg Psychiatry 1978; 41:1013–1015.
31. Shirabe T, Tawara S, Terao A, Araki S. Myxoedematous polyneuropathy: a light and electron microscopy study of peripheral nerve and muscle. J Neurol Neurosurg Psychiatry 1975; 38:241–247.
32. Pollard JD, McLeod JG, Angel Honnibal TG, Verheijden NA. Hypothyroid polyneuropathy: clinical, electro-physiological, and nerve biopsy findings in two cases. J Neurol Sci 1982; 53:461–471.
33. Meier C, Bischoff A. Polyneuropathy in hypothyroidism: clinical and nerve biopsy study of 4 cases. J Neurol 1977; 215:103–114.
34. McComas AJ, Sica REP, McNabb AR, Goldberg WM, Upton ARM. Neuropathy in thyrotoxicosis. N Engl J Med 1973; 289:219–220.
35. Ludin HP, Spiess H, Koenig MP. Neuromuscular dysfunction associated with thyrotoxicosis. Eur Neurol 1969; 2:269–278.
36. Bronsky D, Kaganiec GI, Waldstein SS. An association between the Guillain–Barre syndrome and hyperthyroidism. Am J Med Sci 1964; 247:196–200.
37. Feibel JH, Campa JF. Thyrotoxic neuropathy (Basedow's paraplegia). J Neurol Neurosurg Psychiatry 1976; 39:491–497.
38. Pandit L, Shankar SK, Gayathri N, Pandit A. Acute thyrotoxic neuropathy: Basedow's paraplegia revisited. J Neurol Sci 1998; 155(2):211–214.
39. Fisher M, Mateer JE, Ullrich I, Gutrecht JA. Pyramidal tract deficits and polyneuropathy in hyperthyroidism: combination clinically mimicking amyotrophic lateral sclerosis. Am J Med 1985; 78:1041–1044.
40. Beard L, Kumar A, Estep HL. Bilateral carpal tunnel syndrome caused by Graves' disease. Arch Intern Med 1985; 145:345–346.
41. Ijichi S, Niina K, Tara M. Mononeuropathy associated with hyperthyroidism. J Neurol Neurosurg Psychiatry 1990; 53:1109.
42. Roquer J, Cano JF. Carpal tunnel syndrome and hyperthyroidism: some new observations. J Neurol Sci 1987; 77:237–248.
43. Davidoff LM. Studies in acromegaly III: the anamnesis and symptomatology in 100 cases. Endocrinology 1926; 10:461–483.
44. Low PA, McLeod JG, Turtle JR, Donnelly P, Wright RG. Peripheral neuropathy in acromegaly. Brain 1974; 97(1):139–152.
45. Jamal GA, Kerr DJ, McLellan AR, Weir AI, Davies DL. Generalised peripheral nerve dysfunction in acromegaly: a study by conventional and novel neurophysiological techniques. J Neurol Neurosurg Psychiatry 1987; 50(7):886–894.

46. Dinn JJ, Dinn EI. Natural history of acromegalic peripheral neuropathy. Q J Med 1985; 57(224):833–842.

47. Stewart BM. The hypertrophic neuropathy of acromegaly: a rare neuropathy associated with acromegaly. Arch Neurol 1966; 14(1):107–110.

48. Anagnos A, Ruff RL, Kaminski HJ. Endocrine neuromyopathies. Neurol Clin 1997; 15:673–696.

49. O'Duffy JD, Randall RV, MacCarty CS. Median neuropathy (CTS) in acromegaly: a sign of endocrine overactivity. Ann Intern Med 1973; 78:379–383.

50. Baum H, Ludecke DK, Herrmann HD. Carpal tunnel syndrome and acromegaly. Acta Neurochir 1986; 83:44–45.

51. Sandbank U, Bornstein B, Najanson T. Acidophilic adenoma of the pituitary with polyneuropathy. J Neurol Neurosurg Psychiatry 1974; 37:324–329.

52. Pickett JBE, Layzer RB, Levin SR, Schneider V, Campbell MJ, Sumner AJ. Neuromuscular complications of acromegaly. Neurology 1975; 25:638–645.

53. Jenkins PJ, Sohaib SA, Akker S, Phillips RR, Spillane K, Wass JA, Monson JP, Grossman AB, Besser GM, Reznek RH. The pathology of median neuropathy in acromegaly. Ann Intern Med 2000; 133(3):197–201.

54. Johnston AW. Acroparaesthesiae and acromegaly. Br Med J 1960; 1:1616–1618.

55. Schiller F, Kolb FO. Carpal tunnel syndrome in acromegaly. Neurology 1954; 4:271–282.

56. Luboschitzky R, Barzilai D. Bromocriptine for an acromegalic patient and improvement in cardiac function and carpal tunnel syndrome. J Am Med Assoc 1980; 244:1825–1827.

57. Woltman HW. Neuritis associated with acromegaly. Arch Neurol Psychiatry 1941; 45:680–682.

58. Ruff RL, Weissmann J. Endocrine myopathies. Neurol Clin 1988; 6(3):575–592.

59. Barber J, Butler RC, Davie MW, Sewry CA. Hypoparathyroidism presenting as myopathy with raised creatine kinase. Rheumatology 2001; 40(12):1417–1418.

60. Heckmann JG, Dietrich W, Hohenberger W, Klein P, Hanke B, Neundorfer B. Hypoglycemic sensorimotor polyneuropathy associated with insulinoma. Muscle Nerve 2000; 23:1891–1894.

61. Jaspan JB, Wollman RL, Bernstein L, Rubenstein AH. Hypoglycemic peripheral neuropathy in association with insulinoma: implication of glucopenia rather than hyperinsulinism. Medicine 1982; 61:33–44.

62. Conri C, Ducloux G, Lagueny A, Ferrer M, Vital C. Polyneuropathy in type I multiple endocrine syndrome. Presse Med 1990; 19(6):247–250.

63. Soubrier MJ, Dubost JJ, Sauvezie BJM. POEMS syndrome: a study of 25 cases and a review of the literature. Am J Med 1994; 97:543–553.

64. Nakanishi T, Sobue I, Toyokura Y, Nishitani H, Kuroiwa Y, Satoyoshi E, Tsubaki T, Igata A, Ozaki Y. The Crow–Fukase syndrome: a study of 102 cases in Japan. Neurology 1984; 34:712–720.

65. Feddersen RM, Burgdorf W, Foucar K, Elias L, Smith SM. Plasma cell dyscrasia: a case of POEMS syndrome with a unique dermatologic presentation. J Am Acad Dermatol 1989; 21:1061–1068.

13

Neuropathy and Rheumatologic Disease

Rachel A. Nardin and Seward B. Rutkove
Beth Israel Hospital, Boston, Massachusetts, USA

ABSTRACT

Peripheral neuropathy may occur in nearly all rheumatologic disorders. Vasculitic neuropathy represents the most severe example and is characterized by acute motor and sensory loss in multiple nerve territories associated with prominent pain. Other neuropathic complications occur, including sensory neuronopathy, trigeminal neuropathy, nonvasculitic distal symmetric polyneuropathy, demyelinating polyneuropathy, compression neuropathies, and autonomic neuropathy. Neuropathy usually occurs in the setting of known disease, but may precede rheumatologic symptoms, and the presence of systemic symptoms such as rash, fever, malaise, or renal dysfunction raises the possibility of an associated rheumatologic illness.

Evaluation focuses on electrodiagnostic testing for evidence of primary axon lesions in multiple peripheral nerves (mononeuritis multiplex) or a confluent neuropathy with an asymmetric distribution that suggests a vasculitic neuropathy. Nerve biopsy is definitive for diagnosing vasculitis. Primary demyelinating, compression, and autonomic neuropathies are also identified by electrodiagnostic testing. Treatment depends on the type of neuropathy, and vasculitic neuropathy requires aggressive immunosuppression. Compression neuropathies can be treated conservatively or with surgical decompression. Symmetric polyneuropathies are treated in concert with the underlying rheumatic disease.

1. INTRODUCTION

Rheumatologic diseases represent a variety of syndromes and mechanisms, although most involve some degree of immune dysregulation. Many rheumatologic diseases affect peripheral nerves, giving rise to a spectrum of neuropathies ranging from acute and severe mononeuropathy multiplex to indolent distal symmetric polyneuropathy and compression

Table 13.1 Types of Neuropathy Complicating the Major Rheumatic Diseases

Disease	Neuropathy					
	Sensorimotor	Sensory neuronopathy	Mononeuropathy multiplex	Demyelinating neuropathy	Compressive neuropathies	Trigeminal neuropathy
Vasculitis	+	−	+	−	−	−
RA	+	−	+	−	+	+
Sjögren's	+	+	+	+	+	+
SLE	+	−	+	+	−	+
Scleroderma	+	−	−	−	+	+
MCTD	+	−	−	−	−	+

Note: RA, rheumatoid arthritis; SLE, systemic lupus erythematosus; MCTD, mixed connective tissue disease.

neuropathies (Table 13.1). These neuropathies are most challenging when they are the presenting symptoms of a rheumatologic disease. Given the wide variety of rheumatologic disorders, we have organized our discussion by peripheral nervous system manifestation rather than by rheumatologic disease type. An algorithm assists in the assessment of individuals with known rheumatologic disease who present with involvement of the peripheral nervous system (Fig. 13.1).

2. CLINICAL FEATURES

2.1. Mononeuropathy Multiplex

Mononeuropathy multiplex is a multifocal neuropathy characterized by sensory loss, weakness, and frequently pain, in the distribution of one or more peripheral or cranial nerves. In the setting of known rheumatologic disease, mononeuropathy multiplex is essentially always due to vasculitis, and the onset is typically acute or subacute. Nerve pathology in vasculitis is multifocal nerve ischemia and infarction. Vasculitis usually affects one nerve at a time, in a stepwise fashion, and in 20–40% of patients, nerve involvement is sufficiently discreet that individually involved nerves can be identified clinically. Certain nerves are more commonly involved, perhaps due to restricted collateral blood flow. In the lower extremities, the peroneal division of the sciatic nerve is involved 90% of the time, often in the watershed zone in the mid-thigh (1). In the upper extremity, the ulnar nerve is affected 35–40%, localized most commonly to the upper arm (1). Other nerves include the sural (85%), the posterior tibial nerve (40–70%), and the median nerve (25%) (2–13).

There are frequent exceptions to the classic stepwise presentation. Multiple mononeuropathies may be extensive, and involvement of individual nerves may not be distinguishable clinically (3–5,10–12). In 25–30% of patients, overlap results in a distal, symmetric "stocking-glove" pattern. With questioning, patients may have a history of asymmetric onset or stepwise progression to suggest a vasculitic etiology.

Nerve ischemia affects both motor and sensory and large and small fibers (2,16). However, isolated motor or sensory involvement can occur (4,17). Systemic lupus erythematosis (SLE) and Sjögren's syndrome are also associated with predominantly asymmetric sensory neuropathies with vasculitis of epineurial vessels (14,15). Although burning, dysesthetic pain is common in affected limbs (80%), pain may be absent despite clear motor involvement (16). The typical course is acute or subacute, with steady progression over weeks to months, but occasional patients have an indolent course over years or a stepwise course with quiescent periods of weeks to months. Spontaneous remissions and exacerbations are rare.

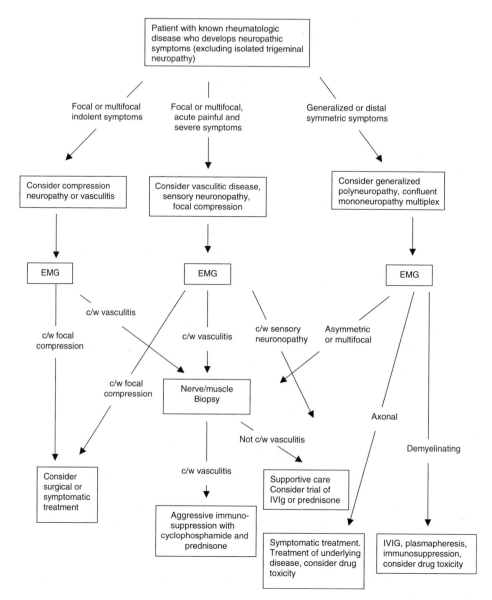

Figure 13.1   Algorithm for evaluation of neuropathic symptoms in patient with known rheumatologic disease.

The term "vasculitis" refers to the pathologic condition of inflammation and necrosis of blood vessel walls. Vasculitis can be primary or secondary. In primary vasculitis, the vasculidesis is the defining feature of the condition. Almost all corrective tissue diseases can cause a secondary vasculitis, or secondary vasculitis can result from exposure to an exogenous antigen such as a drug or infectious agent. The vasculitis involving peripheral nerves can be divided into five main categories based on the size of involved vessels and presumed immunopathologic mechanisms (Table 13.2). As a general rule, an underlying systemic necrotizing vasculitis should be considered in any patient with neuropathy and clinical or laboratory evidence of dysfunction in kidneys, skin, lung, bowel, or liver, particularly if systemic symptoms such as fatigue, anorexia, weight loss, arthralgias, and fevers are also present.

Table 13.2 Classification of the Vasculitides

Vasculitides resulting from immunologic mechanisms
Systemic necrotizing vasculitis
PAN (classic or hepatitis B-associated)
Antineutrophil cytoplasmic antibody (ANCA)-associated
Microscopic polyangiitis
Churg–Strauss syndrome
Wegener's granulomatosis
Vasculitis associated with connective tissue disease
Rheumatoid arthritis
Sjögren's syndrome
Systemic lupus erythematosus
Others
Hypersensitivity vasculitis[a]
Cryoglobulinemic vasculitis[b]
Henoch–Schonlein purpura
Drug-induced vasculitis[b]
Vasculitis associated with malignancy or infection[b]
Giant cell arteritis
Temporal arteritis
Takayasu arteritis
Nonsystemic vasculitic neuropathy
Miscellaneous vasculitides
Behçet's disease
Kawasaki disease
Relapsing polychondritis
Vasculitides resulting from direct infection
Bacterial (syphilis, tuberculosis, Lyme)
Fungal (Cryptococcus, aspergillosis)
Rickettsial (Rocky Mountain spotted fever)
Viral (VZV, CMV, HIV)

[a]Also called cutaneous leukocytoclastic angiitis if skin is the only organ involved.
[b]Also can produce a systemic necrotizing vasculitis.

2.1.1. Systemic Necrotizing Vasculitis

Peripheral nerve involvement occurs in the setting of a heterogeneous group of potentially life-threatening rheumatologic diseases that affect multiple organs, including polyarteritis nodosum (PAN), microscopic polyangiitis, Churg–Strauss syndrome, Wegener's granulomatosis, and vasculitis associated with connective tissue diseases. Most of these disorders involve small- and medium-sized arteries, and all but PAN may involve smaller vessels as well. The incidence of peripheral nerve vasculitis varies: 60% with PAN, 20% with Churg–Strauss syndrome and microscopic polyangiitis, and 15% with Wegener's granulomatosis (18–24).

Systemic symptoms in the systemic vasculitides include fever, fatigue, anorexia, weight loss, and arthralgias. Each rheumatologic disease has a characteristic pattern of organ involvement and laboratory abnormalities. PAN most commonly involves the kidneys, skin, muscle, gastrointestinal tract, and testes. Thirty percent of patients have evidence of hepatitis B infection. Microscopic polyangiitis is typically associated with rapidly progressive glomerulonephritis and palpable purpura, with concurrent pulmonary involvement in 50% of patients (22). Churg–Strauss syndrome is characterized by eosinophilia and asthma, with vasculitis affecting multiple organs, but with a predilection for lung (2,25). Despite the fact that Churg–Strauss syndrome is also known as allergic angiitis and granulomatosis, eosinophilic granulomas are rare in any organ (20%) (25). Wegener's granulomatosis is characterized by granulomas in the respiratory system and prominent involvement of the sinuses, lungs, and kidneys (26,27).

Necrotizing vasculitis can also occur in association with connective tissue diseases, especially RA, and less frequently with Sjögren's syndrome and SLE (28). Vasculitic neuropathy is rare in scleroderma (29–31), Behçet's syndrome (32), and mixed connective tissue disease (33). Nearly 10% of patients with rheumatoid arthritis (RA) develop vasculitic neuropathy, usually in the setting of severe and chronic skin changes, nonarticular manifestations of the disease, and accompanying systemic manifestations such as fever, malaise, weight loss, and cutaneous vasculitis (34,35). The prevalence of vasculitic neuropathy in Sjögren's syndrome is estimated at 5–10% and that in SLE at 5%. The presentation is often a mononeuropathy multiplex (15,36,37), but vasculitic changes have been seen on biopsy in Sjögren's patients with a purely sensory neuropathy and in SLE patients with symmetric motor > sensory neuropathy, and a lumbosacral polyradiculopathy (38).

2.1.2. Hypersensitivity Vasculitis

The term hypersensitivity vasculitis originally described a purely cutaneous vasculitis characterized pathologically by a leukocytoclastic reaction, with a clear history of exposure to a precipitating antigen and clinical resolution within a few weeks. However, the concept has evolved to include a wider range of disorders (Table 13.2), some without clear a precipitant, some with involvement of other organs and requiring immunosuppressive therapy. Vasculitic neuropathy is most common in essential mixed cryoglobulinema (39–41). It is uncommon with other hypersensitivity vasculitides, including the hypersensitivity vasculitis occurring as an immunologic reaction to nearly any type of infection or to a variety of drugs, both illicit (amphetamines, cocaine, and heroin), and prescription (multiple antibiotics, cyclophosphamide, methotrexate, and interferon-alpha) (42,43). Hypersensitivity vasculitis occurs seen as a true paraneoplastic syndrome resulting from an immune response to the tumor with increased frequency in hematologic malignancies, especially hairy cell leukemia (44). The occurrence of hypersensitivity vasculitic neuropathy in association with solid tumors is debated (44–49).

2.1.3. Giant Cell Arteritis

Giant cell arteritis includes Takayasu arteritis and temporal arteritis, which cause giant cell formations in large- and medium-sized arteries. Vasculitis of the peripheral nerves has been reported rarely in temporal arteritis only (50).

2.1.4. Nonsystemic Vasculitic Neuropathy

This is the second most common cause of vasculitic neuropathy. Like PAN, nonsystemic vasculitic neuropathy involves small- and medium-sized arteries of the epineurium and perineurium. As the name implies, clinical involvement is restricted to the peripheral nervous system (4,13), although subclinical involvement of other organs, particularly skeletal muscle, can be demonstrated on biopsy (16,51). Whether this condition is a true organ-specific vasculitis or a restricted form of PAN is unclear. The course of nonsystemic vasculitic neuropathy is more indolent, and the prognosis more benign, than that of PAN.

2.1.5. Vasculitis from Direct Infection

Peripheral nerve vasculitis has been reported in association with many bacterial, fungal, rickettsial, and viral agents (Table 13.2). In cases with herpes zoster and cytomegalovirus infection, the vasculitis may result from direct invasion of the vessel wall, but most cases are thought to be due to secondary deposition of immune complexes in involved vessels.

2.2. Sensory Neuronopathy

Patients with sensory neuronopathy present with paresthesias and dysesthesias involving limbs, trunk, and face. At onset, the distribution of the sensory abnormalities is typically asymmetric and not length-dependent, but often becomes symmetric with disease progression. Loss of proprioception leads to sensory ataxia, and this disorder is also called ataxic sensory neuronopathy. Accompanying autonomic dysfunction is common, causing tonic pupils, orthostatic hypotension, anhidrosis, and facial flushing. Onset varies from acute to chronic. Examination shows prominent large-fiber sensory loss, with less prominent loss of small-fiber sensory modalities. Sensory ataxia, pseudoathetosis, and areflexia are usually seen. Strength is normal (52–55).

2.3. Polyneuropathy

2.3.1. Axonal Polyneuropathy

Symmetric axonal sensorimotor neuropathy is a common manifestation of most rheumatologic diseases. Although such neuropathies may result from chronic vasculitis affecting multiple nerves, differentiating confluent vasculitic mononeuropathies from nonvasculitic sensorimotor neuropathies is not always straightforward. More often, there is no clear vasculitic component. A history of discrete multiple mononeuropathies or a prominent asymmetry supports a vasculitic cause. Nerve biopsy can help with the diagnosis. When a definite distinction between a nonvasculitic sensorimotor neuropathy and a confluent vasculitic mononeuropathy multiplex cannot be made, treatment is guided by the severity and progression of the neuropathy.

Rheumatoid Arthritis. The prevalence of neuropathy in RA varies markedly from 10% to 75% (56,57). This is due in part to different criteria used to assess the presence or absence of neuropathy, with the higher percentage when the diagnosis is based on detailed clinical and electrophysiologic examinations. Patients typically present with distal paresthesias and sensory loss involving all modalities. Neuropathic pain may also be present. In more advanced cases, gait problems may also be present, but these may be difficult to sort out from underlying arthritic problems. Although the neuropathy may present as a symptomatic disorder, it is often found incidentally on examination.

Systemic Lupus Erythematosus. Approximately 5–20% of patients with SLE develop symptoms and signs of a distal symmetric neuropathy (58,59). Mild paresthesias, pain, and sensory loss in the feet are the most common presenting symptoms (14,15). Nerve conduction abnormalities greater than expected for age occurred in 33% of patients followed over a 7 year period (60). There is no clear association between the deteriorating nerve function and medications or other disease-associated factors. GM1 antibodies have also been found to be elevated in SLE patients with and without neuropathy, whereas antisulfatide antibody levels are normal (61). Although biopsy generally reveals distal axonal loss, demyelinating and vasculitic pathology may also occur.

Sjögren's Syndrome. Sjögren's syndrome is strongly associated with a sensory neuronopathy, but a distal sensory neuropathy occurs more frequently, affecting three-quarters of patients (62–64). Patients present with typical distal sensory loss, pain, and paresthesias affecting the feet. This is in contrast to the symptoms of sensory neuronopathy, in which paresthesias affect the arm, trunk, and face with predominantly "large-fiber" symptoms including ataxia. The absence of generalized autonomic manifestations (such as orthostatic hypotension) also suggests neuropathy rather than sensory neuronopathy. Electrodiagnostic tests are helpful in distinguishing the two entities. In Sjögren's-associated neuropathy, abnormalities tend to be distally predominant and relatively symmetric, whereas in sensory neuronopathy, sensory responses are reduced more diffusely and asymmetrically. In some patients, however, differentiating neuropathy from sensory neuronopathy may not be possible, either clinically or electrodiagnostically.

Scleroderma. Neuropathy was initially thought to occur only rarely in scleroderma (65). However, with careful examination and electrodiagnostic testing, it is clear that mild, nonvasculitic neuropathy probably occurs in up to 25% (30,31,66).

Behçet's. Axonal polyneuropathy appears to be exceptionally rare in Behçet's syndrome (67).

Other Diseases. Symmetric neuropathy has been reported in mixed connective tissue disease (68), and in the rare syndrome of relapsing polychondritis (69). We have identified two patients with symptoms of neuropathy in the setting of psoriatic arthritis (unpublished data).

2.3.2. Demyelinating Polyneuropathy

Rare reports of demyelinating neuropathies have been associated with nearly every rheumatologic disease. Chronic inflammatory demyelinating polyradiculoneuropathy (CIDP) has been associated with RA (70). Predominantly demyelinating neuropathy has been reported in Sjögren's and Behçet's syndromes (71–73). SLE appears most strongly associated with demyelinating neuropathies. Acute inflammatory demyelinating polyradiculoneuropathy has occurred as a presenting symptom of SLE (74–76), and there are multiple reports of CIDP associated with SLE (77–80). Drug-induced SLE has also been associated with CIDP (81). The Miller–Fisher syndrome has also been described in SLE (82). Mixed connective tissue disease has also been associated with a CIDP-like neuropathy (83,84). Scleroderma appears to be the only major connective tissue disease with which a demyelinating neuropathy has not been associated.

2.4. Trigeminal Neuropathy

Trigeminal neuropathy, affecting sensory fibers, occurs as a complication of Sjögren's syndrome, SLE, scleroderma, and mixed connective tissue disease (85–87). It is the most common neurological complication of scleroderma and complicates scleroderma more often than other connective tissue diseases (86). When it occurs in association with Sjögren's syndrome, it is usually part of a more widespread sensory neuronopathy (88,89).

Patients with trigeminal neuropathy present with facial numbness involving the second, third, or less commonly, the first division of the nerve. Oropharyngeal involvement is common. Onset is usually gradual, although can be acute or subacute (86,90). More than half of patients eventually have bilateral symptoms and pain is common (91). Motor fibers are usually spared. Symptoms progress for months to a few years and then stabilize, with occasional spontaneous remissions described (86). Other cranial nerves can be affected, and patients with Sjögren's syndrome rarely have a syndrome of cranial polyneuropathy that is self-limited but occasionally recurrent (89).

2.5. Compression Neuropathies

Compression mononeuropathies are more common than vasculitic neuropathies in patients with known rheumatologic disease.

2.5.1. Median Neuropathy

The incidence of carpal tunnel syndrome in RA is 10–40% (92–94). The incidence is 5–20% of patients with Sjögren's syndrome (62,95) and 25% with SLE (96). Compressive neuropathies are attributed to fibrotic changes, calcium deposition, and tophaceous gout (99–101).

2.5.2. Ulnar Neuropathy

RA may predispose to ulnar neuropathy at the elbow, with an incidence of 15–20% (102). Tophaceous gout has been found in the ulnar groove (99) and proximal forearm (103). Proximal ulnar neuropathy can be due to vasculitis and distinguishing between the two can be difficult, but electrodiagnostic studies are helpful.

2.5.3. Peroneal Neuropathy

Peroneal neuropathy at the fibular head occurs rarely in the rheumatologic disorders and often arises as a consequence of prolonged bed rest (104). Peroneal neuropathy has been associated with the formation of Baker's cysts in patients with RA (104). Isolated peroneal neuropathy at the fibular head could be confused with a vasculitic lesion affecting the proximal peroneal nerve, and electrodiagnostic studies are helpful.

2.5.4. Tibial Neuropathy

Tibial neuropathy at the ankle (tarsal tunnel syndrome) is rare, but electrodiagnostic evidence may be found in 10% (105).

2.5.5. Other Compression Neuropathies

A variety of other focal compressive neuropathies have been found in RA, including anterior and posterior interosseous neuropathies, digital neuropathy, and sciatic neuropathy (104,106,107).

2.6. Autonomic Neuropathy

Autonomic neuropathy has been associated with many rheumatologic disorders. Dysfunction in lacrimal and salivary glands in Sjögren's syndrome may include autonomic dysfunction (108). Autonomic dysfunction has been found in RA (109) and SLE (110). Autonomic dysfunction in scleroderma has been related to sympathetic over activity and parasympathetic under activity and possibly associated with secondary cardiac events (111). Abnormalities in sympathetic skin response have also been identified in scleroderma (112). Acute autonomic neuropathy has also been described in mixed connective tissue disease (113). Prominent autonomic symptoms and abnormal testing have also been reported in Behçet's syndrome (114–116).

3. LABORATORY EVALUATION

3.1. Screening Tests without Known Rheumatologic Disease

When a patient presents with an acute picture of mononeuropathy multiplex, suspicion for an underlying rheumatologic disorder is high and a complete work-up, often including tissue biopsy, is warranted. However, in patients who present with more indolent problems, such as distal symmetric neuropathy or compression neuropathies, screening laboratory tests are appropriate and include complete blood count, erythrocyte sedimentation rate, antinuclear antibodies, and rheumatoid factor.

3.2. Evaluation in Patients with Known or Suspected Rheumatologic Disease

3.2.1. Mononeuropathy Multiplex

Diagnostic evaluation centers on determining whether the neuronal injury is vasculitic, and if so, determining the responsible underlying disease. An expanded list of laboratory tests includes serum chemistries, liver and renal function studies, urinalysis, serum auto-antibody assays (Table 13.3), and a chest X-ray. Serologic testing for antineutrophil cytoplasmic antibodies (ANCAs) can also be helpful to diagnose Churg–Strauss syndrome, Wegener's granulomatosis, and microscopic polyangiitis. ANCAs have been divided into c-ANCA, with a cytoplasmic staining pattern, and p-ANCA, with a perinuclear pattern; c-ANCA and p-ANCA are usually directed against proteinase 3 and myeloperoxidase, respectively. c-ANCA is a sensitive and specific marker for Wegener's granulomatosis, whereas p-ANCA has good sensitivity but has poor specificity for Churg–Strauss syndrome and microscopic polyangiitis (121).

Electrodiagnostic studies can demonstrate a pattern consistent with mononeuropathy multiplex, and nerve conduction studies can assist in identifying a nerve appropriate for biopsy (i.e., one which is mildly to moderately affected). Electrodiagnostically, vasculitic mononeuropathy multiplex is an axonal neuropathy involving individual nerves. Nerve conduction studies show reduced motor and sensory amplitudes with normal or mildly slowed conduction velocities. An ischemic "pseudo-conduction block" has been described within 7–10 days of acute ischemic injury, but is transient and disappears with axon degeneration (117–119). Widespread vasculitic neuropathy may appear confluent on electrodiagnostic testing, but disparities in motor or sensory amplitudes, either between individual nerves in a single limb or between the same nerve on both sides, or greater

Table 13.3 Serologic Tests in Rheumatic Diseases

Test	RA	Sjögren's	SLE	Scleroderma	MCTD	WG	PAN	Normals
Rheumatoid factors	80–90	75–90	20–40	25–30	50–60	50–60	15–20	5–20[a]
ANCA	15–25	5–15	10–20	1–5		85–100	5–10	
ANA screen	30–40	80–95	90–100	75–95	95–100		20–25	5–7
Centromere				60–80				
Topoisomerase				20–40				
dsDNA	15–40		60–70					
ssDNA	15–20	10–20	60–70	10–20	10–20			
Histones	15–20		50–70	25–30	10–20			
Smith (Sm)				30–40				
U1-RNP				35–50	5–15			
SS-A (Ro)			60–70	25–40				
SS-B (La)			40–60	10–45				

[a]Prevalence increases with age.

Note: Prevalence as percent of all cases. Nonspecific tests: C3, C4, CH50, absolute eosinophil count.

amplitude reduction in the upper compared to the lower limbs, suggest a multifocal, nonlength-dependent process.

Needle electromyography (EMG) usually reveals evidence of subacute denervation, consisting of fibrillation potentials and positive sharp waves, and decreased motor unit action potential recruitment. If neurogenic injury is <2–3 weeks old, only reduced motor unit potential recruitment will be seen, and if injury is old (chronic) long-duration, polyphasic motor unit action potentials will be seen. Rarely, myopathic motor units are seen suggesting additional involvement of muscle (120). Abnormalities are distributed in a nonlength-dependent fashion, often with significant proximal involvement.

Nerve biopsy should be performed in most patients with suspected vasculitic neuropathy to confirm the diagnosis. Nerve biopsy may not be required in a patient with vasculitis demonstrated on biopsy of an alternative tissue in the setting of a classic, painful, axonal, mononeuropathy multiplex. The diagnostic yield is increased if muscle is also biopsied (10,16). Sural, superficial peroneal, superficial radial, or the intermediate cutaneous nerve of the thigh are candidate nerves.

The pathologic appearance of vasculitis in peripheral nerve varies according to the age of the lesion. T-cell and macrophage infiltration with necrosis of vessel walls is seen in early, active lesions, and these changes are necessary for a definite diagnosis of vasculitis (12,122–124). Epineurial and perineurial vessels are preferentially involved over endoneurial vessels (2–5). Perivascular inflammatory infiltrates alone can occur in other types of neuropathy, and are insufficient for diagnosing vasculitis. Vasculitic changes are associated with axon degeneration and loss, usually of differing severity and extent between adjacent fascicles and within individual fascicles (1,3–5,12,125).

Immunohistochemical staining shows vascular deposits of immunoglobulin and complement in 80% of cases (5,12,13,124). More chronic lesions show thrombosis and vascular recanalization, intimal proliferation, medial hypertrophy, and hemosiderin deposits (126). However, because vasculitis is a multifocal process, an involved vessel may be missed simply due to restricted nerve sampling. The sensitivity of combined nerve and muscle biopsy for vasculitis is 60% (16). In some patients with a suggestive clinical and laboratory picture, a diagnosis must be made presumptively based on less specific biopsy findings which only indirectly suggest vasculitis; these include perivascular inflammation, occlusion of vessels with recanalization, vascular hemosiderin or immunoglobulin deposits, and asymmetric nerve fiber loss (4,13,16,127).

3.2.2. Sensory Neuronopathy

Electrodiagnostic testing shows reduced sensory response amplitudes with normal or minimally slowed conduction velocities, and in more severe cases, responses may be entirely absent. H-reflexes and blink reflexes are typically absent (52–55). Motor nerve conduction studies and F-wave latencies are preserved. Needle EMG is usually normal, although mild denervation may be present (54). Magnetic resonance imaging (MRI) of the cervicothoracic spine may show dorsal column signal abnormalities consistent with degeneration of central dorsal root ganglion projections (128). Nerve biopsy shows loss of large myelinated fibers and scattered perivascular inflammatory cells (52,54). Dorsal root ganglion biopsies can be done in difficult cases; a ganglionopathy with cytotoxic CD^{8+} T cells surrounding neurons is diagnostic of this syndrome (54,55).

Laboratory testing in patients with sensory neuronopathy is directed at confirming Sjögren's syndrome and includes a Schirmer test for reduced tear production or rose bengal staining for keratoconjunctivitis, minor salivary gland biopsy showing mononuclear cell infiltrates, and tests of salivary gland dysfunction such as salivary scintigraphy, parotid sialography, or documentation of reduced unstimulated salivary flow (≤ 1.5 mL in 15 min). Antibodies to Ro/SS-A have a sensitivity of 60–70%, and antibodies to La/SS-B have a sensitivity of 40–60% (129).

3.2.3. Symmetric Polyneuropathy

Electrodiagnostic testing is used to identify the symmetric distribution of the neuropathy and to determine the primary pathology, axonal, or demyelinating.

3.2.4. Trigeminal Neuropathy

This is largely a clinical diagnosis. Electrodiagnostic testing may show abnormal blink reflexes and needle EMG of facial muscles is usually normal (86). MRI helps to exclude alternative causes.

3.2.5. Compression Neuropathy

Nerve conduction studies are used to differentiate focal compression neuropathy from mononeuritis mutiplex.

3.2.6. Autonomic Neuropathy

Bedsides tests for autonomic neuropathy, such as pupillary function and orthostatic blood pressure measurements, can be supplemented by tilt table testing, quantitative sudomotor autonomic reflex testing, and heart rate variability with deep breathing.

4. DIFFERENTIAL DIAGNOSIS

4.1. Vasculitic Neuropathy

Other asymmetric, nonvasculitic neuropathies include multifocal demyelinating neuropathy (Lewis–Sumner syndrome), diabetic or idiopathic lumbosacral radiculoplexopathy, multifocal motor neuropathy, sarcoidosis, Lyme neuropathy, multiple nerve entrapments, malignant infiltration of nerve, and hereditary neuropathy with liability to pressure palsies.

4.2. Sensory Neuronopathy

Other causes of sensory neuronopathy include paraneuplastic syndromes which are frequently associated with anti-Hu antibodies (130), high doses of pyridoxine (131), and monoclonal gammopathies (132).

4.3. Polyneuropathy

Other relatively common causes of neuropathies include diabetes, uremia, and CIDP. Another consideration is medication toxicity. Medications used to treat rheumatologic disease can produce neuropathies including chloroquine, dapsone, tacrolimus (FK-506), thalidomide, gold, D-penicillamine, colchicine, and cyclosporine (133). Most cause an axonal peripheral neuropathy, whereas tacrolimus can produce a predominantly demyelinating disorder.

4.4. Trigeminal Neuropathy

Isolated trigeminal neuropathy occurs rarely as the sole manifestation of other disorders. Brainstem demyelination and infectious processes (Lyme disease, syphilis) should be considered.

4.5. Compression Neuropathies

A differential diagnosis is usually not warranted. In patients who have multiple compressive neuropathies, hereditary neuropathy with predisposition to pressure palsies should be considered.

4.6. Autonomic Neuropathies

Autonomic dysfunction can occur with diabetes. Rare central causes include multiple system atrophy with dysautonomia (Shy–Drager syndrome).

5. MANAGEMENT AND PROGNOSIS

5.1. Mononeuropathy Multiplex

Treatment focuses on the underlying vasculitis and has three main components: removal of antigenic stimuli, immunosuppression, and supportive care. Most vasculitides have no identifiable antigenic stimulus, but possible stimuli include drugs, infectious agents, or concurrent malignancy (134–138).

Immunosuppression is required for almost all patients with vasculitic neuropathy. Corticosteroids alone are appropriate for nonsystemic vasculitic when the neuropathy is mild and relatively stable (13). In the setting of SLE or Sjögren's syndrome and a distal, predominantly sensory neuropathy, corticosteroids alone are also effective. In mild cases, prednisone can be given orally, and in more severe cases corticosteroids can be given as intravenous methylprednisolone (1 gm/day for the first 5–6 days, followed by oral prednisone 1.5 mg/kg per day) (143). After 3–4 weeks of therapy, prednisone is usually switched to an every other day schedule, then gradually tapered by 5 mg every 2–3 weeks. If relapse occurs during tapering, intravenous methylprednisolone or higher doses of oral prednisone can be given.

In more severe cases of systemic vasculitis, addition of a cytotoxic agent, such as cyclophosphamide, is appropriate (139–142). Cyclophosphamide is frequently given concurrently with corticosteroids. Options include oral cyclophosphamide (1.5–2.5 mg/kg per day, or up to 5 mg/kg per day) (140–144), usually continued for at least 1 year after disease stabilization and then tapered over weeks to months. Intravenous pulse cyclophosphamide (15 mg/kg, every 1–4 weeks) has fewer adverse effects than oral delivery, although a higher relapse rate has been reported (20–50%) (145–148). A second approach to minimize the bladder toxicity and other adverse effects of cyclophosphamide is to switch to an alternative immunosuppressant once remission is achieved, usually after 3–6 months (142,149). Small, uncontrolled studies have shown that remission can also be maintained with other immunosuppressive agents including methotrexate (150), cyclosporine (148), and mycophenolate (151).

For refractory disease, intravenous immunoglobulin (IVIG) has been shown effective (152–155). Plasma exchange does not appear to be effective (156) except in some cases of hepatitis B-associated or cryoglobulinemic vasculitis (134,157). Other nonstandard therapies include cyclosporine (158), antithymocyte globulin (159), and monoclonal anti-T-cell antibodies (160). Investigational therapies include interferon-alpha (139), leflunomide (139), tumor necrosis factor antagonists like etanercept (161), anti-adhesion molecule, or anti-T-cell monoclonal antibodies (139,162), and high-dose chemotherapy with autologous stem cell rescue (163).

It is critical for the treating clinician to monitor carefully for medication side effects, which are common with the drugs used to treat vasculitic neuropathy. Up to 70% of vasculitis patients experience treatment-related morbidity due to medication toxicity, opportunistic infections, or treatment-related malignancy (26,147). The most common side effects seen with corticosteroid treatment are hypertension, glucose intolerance, electrolyte imbalance, weight gain, glaucoma, cataracts, osteoporosis, steroid myopathy, and avascular necrosis of the hip and other bones (164). Ideally, patients should have a tuberculin skin test before treatment and receive antituberculous therapy if positive. A low-calorie, low-sodium, low-carbohydrate, high-protein diet will limit weight gain and minimize hypertension and hyperglycemia. Calcium (1000–1500 mg/day) and vitamin D (400–800 IU/day) supplementation, estrogen replacement in postmenopausal women, exercise involving axial stress, and for elderly patients or patients with a low bone density on baseline bone density screening, bisphosphonates (aledronate 5–10 mg/day or 70 mg/week or risedronate 5 mg/day) will limit osteoporosis and reduce the risk of pathologic fracture (165,166). Patients who do suffer a fracture likely merit calcitonin therapy. Pneumocystis carinii pneumonia occurs in up to 20% of vasculitis patients treated with corticosteroids and another cytotoxic agent; in these patients, long-term trimethoprim/sulfamethoxazole prophylaxis three times per week is recommended (147,167,168).

For patients treated with cyclophosphamide, hemorrhagic cystitis occurs in up to 40% of patients; patients should be monitored for microscopic hematuria monthly, should drink at least eight glasses of water/day and urinate frequently (26). There is a 30-fold increased risk of bladder cancer in patients treated with cyclophosphamide compared to controls, with a risk of 5% at 10 years and 16% at 15 years (26,169). Complete blood counts must be monitored monthly due to the risk of bone marrow suppression.

The prognosis for vasculitic neuropathy is dependent on the underlying disease. In nonsystemic vasculitis, mortality is <10%. The neuropathy has a relatively good prognosis, with 75% experiencing a good recovery. Relapses occur in 20% and spread to other organ system in 35% over 5 years (2–7,9,13,170,171). With systemic vasculitis, neuropathy mortality is ∼30%. Significant improvement in the neuropathy occurs in 65% (2–7,9,13,170).

5.2. Sensory Neuronopathy

There are anecdotal reports of improvement of sensory neuronopathy due to Sjögren's syndrome with IVIG (172), prednisone (54), and D-penicillamine (173).

5.3. Symmetric Polyneuropathy

There are no specific treatments for axonal polyneuropathy associated with the rheumatologic diseases, and treatment is directed to the underlying vasculitis. Demyelinating neuropathies may be treated with corticosteroids, plasmapheresis, and IVIG.

5.4. Trigeminal Neuropathy

There is no specific treatment for trigeminal neuropathy, and after a period of progression, deficits usually remain stable or occasionally spontaneously remit (86).

5.5. Compression Neuropathy

Surgical release is appropriate if symptoms are severe or there is axonal damage (99).

5.6. Autonomic Neuropathy

There are no specific treatments for the autonomic neuropathy. Severe orthostasis can be treated with compression stockings, alpha agonists, or fludrocortisone is often very helpful.

6. PATHOGENESIS

6.1. Mononeuropathy Multiplex

Immune-mediated inflammation and necrosis of blood vessel walls results in compromise of the vessel lumen. The nerve ischemia causes axonal degeneration. Unmyelinated fibers are relatively resistant to ischemia, but can be damaged with extensive vasculitis (125). Small blood vessels (50–300 μm) in the vasa nervorum are affected, most prominent in watershed areas between the distributions of major nutrient arteries of proximal nerves (1). Although there is rich anastomotic blood supply of peripheral nerve, the poor auto-regulatory capacity of peripheral nerve and the wide spacing of endoneurial capillaries in the center of nerves compared with other tissues contribute to the susceptibility of peripheral nerve to ischemia (174). True nerve infarcts are rare.

It is likely that several mechanisms trigger and perpetuate the immunologic processes depending on the inciting agent (175). In immune complex-mediated vasculitis, antigen–antibody complexes form in the circulation and deposit in blood vessel walls or antibody may be directed against endothelial cell antigens directly. The immune complexes activate complement, resulting in formation of membrane attack complex, and generate chemotactic factors which attract neutrophils to the vessels, damaging them via toxic oxygen radical formation and release of proteolytic enzymes. This process is termed leukocytoclasia, and hence the term leukocytoclastic vasculitis. This mechanism may be important in vasculitis associated with the connective tissue diseases where multiple auto-antibodies are generated, such as SLE, or the hypersensitivity vasculitis where an exogenous antigen can be identified. Antibody mechanisms may also be important in ANCA-positive vasculitis (176).

Vasculitis may include cell-mediated cytotoxicity. Cytotoxic T-cells are observed in nerve biopsies from patients with vasculitic neuropathy (2,12,124). Cytotoxic T-cells may be directed against endogenous or exogenous antigens expressed by endothelial cells (175).

6.2. Sensory Neuronopathy

In Sjögren's syndrome, sensory neuronopathy results from extraglandular infiltration of dorsal root ganglia by lymphocytes, largely cytotoxic T-cells, with resultant degeneration of sensory neurons (54,55). The trigger of this T-cell-mediated attack on dorsal root ganglia cells is unknown.

6.3. Symmetric Polyneuropathy

Symmetric peripheral neuropathy may develop in the rheumatologic diseases for a number of reasons. In RA, intimal thickening has been found in the endoneurial and epineurial vessels with associated perivascular mononuclear infiltration (177,178). Vasculitis has also been found in some patients with mild sensorimotor neuropathy (35). Anti-ganglioside antibodies have been observed in 40% of patients with RA, and a correlation between the severity of the neuropathy and the level of antibodies was also found (179). Elevations of an antineuroblastoma cell antibody and antibodies to neurofilament polypeptides have also been found in RA patients with a neuropathy (180,181). In SLE, perivascular mononuclear cell infiltration and variable intimal thickening have been described without evidence of frank vasculitis, suggesting involvement of another immune mechanism (15). Although the explanation for neuropathy development in Sjögren's syndrome remains uncertain, some form of small vessel vasculitis has been implicated. Approximately one-third of patients who have evidence for cutaneous vasculitis have a concomitant axonal neuropathy (182). In patients with what appears to be distal symmetric peripheral neuropathy, evidence for a vasculitic component has also been found on biopsy (62,183), although often only evidence for a typical axon loss neuropathy is identified (63,89). In patients with Behçet's, the mechanism of neuropathy remains elusive, but may relate directly to ischemia affecting the distal nerve trunk.

Demyelinating neuropathies in rheumatoid disorders are likely similar to acquired forms and probably involve antibodies against components of myelin.

6.4. Trigeminal Neuropathy

Trigeminal neuropathy is presumed to occur at the level of the trigeminal sensory ganglion. There are no reported pathological studies, but an inflammatory ganglionopathy, as seen in sensory neuronopathy seems most likely.

6.5. Compression Neuropathy

Contributing factors include swelling and inflammation (bursitis and tenosynovitis) in conjunction with postinflammatory effects such as tissue proliferation, fibrosis, and adhesions (104,184). In RA, rheumatoid nodules on tendons in the region of the wrist can contribute (106). Tophi directly compressing the ulnar and median nerves have been reported (99,100,103). Peroneal neuropathies are associated with popliteal (Baker's) cysts (104).

6.6. Autonomic Neuropathy

Autonomic neuropathy probably develops through the same mechanisms that lead to symmetric neuropathies. Tissue fibrosis may have a role in the scleroderma (185).

REFERENCES

1. Dyck P, Conn D, Ozaki H. Necrotizing angiopathic neuropathy: three-dimensional morphology of fiber degeneration related to sites of occluded vessels. Mayo Clin Proc 1972; 47:461–475.
2. Hattori N, Ichimura M, Nagamatsu M, Li M, Yamamoto K, Kumazawa K, Mitsuma T, Sobue G. Clinicopathological features of Churg–Strauss syndrome-associated neuropathy. Brain 1999; 122:427–439.
3. Kissel J, Slivka A, Warmolts J, Mendell J. The clinical spectrum of necrotizing angiopathy of the peripheral nervous system. Ann Neurol 1985; 18:251–257.
4. Dyck P, Benstead T, Conn D, Stevens J, Windebank A, Low P. Nonsystemic vasculitic neuropathy. Brain 1987; 110:843–854.
5. Hawke S, Davies L, Pamphlett R, Guo Y, Pollard J, McLeod J. Vasculitic neuropathy: a clinical and pathological study. Brain 1991; 114:2175–2190.
6. Moore P, Fauci A. Neurologic manifestations of systemic vasculitis: a retrospective study of the clinicopathologic features and responses to therapy in 25 patients. Am J Med 1981; 71:517–524.
7. Chang R, Bell C, Hallett M. Clinical characteristics and prognosis of vasculitic mononeuropathy multiplex. Arch Neurol 1984; 41:618–621.
8. Bouche P, Leger J, Travers M, Cathala H, Castaigne P. Peripheral neuropathy in systemic vasculitis: clinical and electrophysiologic study of 22 patients. Neurology 1986; 36:1598–1602.

9. Harati Y, Niakan E. The clinical spectrum of inflammatory-angiopathic neuropathy. J Neurol Neurosurg Psychiatry 1986; 49:1313–1316.

10. Said G, Lacroix-Ciaudo C, Fujimura H, Blas C, Faux N. The peripheral neuropathy of necrotizing arteritis: a clinicopathological study. Ann Neurol 1988; 23:461–465.

11. Nicolai A, Bonetti B, Lazzarino L, Ferrari S, Monaco S, Rizzuto N. Peripheral nerve vasculitis: a clinico-pathological study. Clin Neuropathol 1995; 14:137–141.

12. Panegyres P, Blumbergs P, Leong A-Y, Bourne A. Vasculitis of peripheral nerve and skeletal muscle: clinicopathological correlation and immuno-pathogenic mechanisms. J Neurol Sci 1990; 100:193–202.

13. Davies L, Spies J, Pollard J, McLeod J. Vasculitis confined to peripheral nerves. Brain 1996; 119:1441–1448.

14. Omdal R, Henriksen OA, Mellgren SI, Husby G. Peripheral neuropathy in systemic lupus erythematosus. Neurology 1991; 41:808–811.

15. McCombe PA, McLeod JG, Pollard JD, Guo YP, Ingall TJ. Peripheral sensorimotor and autonomic neuropathy associated with systemic lupus erythematosus. Clinical, pathological and immunological features. Brain 1987; 110:533–549.

16. Collins M, Mendell J, Periquet M, Sahenk Z, Amato A, Gronseth G, Barohn R, Jackson C, Kissel J. Superficial peroneal nerve/peroneus brevis muscle biopsy in vasculitic neuropathy. Neurology 2000; 55:636–643.

17. Lacomis D, Giuliani M, Steen V, Powell H. Small fiber neuropathy and vasculitis. Arthritis Rheum 1997; 40:1173–1177.

18. Guillevin L, Cohen P, Gayraud M, Lhote F, Jarrousse B, Casassus P. Churg–Strauss syndrome. Clinical study and long-term follow-up of 96 patients. Medicine (Baltimore) 1999; 78:26–37.

19. Guillevin L, Du L, Godeau P, Jais P, Wechsler B. Clinical findings and prognosis of polyarteritis nodosa and Churg–Strauss angiitis: a study in 165 patients. Br J Rheumatol 1988; 27:258–264.

20. Oh S, Herrasa G, Spalding D. Eosinophilic vasculitic neuropathy in the Churg–Strauss syndrome. Arthritis Rheum 1986; 29:1173–1175.

21. Marazzi R, Pareyson D, Boiardi A, Corbo M, Scaioli V, Sghirlanzoni A. Peripheral nerve involvement in Churg–Strauss syndrome. J Neurol 1992; 239:317–321.

22. Guillevin L, Durand-Gasselin B, Cevallos R, Gayraud M, Lhote F, Callard P, Amouroux J, Casassus P, Jarrousse B. Microscopic polyangiitis: clinical and laboratory findings in eighty-five patients. Arthritis Rheum 1999; 42:421–430.

23. Duna G, Galperin C, Hoffman G. Wegener's granulomatosis. Rheum Dis Clin North Am 1995; 21:949–986.

24. Nishino H, Rubino F, Parisi J. The spectrum of neurologic involvement in Wegener's granulomatosis. Neurology 1993; 43:1334–1337.

25. Masi A, Hunder G, Lie J, Michel B, Bloch D, Arend W, Calabrese L, Edworthy S, Fauci A, Leavitt R et al. The American College of Rheumatology 1990 criteria for the classification of Churg–Strauss syndrome. Arthritis Rheum 1990; 33:1094–1100.

26. Hoffman G, Kerr G, Leavitt R, Hallahan C, Lebovics R, Travis W, Rottem M, Fauci A. Wegener granulomatosis: an analysis of 158 patients. Ann Intern Med 1992; 116:488–498.

27. Leavitt R, Fauci A, Bloch D, Michel B, Hunder G, Arend W, Calabrese L, Fries J, Lie J, Lightfoot R. The American College of Rheumatology 1990 criteria for classification of Wegener's granulomatosis. Arthritis Rheum 1990; 33:1101–1107.

28. Bacon P, Carruthers D. Vasculitis associated with connective tissue disorders. Rheum Dis Clin North Am 1995; 21:1077–1096.

29. Dyck P, Hunder G, Dyck P. A case-control and nerve biopsy study of CREST multiple mononeuropathy. Neurology 1997; 49:1641–1645.

30. Hietaharju A, Jaaskelainen S, Kalimo H, Hietarintu M. Peripheral neuromuscular manifestations in systemic sclerosis (scleroderma). Muscle Nerve 1993; 16:1204–1212.

31. Schady W, Sheard A, Hassell A, Holt L, Jayson MI, Klimiuk P. Peripheral nerve dysfunction in scleroderma. Q J Med 1991; 80:661–675.

32. Serdaroglu P, Yazici H, Ozdemir C, Yurdakul S, Bahar S, Aktin E. Neurologic involvement in Behçet's syndrome. A prospective study. Arch Neurol 1989; 46:265–269.

33. Bennett E, O'Connell D. Mixed connective tissue disease: a clinicopathologic study of 20 cases. Semin Arthritis Rheum 1980; 10:25–51.

34. Scott D, Bacon P, Tribe C. Systemic rheumatoid vasculitis: a clinical and laboratory study of 50 cases. Medicine 1981; 60:288–297.

35. Puechal X, Said G, Hilliquin P, Coste J, Job-Deslandre C, Lacroix C, Menkes CJ. Peripheral neuropathy with necrotizing vasculitis in rheumatoid arthritis. A clinicopathologic and prognostic study of thirty-two patients. Arthritis Rheum 1995; 38:1618–1629.

36. Tsokos M, Lazaron S, Moutsopoulos H. Vasculitis in Sjögren's syndrome: histologic classification and clinical presentation. Am J Clin Pathol 1987; 88:26–31.

37. Mellgren S, Conn D, Steven J, Dyck P. Peripheral inflammatory vascular disease in Sjögren's syndrome: association with nervous system complications. Arthritis Rheum 1989; 28:1341–1347.

38. Stefurak TL, Midroni G, Bilbao JM. Vasculitic polyradiculopathy in systemic lupus erythematosus. J Neurol Neurosurg Psychiatry 1999; 66:658–661.

39. Nemni R, Corbo M, Fazio R, Quattrini A, Comi G, Canal N. Cryoglobulinemic neuropathy. A clinical, morphological and immunocytochemical study of 8 cases. Brain 1988; 111:541–552.

40. Gemignani F, Pavesi G, Fiocchi A, Manganelli P, Ferraccioli G, Marbini A. Peripheral neuropathy in essential mixed cryoglobulinemia. J Neurol Neurosurg Psychiatry 1992; 55:116–120.

41. Ferri C, LaCivita L, Cirafisi C, Siciliano G, Longombardo G, Bombardieri S, Rossi B. Peripheral neuropathy in mixed cryoglobulinemia: clinical and electrophysiologic investigations. J Rheumatol 1992; 19:889–895.

42. Calabrese L, Duna G. Drug-induced vasculitis. Curr Opin Rheumatol 1996; 8:34–40.

43. Dubost J, Souteyrand P, Sauvezie B. Drug-induced vasculitides. Baillieres Clin Rheumatol 1991; 5:119–138.

44. Vincent D, Dubas F, Hauw J, Godeau P, Lhermitte F, Buge A, Castaigne P. Nerve and muscle microvasculitis in peripheral neuropathy. A remote effect of cancer? J Neurol Neurosurg Psychiatry 1986; 49:1007–1010.

45. Oh S, Slaughter R, Harrell L. Paraneoplastic vasculitic neuropathy: a treatable neuropathy. Muscle Nerve 1991; 14:152–156.

46. Oh S. Paraneoplastic vasculitis of the peripheral nervous system. Neurol Clin 1997; 15:849–863.

47. Johnson P, Rolak L, Hamilton R, Laguna F. Paraneoplastic vasculitis of nerve: a remote effect of cancer. Ann Neurol 1979; 5:437–444.

48. Kurzrock R, Cohen P, Markowitz A. Clinical manifestations of vasculitis in patients with solid tumors: a case report and review of the literature. Arch Intern Med 1994; 154:334–340.

49. Matsumuro K, Izumo S, Umehara F, Arisato T, Maruyama I, Yonezawa S, Shirahama H, Sato E, Osame M. Paraneoplastic vasculitic neuropathy: immunohistochemical studies on a biopsied nerve and post-mortem examination. J Intern Med 1994; 236:225–230.

50. Caselli R, Daube J, Hunder G, Whisnant J. Peripheral neuropathic syndromes in giant cell (temporal) arteritis. Neurology 1988; 38:685–689.

51. Kissel J, Mendell J. Vasculitic neuropathy. Neurol Clin 1992; 10:761–781.

52. Sobue G, Yasuda T, Kachi T, Sakakibara T, Mitsuma T. Chronic progressive sensory ataxic neuropathy: clinicopathological features of idiopathic and Sjögren's syndrome-associated cases. J Neurol 1993; 240:1–7.

53. Font J, Valls J, Cervera R, Pou A, Ingelmo M, Graus F. Pure sensory neuropathy in patients with primary Sjögren's syndrome: clinical, immunological, and electromyographic findings. Ann Rheum Dis 1990; 49:775–778.

54. Griffin J, Cornblath D, Alexander E, Campbell J, Low P, Bird S, Feldman E. Ataxic sensory neuropathy and dorsal root ganglionitis associated with Sjögren's syndrome. Ann Neurol 1990; 27:305–315.

55. Malinow K, Yannakakis G, Glusman S, Edlow D, Griffin J, Pestronk A, Powell D, Ramsey-Goldman R, Eidelman B, Medsger T et al. Subacute sensory neuronopathy secondary to dorsal root ganglionitis in primary Sjögren's syndrome. Ann Neurol 1986; 20:535–537.

56. Good A, Christopher R, Koepke G, Bender L, Tarter M. Peripheral neuropathy associated with rheumatoid arthritis. Ann Intern Med 1965; 63:87–99.

57. Chamberlain MA, Bruckner FE. Rheumatoid neuropathy. Clinical and electrophysiological features. Ann Rheum Dis 1970; 29:609–616.

58. Feinglass E, Arnett F, Dorsch C, Zizic M, Stevens M. Neuropsychiatric manifestations of systmeic lupus erythematosus: diagnosis, clinical spectrum, and relationship to other features of the disease. Medicine 1976; 55:323–339.

59. Hochberg M, Boyd R, Ahearn J, Arnett F, Bias W, Provost T, Stevens M. Systemic lupus erythematosus: a review of clinico-laboratory features and immunogenetic markers in 150 patients with emphasis on demographic subsets. Medicine (Baltimore) 1985; 64:285–295.

60. Omdal R, Loseth S, Torbergsen T, Koldingsnes W, Husby G, Mellgren SI. Peripheral neuropathy in systemic lupus erythematosus—a longitudinal study. Acta Neurol Scand 2001; 103:386–391.

61. Zeballos RS, Fox RI, Cheresh DA, McPherson RA. Anti-glycosphingolipid autoantibodies in rheumatologic disorders. J Clin Lab Anal 1994; 8:378–384.

62. Mellgren SI, Conn DL, Stevens JC, Dyck PJ. Peripheral neuropathy in primary Sjögren's syndrome. Neurology 1989; 39:390–394.

63. Gemignani F, Marbini A, Pavesi G, Di Vittorio S, Manganelli P, Cenacchi G, Mancia D. Peripheral neuropathy associated with primary Sjögren's syndrome. J Neurol Neurosurg Psychiatry 1994; 57:983–986.

64. Andonopoulos A, Lagos G, Drosos A, Moutsopoulos H. The spectrum of neurological involvement in Sjögren's syndrome. Br J Rheumatol 1990; 29:21–23.

65. Tufanelli D, Winkelmann R. Systemic scleroderma: a clinical study of 727 cases. Arch Dermatol 1961;84:359–371.

66. Lee P, Bruni J, Sukenik S. Neurological manifestations in systemic sclerosis (scleroderma). J Rheumatol 1984; 11:480–483.

67. Ben Taarit C, Turki S, Ben Maiz H. Neurological manifestations in Behcet's disease. Forty observations in a cohort of 300 patients. J Mal Vasc 2002; 27:77–81.

68. Bennett R, Bong D, Spargo B. Neuropsychiatric problems in mixed connective tissue disease. Am J Med 1978; 65:955–962.

69. Isaak BL, Liesegang TA, Michet CJ Jr. Ocular and systemic findings in relapsing polychondritis. Ophthalmology 1986; 93:681–689.

70. McCombe PA, Klestov AC, Tannenberg AE, Chalk JB, Pender MP. Sensorimotor peripheral neuropathy in rheumatoid arthritis. Clin Exp Neurol 1991; 28:146–153.

71. Larrue V, Moulinier L, Arne-Bes MC, Voisin D, Bes A. Chronic inflammatory polyneuropathy and Behçet's syndrome. Presse Med 1987; 16:732–733.

72. Erdem E, Tan E. Peripheral neuropathy in Behcet's disease. Neuromuscul Disord 1999; 9:483.

73. Gross M. Chronic relapsing inflammatory polyneuropathy complicating sicca syndrome [letter]. J Neurol Neurosurg Psychiatry 1987; 50:939–940.

74. Chaudhuri KR, Taylor IK, Niven RM, Abbott RJ. A case of systemic lupus erythematosus presenting as Guillain–Barre syndrome. Br J Rheumatol 1989; 28:440–442.

75. Moreira Filho PF, Nascimento OJ, Cinnicinatus D, Porto FJ, Freitas MR, Santos PC. Guillain–Barre syndrome as a manifestation of systemic lupus erythematosus. Report of a case. Arq Neuropsiquiatr 1980; 38:165–170.

76. Robson MG, Walport MJ, Davies KA. Systemic lupus erythematosus and acute demyelinating polyneuropathy [clinical conference]. Br J Rheumatol 1994; 33:1074–1077.

77. Rechthand E, Cornblath DR, Stern BJ, Meyerhoff JO. Chronic demyelinating polyneuropathy in systemic lupus erythematosus. Neurology 1984; 34:1375–1377.

78. Sigal LH. Chronic inflammatory polyneuropathy complicating SLE: successful treatment with monthly oral pulse cyclophosphamide. J Rheumatol 1989; 16:1518–1519.

79. Sindern E, Stark E, Haas J, Steck AJ. Serum antibodies to GM1 and GM3-gangliosides in systemic lupus erythematosus with chronic inflammatory demyelinating polyradiculoneuropathy. Acta Neurol Scand 1991; 83:399–402.

80. Millette TJ, Subramony SH, Wee AS, Harisdangkul V. Systemic lupus erythematosus presenting with recurrent acute demyelinating polyneuropathy. Eur Neurol 1986; 25:397–402.

81. Sahenk Z, Mendell JR, Rossio JL, Hurtubise P. Polyradiculoneuropathy accompanying procainamide-induced lupus erythematosus: evidence for drug-induced enhanced sensitization to peripheral nerve myelin. Ann Neurol 1977; 1:378–384.

82. Hess DC, Awad E, Posas H, Sethi KD, Adams RJ. Miller–Fisher syndrome in systemic lupus erythematosus. J Rheumatol 1990; 17:1520–1522.

83. Luostarinen L, Himanen SL, Pirttila T, Molnar G. Mixed connective tissue disease associated with chronic inflammatory demyelinating polyneuropathy. Scand J Rheumatol 1999; 28:328–330.

84. Katada E, Ojika K, Uemura M, Maeno K, Mitake S, Tsugu Y, Otsuka Y, Iwase T. Mixed connective tissue disease associated with acute polyradiculoneuropathy. Intern Med 1997; 36:118–124.

85. Farrell DA, Medsger TA. Trigeminal neuropathy in progressive systemic sclerosis. Am J Med 1982; 73:57–62.

86. Hagen N, Stenens J, Michet C. Trigeminal sensory neuropathy associated with connective tissue diseases. Neurology 1990; 40:891–896.

87. Searles R, Mladinich E, Messner R. Isolated trigeminal sensory neuropathy: early manifestation of mixed connective tissue disease. Neurology 1978; 28:1286–1289.

88. Govoni M, Bajocchi G, Rizzo N, Tola M, Caniatti L, Tugnoli V, Colamussi P, Trotta F. Neurological involvement in primary Sjögren's syndrome: clinical and instrumental evaluation in a cohort of Italian patients. Clin Rheumatol 1999; 18:299–303.

89. Grant IA, Hunder GG, Homburger HA, Dyck PJ. Peripheral neuropathy associated with sicca complex. Neurology 1997; 48:855–862.

90. Lecky BR, Hughes RA, Murray NM. Trigeminal sensory neuropathy. A study of 22 cases. Brain 1987; 110:1463–1485.

91. Tajima Y, Mito Y, Owada Y, Tsukishima E, Moriwaka F, Tashiro K. Neurological manifestations of primary Sjögren's syndrome in Japanese patients. Intern Med 1997; 36:690–693.

92. Smukler N, Patterson J, Lorenz H, Weiner L. The incidence of carpal tunnel syndrome in patients with rheumatoid arthritis. Arthritis Rheum 1963; 6:298–299.

93. Barnes C, Currey H. Carpal tunnel syndrome in rheumatoid arthritis; a clinical and electrodiagnostic survey. Ann Rheum Dis 1967; 26:226–233.

94. Chamberlain M, Corbett M. Carpal tunnel syndrome in early rheumatoid arthritis. Ann Rheum Dis 1970; 29:149–152.

95. Mauch E, Volk C, G K, Krapf H, Kornhuber H, Laufen H, Hummel K. Neurological and neuropsychiatric dysfunction in primary Sjögren's sydnrome. Acta Neurol Scand 1994; 89:31–35.

96. Machet L, Vaillant L, Machet M, Esteve E, Muller C, Khallouf R, Lorette G. Carpal tunnel syndrome and systemic sclerosis. Dermatology 1992; 185:101–103.

97. Sidiq M, Kirsner A, Sheon R. Carpal tunnel syndrome: first manifestation of systemic lupus erythematosus. J Am Med Assoc 1992; 222:1416–1417.

98. Omdal R, Mellgren SI, Husby G, Salvesen R, Henriksen OA, Torbergsen T. A controlled study of peripheral neuropathy in systemic lupus erythematosus. Acta Neurol Scand 1993; 88:41–46.

99. Akizuki S, Matsui T. Entrapment neuropathy caused by tophaceous gout. J Hand Surg [Br] 1984; 9:331–332.

100. Janssen T, Rayan GM. Gouty tenosynovitis and compression neuropathy of the median nerve. Clin Orthop 1987:203–206.

101. Vincent FM, Van Houzen RN. Trigeminal sensory neuropathy and bilateral carpal tunnel syndrome: the initial manifestation of mixed connective tissue disease. J Neurol Neurosurg Psychiatry 1980; 43:458–460.

102. Hanna B, Robertson F, Ansell B, Maudsley R. Nerve entrapment at the elbow in rheumatoid arthritis. Rheumatol Rehabil 1975; 14:212–217.

103. Wang HC, Tsai MD. Compressive ulnar neuropathy in the proximal forearm caused by a gouty tophus. Muscle Nerve 1996; 19:525–527.

104. Nakano K. The entrapment neuropathies of rheumatoid arthritis. Orthop Clin North Am 1975; 6:837–860.

105. McGuigan L, Burke D, Fleming A. Tarsal tunnel syndrome and peripheral neuropathy in rheumatoid disease. Ann Rheum Dis 1983; 42:128–131.

106. Dawson D, Hallett M, Wilbourn A. Entrapment Neuropathy. Philadelphia: Lippincott-Raven, 1999.

107. Westkaemper JG, Varitimidis SE, Sotereanos DG. Posterior interosseous nerve palsy in a patient with rheumatoid synovitis of the elbow: a case report and review of the literature. J Hand Surg [Am] 1999; 24:727–731.

108. Wright RA, Grant IA, Low PA. Autonomic neuropathy associated with sicca complex. J Auton Nerv Syst 1999; 75:70–76.

109. Tan J, Akin S, Beyazova M, Sepici V, Tan E. Sympathetic skin response and R–R interval variation in rheumatoid arthritis. Two simple tests for the assessment of autonomic function. Am J Phys Med Rehabil 1993; 72:196–203.

110. Lagana B, Tubani L, Maffeo N, Vella C, Makk E, Baratta L, Bonomo L. Heart rate variability and cardiac autonomic function in systemic lupus erythematosus. Lupus 1996; 5:49–55.

111. Dessein PH, Joffe BI, Metz RM, Millar DL, Lawson M, Stanwix AE. Autonomic dysfunction in systemic sclerosis: sympathetic overactivity and instability. Am J Med 1992; 93:143–150.

112. Raszewa M, Hausmanowa-Petrusewicz I, Blaszczyk M, Jablonska S. Sympathetic skin response in scleroderma. Electromyogr Clin Neurophysiol 1991; 31:467–472.

113. Edelman J, Gubbay S, Zilko P. Acute pandysautonomia due to mixed connective tissue disease. Aust NZ J Med 1981; 11:68–70.

114. Bayramlar H, Hepsen IF, Uguralp M, Boluk A, Ozcan C. Autonomic nervous system involvement in Behçet's disease: a pupillometric study. J Neuroophthalmol 1998; 18:182–186.

115. Tellioglu T, Robertson D. Orthostatic intolerance in Behçet's disease. Auton Neurosci 2001; 89:96–99.

116. Aksoyek S, Aytemir K, Ozer N, Ozcebe O, Oto A. Assessment of autonomic nervous system function in patients with Behçet's disease by spectral analysis of heart rate variability. J Auton Nerv Syst 1999; 77:190–194.

117. Briemberg H, Levin K, Amato A. Multifocal conduction block in peripheral nerve vasculitis. J Clin Neuromuscul Disord 2002; 3:153–158.

118. Jamieson P, Guiliani M, Martinez A. Necrotizing angiopathy presenting with multifocal conduction blocks. Neurology 1991; 41:442–444.

119. McCluskey L, Feinberg D, Cantor C, Bird S. "Pseudo-conduction block" in vasculitic neuropathy. Muscle Nerve 1999; 22:1361–1366.

120. Battaglia M, Mitsumoto H, Wilbourn A, Estes M. Utility of electromyography in the diagnosis of vasculitic neuropathy. Neurology 1990; 40(suppl 1):427.

121. Bajema I, Hagen E. Evolving concepts about the role of antineutrophil cytoplasm autoantibodies in systemic vasculitides. Curr Opin Rheumatol 1999; 11:34–40.

122. Lie J. Histopathological specificity of systemic vasculitis. Rheum Dis Clin North Am 1995; 21:883–909.

123. Englehardt A, Lorler H, Neundorfer B. Immunochemical findings in vasculitic neuropathies. Acta Neurol Scand 1993; 87:318–321.

124. Kissel J, Riethman J, Omerza J, Rammohan K, Mendell J. Peripheral nerve vasculitis: immune characterization of the vascular lesions. Ann Neurol 1989; 25:291–297.

125. Fujimura H, LaCroix C, Said G. Vulnerability of nerve fibers to ischaemia: a quantitative light and electron microscopic study. Brain 1991; 114:1929–1942.

126. Lie J. Systemic and isolated vasculitis: a rational approach to classification and pathologic diagnosis. Pathol Annu 1989; 24:25–114.

127. Claussen G, Thomas T, Goyne C, Vazquez L, Oh S. Diagnostic value of nerve and muscle biopsy in suspected vasculitis cases. J Clin Neuromuscul Disord 2000; 1:117–123.

128. Lauria G, Pareyson D, Grisoli M, Sghirlanzoni A. Clinical and magnetic resonance imaging findings in chronic sensory ganglionopathies. Ann Neurol 2000; 47:104–109.

129. Vitali C, Bombardieri S, Moutsopoulos H, Balestrieri G, Bencivelli W, Bernstein R, Bjerrum K, Braga S, Coll J, de Vita S et al. Preliminary criteria for the classification of Sjögren's syndrome. Arthritis Rheum 1993; 36:340–347.

130. Chalk D, Lennon V, Stevens J, Windebank A. Seronegativity for type 1 antineuronal nuclear antibodies ("anti-Hu") in subacute sensory neuronopathy patients without cancer. Neurology 1993; 43:2209–2211.

131. Schaumburg H, Kaplan J, Windebank A, Vick N, Rasmus S, Pleasure D, Brown MJ. Sensory neuropathy from pyridoxine abuse. A new megavitamin syndrome. N Engl J Med 1983; 309:445–448.

132. Dalakas M. Chronic idiopathic ataxic neuropathy. Ann Neurol 1986; 19:545–554.

133. Kissel J, Collins M. Vasculitic neuropathies and neuropathies of connective tissue diseases. In: Katirji B, Kaminski H, Preston D, Ruff R, Shapiro B, eds. Neuromuscular Disorders in Clinical Practice. Boston: Butterworth–Heinemann, 2002:669–702.

134. Guillevin L, Lhote F, Cohen P, Sauvaget F, Jarrousse B, Lortholary O, Noel L, Trepo C. Polyarteritis nodosa related to hepatitis B virus: a prospective study with long-term observation of 41 patients. Medicine 1995; 74:238–253.

135. Maclachlan D, Battegay M, Jacob A, Tyndall A. Successful treatment of hepatitis B-associated polyarteritis nodosa with a combination of lamivudine and conventional immunosuppressive therapy: a case report. Rheumatology 2000; 39:106–108.

136. Boonyapisit K, Katirji B. Severe exacerbation of hepatitis C-associated vasculitic neuropathy following treatment with interferon alpha: a case report and literature review. Muscle Nerve 2002; 25:909–913.

137. Khella S, Frost S, Hermann G, Leventhal L, Whyatt S, Sajid M, Scherer S. Hepatitis C infection, cryoglobulinemia, and vasculitic neuropathy: treatment with interferon alfa: case report and literature review. Neurology 1995; 45:407–411.

138. Misiani R, Bellavita P, Fenili D, Vicari O, Marchesi D, Sironi P, Zilio P, Vernocchi A, Massazza M, Vendramin G et al. Interferon alfa-2a therapy in cryoglobulinemia associated with hepatitis C virus. N Eng J Med 1994; 330:751–756.

139. Gross W. New concepts in treatment protocols for severe systemic vasculitis. Curr Opin Rheumatol 1999; 11:41–46.

140. Fauci A, Haynes B, Katz P, Wolff S. Wegener's granulomatosis: prospective and therapeutic experience with 85 patients for 21 years. Ann Intern Med 1983; 98:76–85.

141. Langford C, Klippel J, Balow J, James S, Sneller M. Use of cytotoxic agents and cyclosporine in the treatment of autoimmune disease. Part 2: inflammatory bowel disease, systemic vasculitis, and therapeutic toxicity. Ann Intern Med 1998; 129:49–58.

142. Jayne D. Evidence-based treatment of systemic vasculitis. Rheumatology 2000; 39.

143. Guillevin L, Rosser J, Cacoub P, Mousson C, Jarrousee B. Methylprednisolone in the treatment of Wegener's granulomatosis, polyarteritis nodosa and Churg–Strauss angiitis. APMIS 1990; 19(suppl):52–53.

144. Fauci A, Katz P, Haynes B, Wolff S. Cyclophosphamide therapy of severe necrotizing vasculitis. N Engl J Med 1979; 301:235–238.

145. Adu D, Pall A, Luqmani R, Richards N, Howie A, Emery P, Michael J, Savage C, Bacon P. Controlled trial of pulse versus continuous prednisolone and cyclophosphamide in the treatment of vasculitis. Q J Med 1997; 90:401–409.

146. Gayraud M, Guillevin L, Cohen P, Lhote F, Cacoub P, Deblois P, Godeau B, Ruel M, Vidal E, Piontud M, Ducroix J, Lassoued S, Christoforov B, Babinet P. Treatment of good-prognosis polyarteritis nodosa and Churg–Strauss syndrome: comparison of steroids and oral or pulse cyclophosphamide in 25 patients. French Cooperative Study Group for Vasculitides. Br J Rheumatol 1997; 36:1290–1297.

147. Guillevin L, Cordier J-F, Lhote F, Cohen P, Jarrousse B, Royer I, Lesavre P, Jacquot C, Bindi P, Bielefeld P, Desson J, Detree F, Dubois A, Hachulla E, Hoen B, Jacomy D, Seigneuric C, Lauque D, Stern M, Longy-Boursier M. A prospective, multicenter, randomized trial comparing steroids and pulse cyclophosphamide versus steroids nd oral cyclophosphamide in the treatment of generalized Wegener's granulomatosis. Arthritis Rheum 1997; 40:2187–2198.

148. Haubitz M, Koch K, Brunkhorst R. Cyclosporin for the prevention of disease reactivation in relapsing ANCA-associated vasculitis. Nephrol Dial Transplant 1998; 13:2074–2076.

149. Jayne D, Gaskin G. Randomized trial of cyclophosphamide versus azathioprine during remission in ANCA-associated vasculitis (CYCAZAREM). J Am Soc Nephrol 1999; 10:105A.

150. Langford C, Talar-Williams C, Barron K, Sneller M. A staged approach to the treatment of Wegener's granulomatosis: induction of remission with glucocorticoids and daily cyclophosphamide switching to methotrexate for remission maintenance. Arthritis Rheum 1999; 42:2666–2673.

151. Nowack R, Gobel U, Klooker P, Hergesell O, Andrassy K, van der Woude F. Mycophenolate mofetil for maintenance therapy of Wegener's granulomatosis and microscopic polyangiitis: a pilot study in 11 patients with renal involvement. J Am Soc Nephrol 1999; 10:1965–1971.

152. Jayne D, Chapel H, Adu D, Misbah S, O'Donoghue D, Scott D, Lockwood C. Intravenous immunoglobulin for ANCA-associated systemic vasculitis with persistent disease activity. Q J Med 2000; 93:433–439.

153. Jayne D, Lockwood C. Pooled intravenous immunoglobulin in the management of systemic vasculitis. Adv Exp Med Biol 1993; 336:469–472.

154. Richter C, Schnabel A, Csernok E, De Groot K, Reinhold-Keller E, Gross W. Treatment of anti-neutrophil cytoplasmic antibody (ANCA)-associated vasculitis with high-dose intravenous immunoglobulin. Clin Exp Immunol 1995; 101:2–7.

155. Levy Y, Sherer Y, George J, Langevitz P, Ahmed A, Bar-Dayan Y, Fabbrizzi F, Terryberry J, Peter J, Shoenfeld Y. Serologic and clinical response to treatment of systemic vasculitis and associated autoimmune disease with intravenous immunoglobulin. Int Arch Allergy Immunol 1999; 119:231–238.

156. Guillevin L, Lhote F, Cohen P, Jarrousse B, Lortholary O, Genereau T, Leon A, Bussel A. Corticosteroids plus pulse cyclophosphamide and plasma exchanges versus corticosteroids plus pulse cyclophosphamide alone in the treatment of polyarteritis nodosa and Churg–Strauss syndrome patients with factors predicting poor prognosis. Arthritis Rheum 1995; 38:1638–1645.

157. Lamprecht P, Gause A, Gross W. Cryoglobulinemic vasculitis. Arthritis Rheum 1999; 42:2507–2516.

158. Georganas C, Ioakimidis D, Iatrou C, Vidalaki B, Iliadou K, Athanassiou P, Kontomerkos T. Relapsing Wegener's granulomatosis: successful treatment with cyclosporin-A. Clin Rheumatol 1996; 15:189–192.

159. Hagen E, de Keizer R, Andrassy K, van Boven W, Bruijn J, van Es L, van der Woude F. Compassionate treatment of Wegener's granulomatosis with rabbit anti-thymocyte globulin. Clin Nephrol 1995; 43:351–359.

160. Lockwood C, Thiru S, Isaacs J, Hale G, Waldmann H. Long-term remission of intractable systemic vasculitis with monoclonal antibody therapy. Lancet 1993; 341:1620–1622.

161. Stone J, Uhlfelder M, Hellman D, Crook S, Bedocs N, Hoffman G. Etanercept in Wegener's granulomatosis: a six-month open-label trial to evaluate safety. Arthritis Rheum 2000; 43(suppl):S404.

162. Lockwood C, Elliot J, Brettman L, Hale G, Rebello P, Frewin M, Ringler D, Merrill C, Waldmann H. Anti-adhesion molecule therapy as an interventional strategy for autoimmune inflammation. Clin Immunol 1999; 93:93–106.

163. Tyndall A, Fassas A, Passweg J, Ruiz de Elvira C, Attal M, Brooks P, Black C, Durez P, Finke J, Forman S, Fouillard L, Furst D, Holmes J, Joske D, Jouet J, Kotter I, Locatelli F,

Prentice H, Marmont A, McSweeney P, Musso M, Peter H, Snowden J, Sullivan K, Gratwohl A et al. Autologous haematopoietic stem cell transplants for autoimmune disease: feasibility and transplant-related mortality. Bone Marrow Transplant 1999; 24:729–734.

164. Boumpas D. Glucocorticoid therapy for immune diseases: basic and clinical correlates. Ann Intern Med 1993; 119:1198–1208.

165. Dalakas M. Pharmacologic concerns of corticosteroids in the treatment of patients with immune-related neuromuscular diseases. Neurol Clin 1990; 8:93–118.

166. Eastell R, Reid D, Compston J, Cooper C, Fogelman I, Francis R, Hosking D, Purdie D, Ralston S, Reeve J, Russell R, Stevenson J, Torgerson D. A UK Consensus Group on management of glucocorticoid-induced osteoporosis: an update. J Intern Med 1998; 244:271–292.

167. Ognibene F, Shelhamer J, Hoffman G, Kerr G, Reda D, Fauci A, Leavitt R. *Pneumocystis carinii* pneumonia: a major complication of immunosuppressive therapy in patients with Wegener's granulomatosis. Am J Respir Crit Care Med 1995; 151:795–799.

168. Chung J, Armstrong K, Schwartz J, Albert D. Cost-effectiveness of prophylaxis against *Pneumocystis caranii* pneumonia in patients with Wegener's granulomatosis undergoing immunosuppressive therapy. Arthritis Rheum 2000; 43.

169. Talar-Williams C, Hijazi Y, Walther M, Linehan W, Hallahan C, Lubensky I, Kerr G, Hoffman G, Fauci A, Sneller M. Cyclophosphamide-induced cystitis and bladder cancer in patients with Wegener granulomatosis. Ann Intern Med 1996; 124:477–484.

170. Singhal BS, Khadilkar SV, Gursahani RD, Surya N. Vasculitic neuropathy: profile of twenty patients. J Assoc Physicians India 1995; 43:459–461.

171. Said G. Necrotizing peripheral nerve vasculitis. Neurol Clin 1997; 15:835–848.

172. Molina JA, Benito-Leon J, Bermejo F, Jimenez-Jimenez FJ, Olivan J. Intravenous immunoglobulin therapy in sensory neuropathy associated with Sjögren's syndrome. J Neurol Neurosurg Psychiatry 1996; 60:699.

173. Asahina M, Kuwabara S, Nakajima M, Hattori T. D-penicillamine treatment for chronic sensory ataxic neuropathy associated with Sjögren's syndrome. Neurology 1998; 51:1451–1453.

174. McManis P, Low P, Lagerund T. Microenvironment of nerve: blood flow and ischemia. In: Dyck P, Thomas P, eds. Peripheral Neuropathy. Philadelphia: WB Saunders, 1993:453–475.

175. Jennette J, Falk R, Millin D. Pathogenesis of vasculitis. Semin Neurol 1994; 14:291–299.

176. Ben-Baruch A, Michiel D, Oppenheim J. Signals and receptors involved in recruitment of inflammatory cells. J Biol Chem 1995; 270:11703–11706.

177. Conn DL, McDuffie FC, Dyck PJ. Immunopathologic study of sural nerves in rheumatoid arthritis. Arthritis Rheum 1972; 15:135–143.

178. Weller RO, Bruckner FE, Chamberlain MA. Rheumatoid neuropathy: a histological and electrophysiological study. J Neurol Neurosurg Psychiatry 1970; 33:592–604.

179. Salih AM, Nixon NB, Gagan RM, Heath P, Hawkins CP, Dawes PT, Mattey DL. Anti-ganglioside antibodies in patients with rheumatoid arthritis complicated by peripheral neuropathy. Br J Rheumatol 1996; 35:725–731.

180. Salih AM, Nixon NB, Dawes PT, Mattey DL. Prevalence of antibodies to neurofilament polypeptides in patients with rheumatoid arthritis complicated by peripheral neuropathy. Clin Exp Rheumatol 1998; 16:689–694.

181. Salih AM, Nixon NB, Dawes PT, Mattey DL. Antibodies to neuroblastoma cells in rheumatoid arthritis: a potential marker for neuropathy. Clin Exp Rheumatol 2000; 18:23–30.

182. Molina R, Provost T, Alexander E. Peripheral neuropathy in primary Sjögren's syndrome. Arthritis Rheum 1985; 28:1341–1347.

183. Kaplan JG, Rosenberg R, Reinitz E, Buchbinder S, Schaumburg HH. Invited review: peripheral neuropathy in Sjögren's syndrome. Muscle Nerve 1990; 13:570–579.

184. Balagtas-Balmaseda O, Grabois M, Balmaseda P, Lidsky M. Cubital tunnel syndrome in rheumatoid arthritis. Arch Phys Med Rehabil 1983; 64:163–166.

185. Straub RH, Zeuner M, Lock G, Rath H, Hein R, Scholmerich J, Lang B. Autonomic and sensorimotor neuropathy in patients with systemic lupus erythematosus and systemic sclerosis. J Rheumatol 1996; 23:87–92.

14

Neuropathy Associated with Cancer

David R. Renner and Deborah T. Blumenthal
University of Utah, Salt Lake City, Utah, USA

ABSTRACT

All portions of the peripheral nervous system may be involved in the setting of cancer, including cranial nerves, brachial and lumbar plexus, peripheral nerves, and neuromuscular junction. Causes include direct effects of the tumor, secondary effects or treatment, remote effects (paraneoplastic), and secondary effects from organ and metabolic failures. Recognizing involvement and distinguishing between causes can be challenging, but is important for optimal treatment. This chapter reviews the spectrum of peripheral nerve involvement based on underlying mechanisms.

1. INTRODUCTION

Patients with systemic malignancies may develop peripheral neuropathies either by direct effect through invasion or compression of nerve structures, iatrogenic effect of treatment (chemotherapy, radiation, and transplantation), and immune-mediated paraneoplastic effect, or indirect effect of the cancer from organ failure or secondary metabolic derangements. In some instances, no underlying etiology is identified, and the peripheral neuropathy is considered cryptogenic (Table 14.1). Cardinal features of neuropathy (paresthesias, weakness, cranial nerve dysfunction, and dysautonomia) are not unique to cancer-related neuropathies. All divisions of the peripheral nervous system may become involved in systemic malignancies, including the cranial nerves, spinal nerve roots, plexuses, sensory and/or motor nerves, and the neuromuscular junction. However, the location and biology of the primary neoplasm, the type of antineoplastic therapy, and the spectrum of associated paraneoplastic syndromes are factors when addressing neuropathy in a patient with cancer (1). Although the incidence of clinically recognizable peripheral neuropathy in cancer patients is low (0.5–5%), electrophysiologic studies reveal a higher incidence (30–40%) of subclinical disease (2–7). The type of malignancy, stage and location of the cancer, duration of the disease, nutritional status of the patient, concurrent metabolic abnormalities, and the potential neurotoxicity of therapy influence the incidence of peripheral neuropathy (8). Once suspected by history and clinical examination, the diagnosis and etiology of neuropathy can be confirmed by electrodiagnostic tests, imaging, biopsy, or by antibodies associated with paraneoplastic syndromes in either serum or cerebrospinal fluid (CSF).

    This chapter addresses neuropathies related to cancer, grouped into three major categories: (i) direct infiltration or compression; (ii) toxicities of cancer therapy; and (iii) immune-mediated paraneoplastic neuropathy syndromes.

Table 14.1   Etiology of Neuropathy in Patients with Systemic Malignancy

Direct effect of malignancy
   Diffuse/restricted invasion or compression of nerve roots, brachial or
      lumbosacral plexuses, or peripheral and cranial nerve
Iatrogenic effect of treatment
   Neurotoxicity of chemotherapeutic and immunosuppressive agents
   Neurotoxicity of radiation
   Surgery
   Infection
   Alteration of immune system after bone marrow transplantation
Paraneoplastic effect
Indirect effect of malignancy
   Organ failure
   Malnutrition
   Malabsorption
   Critical Illness
Cryptogenic

2.   NEUROPATHY FROM DIRECT TUMOR INVOLVEMENT

2.1.   Cranial Neuropathies

2.1.1.   Clinical Features

Cranial neuropathies are often the product of skull-based and leptomeningeal metastases, though they can also be related to opportunistic infections, late effects of radiation therapy, or nonmalignant processes. Although most skull-based metastases are from breast cancer, other neoplasms include lymphoma, lung, head and neck carcinoma, thyroid, renal, melanoma, and prostate cancers (9). Presenting symptoms include headache, nausea, blurred or decreased vision, diplopia, abnormal facial sensation and pain, chin numbness, impaired hearing, hoarseness, dysphagia, retro-auricular pain, dysarthria, and occasionally syncope.

   The most common cranial nerve affected (regardless of tumor type) is the abducens nerve (CN VI), followed by the oculomotor (CN III), trigeminal (CN V), and hypoglossal (CN XII) (9). Melanoma, and head and neck (squamous cell) carcinoma can be *neurotropic*, and progress along the course of cranial nerves (trigeminal, facial) from their primary site. Lymphoma frequently involves cranial nerves as they exit the subarachnoid spaces peripherally. Leptomeningeal disease commonly presents with one or more cranial neuropathies.

   Olfactory Nerve (CN I).   Hyposmia and anosmia, and occasionally dysgeusia can result from olfactory groove compression, most commonly with inferiofrontal tumors such as meningioma, esthesioneuroblastoma, or from direct extension to the olfactory nerve by nasopharyngeal carcinoma.

   Optic Nerve (CN II).   Loss of visual acuity and eventual blindness can occur from optic neuropathy related to leptomeningeal disease. Elevated intracranial pressure from space-occupying intracranial tumors can produce papilledema and subsequent visual scotoma. Monocular visual loss may occur with optic nerve gliomas and nerve sheath meningiomas.

   Oculomotor Nerve (CN III).   Patients may complain of blurred or double vision with oculomotor paresis (ipsilateral midriasis with ptosis and an eye that looks down and out in primary gaze). Breast, lung, and prostrate cancer are most common, with initial involvement of bone and extension into the cavernous sinus. CN IV, VI, and V-1 and V-2 pass through the cavernous sinus, and may also be involved.

Trochlear Nerve (CN IV). Double vision may result from trochlear nerve involvement in cavernous sinus syndrome, in association with other cranial neuropathies from nerves passing through the cavernous sinus.

Trigeminal Nerve (CN V). Proptosis, chemosis, and hyperesthesia, the *orbital syndrome*, involves V-1. Mental or inferior alveolar nerve neuropathy, *numb chin syndrome*, is commonly due to neoplastic involvement.

Abducens Nerve (CN VI). This is the most commonly involved cranial nerve, presenting with double vision. Its vulnerability is due to its long intracranial course, its vulnerability to compression, changes in intracranial pressure, and irritation from leptomeningeal processes.

Facial Nerve (CN VII). Progressive facial pain and weakness distinguishes cancer-related facial neuropathy from acute weakness in idiopathic Bell's palsy. Leptomeningeal disease usually involves multiple nerves. Parotid gland malignancies impinge upon the nerve in 5–25% of cases (10). Dysgeusia may result from facial nerve branch injury secondary to radiation and may be permanent in patients treated with high doses (>50 Gy) for head and neck tumors (11). Decreased salivary gland secretion from radiation can result in xerostomia leading to an increased incidence of dental caries.

Vestibulocochlear Nerve (CN VIII). Tumors in the cerebellopontine angle are typically benign. Metastatic lesions can also reach this area and involve the eighth nerve, as well as the nearby facial and trigeminal nerves. Presenting symptoms include disequilibrium, ear fullness, vertigo, tinnitus, and hearing loss.

Glossopharyngeal Nerve (CN IX) and Vagus Nerve (CN X). Hoarseness and dysphagia are common presenting symptoms. Esophageal metastases can involve the glossopharyngeal or vagal nerve branches, and cause *swallow syncope*. The *jugular foramen syndrome* is more common, and may produce *glossopharyngeal neuralgia*. Other tumors include schwannomas of the glossopharyngeal nerve, metastases (melanoma, renal cell, and prostate), meningiomas, and glomus tumors (12).

Spinal Accessory Nerve (CN XI). Weakness occurs in the sternocleidomastoid and trapezius muscles. This nerve is rarely compromised by tumor, but may be injured during radical and modified radical neck dissections and lymph node biopsy surgery.

Hypoglossal Nerve (CN XII). Tongue weakness with deviation to the affected side and lingual dysarthria and dysphagia are common symptoms of hypoglossal neuropathy (13). Tumors at the base of the skull/clivus (most commonly metastases) may impinge on the hypoglossal foramina. Cancers of the head and neck (typically nasopharyngeal carcinoma) can affect the nerve either by erosion into the hypoglossal canal, or by perineural infiltration.

2.1.2. Evaluation

Suspicion should be high for metastatic disease when a cranial neuropathy occurs in the setting of a known malignancy. Skull-based and leptomeningeal processes usually result in multiple cranial neuropathies. Computed tomography (CT) scanning with bone windows is helpful in the evaluation of osseous metastases. A bone scan may reveal abnormal uptake in the skull base or mandible. High-resolution magnetic resonance imaging (MRI) is used to investigate infiltrative or compressive lesions. MRI with gadolinium enhancement and fine cuts through the skull base may reveal abnormal enhancement of nerves either at their origin or along their course. MR neurography can be helpful if the nerve has been clinically localized. Nerve conduction studies (NCS) of the facial nerve (CN VII) may reveal decreased compound muscle action potential (CMAP) amplitude. Blink reflex studies may show absent or prolonged R1 and R2 if CN V or VII are involved. Needle electromyography (EMG) can be used to evaluate muscle supplied by affected cranial nerves. Denervation will be evident by increased insertional activity, sustained positive waves and fibrillation potentials. Voluntary motor units show reduced recruitment and varying degrees of waveform complexity dependent upon the chronicity of the lesion (14).

Serologic testing may identify serum markers associated with the primary neoplasm, and a rising serum marker level can support clinical suspicion of active metastatic involvement. Active systemic lymphoma (but not primary CNS lymphoma) may be associated with rising lactate dehydrogenase enzymes (15).

2.1.3. Differential Diagnosis

CNS structures are more vulnerable to radiation injury than peripheral nerves. Cranial nerves are more resistant than brachial plexus nerves, but cranial neuropathies can occur in patients who have had external beam treatment to the head and neck (16,17). The five lowest cranial nerves are most frequently affected because of their proximity to sites of cancer included in radiation portals (18). Radiation-related cranial neuropathies can be distinguished from other causes when myokymic discharges are observed on needle EMG.

Cranial nerves may be affected by infectious processes in the setting of immunosuppression from cancer and chemotherapy. Varicella-zoster virus infection occurs more frequently in patients with systemic cancer, most notably lymphoma. Although the infection usually presents with dysesthesias, hyperpathia, allodynia, and vessicular eruption following a dermatome distribution, facial weakness occurs in 10% (19). Weakness usually presents acutely over hours to subacutely over days, and may lag behind the rash by up to 5 months (20).

2.1.4. Management and Prognosis

Most osseous metastases respond to focal irradiation, but the neuropathy may not fully respond, although early treatment is associated with overall better functional recovery. Focal irradiation may also slow progression of involvement to neighboring nerves (21).

Diplopia may be managed with alternating eye patching or prisms. Painful dysesthesias from trigeminal and glossopharyngeal neuralgias respond to tricyclic antidepressants, conventional and atypical antiseizure medications, and occasionally high dose NSAIDs or opiates. Facial weakness from facial neuropathy may cause xerophthalmia and exposure keratoconjunctivitis, and lubricating gels and nocturnal eye patching should be used. Vestibular rehabilitation protocols can help with peripherally mediated disequilibrium/vertigo. Lower peripheral cranial nerve lesions may produce dysphagia and dysarthria, predisposing patients to aspiration pneumonia. In these instances, speech pathology can suggest swallowing strategies.

2.2. Radiculopathies

2.2.1. Clinical Features

Mono- or polyradiculopathies are caused by metastases or local spread to epidural or paravertebral spaces. Damage is due to direct invasion or indirect compression of neural structures. The incidence of epidural metastases in patients with systemic cancer is 1–5%, and the most common tumors are breast, lung, and prostate, multiple myeloma and other lymphoproliferative disorders. The thoracic spine is the most frequent site of epidural cord or root compression, followed by the lumbosacral spine and cervical spine (22).

Back pain is a common symptom in cancer patients: one-third have vertebral metastases without epidural or nerve involvement, and one-third have epidural tumor (23). Symptoms of spinal nerve root involvement include lateralized back pain exacerbated by provocative maneuvers producing dural tension, lateralized sensory dysesthesias (electric jolt, tingling numbness, or nonspecific pain), and weakness in the involved myotome. Signs include abnormal sensation in a dermatomal distribution, but weakness is less common. A reduced tendon reflex in the suspected nerve root distribution is supportive. Lesions may also produce a myeloradiculopathy, manifested clinically by lower motor neuron findings at the level of the compression, and upper motor neuron signs below the level of compression.

2.2.2. Evaluation

Acute lesions should be evaluated with imaging studies. A myeloradiculopathy is a neurologic emergency, and careful neurologic examination for signs of myelopathy is imperative. Chronic lesions should follow a step-wise plan.

Electrodiagnostic studies can localize the level of spinal roots involved in chronic disorders. NCS will rarely show reduced sensory nerve action potentials (SNAP) and CMAP amplitudes, or reduced conduction velocities. Prolonged or absent F-wave responses in the involved segments may be an early indicator of nerve root involvement (24). Needle EMG of paraspinal and limb muscles is the most sensitive indicator of nerve root dysfunction (25). Abnormal spontaneous activity is indicative of denervation. Myokymia in the setting of radiation therapy supports radiation-induced nerve damage, as opposed to neoplastic involvement (26).

When a lesion has been localized to a specific nerve root, imaging studies can help determine the etiology and extent of the lesion. Spinal cord tumors and masses can be classified into three catagories (Table 14.2) (27). Extradural lesions often displace dura and cord away from the pedicle or vertebral body, resulting in indistinct margins on imaging and a feathering on myelography (28). Intradural metastases are rare. *Drop metastases* occur with specific intracranial tumors, most notably medulloblastoma, ependymoma, and germ cell tumors (29). Intradural extramedullary lesions are best evaluated

Table 14.2 Spinal Cord Tumor/Mass Classification by Location (27)

Extradural lesions
  Osseous spine
  Epidural space
  Paraspinous soft tissues
Intradural extramedullary lesions
  Nerve roots
  Leptomeninges
  CSF spaces
Intramedullary lesions
  Cord parenchyma
  Piamater

---

with myelography or MRI. Classic findings include a capping-type defect on myelography, displacement of the cord away from the dural margin, widening of the subarachnoid space on the side of the lesion, and usually in the absence of any bony abnormality (with the exception of *dumbell* lesions). Contrast enhanced MRI is generally the imaging procedure of choice, whereas CT-myelography is appropriate when MRI is contra-indicated.

Most metastases are osteolytic, although breast and prostate cancer can produce osteoblastic or osteosclerotic lesions (30). These lesions are evident on plain films when 40–50% of bone area is involved. CT-myelography is useful for identifying mass effect from tumor, and determining whether CSF blockage has occurred. Bone scintigraphy is sensitive in detecting altered local bone metabolism. Single photon emission computed tomographic imaging may differentiate between benign and malignant lesions. Non-enhanced CT scans can identify both osteolytic or osteoblastic lesions, and intrathecal contrast is necessary to precisely evaluate the epidural space. MRI can delineate epidural from paraspinous soft tissue involvement, and spinal cord involvement. Lytic lesions are often multifocal, and are characterized by low signal on T1-weighted, and high signal on T2-weighted sequences. Sclerotic lesions are hypo-intense on both T1- and T2-weighted sequences. Contrast enhancement may be required to evaluate for metastatic disease. Lesion degree and pattern of enhancement varies among tumor types. MRI standard sequences, along with fat suppression sequences and precontrast enhanced scans, may further clarify tumor characteristics.

2.2.3. *Differential Diagnosis*

Extramedullary spine lesions can be either intradural or extradural. Metastatic masses are the most common extramedullary, extradural neoplasm, whereas primary extramedullary, extradural malignant neoplasms such as chordomas, lymphomas, and sarcomas are uncommon. In adults, almost half of all spine metastases with epidural cord compression are from breast, lung, or prostate cancers, whereas primary tumors are from lymphoma, renal cancer, multiple myeloma, melanoma, and sarcoma.

The most common CNS primary tumors that metastasize to the subarachnoid space are grade 3 and 4 astrocytomas (anaplastic astrocytomas and glioblastoma multiformae, respectively), ependymomas, and primitive neuro-ectodermal tumors/medulloblastomas, and less commonly choroid plexus papillomas and carcinomas, germinomas, and pineal tumors (pinealblastomas) (31).

Nerve sheath tumors (schwannomas, neurofibromas, and ganglioneuromas) and meningiomas account for 80–90% of all intradural extramedullary masses. They have a predilection for the dorsal sensory nerve roots, and therefore they often manifest with radicular symptoms that mimic those associated with the uncommon intradural disc herniation syndrome. Enlarged nerve roots may extend intradurally, as seen in Dejerine–Sottas disease, Charcot–Marie–Tooth disease, Guillain–Barré Syndrome, nonHodgkins lymphoma, hexane toxicity, carcinomatous meningitis, lymphoma, and leukemia. The most common intradural extramedullary lesion is a meningioma, classically seen in middle aged females and most commonly localized to the thoracic spine. Almost all are benign and occur in isolation. Occasionally, they can occur both intradurally and extradurally, and when present, give a dumbell appearance on imaging. Conus and filum terminale ependymomas can look identical to schwannomas.

Neurologic symptoms and signs in a multifocal root pattern raise suspicion for neoplastic meningitis. Neoplastic meningitis presents with cauda equine syndrome (uncommonly mimicking Guillain–Barré Syndrome) or mononeuritis multiplex.

2.2.4.   Management and Prognosis

Treatment for focal lesions is similar to that for cranial nerve involvement. Treatment of systemic disease may not produce relief of symptoms, and is often supplemented by palliative treatment (focal radiation). When neoplastic radiculopathy occurs with spinal cord compression, urgent irradiation is indicated.

2.3.   Plexopathies (Brachial and Lumbosacral)

2.3.1.   Clinical Features

Brachial Plexopathies.   Primary nerve tumors surround the nerve and are slow growing. Secondary tumors more commonly infiltrate nerves, and the primary tumor is usually known. Pancoast tumors are an exception, and represent the presenting symptom of nonsmall cell carcinoma of the lung with invasion of C8 and T1 spinal nerves. Overall, the lower trunk is affected in 60% (because of its proximity to the axillary lymph nodes and direct invasion from the apex of the lung), the upper and middle trunks in 10%, and all trunks in 30% (32). Presenting symptoms of middle trunk lesions are dysesthesias and anesthesia in the medial hand and forearm. Lower trunk lesions present with intrinsic hand weakness, sensory loss in the distribution of the medial hand, forearm, posteromedial arm and axilla. Horner's syndrome may be present. Posterior cord lesions present with weakness of elbow, wrist, and finger extension. Upper trunk lesions present with weakness of arm abduction and elbow flexion. Muscle atrophy and fasiculations may be seen in long-standing axonal brachial plexopathies. Sensory findings are less reliable in localizing plexus injuries, and deep tendon reflexes may be depressed or even absent (8).

Lumbosacral Plexopathies.   Lumbosacral plexopathies are twice as common as brachial plexopathies, and are often the result of direct tumor extension or infiltration from pelvic and abdominal cancer. Pain is the most common presenting symptom, which is typically worse at night while lying down, and ameliorated with standing or walking. With progression, weakness may ensue, and L4–S2 muscles are more commonly affected. There may be associated reflex asymmetries. Sympathetic ganglia are rarely involved from extension to retroperitoneal and para-aortic areas, but can produce a painful, warm, anhidrotic foot (*dry foot syndrome*) (33).

2.3.2.   Evaluation

When a Pancoast tumor is suspected, plain film chest x-rays or CT of the chest and thorax are appropriate imaging modalities. For other brachial plexopathies, cervical spine MRI without and with contrast may be needed to ensure that a cervical polyradiculopathy is not mimicking a plexopathy. For lumbosacral plexopathies, routine x-rays of the lumbo-sacral spine are appropriate to exclude pathologic fracture or osseous destruction producing a mono- or polyradiculopathy. Bone scans may provide corroborative information, revealing increased uptake at areas of involvement. MRI of the intradural spinal nerves of the cauda equina can reveal a cauda equine syndrome or arachnoiditis. When electrodiagnostic testing localizes the lesion, MR-neurography may determine whether the lesion is externally compressing or locally infiltrating the plexus.

Electrodiagnostic testing is helpful in defining a plexus lesion. NCS may demonstrate reduced or absent sensory responses. Conduction velocities are usually preserved, but F-waves may be prolonged or absent. Needle EMG is the most sensitive indicator of denervation, and can be used to determine that the distribution of axonal damage is consistent with a plexopathy (8,34) (Table 14.3).

Table 14.3 High Yield Brachial Plexus Injury Study (8)

Suspected site of plexus lesion		SNAP/MUAP
Lateral cord		
	SNAP:	lateral antebrachial cutaneous sensory nerve
	SNAP:	median sensory nerve
	MUAP:	musculocutaneous motor nerve
Posterior cord		
	SNAP:	radial sensory nerve
	MUAP:	radial motor nerve
	MUAP:	axillary motor nerve
Medial cord		
	SNAP:	ulnar sensory nerve
	SNAP:	medial antebrachial cutaneous sensory nerve
	MUAP:	ulnar motor nerve
	MUAP:	median motor nerve

Note: MUAP, motor unit action potential.

2.3.3. Differential Diagnosis

Primary nerve tumors are most commonly benign, and include schwannomas or neuro-fibromas, and less common lipomas, ganglioneuromas, desmoids, lymphangiomas, and myoblastomas. Secondary tumors are most commonly from breast, lung, colon, uterine, cervical, and prostrate primary sources. Lymphomas may be *neurotropic*, and infiltrate along the nerve course to involve the brachial plexus (35) (Fig. 14.1).

Parsonage–Turner Syndrome (idiopathic brachial plexitis) traditionally presents with acute onset of shoulder pain that subsides over weeks, and segues into weakness and atrophy of proximal, and less distal, muscles. It is unclear whether Parsonage–Turner Syndrome is more common in lymphoma.

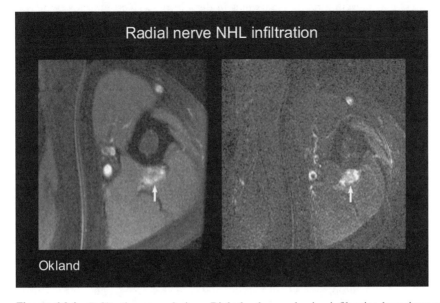

Figure 14.1 Infiltrating nerve lesions. Right lumbosacral spine infiltrating hyperintense mass.

Herniated discs in the lumbosacral region tend to involve L5–S1 and L4–L5 nerve roots, producing pain and lower motor neuron weakness, and hypo- to areflexia. Diabetic proximal neuropathy (diabetic amyotrophy) is a syndrome with similar clinical features to Parsonage–Turner syndrome, but in the lower extremity. Diffuse infiltration of the psoas muscle by cancer can produce anterior thigh pain and a tendency to keep the hip flexed, with pain provoked by leg extension (*malignant psoas syndrome*).

2.3.4. *Management and Prognosis*

Focal radiation can palliate symptoms, and may restore or stabilize function. Pain management may require narcotic analgesics and centrally acting drugs. Corticosteroids may be used to temporize symptoms. Weakness may reduce independence of function, and physical and occupational therapy may be useful for home safety assessment, orthotics, and rehabilitation. Prognosis is dependent upon the nature of the underlying cancer.

2.4. Peripheral Neuropathies (Polyneuropathies and Mononeuropathies)

2.4.1. *Clinical Features*

Polyneuropathies secondary to cancer or its treatment are initially perceived as dysesthesia, hypoesthesia, or anesthesia, starting in the feet. With time, sensory complaints may include hyperpathia or allodynia. Progression of the neuropathy follows a stocking and glove distribution, reflecting the length of nerves involved. Less common are complaints of weakness in the feet, with a tendency to catch the toes when ambulating on uneven surfaces because of weakness in ankle dorsiflexion. Mononeuropathies due to direct tumor infiltration or compression of a nerve begin as pain, dysesthesias, and weakness in the distribution of a peripheral nerve. Occasionally, referred pain can be experienced.

Physical examination findings in polyneuropathies are reduced temperature and vibration indiscrimination prior to involvement of light touch, pinprick, and proprioception. Weakness and muscle atrophy occur first in distally innervated muscles (extensor digitorum brevis and anterior tibialis). When intrinsic foot muscles become weak and atrophic, the normal architecture of the foot can change, producing high arches, collapsing arches when standing, and hammer toes. Deep tendon reflexes are hypo-active or absent in a distal to proximal distribution. Patients with polyneuropathies may give mute responses when assessing for the Babinski response because of interruption of the afferent limb of the muscle stretch reflex.

Physical examination findings in mononeuropathies are sensory abnormalities and weakness confined to the peripheral nerve sensory distribution, although at times this may be difficult to ascertain. When weak muscles are superficial, atrophy and fasciculations may be observed. The deep tendon reflexes may become reduced or absent if the mononeuropathy in question carries a reflex arc.

2.4.2. *Evaluation*

NCS and needle EMG can accurately define which nerves are involved, as well as characterize the neuropathy (axonal vs. demyelinating), and indicate the degree of severity of denervation, all of which may provide information for rehabilitation potential.

Primary axonal neuropathies result in reduction of absent SNAP and CMAP amplitudes, with relative preservation of conduction velocities, distal latencies, and late responses (F-waves). Primary demyelinating neuropathies are characterized by prolonged distal latencies, slowed conduction velocities, and prolonged or absent late responses. Waveforms show abnormal temporal dispersion, and possibly conduction block. Needle EMG evidence of axonal loss is increased insertional activity, sustained positive waves, and fibrillation potentials. Motor units show reduced recruitment and increased amplitude to a degree dependent upon the severity of axonal loss. These EMG abnormalities may occur in primary demyelinating neuropathies because they frequently include some degree of axonal damage.

Electrodiagnostic studies can confirm involvement of specific nerves. In these situations, sensory responses are reduced or absent, and needle EMG shows evidence for denervation confined to muscles innervated by the suspected nerve.

MR neurography can be used to image individual nerves in question. When infiltration of nerve is considered, nerve biopsy may be useful. In individuals with preserved reflexes, distal painful pin prick dysesthesias, and normal electrodiagnostic testing, skin biopsy is useful to assess for the presence of a small fiber neuropathy via analysis of the intra-epidermal nerve fiber density.

Even when an underlying cancer has been well established and it is presumed that a patient's neuropathy is cancer related, it is appropriate to evaluate for reversible causes of peripheral neuropathies to ensure that a patient does not harbor more than one etiology for the neuropathy. This includes testing for B12, thyroid stimulating hormone and for T4, RPR, serum protein electrophoresis with immunofixation, fasting blood sugar and 2-h oral glucose tolerance test, and ESR and a urinalysis for microhematuria.

2.4.3. Differential Diagnosis

Other metabolic and systemic causes for peripheral neuropathy, including unsuspected diabetes or impaired glucose tolerance, should be excluded (36). Azotemia, malnutrition, metabolic derangements, hypoxemia, toxic metabolite accumulations from hepatic insufficiency, and medication related etiologies are common in cancer patients. In individuals hospitalized for acute illness requiring the use of glucocorticoid steroids without or with chemical paralytics, critical illness neuropathy/myopathy may present as a new-onset subacute progressive weakness and dysesthesias. Cancer therapy treatments, including medications and radiation, must be considered. Suspicion for a paraneoplastic neuropathy is frequently raised, but it is very rare (see subsequently).

Lymphomatous neuropathy (lymphomatosis) is the direct infiltration of neoplastic cells into peripheral nerves. It is most common in patients with B-cell lymphomas, and is diagnosed by nerve biopsy. It presents as a relatively asymmetric, slowly progressive, painful axonal sensorimotor neuropathy (or polyradiculoneuropathy). Acute inflammatory demyelinating polyradiculoneuropathy (AIDP) or the Guillain–Barré Syndrome, and chronic inflammatory demyelinating polyradiculoneuropathy (CIDP) are seen with Hodgkins and nonHodgkins lymphoma. Overall, the etiology of most distal predominant sensorimotor axonal peripheral neuropathies in patients with malignancy remains unknown.

2.4.4. Management and Prognosis

Recovery is dependent upon identifying and stopping the underlying cause, and these two factors are frequently elusive. The degree of recovery is primarily a function of the degree of axonal damage. Motor nerves undergo collateral re-innervation, which can preserve strength. Axonal regeneration is slow, and frequently incomplete under the best of circumstances.

The list of directly treatable neuropathies is short. B12 replacement may result in a return of proprioceptive discrimination, but the degree of neurologic damage determines whether permanent underlying disability remains. Paraneoplastic neuropathies may improve upon treatment of the underlying cancer. Acquired inflammatory neuropathies (AIDP and CIDP) may respond to immune-mediated therapies such as prednisone, IVIg, and plasmaphoresis. Lymphomatosis is best treated by chemotherapies directed at the underlying malignancy.

Management of sensory symptoms involves pharmacologic masking of positive symptoms with medications that include tricyclic antidepressants, centrally acting anti-seizure medications such as gabapentin, lamotrigine, and tiagabine. Topical lidocaine gels, and occasionally opioid analgesics may be required for pain control. Distal motor weakness is treated symptomatically with the use of ankle–foot orthoses. Muscle cramps may be treated with quinine sulfate.

3. NEUROPATHY SECONDARY TO CANCER TREATMENT

3.1. Surgical Injury

Peripheral nerve injuries may occur during the surgical treatment of cancers. The brachial plexus can be injured during breast reconstructive surgery involving pedicle TRAM flaps and tissue expansion (37). Postmastectomy lymphedema can cause nerve compression syndromes involving the brachial plexus and median nerve in the carpal tunnel (38). The spinal accessory nerve is often damaged in the course of radical neck dissection, or cervical node dissection, or biopsy. Pelvic surgeries for rectal and gynecologic cancers can injure the pelvic and pudendal nerves and cause urinary sphincter dysfunction and incontinence (39).

3.2. Chemotherapy

A number of chemotherapeutic agents are toxic to peripheral nerves, but only vincristine, cisplatin (Oxaliplatin), taxol, and thalidomide are discussed.

The vinca alkaloids include vincristine and vinblastine, which bind to tubulin and prevent microtubule formation and metaphase arrest. Neurotoxicity is less common with vinblastine, but sensorimotor neuropathy is dose-limiting for vincristine. Symptoms begin with distal numbness and tingling, muscle cramps, loss of tendon reflexes, and weakness of distal muscles (wrist extension and ankle dorsiflexion). Symptoms may progress over several weeks to months after the treatment, a phenomenon known as *coasting*. Unilteral or focal neuropathies also occur. Autonomic nerve involvement is noted in over one-third of patients.

Cisplatin is a heavy metal compound that binds to DNA bases and disrupts function. The drug enters and accumulates in the dorsal root ganglion and peripheral nerves, causing sensory nerve toxicity. It can also cause CNS toxicity and ototoxicity. Intra-arterial infusions for head and neck cancers have been associated with cranial neuropathies (CN VII–XII) (40). Peripheral neuropathy can occur at doses of $200 \, mg/m^2$, and is expected at doses $>400 \, mg/m^2$. The neuropathy initially involves the distal extremities, with numbness and tingling. Pin prick and temperature discrimination are spared, although proprioceptive loss can be significant, producing sensory ataxia. Strength is typically preserved. Symptoms may worsen for several months (coasting) after treatment stops. Neuropathy improves, and may even resolve over months. Histologic examination of affected nerve reveals axonal loss with secondary demyelination. The ventral root is classically spared. Protective agents, including amifostine (a thiophosphate cytoprotectant), have been used, but there is no effective treatment once the neuropathy has developed (41).

Oxaliplatin (Eloxatin) is a new platinum compound that inhibits DNA synthesis by causing inter- and intrastrand DNA crosslinks. It is not associated with nephrotoxicity or ototoxicity. However, it can cause a cold-sensitive, hyperpathic sensory neuropathy that is a dose-limiting toxicity, but appears to be largely reversible once therapy is stopped. The mechanism may be an increase in the refractory period of peripheral nerves via voltage-gated Na^+ channels. An acute laryngeal reaction can be seen, also cold-triggered and probably more prevalent in the winter in colder regions (42).

Paclitaxel (Taxotere) and docetaxel (Taxol) are agents that affect microtubule structure by promoting polymerization. The most commonly associated neuropathy seen is a sensory type, but reversible motor neuropathy occurs. Electrodiagnostic studies suggest either a distal axonopathy, or denervation of proximal muscles innervated by the anterior horn cell or nerve root, although more than one mechanism may be involved.

The peripheral sensory neuropathy seen with paclitaxel occurs in doses >200 mg/m^2, and increases with cumulative dose. When weakness occurs, it is usually distal predominant, although can be occasionally proximal or generalized. Sensory neuropathy from docetaxel is less common (doses 50–720 mg/m^2), although is more often seen in patients previously treated with cisplatin. Weakness is rare, is felt to be idiosyncratic, and can occur at any stage of the treatment (43). Severe neuropathy may be seen with cumulative doses >600 mg/m^2 (44). Nerve biopsies show an axonal neuropathy with preferential loss of large myelinated fibers (45).

Thalidomide works through complex effects on tumor angiogenesis, the immune system, and adhesion molecules. A peripheral neuropathy occurs in 25% of patients treated with doses of 400–800 mg, and older patients may be more susceptible to toxic effects. The neuropathy is characterized as a distal axonopathy involving large diameter motor and sensory fibers, and may be permanent. Paresthesias in the feet are the most common clinical manifestation, but hyperesthesia and a sensation of tightness in the feet are also described. Muscle cramps, intrinsic muscle weakness, and decreased stretch reflexes can follow. Fifty percent of patients report subjective symptoms of neuropathy without objective evidence on electrophysiologic studies. The neuropathic symptoms appear to be related to dose and duration of treatment.

3.3. Radiation Injury

Any part of the nervous system exposed to ionizing radiation can be damaged. Damage is caused by the breaking DNA strands, which leads to cell death. Radiation-induced damage is dependent upon the dose reaching nervous tissue.

Optic neuropathy develops between 7 months to 2 years after radiation treatment. Axonal loss, demyelination, gliosis, and vessel hyalinization cause visual loss that is not reversible. Optic nerves can be spared by shielding the eyes, but some damage occurs with whole-brain radiation. Dysgeusia may result from facial nerve branch injury secondary to radiation and may be permanent in patients treated with high doses (>50 Gy) for head and neck tumors. Decreased salivary gland secretion from radiation can result in xerostomia and dental caries, which may be amenable to pilocarpine. Radiation injury to the peripheral nerves and brachial and lumbosacral plexuses is dose-limiting for treatment of many tumors.

Radiation-induced plexopathy occurs typically one or more years following treatment, although as soon as 4–7 months after intra-operative pelvic irradiation

(Table 14.4). A multilevel lower motor neuron lumbosacral polyradiculopathy or cauda equina syndrome may occur months to decades after para-aortic radiation for malignant testicular cancers and lymphoma (26).

3.4. Management and Prognosis

Delayed radiation therapy injury is typically irreversible, although treatment with anti-coagulation, anti-oxidant therapy, and hyperbaric oxygen, may slow or halt the progression of injury, or even reverse the damage. Urinary incontinence from lower sacral nerve involvement may warrant pharmacologic treatment, and possible suprapubic catheterization to prevent repeated overflow incontinence with recurrent urinary tract infections. Dysesthesias and pain can be treated with anticonvulsants, topical analgesic preparations such as lidocaine gel, and rarely opioids may be utilized.

4. PARANEOPLASTIC SYNDROMES

4.1. Paraneoplastic Neuropathies and Neuronopathies

4.1.1. Clinical Features

A paraneoplastic syndrome is a disorder associated with neoplasia, but not caused by direct tumor invasion or metastases. Neurologic syndromes attributable to toxicity from cancer therapy (i.e., chemotherapy and radiation therapy), cerebrovascular effect, infection, toxic/metabolic insult, or coagulopathy from malignancy are not included. Only syndromes involving the peripheral nervous system will be discussed in this section (Table 14.5).

Syndromes affecting peripheral nerve include sensory neuronopathy, acute and chronic demyelinating polyneuropathy, multifocal motor neuropathy, mononeuritis multiplex, small fiber painful/autonomic neuropathy, distal sensorimotor axonal polyneuropathy, Lambert–Eaton myasthenic syndrome, and myasthenia gravis.

Sensory neuronopathies produce symptoms of burning dysesthesias, aching, and lancinating pain. The distribution tends to involve the torso and face early in the course of symptoms, distinguishing it from length-dependent peripheral neuropathy. The dense loss of sensation often leads to a de-afferented sensory state, and patients may complain of imbalance and frequent falls, but rarely of weakness. Physical examination reveals disproportionate indiscrimination of vibration and proprioception, though all sensory modalities are usually affected. Tendon reflexes are reduced or absent in affected limbs. True weakness is rarely observed, but rather there is a *motor impersistence* with difficulty in sustaining effort against manual motor testing when the limb being tested is not visualized. The loss of sensory input may further lead to an altered sensorium (encephalopathy). Uncommon findings include ocular dysmotility, dysarthria, dysphagia, cerebellar ataxia, corticospinal tract findings, asymmetric lower motor neuron weakness, or autonomic findings (32). Although sensory neuronopathies tend to occur in isolation, other paraneoplastic disorder, such as Lambert–Eaton myasthenic syndrome, motor neuronopathy, and peripheral nerve vasculitis, may occur in combinations.

Acute and chronic demyelinating polyneuropathies produce length-dependent tingling dysesthesias, hyperpathia, and occasionally allodynia. The clinical distinction between acute and chronic demyelinating polyneuropathies is based upon the duration of symptom progression. Chronic neuropathies progress over the course of ≥6 weeks, whereas acute demyelinating neuropathies reach peak disability by 4 weeks. Physical examination in both disorders is notable for distal predominant loss of sensory

Table 14.4 Normal Tissue Tolerance to Therapeutic Irradiation

Organ	TD 5/5 volume			TD 50/5 volume			Endpoint
	1/3	2/3	3/3	1/3	2/3	3/3	
Brain	6000	5000	4500	7500	6500	6000	Necrosis / Infarction
Brain stem	6000	5300	5000	–	–	6500	Necrosis / Infarction
Optic nerve I & II	No partial volume		5000	No partial volume		6500	Blindness
Chiasm	No partial volume		5000	No partial volume		6500	Blindness
Spinal cord	5 cm/5000	10 cm/5000	20 cm/4700	5 cm/7000	10 cm/7000	20 cm/–	Myelitis / Necrosis
Cauda equina	No volume effect		6000	No volume effect		7500	Clinically apparent nerve damage
Brachial plexus	6200	6100	6000	7700	7600	7500	Clinically apparent nerve damage
Eye lens I and II	No partial volume		1000	–	–	1800	Cataract requiring intervention
Eye retina I and II	No partial volume		4500	–	–	6500	Blindness
Ear mid/external	3000	3000	3000	4000	4000	4000	Acute serous otitis
Ear mid/external	5500	5500	5500	6500	6500	6500	Chronic serous otitis

Table 14.5 Neuromuscular Paraneoplastic Clinical Syndromes and Associated Tumors

Clinical syndrome	Associated tumor(s)
Sensory neuronopathy	Small cell lung carcinoma
Acute demyelinating polyneuropathy	Hodgkin lymphoma
	Variety of solid tumors (rare)
Chronic demyelinating polyneuropathy	Osteosclerotic myeloma
	POEMS syndrome
	Other plasma cell dyscrasias
Multifocal motor neuropathy	Plasma cell dyscrasias
Mononeuritis multiplex	Variety of solid tumors
	Cryoglobulinemia
Small fiber painful/autonomic neuropathy	Amyloidosis
	Plasma cell dyscrasias
Distal sensorimotor axonal polyneuropathy	Variety of solid tumors
	Plasma cell dyscrasias

discrimination affecting all sensory modalities, and weakness affecting both distal and proximal musculature. Muscle atrophy is more common in axonal sensorimotor polyneuropathies, but the distinction between axonal and demyelinating polyneuropathies cannot be made on physical examination alone, but is aided by electrodiagnostic studies.

Patients with multifocal motor neuropathy have progressive or step-wise loss of strength in muscles confined to a single peripheral nerve distribution in any limb. There is atrophy and fasciculations in these involved muscles, and tendon reflexes are reduced or absent. Mononeuritis multiplex includes sensory or mixed nerves. Physical examination findings of weakness and sensory loss are confined to single nerves.

4.1.2. Laboratory Evaluation

Symptoms of paraneoplastic syndromes frequently develop months to years before discovery of cancer. Paraneoplastic neuromuscular syndromes are not clinically distinguishable from those of nonparaneoplastic origin, thus complicating their recognition. When a paraneoplastic syndrome is suspected, antineuronal antibodies may be assayed (Table 14.6). Although antibody panels are commercially available, they should not be relied upon, because not all patients with paraneoplastic syndromes express antineuronal antibodies. In addition, there is clinical heterogeneity within most syndromes. Accordingly, clinical examination and testing should be pursued simultaneously with antibody testing.

In sensory neuronopathy NCS reveal reduced or absent SNAPs in a non-length dependent fashion, with preservation of motor potentials, latencies, and conduction velocities. Demyelinating polyneuropathies show prolonged distal latencies, markedly slow conduction velocities, and prolonged F-wave latencies. This is in contrast to distal predominant sensorimotor axonal polyneuropathies, whereby sensory nerve and motor unit action potentials are low in amplitude, with preservation of distal latencies, conduction velocities, and late responses.

Multifocal motor neuropathy is characterized by an abrupt drop in CMAP amplitudes by $>50\%$, with preservation of conduction velocities, distal latencies, and late responses. This is in contrast to mononeuritis multiplex, whereby both SNAP and CMAP have low amplitudes with preservation of conduction velocities, distal latencies, and late responses. Painful small fiber peripheral neuropathies may have normal sensory and motor responses. Testing for Lambert–Eaton myasthenic syndrome and

Table 14.6 Paraneoplastic Disorders and Autoantibodies (37)

Clinical syndrome	Associated tumor(s)	Auto-antibodies
Multifocal encephalomyelitis/ sensory neuronopathy	Small cell lung carcinoma	Anti-Hu (ANNA-1)
		Anti-CV2
		Anti-Amphiphysin
Cerebellar degeneration	Breast, ovarian, adnexal	Anti-Yo
	Small cell lung carcinoma	Anti-Ri (ANNA-2)
	Hodgkin lymphoma	Anti-Hu
	Various carcinomas	Anti-CV2
		PCA-2
		Anti-Tr
		Anti-mGluR1
		Anti-MA
Limbic encephalopathy	Small cell lung carcinoma	Anti-Hu
		Anti-CV2
		PCA-2
	Testicular germ cell tumors	Anti-Hu
		Anti-CV2
		PCA-2
	Testicular germ cell tumors	Anti-amphiphysin
		Anti-Ta
	Breast carcinoma	Anti-voltage gated
	Thymoma	Potassium channel
Opsoclonus/myoclonus	Breast, ovarian carcinomas	Anti-Ri
		Anti-Hu
	Small cell lung carcinoma	Anti-Hu
	Neuroblastoma	Anti-Hu
	Testicular	Anti-Ta
Stiff person syndrome	Small cell lung carcinoma	Anti-amphiphysin
	Breast carcinoma	Anti-amphiphysin
		Anti-GAD
Retinal degeneration	Small cell lung carcinoma	Anti-recoverin
	Melanoma	Anti-bipolar cell
Neuromyotonia	Thymoma	Anti-voltage gated potassium channel
Lambert–Eaton myasthenic syndrome	Small cell lung carcinoma	Anti-voltage gated calcium channel

myasthenia gravis entails repetitive nerve stimulation at both high and low frequencies, and occasionally single fiber EMG measurement of jitter.

Patients with associated Sicca syndrome (xerophthalmia, xerostomia) should be interrogated for Sjögren's syndrome via an extractable nuclear antigen panel, as subacute sensory neuronopathies have been described in these patients. Ultimately, a dorsal root ganglion biopsy may prove diagnostic. In those with a history of smoking, routine chest imaging is appropriate. Suspicious pulmonary parenchymal or bronchial masses can be biopsied by CT-guided biopsy, video assisted thoracoscopy, or via mediastinoscopy/ bronchoscopy. Sensory neuronopathy is associated with paraneoplastic encephalomyeloneuritis, and MRI of the brain with and without contrast can be helpful in making the diagnosis. CSF analysis in patients with a pleocytosis often benefit from a high volume tap for spin-down cytology, in addition to flow cytometry for lymphoma markers.

4.1.3. Differential Diagnosis

The differential diagnosis of paraneoplastic neuromuscular disorders depends upon whether a diagnosis of cancer is established. In patients with an established diagnosis of cancer, chemotherapy neurotoxicity should be considered as potential etiologies, with particular attention to prior cisplatin and carboplatin therapy. Coasting phenomena can occur weeks to months following platin therapy. Sensory neuropathies are more likely to occur when these medications are paired with taxol (paclitaxel) and docetaxel (taxotere), and are likely mediated by both cumulative drug dose and single dose intensity. Chronic sensory neuropathies have been described in patients with IgM paraproteinemia and polyclonal hypergammaglobulinemia, some of which possess concomitant elevated antibody titers against chondroitin sulfate, sulfatide, and disialogangliosides. Subacute sensory neuropathies may produce the presenting symptoms heralding a diagnosis of Sjögren's syndrome, and thus warrant continued queries for Sicca syndrome. HIV infection can produce dorsal root ganglionitis and dorsal column degeneration, thus warranting ELISA testing with Westernblot confirmation. Pyridoxime hypervitaminosis (vitamin B6) causes a subacute sensory neuropathy, although the presenting symptoms of vibratory and proprioceptive loss tends to occur in a distal-predominant manner with associated Lhermitte's symptom (because of both central dorsal column and peripheral nerve involvement).

4.1.4. Management and Prognosis

Management involves identification of the occult cancer, its treatment, and suppression of the autoimmune-mediated cascade producing peripheral nerve dysfunction. Suppression of the autoimmune-mediated cascade is recommended in patients with a clinical diagnosis of a sensory neuronopathy and documented serum anti-Hu antibodies, even in the absence of detectable neoplasm. Although no concensus exists regarding the best way to treat these patients, therapies tend to initiate high dose steroid treatment (prednisone 1 mg/kg PO QD).

Most patients with a sensory neuronopathy experience deterioration over the course of weeks to months, with subsequent stabilization at a level of significant disability. However, some experience a progressive or a step-wise loss of function. In patients who seem to pass away from their neuropathy, as opposed to the cancer, a dysautonomia is believed to be the etiology of sudden death in a minority of patients.

5. OTHER

5.1. Organ Failure and Metabolic Derangements

Various organs may be affected by cancer or therapy-related side effects, or by opportunistic infection. End organ dysfunction may ultimately cause peripheral nerve damage through the accumulation of toxic substances (in the case of both liver and kidney damage), and through the accumulation of metabolic substrates (hyperglycemia and malnutrition in pancreatic illness).

6. CRYPTOGENIC ETIOLOGIES

When a cancer patient develops neuropathy, there is a tendency to assume that it must be somehow related to the cancer or its therapy. Unfortunately, despite an aggressive search for a parsimonious etiology to unite the neuropathy and a cancer, or to another cause, one is often not found, and the neuropathy is said to be *cryptogenic*.

REFERENCES

1. Ampil FL. Radiotherapy for carcinomatous brachial plexopathy. A clinical study of 23 cases. Cancer 1985; 56(9):2185–2188.
2. Croft PB, Wilkinson M. Carcinomatous neuromyopathy. Its incidence in patients with carcinoma of the lung and carcinoma of the breast. Lancet 1963; 1:184–188.
3. Croft PB, Wilkinson M. The incidence of carcinomatous neuromyopathy in patients with various types of carcinoma. Brain 1965; 88:427–434.
4. McLeod JG. Peripheral neuropathy associated with lymphomas, leukemias and polycythemia vera. In: Dyck PJ, Thomas PK, Griffin JW et al., eds. Peripheral Neuropathy. 3rd ed. Philadelphia: WB Saunders, 1993b:1591–1598.
5. Moody JF. Electrophysiologic investigations into the neurological complications of carcinoma. Brain 1965; 88:1023–1036.
6. Trojaborg W, Frantzen E, Andersen I. Peripheral neuropathy and myopathy associated with carcinoma of the lung. Brain 1969; 92:71–82.
7. Paul T, Katiyar BC, Misra S, Pant GC. Carcinomatous neuromuscular syndromes. A clinical and quantitative electrophysiological study. Brain 1978; 101:53–63.
8. Amato AA, Collins MP. Neuropathies associated with malignancy. Semin Neurol 1998; 18(1):125–144.
9. Gupta SR, Zdonczyk DE, Rubino FA. Cranial neuropathy in systemic malignancy in a VA population. Neurology 1990; 40:997–999.
10. Batsakis JG. Nerves and neurotropic carcinomas. Ann Otol Rhinol Laryngol 1985; 94:426–427.
11. Giese WL, Kinsella TJ. Radiation injury to peripheral and cranial nerves. In: Gutin PH, Leibel SA, Sheline GE, eds. Radiation Injury to the Nervous System. New York: Raven Press, 1991:383–403.
12. Robbins KT, Fenton RS. Jugular foramen syndrome. J Otolaryngol 1980; 9:505–516.
13. Chong VF, Fan YF. Hypoglossal nerve palsy in nasopharyngeal carcinoma. Eur Radiol 1998; 8: 939–945.
14. Collins MP, Amato AA. Peripheral Nervous System Diseases Associated with Malignancy. In: Pyck PJ, Thomas PK, Griffin JW, Low PA, Poduslo JF, eds. Peripheral Neuropathy. 3rd ed. Philadelphia: WB Saunders, 1993:1188.
15. Fasola G, Fanin R, Gherlinzoni F et al. Serum LDH concentration in nonHodgkin's lymphomas. Relationship to histologic type, tumor mass, and presentation features. Acta Haematol 1984; 72:231–238.
16. Thomas PK, Holdorff B. Neuropathy due to physical agents. In: Dyck PJ, Thomas PK, Griffin JW, eds. Peripheral Neuropathy. 3rd ed. Philadelphia: WB Saunders, 1993:990–1013.
17. Berger PS, Bataini JP. Radiation-induced cranial nerve palsy. Cancer 1977; 40:152–155.
18. Chew NK, Sim BF, Tan CT et al. Delayed post-irradiation bulbar palsy in nasopharyngeal carcinoma. Neurology 2001; 57:529–531.
19. Haanpaa M, Hakkinen V, Nurmikko T. Motor involvement in acute herpes zoster. Muscle Nerve 1997; 14:1043–1049.
20. Merchunt MP, Gruener G. Segmental zoster paresis of limbs. Electromyogr Clin Electrophysiol 1996; 36:369–375.
21. Pollock BE, Brown PD, Foote RL, Stafford SL, Schomberg PJ. Properly selected patients with multiple brain metastases may benefit from aggressive treatment of their intracranial disease. J Neuro Oncol 2003; 61(1):73–80.
22. Chamberlain MC, Kormanik PA. Epidural spinal cord compression: a single institution's retrospective experience. Neuro Oncol 1999; 1(2):120–123.
23. Clouston PD, DeAngelis LM, Posner JB. The spectrum of neurological diseases in patients with systemic cancer. Ann Neurol 1992; 31:268–273.
24. Argov Z, Siegel T. Leptomeningeal metastases: peripheral nerve and root involvement: clinical and electrophysiological study. Ann Neurol 1985; 17:593–597.

25. Kaplan JG, Portenoy RK, Pack DR, DeSouza T. Polyradiculopathy in leptomeningeal metastasis: the role of EMG and late response studies. J Neuro Oncol 1990; 9:219–224.
26. Lamy C, Mas JL, Varet B et al. Postradiation lower motor neuron syndrome presenting as monomelic amyotrophy. J Neurol Neurosurg Psychiatry 1991; 54:648–649.
27. Osborn AG. Diagnostic Neuroradiology. Chapter 21. St. Louis: Mosby, 1994:876.
28. Kirkwood JR. Essentials of Neuroimaging. Chapter 13. New York: Churchill Livingstone, 1990:412.
29. Kirkwood JR. Essentials of Neuroimaging. Chapter 13. New York: Churchill Livingstone, 1990:414.
30. Osborn AG. Diagnostic Neuroradiology. Chapter 21. St. Louis: Mosby, 1994:894.
31. Schunknecht B, Hubner P, Buller B, Nadjmi M. Spinal leptomeningeal neoplastic disease. Eur Neurol 1992; 32:11–16.
32. Posner JB. Neurologic Complications of Cancer. Philadelphia: FA Davis, 1995.
33. Aguilera Navarro JM, Lopez Domingues JM, Gil Neciga E, Gil Peralta A. Neoplastic lumbosacral plexopathy and "hot foot." Neurologia 1993; 8(8):271–273.
34. Harper CM, Thomas JE, Cascino TL, Litchy WJ. Distinction between neoplastic and radiation-induced brachial plexopathy, with emphasis on the role of EMG. Neurology 1989; 39:502–506.
35. Stubgen JP, Elliot JJ. Malignant radiculopathy and plexopathy. In: Vecht CJ, ed. Handbook of Clinical Neurology. Vol. 25 (69), part III. New York: Elsevier Science, 1997:71–103.
36. Singleton JR, Smith AG, Bromberg MB. Painful sensory polyneuropathy associated with impaired glucose tolerance. Muscle Nerve 2001; 24(9):1225–1228.
37. Ganel A, Engel J, Sela M, Brooks M. Nerve entrapments associated with postmastectomy lymphedema. Cancer 1979; 44:2254–2259.
38. Godfrey PM, Godfrey NV, Fast A, Kemeny M. Bilateral brachial plexus palsy after immediate breast reconstruction with TRAM flaps. Palst Reconstr Surg 1994; 93:1078–1079.
39. Hoffman MS, Roberts WS, Cavanagh D. Neuropathies associated with radical pelvic surgery for gynecologic cancer. Gynecol Oncol 1988; 31:462–466.
40. Frustaci S, Barzan L, Comoretto R et al. Local neurotoxicity after intra-arterial cisplatin in head and neck cancer. Cancer Treat Rep 1987; 71:257–259.
41. DiPaola RS, Schuchter L. Neurologic protection by amifostine. Semin Oncol 1999; 26:82–88.
42. Adelsberger H, Quasthoff S, Grosskreutz J et al. The chemotherapeutic oxaliplatin alters voltage-gaited Na^+ channel kinetics on rat sensory neurons. Eur J Pharmacol 2000; 406:25–32.
43. Freilich RJ, Balmaceda C, Seidman AD et al. Motor neuropathy due to docetaxel and paclitaxel. Neurology 1996; 47:115–118.
44. Hilkens PH, Verweij J, Vecht CJ et al. Clinical characteristics of severe peripheral neuropathy induced by docetaxel (Taxotere). Ann Oncol 1997; 8:187–190.
45. Fazio R, Quattrini A, Bolognesi et al. Docetaxel neuropathy: a distal axonopathy. Acta Neuropathol 1999; 98:651–653.

15

Paraproteinemias and Acquired Amyloidosis*

Mark E. Landau and William W. Campbell
Walter Reed Army Medical Center, Washington DC, USA

ABSTRACT

Approximately 10% of individuals with an idiopathic polyneuropathy harbor a monoclonal protein (M-protein) in serum or urine. In some instances, the M-protein is etiopathogenic, whereas in others it may be an epiphenomenona. An M-protein may be seen in demyelinating or axonal polyneuropathies. Serum and urine protein electrophoresis are the most common means for detecting an M-protein, but immunofixation electrophoresis provides the highest sensitivity and specificity. This chapter discusses the various disease entities associated with M-proteins and polyneuropathy, the most common being

---

*The opinions or assertions contained herein are the private views of the authors and are not to be construed as official or as reflecting the views of the Department of the Army or the Department of Defense.

monoclonal gammopathy of undetermined significance. Optimal diagnosis and management occurs when a solid working relationship is formed with a hematology consultant.

1. INTRODUCTION

The paraproteinemias, also called monoclonal gammopathies and plasma cell dyscrasias, are a group of heterogeneous clinical diseases and syndromes that have in common a monoclonal immunoglobulin in serum or urine. Proliferation of a single plasma cell clone in bone marrow is responsible for production of the monoclonal immunoglobulin. Any monoclonal protein is usually referred to as an M-protein, regardless of its immunoglobulin type, and "M" means monoclonal and has nothing to do with IgM. Other terms are also used and include M-protein, M-component, M-spike, and paraprotein. The M-protein consists of two heavy polypeptide chains and two light chains. The M-protein is called IgG, IgA, IgM, IgD, or IgE when the heavy chain is γ, α, μ, δ, or ε, respectively. The light chain may be either κ or λ. In a polyclonal gammopathy, there is an increase of one or more heavy chains and both light chains and indicates a reactive or inflammatory process. A monoclonal gammopathy is indicative of a malignant or potentially malignant process. The paraproteinemias associated with peripheral neuropathy (PN) are listed in Table 15.1.

Various methods are available to detect the M-protein, including serum protein electrophoresis (SPEP), urine protein electrophoresis (UPEP), immunoelectrophoresis (IEP), and immunofixation electrophoresis (IFE). These techniques vary in regard to the expense, skill, and intensity of labor involved. High-resolution SPEP can detect up to 96% of small M-spikes, whereas low-resolution techniques may only detect 28–60% (1). IFE is the most sensitive and critical in differentiating a monoclonal from a polyclonal gammopathy, but is more expensive and may not be readily available. Laboratories may not want to perform an IFE in the setting of a normal SPEP, but routine SPEP may miss small M-spikes, particularly when they migrate outside the gamma region into the alpha or beta region. In certain situations, the clinician should insist upon an IFE despite a normal SPEP (Table 15.2). An SPEP prior to the IFE helps ensure an optimal dilution of the serum. Urine for detection of monoclonal light chains should be performed from 24 h samples and may be positive when no serum M-spike is detected (2).

The presence of a M-protein is not necessarily indicative of disease as it may be detected in otherwise asymptomatic individuals. Epidemiologic studies indicate that a M-protein is found in ~1% of individuals >25 years and 3% of those >70 years (3). The association of monoclonal gammopathies and peripheral neuropathies cannot be

Table 15.1 Monoclonal Gammopathies Associated with Peripheral Neuropathies

---

Monoclonal gammopathy of undetermined significance
  IgM with anti-MAG—distal demyelinating neuropathy
  IgM without anti-MAG—axonal, distal demyelinating, or CIDP neuropathy
  IgG or IgA—CIDP-like or small fiber axonal
Light chain amyloidosis
Multiple myeloma
Osteosclerotic myeloma
Waldenström's macroglobulinemia
Cryoglobulinemia

Table 15.2 When to Order an IFE

Electrodiagnosis indicative of a demyelinating polyneuropathy
Hypergammaglobulinemia on SPEP without M-spike
Evidence of a small sensory fiber polyneuropathy early in the clinical course
Evidence of systemic disease (cardiac conduction defect, liver, renal, or
dermatological abnormalities)

explained by chance alone. Although, up to 3% of all patients >70 years have a detectable serum M-protein, as many as 10% of patients with an otherwise idiopathic PN have detectable levels (4). Upon detection of an M-protein, a full hematological evaluation, including bone marrow biopsy and skeletal survey, is indicated. If no underlying etiology is found on initial evaluation, then the diagnosis of monoclonal gammopathy of undetermined significance (MGUS) is made. These patients are at risk for developing multiple myeloma (MM), Waldenströms macroglobulinemia (WM), light chain amyloidosis (AL), or other proliferative disease and must be carefully followed. Longitudinal studies show that up to 30% of patients with MGUS will develop one of these disorders, if followed for ≥25 years (5). There are no initial laboratory or clinical features that predict which patients are at risk. When levels of the M-protein are >3 g/dL, MM is more likely to be found at initial evaluation.

The pathogenetic role of the immunoglobulin in neuropathy is not always clear. In some instances, the M-spike may represent an epiphenomenon, as in the cases of chronic inflammatory demyelinating polyneuropathy (CIDP) associated with an IgG-MGUS. Evidence for a causative role of the M-protein exists in some cases of IgM-MGUS, where pathologic studies show antibody to myelin-associated glycoprotein (anti-MAG) to intercalated between the myelin lamellae on EM studies (6). The discovery of other antibodies that recognize nerve proteins, such as anti-SGPG (sulfated glucuronyl-paragloboside), anti-Gd1b (diasialyl ganglioside), anti-GM1 (ganglioside-monosialic), anti-chondroitin sulfate C, and others, supports a pathogenetic role in neuropathy (7).

The neurologist's goal is to determine an etiology for a neuropathy based on clinical presentation, but the literature mainly describes only clinical syndromes related to specific monoclonal antibodies, and there is rarely a distinct phenotypic presentation associated with a particular serological finding. For instance, an IgG M-protein may be seen in MM where the neuropathy is generally an axonal motor and sensory polyneuropathy, in AL where the neuropathy is typically a small fiber sensory and autonomic neuropathy, or in MGUS where there are a variety of clinical presentations. These factors preclude a rigid clinical approach to neuropathy patients with M-spikes.

2. MONOCLONAL GAMMOPATHY OF UNDETERMINED SIGNIFICANCE (MGUS)

MGUS is characterized by the presence of a serum M-protein <3 g/dL, <5% plasma cells in the bone marrow, no or minimal Bence Jones protein in the urine, absence of lytic bone lesions, and no related anemia, hypercalcemia, or renal failure. Of patients with a PN and monoclonal gammopathy, approximately two-thirds fall into this category. In patients with MGUS and a neuropathy, 60% are IgM, 30% IgG, and 10% IgA. In patients without neuropathy, the most common subclass is IgG (8). There is pathological

Table 15.3 Chronic Acquired Dysimmune Polyneuropathies

Chronic inflammatory demyelinating polyneuropathy
1. Iatrogenic
2. Concurrent illnesses
   a. MGUS—IgG >IgM λ
   b. Osteosclerotic myeloma
   c. Lymphoma
   d. HIV
   e. Diabetes mellitus
Distal acquired demyelinating symmetric neuropathy (DADS)
1. DADS-M (M-protein identified)—IgM κ
   a. Anti-MAG activity
   b. No anti-MAG
2. DADS-I (no M-protein)
Multifocal motor neuropathy
Multifocal acquired demyelinating sensory and motor neuropathy

and immunological evidence to support a causal role of the immunoglobulin when IgM is present.

Clinical, electrophysiological, and immunological data from patients with MGUS correlate imperfectly, defying simplistic classification. There is significant overlap of these neuropathies with chronic acquired dysimmune polyneuropathies (CADP) and multiple nomenclatures exist to describe similar yet not necessarily distinct entities (Table 15.3). CIDP is associated with the M-protein ~20% of the time, and the term CIDP–MGUS encompasses all patients with CIDP, or its clinical variants, who harbor an IgM, IgG, or IgA subclass (9). Studies that compared idiopathic CIDP (CIDP-I) with CIDP–MGUS demonstrated a more indolent course, less functional impairment, and less severe weakness, but greater imbalance, leg ataxia, and vibration loss in the MGUS group (10). The term distal acquired demyelinating symmetric neuropathy (DADS) has been proposed to distinguish this phenotypic variation (11). DADS-M is associated with a M-protein (IgM κ in 90% and IgG in the remainder). DADS-I refers to patients with similar clinical manifestations, but no monoclonal gammopathy. DADS-I may be more responsive to immunosuppressive agents than DADS-M. It has been suggested that the term CIDP be applied to patients with predominantly motor manifestations in a proximal and distal distribution, and note that particular patients with an M-protein usually have IgG. The various MGUS neuropathies have been described primarily from the vantage point of the immunoglobulin subtype.

2.1. IgM-MGUS

Neuropathies associated with IgM-MGUS are relatively homogeneous. Most have anti-MAG antibodies, and may be referred to as anti-MAG neuropathy or Latov's syndrome, emphasizing the pathophysiology (12). The other nomenclature is DADS-M emphasizing the clinical and electrophysiologic data (11). The typical patient is an older man who presents with distal, ascending parasthesias, numbness, and sensory ataxia. Pain is relatively uncommon and weakness is confined to the distal muscles. Examination discloses distal joint position and vibration sensation decreased to a greater degree than pain and temperature and a positive Romberg test. Autonomic involvement is rare and helpful in excluding amyloidosis. Atrophy and weakness are confined to the distal lower extremities. Early in the course, the illness may resemble a pure sensory neuropathy. Reflexes are markedly decreased or absent in the lower extremities and mildly decreased in the arms. Nerves may be thickened and firm to palpation. A postural upper extremity tremor may be present in many (13). The disease is chronic, progressing over months to years.

Electrophysiological testing reveals a demyelinating polyneuropathy, with prolonged distal latencies, decreased nerve conduction velocities (NCVs), and conduction blocks (14). The terminal latency index, which compares the NCV of a distal segment of a nerve to a proximal segment, is decreased, indicative of greater degrees of demyelination in the more distal segments (15). Sensory potentials are usually absent in the legs and diminutive in the arms. Cerebrospinal fluid shows a high protein concentration and normal cell count. Approximately two-thirds of patients have anti-MAG antibodies, a glycoprotein constituent of peripheral and central nervous system myelin with neural adhesion properties (11).

Nerve pathology reveals a characteristic wide spacing between the myelin lamellae and, immunopathological studies show IgM binding to myelin sheaths (16). Furthermore, the anti-MAG antibody has been found to be intercalated between densely packed layers of myelin (17). Induction of a similar neuropathic picture in animal models through passive transfer of anti-MAG serum or by direct intraneural injection of anti-MAG also support a causative role for the antibody (18,19).

Rarely, a patient's serum may be positive for anti-MAG antibodies when no M-spike is present on IEP, although this would not technically represent an MGUS (20). Thus, it is appropriate in the clinical setting of a predominantly distal demyelinating features on electrodiagnostic studies to test serum for MAG antibodies, even in the presence of a normal IFE.

The incidence of this syndrome, even in major medical centers, is low. Therefore large, randomized, controlled trials do not exist, limiting treatment recommendations. Further, the slow progression of the neuropathy influences management. When symptoms are mild, benefits of immunologic therapy are likely outweighed by the risks. The time to initiate therapy is done on a case-by-case basis. Long-term prognosis is favorable, and therapies may only be effective in half of the patients (21). Treatment modalities include intravenous immunoglobulin (IVIg), plasma exchange (PE), cyclophosphamide, prednisone, chlorambucil, and interferon α (11,22–25). There is no literature on the use of mycophenolate mofetil. Patients treated with PE may show fluctuations in symptoms and signs that correlate with serum IgM levels, supporting a causal role of the paraprotein (26).

Approximately one-third of patients with IgM-MGUS do not have anti-MAG antibodies. Detailed electrodiagnostic, clinical, and immunological studies have been performed to determine whether patients with anti-MAG antibody differ from those without. Anti-MAG antibody negative patients tend to be more heterogeneous with respect to the clinical and electrodiagnostic features and differ from anti-MAG antibody positive patients (12,13,27,28). Patients with demyelination, irrespective of the presence or absence of anti-MAG, were clinically indistinguishable, with sensory greater than motor manifestations, and these have been classified as DADS-M (11).

2.2. IgG- and IgA-MGUS

There is less evidence implicating IgG- or IgA-MGUS immunoglobulins in the pathogenesis of the neuropathy. Anti-MAG antibodies are rarely found. It is not clear that the PN in patients with IgG or IgA differ from those with IgM gammopathy (27–29). Some patients with IgG- or IgA-MGUS neuropathy are indistinguishable from idiopathic CIDP and do not differ in response to therapy. Progression may be subacute, chronic, or relapsing and remitting, with greater motor than sensory symptoms. Weakness is symmetric, affecting proximal and distal muscles. Other patients may have an axonal polyneuropathy that is chronic and mild. These patients tend to be older and have predominantly sensory symptoms with dysesthesias and autonomic dysfunction, resembling the idiopathic sensory neuropathy seen in the elderly. These symptoms are similar to those in amyloidosis, but progress at a slower rate. However, features such as anemia, elevated sedimentation rate, proteinuria, and cardiac conduction abnormalities should raise suspicion for amyloidosis.

Treatment recommendations for neuropathies associated with a MGUS are limited. Dyck et al. (30) performed a controlled trial comparing PE and sham exchanges on 39 patients with polyneuropathy and MGUS. Testing for MAG antibody was not performed. They concluded that PE appeared to be efficacious, particularly for IgG- or IgA-MGUS and less so for IgM-MGUS. As stated earlier, there is clinical and electrodiagnostic heterogeneity within each of these subtypes, and to what degree any of these factors played a role is unknown. If a patient has clinical and electrodiagnostic criteria consistent with CIDP, then they should be treated the same, regardless of the presence of an IgG- or IgA-MGUS (9). Using strict electrodiagnostic criteria, Gorson and Ropper (31) performed a study of patients with MGUS and polyneuropathy comparing axonal vs. demyelinating subtypes. Fewer patients with an axonal polyneuropathy responded to immunomodulatory treatment.

3. CRYOGLOBULINEMIA

Cryoglobulins are immunoglobulins that precipitate when cooled. They may be formed by one immunoglobulin class or from the interaction of two or more different isotypes (32,33). Type I cryoglobulins are isolated monoclonal immunoglobulins, usually IgG or IgM, and self-aggregate. Type II cryoglobulins have rheumatoid factor (RF) activity, and monoclonal IgM, more commonly than IgG or IgA, and are directed against a polyclonal immunoglobulin, usually IgG. Type III cryoglobulins consist of a polyclonal RF, usually IgM, and other immuoglobulins. Types II and III are referred to as mixed cryoglobulins. RF is present in >87% of patients with mixed cryoglobulinemia. The presence of cryoglobulins does not necessarily establish disease, as approximately one-half of normal patients have detectable, albeit low, levels.

Cryoglobulinemia is defined as having a cryocrit >1% for at least 6 months, a positive serum RF, and at least two of the following: purpura, weakness, arthralgia, or C4 <8 mg/dL. It is considered to be essential cryoglobulinemia when no underlying condition exists and secondary when associated with connective tissue disease, chronic liver disease, a lymphoproliferative disorder, or infection. The most characteristic clinical manifestations of cryoglobulinemia are those related to cold sensitivity, usually affecting acral and dependent regions of the body, such as Raynaud's phenomenon, petechiae, and purpuric eruptions (34). Other possible manifestations include ulcerations, gangrene, oronasal and retinal hemorrhages, liver abnormalities, and a membranoproliferative glomerulonephritis (32).

Clinical peripheral nerve involvement is noted in 17–56% of patients with cryoglobulinemia (32,35,36). Electrophysiological evidence of nerve involvement can be detected in 80% and is typically axonal (37). Clinical features are a progressive, distal, sensory greater than motor, polyneuropathy. Asymmetry is common early on. Dysesthetic pain is the most common complaint (38). The neuropathy may not progress significantly when other aspects of the disease are well controlled (39). Other presentations include mononeuritis multiplex and subacute sensory ataxia (40). The main pathological abnormalities are axonal degeneration with few signs of axonal regeneration (41). Proposed pathogenetic factors include ischemia related to thrombosis or increased blood viscosity, immunologically mediated damage, or cellular infiltration.

Proper collection and processing of serum is critical for detection of cryoglobulins (32). A minimum of 10–20 cc of blood must be allowed to clot at 37°C for 30–60 min. Following centrifugation, the supernatant is kept at 4°C and inspected daily for up to 1 week for cryoprecipitate. If cryoprecipitate forms, it should be resolubilized at 37°C to prove it is a cryoglobulin. Other laboratory abnormalities in essential cryoglobulinemia include a polyclonal hypergammaglobulinemia on SPEP (only 15% of patients have a visible M-spike), anemia, elevated erythrocyte sedimentation rate (ESR), depression of the complement factors C1q and C4, and abnormal liver function tests. Antibodies to hepatitis C virus (HCV) have been found in >50% of patients with types II and III cryoglobulins. Treatments have included corticosteroids, cyclophoshamide, and PE. Interferon A can also be used when anti-HCV antibodies are found.

4. WALDENSTRÖM'S MACROGLOBULINEMIA

Waldenström's macroglobulinemia (WM) is a rare disease characterized by diffuse proliferation of small lymphocytes, plasmacytoid lymphocytes, and plasma cells in bone marrow (42). An IgM M-protein is present in serum. The term "macroglobulin" refers to the high molecular weight of IgM. Direct tumor infiltration and effects of high circulating levels of IgM contribute to clinical manifestations. Although the malignant cells divide slowly, they can disseminate throughout the lymphatic system. Monoclonal IgM can form complexes with other serum proteins resulting in vascular damage in skin or glomeruli. Alternatively, it can act as an autoantibody that attaches to antigens in the nervous system, skin, or skeletal muscle.

Clinical manifestations of WM include weakness, fatigue, nasal and oral bleeding, impaired vision, splenomegaly, and lymphadenopathy. A hyperviscosity syndrome occurs in one-third of patients, causing bleeding tendencies, headache, tinnitus, vertigo, decreased hearing, ataxia, or blurred vision. Fundoscopy reveals distended retinal veins, hemorrhages, or papilledema. PN occurs in ~50% of patients and can be the presenting feature (43). Less common manifestations include lytic bone lesions, amyloidosis, renal, and pulmonary involvement.

The neuropathic manifestations are similar to those seen in IgM-MGUS, including anti-MAG antibodies detectable in 50% (43). Clinically, the neuropathy follows a chronic and slowly progressive course, with distal numbness and parasthesias to a greater degree than distal weakness, sensory ataxia, and tremor. Pain is uncommon. In patients without anti-MAG activity, the clinical manifestations do not differ from those with anti-MAG, but the electrophysiologic findings are less homogeneous, with demyelinating and axonal features. Morphologic studies show demyelination and remyelination. Amyloid deposition and cryoglobulins can also occur, and amyloid should be suspected with the development of dysautonomia. Subclinical, electrophysiologic evidence of neuropathy can also be seen. There is no correlation between the IgM level and the presence oseverity of a neuropathy.

Laboratory abnormalities include anemia, Bence Jones proteinuria, elevated β-2 microglobulin, and hyperviscosity. The IgM immunoglobulins may behave as a cryoglobulin. The median survival is ~5 years, with at least 20% of patients surviving >10 years. Death is due to the complications of a heavily infiltrated bone marrow or transformation to other malignancies such as lymphoma or acute lymphoblastic leukemia.

Primary therapy for WM consists of cytotoxic agents. Patients are often diagnosed in an asymptomatic stage, and the course may be indolent for years, and therapy is typically withheld until complications develop. In patients whose neuropathy features predominate, immunosuppressive therapy with prednisone, chlorambucil, IVIg, or plasmapheresis can be considered (44). There is one published case of a successful response to autologous bone marrow transplantation (45).

5. LIGHT CHAIN AMYLOIDOSIS

AL is a monoclonal plasma cell disorder closely related to MM with some patients fulfilling diagnostic criteria for MM. The amyloid diseases are characterized by the accumulation of insoluble protein fibrils in the extracellular spaces of various organs. Twenty different types of fibrils have been described in human amyloidosis, each with a different clinical picture (46). In AL, the fibril protein is an immunoglobulin light chain or light chain fragment. Rarely, the fibril deposits consist of the heavy chain component (AH). AL and AH are also referred to as immunoglobulin-related amyloidosis. Prior to the description of the fibril component, AL was called primary systemic amyloidosis or when the burden of monoclonal plasma cells was large, myeloma-associated amyloidosis. AL is a systemic disorder with cardiac, gastrointestinal, renal and pulmonary manifestations in addition to a PN. The incidence is $\sim 1/100,000$ per year (47). The clinical presentation is variable depending on which manifestations predominate. Seventy percent of patients are men, with a median age of 64 (47). Prognosis is poor with the median duration of survival 13–25 months (47,48), and only 7% of patients survive >5 years. Serum elevations of β-2 microglobulin are associated with particularly poor prognosis (49). Rarely, survival >10 years occurs. Prolonged survival is generally seen in younger patients with a high initial platelet count (50). Patients who present with a PN tend to have a somewhat longer median survival (25–35 months) (47,51,52). Death is due to systemic involvement and not due to the PN.

PN occurs in $\sim 17\%$ and may be the presenting abnormality (47,53). Small myelinated and unmyelinated fibers that subserve pain and temperature are commonly affected to a greater extent than larger myelinated sensory and motor fibers (54). Usual symptoms are numbness, parasthesias, and dysesthesias in the distal lower extremities. Dysesthesias may be incapacitating, precluding weight bearing, and requiring narcotic medications. Weakness and atrophy are milder, limited to distal lower extremities, and occur later in the course of the illness. Autonomic fibers are also significantly involved and patients can have distressing orthostatic hypotension. Other autonomic features include bowel or bladder dysfunction, impotence, xerostomia, and anhidrosis. Superimposed carpal tunnel syndrome (CTS) due to deposition of amyloid into the flexor retinaculum is not uncommon. CTS may occur prior to the other manifestations of the PN.

Electrodiagnostic testing reveals symmetric axonal degeneration with small or absent sensory nerve action potentials (SNAPs) and decreased compound muscle action potentials (CMAPs). Conduction velocities and distal latencies are minimally affected. Needle EMG discloses distal denervation. Autonomic testing may show absent sympathetic skin responses and fixed heart rate. Rarely, amyloid neuropathy simulates lower motor neuron disease (55) or causes a myopathy associated with skeletal muscle pseudohypertrophy and macroglossia (56). In the latter, serum creatine kinase is normal and needle EMG discloses small, short duration, polyphasic units.

AL should be suspected in patients presenting with symptoms of a small fiber sensory neuropathy. Many patients with AL have constitutional symptoms such as weight loss, fatigue, and postural lightheadedness. Non-neurological signs include periorbital and facial purpura, peripheral edema from cardiac or renal disease, and hepatomegaly. Laboratory clues to the diagnosis include anemia or pancytopenia, elevated ESR, and proteinuria. Other organ involvement, such as cardiac failure, nephrotic syndrome, and a malabsorption syndrome, should raise further suspicion. A classic pattern on ECG is a low voltage QRS complex in the limb leads due to infiltration of amyloid in cardiac conduction tissue. A M-spike is noted in the urine or serum of 90% of patients (47). Serum IEP showed an M-spike in 70%, an intact immunoglobulin (usually IgG) in 50%, and a free monoclonal light chain in 25% (usually λ). The median M-spike is 1.4 g/dL and rarely >3.0 g/dL. The M-spike may be detected in the urine when the serum is negative, supporting the need to order UPEP. CSF protein is moderately elevated in most (average 66 mg/dL). CSF is acellular in most, but a modest pleocytosis can be observed (up to 19 cells/mm^3) (54).

Definitive diagnosis is histological. Amyloid can be found in epineurium and epineural blood vessels or in endoneurium between the nerve fibers. Congo red staining reveals apple-green birefringence under polarized light, and electron microscopy identifies β-pleated fibrils. The sensitivity of nerve biopsy ranges from 33% to 90% (47,54,57). One factor for lower sensitivities in some patients is the timing of the biopsy relative to the pattern of amyloid deposition. Proximal portions of the nervous system are thought to be involved first, and a negative study should not preclude biopsy of the contralateral sural nerve or other tissues based on clinical circumstances. The sensitivity of rectal and fat pad biopsy is $\sim$70–80%. Muscle is another tissue to consider, and amyloid deposits may be found in or around blood vessel walls or in connective tissue, but not within muscle fibers (58). The selection of the biopsy site is dictated by evidence of clinical involvement.

There are currently no medications that have proven successful in stopping the relentless progression of the disease. Combination therapy with melphalan and prednisone has prolonged survival (59). High-dose dexamethasone has been occasionally beneficial in untreated and previously treated patients (60). Iododoxorubicin, a molecule that binds to and solubilizes amyloid fibrils, is undergoing clinical investigation (61).

6. MULTIPLE MYELOMA

MM is a neoplastic disorder characterized by the infiltration of malignant plasma cells in the bone marrow. Onset is usually in the third to fifth decade of life. Clinical evidence of a PN is noted in $\sim$3–5% of patients (62). On the other hand, electrophysiological evidence of neuropathy is present in up to 39% (63). Other neurological manifestations are more common, including radiculopathy and myelopathy from vertebral bone infiltration and those secondary to hypercalcemia. Non-neurological manifestations include bone pain, renal disease, elevated ESR, pancytopenia, and a high incidence of infections. Major criteria for diagnosis include a plasmacytoma, bone marrow infiltration of plasma cells $>30\%$, serum IgG >3.5 g/dL, serum IgA >2.0 g/dL, and urine protein >1.0 g/24 h (64). Other criteria include lytic bone lesions and a reciprocal decrease in the levels of the nonmonoclonal immunoglobulins.

Neuropathy in MM is uncommon and usually is mild, with distal sensory and motor manifestations (63). Sensory symptoms are symmetric, most prominently in the distal lower extremities. The course is slowly progressive and tends to parallel the progression of the MM. Primarily axonal features are noted electrodiagnostically and pathologically (63,65). The neuropathy is usually not disabling, but can herald the onset of MM. Less common is a sensory neuropathy manifested by disabling proprioception and vibration loss. Symptoms progress subacutely over months and then tend to stabilize without improvement or worsening. Least common is a subacute or chronic demyelinating poly-radiculoneuropathy manifested by symmetric progression of weakness both distally and proximally. Approximately one-third of patients with MM and neuropathy have evidence of amyloid deposition, similar to patients with AL (63). In these cases, it is commonly stated that MM can be associated with mononeuritis multiplex because of painful, asymmetric neuropathic signs and symptoms, but these are more likely secondary to lytic bone lesions and polyradiculopathy.

7. OSTEOSCLEROTIC MYELOMA

Osteosclerotic myeloma (OSM) represents <3% of all cases of myeloma (63). It has a more indolent course, bone marrow is not infiltrated by plasma cells, the concentration of the M-spike is low, and anemia, renal disease, and hypercalcemia are uncommon. However, PN is noted in ~50% of cases. OSM is due to a plasmacytoma that is usually found in a sclerotic bone lesion, otherwise proliferation of plasma cells is confined to the lymph nodes. Sclerotic lesions may be solitary or multiple and are typically located in the spine, ribs, or pelvis, with relative sparing of the skull and distal long bones.

The neuropathy is relatively homogeneous with motor manifestations dominating (66). Patients present with progressive, symmetric weakness beginning distally and spreading proximally. Symptoms progress over months to years. Sensory ataxia with imbalance, distal hypesthesias, and parasthesias occurs, but to a lesser extent than weakness. Other manifestations include an action tremor and palpable nerves. The clinical and electrodiagnostic phenomena are not distinctly different from idiopathic CIDP. CSF is acellular with an elevated protein. Somatosensory evoked potentials show proximal abnormalities, suggesting that the syndrome is a polyradiculoneuropathy (67). The neuropathy does not respond to conventional immunotherapy, but does remit with radiation of the tumor.

The diagnosis of OSM may be difficult. A serum M-spike of low concentration, usually IgG or IgA with the light chain more commonly λ, is noted in ~75% of patients (66). A skeletal bone survey is necessary to detect the sclerotic lesions. Radioisotope bone scanning is not helpful. Often the tumors are inadvertently ascribed to benign processes such as fibrous dysplasia or vertebral hemangioma. In the appropriate clinical setting, biopsy of such lesions is necessary. Radiation therapy effectively treats solitary lesions, with subsequent improvement of the neurological manifestations and decreased titers of the M-spike. Patients must be followed after treatment, as return of the neurological symptoms or elevations of the M-spike can signify tumor recurrence. Multiple lesions are more difficult to treat due to radiation therapy dose limitations. Chemotherapy is less effective in treating the tumors or the neuropathy.

OSM may also be associated with a systemic process that is referred to as either the POEMS (polyneuropathy, organomegaly, endocrinopathy, M-proteins, and skin changes) syndrome (68) or the Crow–Fukase syndrome (69). Again, the polyneuropathy is CIDP-like. Organomegaly can be noted in the liver, spleen, or lymph nodes. Endocrine abnormalities include glucose intolerance, hypothyroidism, gynecomastia, amenorrhea, or impotence. Dermatologic manifestations include hypertrichosis, hyperpigmentation, clubbed fingers, and sclerodermatous changes. Edema is very common and can be severe. Patients may have ascites or anasarca. Ocular complications such as optic disc swelling, preretinal hemorrhages, or uveitis also occur. Patients can have any number of manifestations, but rarely fulfill all criteria for POEMS (70). Approximately 90% of patients will have a detectable M-spike, either IgA or IgG (70). The course of the illness is slowly progressive, with median survival of 33 months and death in >50% of patients. Long-term treatment with melphalan and prednisolone may be effective in a few patients (71).

A related neoplasm, angiofollicular lymph node hyperplasia, or Castleman's disease may be associated with the same systemic manifestations as OSM. It also causes a primarily demyelinating motor greater than sensory polyneuropathy, associated with an IgG or IgA M-spike and λ light chains (72).

8. CLINICAL EVALUATION

The clinical manifestations of peripheral neuropathies associated with monoclonal gammopathies are diverse. Routine screening with SPEP and 24 h UPEP is recommended for all patients having a PN without an obvious etiology. SPEP is not the most sensitive test for detecting a M-spike, but it is the cheapest and most readily available. The clinician must decide when to order the more sensitive, but also more expensive, IFE when the SPEP is negative. Suggestions are listed in Table 15.2. When a M-spike is detected, all patients should have a hematology consultation and skeletal survey. Further workup is dependent upon the clinical and electrodiagnostic data.

1. CIDP presentation: IFE is necessary if SPEP/UPEP is negative. When a M-spike is found, the differential diagnosis includes CIDP–MGUS and OSM. A skeletal survey is necessary for detecting sclerotic lesions, and a nuclear bone scan is insensitive. Evidence of the Crow–Fukase syndrome (POEMS) must be sought by clinical evaluation. Serum anti-MAG is recommended if the M-spike is IgM. CIDP–MGUS is managed the same as CIDP-I, except that periodic re-evaluations for OSM are required.

2. DADS presentation: IFE is necessary if SPEP/UPEP is negative. DADS-M can be seen in MGUS or in WM, and bone marrow biopsy is the most useful tool to differentiate between them. Other laboratory abnormalities in WM include anemia, elevated β-2 microglobulin, and hyperviscosity. Testing serum for anti-MAG is recommended regardless of the presence or absence of a M-spike.

3. Axonal neuropathy involving unmyelinated and small sensory fibers and autonomic fibers: IFE not required when SPEP/UPEP is negative unless other clinical features suggest cryoglobulinemia or AL. If an M-spike is detected, serum evaluation for cryoglobulins, RF, ESR, complement levels, and HCV are recommended. Sural nerve, rectal or fat pad biopsy is also recommended. The absence of a M-spike does not obviate the need for biopsy under the appropriate clinical settings.

4. Axonal, sensory, and motor neuropathy: IFE not needed when SPEP/UPEP is negative. If positive, skeletal survey for osteolytic lesions and hematologic consultation recommended.

REFERENCES

1. Keren DF. Procedures for the evaluation of monoclonal immunoglobulins. Arch Pathol Lab Med 1999; 123:126–132.
2. Kyle RA, Gertz MA. Primary systemic amyloidosis: clinical and laboratory features in 474 cases. Semin Hematol 1995; 32:45–59.

3. Kyle RA, Finklestein S, Elveback LR, Kurland LT. Incidence of monoclonal proteins in a Minnesota community with a cluster of multiple myeloma. Blood 1972; 40:719–724.

4. Kelly JJ Jr, Kyle RA, O'Brien PC, Dyck PJ. Prevalence of monoclonal protein in peripheral neuropathy. Neurology 1981; 31:1480–1483.

5. Kyle RA, Therneau TM, Rajkumar SV, Offord JR, Larson DR, Plevak MF, Melton LF. A long-term study of prognosis in monoclonal gammopathy of undetermined significance. N Engl J Med 2002; 346:564–569.

6. Trojaborg W, Hays AP, Van Den Berg L, Younger DS, Latov N. Motor conduction parameters in neuropathies associated with anti-MAG antibodies and other types of demyelinating and axonal neuropathies. Muscle Nerve 1995; 18:730–735.

7. Nobile-Orazio E, Manfredini E, Carpo M, Meucci N, Monaco S, Ferari S, Boneti B, Cavaletti G, Gemignani F, Durelli L, Barbieri S, Allaria S, Sgarzi M, Scarlato G. Frequency and clinical correlates of anti-neural IgM antibodies in neuropathy associated with IgM monoclonal gammopathy. Ann Neurol 1994; 36:416–424.

8. Ropper AH, Gorson KC. Neuropathies associated with paraproteinemia. N Engl J Med 1998; 338:1601–1607.

9. Gorson KC, Allam G, Ropper AH. Chronic inflammatory demyelinating polyneuropathy: clinical features and response to treatment in 67 consecutive patients with and without a monoclonal gammopathy. Neurology 1997; 48:321–328.

10. Simmons Z, Albers JW, Bromberg MB, Feldman EL. Presentation and initial clinical course in patients with chronic inflammatory demyelinating polyradiculoneuropathy: comparison of patients without and with monoclonal gammopathy. Neurology 1993; 43:2202–2209.

11. Katz JS, Saperstein DS, Gronseth G, Amato AA, Barohn RJ. Distal acquired demyelinating symmetric neuropathy. Neurology 2000; 54:615–620.

12. Kelly JJ. Neuropathies of monoclonal gammopathies of undetermined significance. Hematol Oncol Clin North Am 1999; 13:1203–1210.

13. Chassande B, Leger J, Younes-Chennoufi AB, Bengoufa D, Maisonobe T, Bouche P, Baumann N. Peripheral neuropathy associated with IgM monoclonal gammopathy: correlations between M-protein antibody activity and clinical/electrophysiological features in 40 cases. Muscle Nerve 1998; 21:55–62.

14. Kelly JJ. The electrodiagnostic findings in polyneuropathies associated with IgM monoclonal gammopathies. Muscle Nerve 1990; 13:1113–1117.

15. Kaku DA, England JD, Sumner AJ. Distal accentuation of conduction slowing in polyneuropathy associated with antibodies to myelin-associated glycoprotein and sulphated glucornyl paragloboside. Brain 1994; 117:941–947.

16. Vital A, Vital C, Julien J, Baquey A, Steck AJ. Polyneuropathy associated with IgM monoclonal gammopathy. Immunological and pathological study in 31 patients. Acta Neuropathol 1989; 79:160–167.

17. Nemni R, Galassi G, Latov N, Sherman WH, Olarte MR, Hays AP. Polyneuropathy in nonmalignant IgM plasma cell dyscrasia: a morphological study. Ann Neurol 1983; 14:43–54.

18. Tatum AH. Experimental paraprotein neuropathy, demyelination by passive transfer of human IgM anti-myelin-associated glycoprotein. Ann Neurol 1993; 33:502–506.

19. Hays AP, Latov N, Takatsu M, Sherman WH. Experimental demyelination of nerve induced by serum of patients with neuropathy and an anti-MAG IgM M protein. Neurology 1987; 37:242–256.

20. Nobile-Orazio E, Latov N, Hays AP, Takatsu M, Abrams GM, Sherman WH, Miller JR, Messito MJ, Saito T, Tahmoush A. Neuropathy and anti-MAG antibodies without detectable serum M-protein. Neurology 1984; 34:218–221.

21. Nobile-Orazio E, Meucci N, Baldini L, Di Troia A, Scarlato G. Long-term prognosis of neuropathy associated with anti-MAG IgM M-proteins and its relationship to immune therapies. Brain 2000; 123:710–717.

22. Haas DC, Tatum AH. Plasmapheresis alleviates neuropathy accompanying IgM anti-myelin associated glycoprotein paraproteinemia. Ann Neurol 1988; 23:394–396.

23. Blume G, Pestronk A, Goodnough LT. Anti-MAG antibody associated polyneuropathies: improvement following immunotherapy with monthly plasma exchange and IV cyclophosphamide. Neurology 1995; 45:1577–1580.

24. Nobile-Orazio E, Baldini L, Barbieri S, Marmiroli P, Spagnol G, Francomano E, Scarlato G. Treatment of patients with neuropathy and anti-MAG IgM M-proteins. Ann Neurol 1988; 24:93–97.

25. Mariette X, Chastang C, Clavelou P, Louboutin JP, Leger JM, Brouet JC. A randomized clinical trial comparing interferon-α and intravenous immunoglobulin in polyneuropathy associated with monoclonal IgM. J Neurol Neurosurg Psychiatry 1997; 63:28–34.

26. Sherman WH, Olarte MR, McKiernan G, Sweeney K, Latov N, Hays AP. Plasma exchange treatment of peripheral neuropathy associated with plasma cell dyscrasia. J Neurol Neurosurg Psychiatry 1984; 813–819.

27. Suarez GA, Kelly JJ. Polyneuropathy associated with monoclonal gammopathy of undetermined significance: further evidence that IgM-MGUS neuropathies are different than IgG-MGUS. Neurology 1993; 43:1304–1308.

28. Gosselin S, Kyle RA, Dyck PJ. Neuropathy associated with monoclonal gammopathies of undetermined significance. Ann Neurol 1991; 30:54–61.

29. Simovic D, Gorson KC, Ropper AH. Comparison of IgM-MGUS and IgG-MGUS polyneuropathy. Acta Neurol Scand 1998; 97:194–200.

30. Dyck PJ, Low PA, Windebank AJ, Jaradeh SS, Gosselin S, Bourque P, Smith BE, Kratz KM, Karnes JL, Evans BA, Pineda AA, O'Brien PC, Kyle RA. Plasma exchange in polyneuropathy associated with monoclonal gammopathy of undetermined significance. N Engl J Med 1991; 325:1482–1486.

31. Gorson KC, Ropper AH. Axonal neuropathy associated with monoclonal gammopathy of undetermined significance. J Neurol Neurosurg Psychiatry 1997; 63:163–168.

32. Dispenzieri A, Gorevic PD. Cryoglobulinemia. Hematol Oncol Clin North Am 1999; 13:1315–1349.

33. Brouet JC, Clauvel JP, Danon F, Klein M, Seligmann M. Biologic and clinical significance of cryoglobulins. A report of 86 cases. Am J Med 1974; 57:775–788.

34. Logothetis J, Kennedy WR, Ellington A, Williams RC. Cryoglobulinemic neuropathy. Incidence and clinical characteristics. Arch Neurol 1968; 19:389–397.

35. Cavaletti G, Petruccioli MG, Crespi V, Pioltelli P, Marmiroli P, Tredici G. A clinicopathological and follow up study of 10 cases of essential type II cryoglobulinaemic neuropathy. J Neurol Neurosurg Psychiatry 1990; 53:886–889.

36. Logothetis J, Kennedy WR, Ellington A, Williams RC. Cryoglobulinemic neuropathy. Arch Neurol 1968; 19:389–397.

37. Ferri C, La Civita L, Cirafisi C, Siciliano G, Longombardo G, Bombardieri S, Rossi B. Peripheral neuropathy in mixed cryoglobulinemia: clinical and electrophysiologic investigations. J Rheumatol 1992; 19:889–895.

38. Garcia-Bragado F, Fernandez JM, Navarro C, Villar M, Bonaventura I. Peripheral neuropathy in essential mixed cryoglobulinemia. Arch Neurol 1988; 45:1210–1214.

39. Crespi V, Cavaletti G, Pioltelli P, Zincone A, Tredici G, Mamiroli P, Petruccioli MG. Cryoglobulinaemic neuropathy: lack of progression in patients with good hematological control. Acta Neurol Scand 1995; 92:372–375.

40. Lippa CF, Chad DA, Smith TW, Kaplan MH, Hammer K. Neuropathy associated with cryoglobulinemia. Muscle Nerve 1986; 9:626–631.

41. Nemni R, Corbo M, Fazio R, Quattrini A, Comi G, Canal N. Cryoglobulinaemic neuropathy: a clinical, morphological and immunocytochemical study of 8 cases. Brain 1988; 111:541–552.

42. Dimopoulos MA, Galani E, Matsouka C. Monoclonal gammopathies and related disorders: Waldenström's macroglobulinemia. Hematol Oncol Clin North Am 1999; 13:1351–1366.

43. Nobile-Orazio E, Marmiroli P, Baldini L, Spagnol G, Barbieri S, Moggio M, Polli N, Polli E, Scarlato G. Peripheral neuropathy in macroglobulinemia: incidence and antigen-specificity of M proteins. Neurology 1987; 37:1506–1514.

44. Dalakas MC, Flaum MA, Rick M, Engel WK, Gralnick HR. Treatment of polyneuropathy in Waldentström's macroglobulinemia: role of paraproteinemia and immunologic studies. Neurology 1983; 33:1406–1410.

45. Rudnicki SA, Harik SI, Dhodapkar M, Barlogie B, Eidelberg D. Nervous system dysfunction in Waldenström's macroglobulinemia: response to treatment. Neurology 1998; 51:1210–1213.

46. Westermark P, Araki S, Benson MD. Nomenclature of amyloid fibril proteins. Report from the meeting of the International Nomenclature Committee on Amyloidosis, Aug 8–9, 1998. Part 1. Amyloid 1999; 6:63–66.

47. Kyle RA, Gertz MA. Primary systemic amyloidosis: clinical and laboratory features in 474 cases. Semin Hematol 1995; 32:45–59.

48. Gertz MA, Kyle RA. Amyloidosis: prognosis and treatment. Semin Arthritis Rheum 1994; 24:124–138.

49. Gertz MA, Kyle RA, Greipp PR, Katzmann JA, O'Fallon WM. Beta 2-microglobulin predicts survival in primary systemic amyloidosis. Am J Med 1990; 89:609–614.

50. Kyle RA, Gertz MA, Greipp PR, Witzig TE, Lust JA, Lacy MQ, Therneau TM. Long-term survival (10 years or more) in 30 patients with primary amyloidosis. Blood 1999; 93:1062–1066.

51. Duston MA, Skinner M, Anderson J, Cohen AS. Peripheral neuropathy as an early marker of AL amyloidosis. Arch Intern Med 1989; 149:358–360.

52. Rajkumar SV, Gertz MA, Kyle RA. Prognosis of patients with primary systemic amyloidosis who present with dominant neuropathy. Am J Med 1998; 104:232–237.

53. Kyle RA, Bayrd ED. Amyloidosis: review of 236 cases. Medicine (Baltimore) 1975; 54:271–299.

54. Kelly JJ, Kyle RA, O'Brien PC, Dyck PJ. The natural history of peripheral neuropathy in primary systemic amyloidosis. Ann Neurol 1979; 6:1–7.

55. Quattrini A, Nemni R, Sferrazza B, Ricevuti G, Dell'Antonio G, Lazzerini A, Iannaccone S. Amyloid neuropathy simulating lower motor neuron disease. Neurology 1998; 51:600–602.

56. Whitaker JN, Hashimoto K, Quinones M. Skeletal muscle pseudohypertrophy in primary amyloidosis. Neurology 1977; 27:47–54.

57. Simmons Z, Blaivas M, Aguilera AJ, Feldman EL, Bromberg MB, Towfighi J. Low diagnostic yield of sural nerve biopsy in patients with peripheral neuropathy and primary amyloidosis. J Neurol Sci 1993; 120:60–63.

58. Trotter JL, Engel WK, Ignaczak TF. Amyloidosis with plasma cell dyscrasia: an overlooked cause of adult onset sensorimotor neuropathy. Arch Neurol 1977; 34:209–214.

59. Kyle RA, Gertz MA, Greipp PR, Witzig TE, Lust JA, Lacy MQ, Therneau TM. A trial of three regimens for primary amyloidosis: colchicines alone, melphalan and prednisone, and melphalan, prednisone, and colchicines. N Engl J Med 1997; 336:1202–1207.

60. Gertz MA, Lacy MQ, Lust JA, Greipp PR, Witzig TE, Kyle RA. Phase II trial of high-dose dexamethasone for untreated patients with primary systemic amyloidosis. Med Oncol 1999; 16:104–109.

61. Gianni L, Bellotti V, Gianni AM, Merlini G. New drug therapy of amyloidosis: resorption of AL-Type Deposits with 4'-Iodo-4'-deoxydoxorubicin. Blood 1995; 3:855–861.

62. Kelly JJ, Kyle RA, Miles JM, O'Brien PC, Dyck PJ. The spectrum of peripheral neuropathy in myeloma. Neurology 1981; 31:24–31.

63. Walsh JC. The neuropathy of multiple myeloma: an electrophysiological and histological study. Arch Neurol 1971; 25:404–414.

64. Grethlein S. Multiple myeloma. EMedicine J 2004. Available at www.emedicine.com/med/topic1521.htm.

65. Maurice V, Banker BQ, Adams RD. The neuropathy of multiple myeloma. J Neurol Neurosurg Psychiatry 1958; 21:73–88.

66. Kelly JJ, Kyle RA, Miles JM, Dyck PJ. Osteosclerotic myeloma and peripheral neuropathy. Neurology 1983; 33:202–210.

67. Shibasaki H, Ohnishi A, Kuroiwa Y. Use of SEPs to localize degeneration in a rare polyneuro-pathy: studies on polyneuropathy associated with pigmentation, hypertrichosis, edema, and plasma cell dyscrasia. Ann Neurol 1982; 12:355–360.
68. Bardwick PA, Zvaifler NJ, Gill GN, Newman D, Greenway GD, Resnick DL. Plasma cell dyscrasia with polyneuropathy, organomegaly, endocrinopathy, M-proteins, and skin changes: the POEMS syndrome. Report on two cases and a review of the literature. Medicine 1980; 59:311–324.
69. Nakanishi T, Sobue I, Toyokura Y, Nishitani H, Kuroiwa Y, Satoyoshi E, Tsubake T, Igata A, Ozaki Y. The Crow–Fukase syndrome: a study of 102 cases in Japan. Neurology 1984; 34:712–720.
70. Miralles GD, O'Fallon JR, Talley NJ. Plasma-Cell dyscrasia with polyneuropathy: the spectrum of POEMS Syndrome. N Engl J Med 1992; 327:1919–1923.
71. Kuwabara S, Hattori T, Shimoe Y, Kamitsukasa I. Long term melphalan-prednisolone chemotherapy for POEMS syndrome. J Neurol Neurosurg Psychiatry 1997; 63:385–387.
72. Donaghy M, Hall P, Gawler J, Gregson NA, Leibowitz S, Jitpimolmard S, King RH, Thomas PK. Peripheral neuropathy associated with Castleman's disease. J Neurol Sci 1989; 89:253–267.

16

Peripheral Neuropathy in HIV Infection

Lydia Estanislao and David Simpson
Mount Sinai Medical Center, New York, New York, USA

ABSTRACT

Peripheral nerves are the most frequently affected portion of the nervous system in HIV-infected individuals. Distal symmetric polyneuropathy (DSP) is the most common form of neuropathy, occurring in $\sim$30% of individuals. It can occur as a result of the HIV infection, usually in intermediate to advanced stages. A variety of neuropathies, some similar to DSP, may occur as a toxic effect of medications. These include the dideoxynucleoside antiretroviral drugs and others used to treat associated infections. Correction of any underlying medical disease aggravating or unmasking DSP (e.g., diabetes mellitus), dose reductions or cessation of offending drugs, virologic suppression, and adequate pain control are mainstays of management.

Mononeuropathy multiplex and inflammatory demyelinating polyneuropathy may occur during early stages of HIV infection, implicating immune-mediated mechanisms, or in advanced disease, more often associated with opportunistic infections such as cytomegalovirus (CMV). Diagnosis and management are dictated by the stage of HIV infection. A progressive and potentially fatal polyradiculopathy may result from CMV infection in advanced AIDS.

1. INTRODUCTION

The life expectancy of HIV-infected patients has increased as a result of highly active antiretroviral therapy (HAART). Consequently, patients and physicians are dealing with neurologic complications from the HIV disease, from concurrent diseases, and from drugs used to treat it. Peripheral neuropathy is the most common HIV-associated neurologic complication (1,2). Several forms of neuropathy may occur, depending on the level of immunosuppression and the presence of risk factors. In this chapter, the different forms of neuropathy occurring in HIV-infected individuals are reviewed, including distal symmetrical polyneuropathy (DSP) caused by the HIV infection or HAART drugs toxicity, inflammatory demyelinating polyneuropathy (IDP), progressive polyradiculopathy (PP), and mononeuropathy multiplex (MM). The epidemiology, pathogenesis, clinical features, and management of each type is discussed.

2. DISTAL SYMMETRICAL POLYNEUROPATHY

2.1. Epidemiology

DSP is the most common neuropathy. When both symptomatic and asymptomatic forms are combined, DSP occurs in one-third of HIV-positive patients (3–5). Advanced disease stage is the most important risk factor (5–8). Plasma HIV viral load is predictive of the development and severity of DSP (8). HIV RNA levels >10,000 copies/mL are associated with a 2.3-fold greater hazard of developing a neuropathy, and HIV viral load is correlated with severity of pain and quantitative sensory test (QST) abnormalities (9). Other risk factors include diabetes mellitus, alcohol abuse, illicit drug abuse, older age, and other neurologic disorders.

2.2. Clinical Manifestations and Examination Findings

DSP presents with symmetric dysesthesias, paresthesias, or numbness in the legs which may progress to above the ankles. The pain is often characterized as burning, and may be so intense that gait is altered to avoid pressure on the soles of the feet (10). The soft touch of socks or bed sheets may be very painful.

Decreased sensory perception to pinprick and temperature is found in the distal lower extremities and, in advanced stages, in the distal upper extremities. Joint position sense is usually preserved, except in severe cases. Ankle reflexes are absent or depressed compared with knee reflexes. However, in the setting of a coexisting HIV-associated myelopathy, knee reflexes may be hyperactive, whereas ankle reflexes will be normal or minimally depressed. Muscle weakness involving only distal intrinsic muscles of the feet may occur late in the disease.

2.3. Laboratory and Electrophysiologic Findings

Laboratory investigations are usually uninformative, but it is prudent to look for reversible cause of neuropathy, including serum vitamin B12 and glucose levels and 2 h glucose tolerance test. Cerebrospinal fluid (CSF) analysis is usually not necessary, unless there is suspicion of an infectious process. Nerve biopsy is rarely necessary except in cases with atypical features. Skin biopsy for intraepidermal nerve fiber density analysis provides a minimally invasive marker of nerve loss, particularly when nerve conduction studies are normal (11).

The electrophysiologic features are those indicative of distal and symmetrical degeneration of sensory and motor axons. Nerve conduction studies usually reveal reduced or absent sural nerve responses (12–14). However, DSP may be associated with normal sural nerve studies because of preferential small fiber loss (12,14–16). Less commonly, sensory nerve action potential (SNAP) or compound motor action potential (CMAP) of the median or ulnar nerves are reduced. F-waves are only mildly prolonged, consistent with axonal neuropathy. Electromyography may show active or chronic denervation with reinnervation in very distal muscles.

2.4. Pathology

Pathologic evidence for DSP is found in nearly all patients dying with AIDS. The pattern of fiber loss is predominantly distal, and distal axonal degeneration may affect both central and peripheral projections of dorsal root ganglion cells (17). Loss of dorsal root ganglion cells and mononuclear infiltration is usually mild when compared with the degree of axonal degeneration and inflammation noted in distal nerves (17,18).

The most common nerve biopsy finding is degeneration of myelinated and unmyelinated axons (18,19). Mild epineural and endoneural perivascular mononuclear inflammation is observed in up to two-thirds of specimens (18–20). T-lymphocytes and activated macrophages, with suppressor/cytotoxic cells (CD8) predominating over helper/inducer (CD4) cells endoneurially are observed (18). No deposition of immunoglo-bulin, complement, or fibrin is observed. Demyelination is occasionally observed, but does not appear to be macrophage-mediated or follow a segmental pattern (18–22).

2.5. Pathogenesis

The pathogenesis is not known. HIV infection appears to be a factor because aggressive antiretroviral therapy and suppression of plasma HIV-1 viral burden improves sensory function in HIV-infected patients, as measured by QST, but it is not clear if this represents a direct or indirect mechanism (23). There has been no consistent demonstration of HIV in dorsal root ganglion cells, nerve roots or peripheral nerves (16,18,19,24), and a paucity of evidence for significant *in vivo* infection of neurons. Possible indirect mechanisms include cytokine dysregulation and immunologic dysfunction. Elevated levels of tumor necrosis factor-α, interleukin-1, and interleukin-6 have been identified in peripheral nerve and dorsal root ganglia of patients with AIDS (3,14,18,19,21,25–27), and their expression may be induced though low levels of HIV-1 replication acting on cytotoxic T-lymphocytes, resulting in degeneration of sensory neurons within the dorsal root ganglion (27).

Paraproteinemia may be a factor in some cases, with reactivity of IgM and IgG against myelin proteins identified in a majority of tested samples from HIV-infected individuals (28). High titers of antisulfatide antibodies have been found which show immunofluorescence at paranodal regions (29,30).

Cytomegalovirus (CMV) inclusions or antigens have been identified in peripheral nerve, nerve roots, and dorsal root ganglion cells of some patients with DSP (17–19,24). Although some patients with painful neuropathy, particularly in advanced disease stages, have an underlying systemic CMV infection (31), there is no compelling evidence that direct CMV infection causes DSP and accounts for DSP in patients with early HIV infection.

2.6. Treatment

Control of pain is the primary treatment goal. Of note, up to 85% of patients with AIDS-related pain are under treated (32). Guidelines established by the world Health Organization (WHO) to manage cancer pain can be adapted for HIV-associated DSP (33). In addition to the use of mild analgesics, adjunctive analgesic medications may necessary. These include tricyclic antidepressants amitriptyline or desipramine and gaba-pentin and lamotrigine. Topical anesthetic agents may also be used (lidocaine patch or gel or capsaicin). Narcotic analgesics are often necessary to control pain in severe cases.

The efficacy of various modalities has been studied in randomized clinical trials (Table 16.1). Lamotrigine and recombinant human nerve growth factor (NGF) are most promising (34,35). NGF is not available for clinical use. Lamotrigine has been effective in pain reduction in two placebo-controlled trails of HIV DSP (34). In the recent larger trial, lamotrigine's superiority was demonstrated only in the strata of subjects receiving ARV, due to the large placebo response in the strata with primary HIV DSP (36). Successful HAART may have a beneficial effect on non-ARV-associated DSP. A pilot study has shown improvement in quantitative thermal testing results in subjects fol-lowed up prospectively after initiation of HAART (23). In cases of ARV-associated DSP (as discussed subsequently), ARV dose reduction or substitution of a less neurotoxic ARV without sacrificing virologic control may be sufficient to alleviate symptoms. In cases in which alternative non-neurotoxic ARV agents are not available due to resistance or

Table 16.1 Summary of Randomized Clinical Trials of Efficacy and/or Safety of Agents for DSP Pain in HIV-Infected Patients

Study and number of study subjects	Reference	Outcome/s measured	Results
Peptide T vs. placebo, $n = 81$ (40/41)	Simpson et al. (37)	Primary: change in modified Gracely pain scale	(−) Significant difference
		Secondary: change in neurological exam, neuropsychiatric exam, electrophysiologic studies, global evaluation, and CD4 counts	(−) Significant difference
		Safety: adverse events	
Amitriptyline vs. mexiletine vs. placebo, $n = 145$ (48/47/50)	Kieburtz et al. (38)	Primary: change in Gracely pain scale at baseline and end of study	(−) Significant difference
		Secondary: change in mood, quality-of-life measures, requirement for additional analgesic agents	(−) Significant difference
			(−) Significant difference
		Safety: frequency and severity of clinical adverse experience and laboratory test abnormalities	(−) Significant difference
Mexiletine vs. placebo, $n = 19$ (9/10)	Kemper et al. (39)	Primary: visual analogue rating scale (VAS)	(−) Significant difference
		Safety: frequency of dose-limiting adverse events	(+) Significant difference mexiletine > placebo
Acupuncture vs. amitriptyline, $n = 250$	Shlay et al. (40)	Primary: change in Gracely pain scale	(−) Significant difference
		Secondary: change in quality-of-life measures, neurological examination, and discontinuation of study treatments	(−) Significant difference
NGF (2 doses) vs. placebo, $n = 270$ (90/90/90)	McArthur et al. (35)	Primary: change in Gracely pain scale	(+) Significant difference
		Secondary: practitioner and patient assessment of global improvement, change in neurological exam, use of prescription analgesics, and QST	(+) Significant difference
			(−) difference
		Subset: change in epidermal nerve fiber density as determined by punch skin biopsy	(−) Significant difference
Lamotrigine vs. placebo, $n = 29$ (9/20)	Simpson et al. (34)	Primary: change in modified Gracely pain scale: average daily pain and worst pain	(+) Significant difference
		Secondary: change in neurological exam, use of concomitant analgesics, global pain relief	(−) Significant difference
Lamotrigine vs. placebo, $n = 227$ (ddrug = 92:62/30 w/o ddrug = 135:88/47)	Simpson et al. (36)		(−) Significant difference
		Primary: Gracely pain scale; visual analogue scale; McGill pain assessment; patient and clinical global impression of change	(+) Significant difference in all three measures in those with drug neuropathy

toxicity, and substitution is not possible without jeopardizing virologic control, symptomatic analgesic treatment while continuing the neurotoxic ARV may be appropriate.

3. TOXIC NEUROPATHY

3.1. Antiviral Drugs

Medications used to treat HIV infection may cause a DSP indistinguishable from that caused by the infection itself. Among the currently approved antiretrovirals, only the dideoxynucleosides analogs (d-drugs) are clearly neurotoxic. These include didanosine (ddI), zalcitabine (ddC), and stavudine (d4T) (41–45). DSP associated with dideoxynucleoside analogs is clinically and electrophysiologically similar to DSP associated with HIV. Although the symptoms and signs of DSP associated with neurotoxicity bear a temporal relationship to the drug, it is often difficult to determine the date of symptom onset relative to the frequent changes in a patient's antiretroviral regimen. Accordingly, the incidence of d-drug-induced DSP is difficult to determine.

The pathogenesis of toxic DSP is not known. One hypotheses is that ddC, containing a cytosine base, interferes with the production of sphingomyelin via the formation of a ddC-diphospho-choline metabolite (46). However, a similar toxicity is observed with d4T and ddI that do not contain a cytosine base. *In vitro* and animal experiments suggest that inhibition of mitochondrial DNA synthesis, particularly the potent inhibition of DNA polymerase-γ, may contribute to neurotoxicity (47–51).

The mechanism responsible for the antiviral activity of these drugs is the same one implicated in the pathogenesis. Nucleoside analogs, when phosphorylated to their active triphosphate form, are incorporated into the HIV DNA, resulting in inhibition of the reverse transcriptase and subsequent chain termination. The same phophorylated analogs may be used by mammalian mitochondrial DNA polymerase-γ resulting in disruption of the normal mitochondria (52). The delayed onset of symptoms may be due to the gradual decline of mitochondrial DNA levels, and the coasting phenomenon may result from abnormal signaling as mitochondrial DNA is gradually restored during recovery (53).

Neurotoxicity may also occur from depletion of acetyl-L-carnitine. Acetyl-L-carnitine may promote peripheral nerve regeneration following injury by causing the release of NGF (54). Carnitine depletion causes a disruption of mitochondrial metabolism with resultant toxic accumulation of fatty acids (55). Lower levels of acetyl-L-carnitine were found in some HIV-infected patients taking dideoxynucleosides with peripheral neuropathy, but correlations of serum carnitine levels with measures of neuropathy severity are poor (56,57).

3.2. Thalidomide

Symptoms include painful paresthesias of feet and hands with hyperesthesia and numbness. Thalidomide neuropathy may not be reversible after dose reduction or drug withdrawal. Damage to dorsal root ganglia and posterior columns may explain incomplete reversibility of symptoms. The incidence of thalidomide neuropathy, thalidomide varies from 1% to 70% (58). Although thalidomide neurotoxicity is a concern in HIV-infected patients, placebo-controlled studies in HIV-associated aphthous ulcers have not demonstrated an increased incidence of peripheral neuropathy (59).

3.3. Isoniazid

Isoniazid (INH) is used in mycobacterial infections. INH produces a predominantly sensory, distal symmetric peripheral neuropathy (60–62). INH competitively inhibits coenzymes derived from pyridoxine (63–65), causing reduced synthesis of several neurotransmitters, including serotonin and GABA (66). Supplementation with low dose pyridoxine (0–50 mg/day) prevents INH neuropathy. Pyridoxine may interfere with the antimicrobial activity of INH (67) and in high doses, may in itself cause a neuropathy (68–70).

3.4. Pyridoxine

Pyridoxine is neurotoxic when given in doses >200 mg/day. Symptoms include numbness and tingling, and are often reversible after discontinuation of the vitamin, although a coasting period during which they may intensify for 2–3 weeks after discontinuation may be observed (70). The neuropathy is thought to result from competitive inhibition of the more active form, pyridoxal phosphate, by the less active form, pyridoxine. Saturation of the activating enzymes results in paradoxical deficiency of pyridoxine (69).

3.5. Ethambutol

Ethambutol, an anti-tuberculosis bacteriostatic drug, causes both a distal sensory neuropathy and an optic neuropathy. DSP may occur with doses of 20 mg/kg or more. Neuropathy is less common than optic neuropathy, but can be disabling (71), and may herald the onset of optic neuropathy (72). Ethambutol can aggravate neurotoxicity of other drugs commonly used in combination (e.g., INH). Discontinuation of ethambutol is generally followed by prompt improvement of symptoms.

3.6. Metronidazole

Metronidazole is an antimicrobial used to treat anaerobic infections. DSP has been reported with doses of 1.5 gm/day or drug usage >1 month (73–75). Symptoms include numbness, painful paresthesias and dysesthesias in a stocking, and glove distribution. A proposed mechanism is binding of the drug to ribonucleic acid (RNA) in nerve cells causing inhibition of neuronal protein synthesis leading to peripheral axonal degeneration (76). Metronidazole neuropathy is generally reversible after dose reduction or withdrawal, but coasting has been reported (77).

3.7. Dapsone

Dapsone is used for prophylaxis for *Pneumocystis carinii* pneumonia in patients with sulfonamide intolerance (78). Unlike other toxic neuropathies, dapsone-induced peripheral neuropathy involves primarily motor nerves with less prominent sensory symptoms (79–85). Progressive muscle weakness of both proximal and distal muscles occurs in upper and lower extremities. Electrophysiologic findings demonstrate motor axonopathy. Symptoms begin from 6 weeks to several years after initiation of the drug, and are associated with cumulated doses from 4 g to 600 g. Withdrawal of the drug results in improvement of symptoms. The mechanism is not known, but may represent an idiosyncratic reaction, or occur in individuals who have slow acetylation (84).

3.8. Vincristine

Vinca alkaloids are used as chemotherapy for AIDS-related lymphoma and Kaposi's sarcoma. DSP is a major dose-limiting effect, occurring with a cumulative dose of 15–20 mg, and particularly with vincristine (86). Symptoms are distal paresthesias, with reduced or absent ankle reflexes in early stages, and objective sensory findings and motor weakness in later stages. Cranial neuropathies and autonomic dysfunction may also occur (86–88). Vincristine neurotoxicity is thought due to impaired microtube assembly, resulting in disruption of axonal transport.

3.9. Hydroxyurea

Hydroxyurea is an adjunctive agent for HIV infection. It is neurotoxic, particularly when used in combination with ddI and d4T (89). The high incidence of neuropathy has lead to reduced use of hydroxyurea.

4. INFLAMMATORY DEMYELINATING POLYNEUROPATHY

4.1. Epidemiology

IDP occurs in acute and chronic forms. The prevalence of IDP in HIV patients is unknown, but the acute form often presents at the time of HIV seroconversion or primary infection.

4.2. Clinical Manifestations and Examination Findings

The clinical features of the acute form in HIV-positive patients are similar to acute inflammatory demyelinating polyradiculoneuropathy (AIDP), or Guillain–Barré syndrome in non-HIV-infected patients (90). There is rapidly progressive limb weakness and generalized areflexia in a symmetric distribution. Sensory symptoms are mild or absent. Cranial nerve involvement is common, but autonomic dysfunction is rare. Recovery begins within 2–4 weeks from the nadir. Chronic inflammatory demyelinating polyradiculoneuropathy (CIDP) has a slower course, progressing over weeks to months, and usually has a less favorable long-term prognosis.

4.3. Laboratory and Electrophysiologic Findings

CSF analysis reveals a cytoalbumin dissociation typical of that seen in non-HIV-infected AIDP patients, but a lymphocytic pleocytosis (10–50 cells/mm^3) is more common in HIV-infected patients (10). In advanced HIV disease, search for opportunistic infections, notably CMV, should be considered.

Electrophysiologic findings are similar to those reported in non-HIV-uninfected patients, and are consistent with a primary demyelinating neuropathy (REF). These include markedly reduced SNAP and CMAP response amplitudes, prolonged distal and F-wave latencies, and decreased conduction velocities with evidence for conduction block. Superimposed axonal loss may coexist, particularly in CIDP.

4.4. Pathogenesis

IDP is likely immune-mediated, particularly early in the course of HIV infection, when CD4 lymphocyte counts are relatively high. In patients with CD4 counts <100 cells/mm^3, CMV infection may cause IDP and should be considered in these cases (91). IDP associated with CMV infection may include more severe sensory involvement (92). Other laboratory abnormalities that parallel the course of the disease in IDP include increased CSF levels of soluble CD8 and neopterin and anti-peripheral nerve myelin antibody titers (93).

4.5. Treatment

Case series indicate responsiveness to immunomodulating therapy, including as cortico-steroids, intravenous immunoglobulin (0.5–1.0 gm/kg for 2 days), or plasmapheresis (four to five exchanges). In patients with advanced HIV infection, antiviral therapy against CMV may be indicated.

5. PROGRESSIVE POLYRADICULOPATHY

5.1. Epidemiology

PP usually occurs in advanced AIDS as a complication of CMV infection. The use of HAART is associated with a reduction in both the incidence of systemic CMV infection and PP. Less common causes of PP should therefore be considered, including neurosyphilis, herpes radiculitis, tuberculous radiculopathy, and lymphomatous meningoradiculopathy.

5.2. Clinical Manifestations and Examination Findings

The primary manifestations of PP are lower extremity pain and weakness which may pro-gress rapidly to flaccid paraparesis with sphincter dysfunction (urinary retention or incon-tinence). Examination findings are weakness in a cauda equina distribution, areflexia in the legs, sensory loss, and occasionally a thoracic sensory level (94).

5.3. Laboratory and Electrophysiologic Data

Contrast-enhanced lumbar spine MRI may reveal increased T2 signal of the cauda equina and enhanced, thickened, and clumped lumbosacral roots. In CMV polyradiculopathy, CSF shows marked polymorphonuclear pleocytosis (mean, 651 cells $\pm$ 1053 $\times$ 10^6/L), elevated protein (mean, 2.28 $\pm$ 1.78 g/L), and decreased glucose (mean CSF : plasma glucose ratio, 0.48 $\pm$ 0.17). Detection of CMV by polymerase chain reaction (PCR) analysis of CSF has 92% sensitivity and 94% specificity in CMV-associated PP (95–97). For most of the other etiologies of PP, CSF reveals predominantly lymphocytic pleo-cytosis, and CSF should be assayed for varicella-zoster virus (VZV) PCR, TB PCR, VDRL, and cytology.

Electrophysiologic evaluation reveals evidence of a lumbosacral polyradiculopathy. Nerve conduction studies reveal diminished CMAP amplitude, but conduction velocity is normal. SNAP amplitude is normal. Electromyography reveals widespread denervation which helps differentiate PP from MM or IDP.

5.4. Pathogenesis

PP is due to opportunistic infections while CMV is the most common pathogen; with the advent of HAART, other etiologies have been identified, such as treponema pallidum, herpes zoster, herpes simplex 2, mycobacterium tuberculosis, and lymphoma, and should be considered. Early recognition and treat is important to minimize irreversible nerve root damage.

5.5. Treatment

PP secondary to CMV is a neurologic emergency, because untreated mortality is 100%. Combination therapy with ganciclovir and foscarnet may be more effective (98). Therapy appropriate for other etiologies include penicillin for syphilitic radiculopathy, acyclovir for zoster radiculitis, anti-tuberculosis regimen for tuberculosis radiculopathy, and radiotherapy and/or chemotherapy for lymphomatous radiculitis.

6. MONONEUROPATHY MULTIPLEX

6.1. Epidemiology

MM can be seen early in the course of HIV infection when CD4 counts are >200 cells/μL (99). When MM occurs late in the course of HIV infection, it may be a result of CMV infection (100). A Sjögren's syndrome-like disease is a rare cause of MM and other peripheral neuropathies in HIV. It is associated with a diffuse interstitial lymphocytic syndrome (101).

6.2. Clinical Manifestations and Examination Findings

MM is an accumulation of mononeuropathies, frequently presenting as a wrist drop (radial nerve palsy) or foot drop (peroneal neuropathy). There may also involvement of cutaneous nerves with paresthesias and numbness in patchy areas in the trunk or extremities, or with facial or extraocular muscle weakness (cranial neuropathies) (102).

6.3. Laboratory and Electrophysiologic Findings

CSF in HIV-associated MM is frequently abnormal, but findings are nonspecific, and include elevated protein and mild mononuclear pleocytosis. When MM occurs in late-stage of AIDS, PCR for CMV should be performed on CSF. Electrophysiologic studies are helpful to document asymmetric axonal damage with reduced CMAP and SNAP amplitudes. Electromyography shows neurogenic denervation in the distribution of individual nerves. Nerve biopsy findings range from axonal degeneration with or without endoneural and epineural perivascular inflammatory infiltrates in early-onset MM, to numerous polymorphonuclear infiltrates with mixed axonal and demyelinative lesions in late-onset MM. Vasculitis has been noted in several cases (103). CMV inclusions are detected in peripheral nerve and in some cases of late-onset MM.

6.4. Pathogenesis

Early-onset MM is thought to be mediated by immune mechanisms and is usually a self-limited disease (4,104). In the setting of advanced HIV disease, concurrent CMV infection is implicated (105).

6.5. Treatment

Early-onset MM may resolve spontaneously within weeks to several months (4,104). For patients with progressive MM or who have incomplete recovery, immunomodulatory therapies including corticosteroids, plasmaphoresis, and IVIG have all been shown to be effective in uncontrolled reports. In late-onset MM occurring in advanced HIV infection, empiric therapy for CMV with ganciclovir, foscarnet or cidofovir should be considered.

Table 16.2 Types of Peripheral Neuropathy in HIV Infection

Neuropathy type and CD4 stage of occurrence	Clinical manifestations	Neurological signs	Diagnostic studies	Treatment
DSP CD4 <200	Paresthesias, dysesthesia, distal weakness in severe cases (and in dapsone neuropathy)	Sensory (pinprick and vibration) deficits, stocking and glove distribution, depressed distal reflexes	EMG/NCV: abnormal sensory nerve amplitudes, distal axonopathy	Analgesics (primary and adjuvant), neurotoxic drug withdrawal or dose-reduction; adequate virologic suppression
IDP Early: CD4 >200 Late: CD4 <100	Progressive weakness, paresthesias	Weakness, mild sensory deficits, areflexia	CSF: lymphocytic pleocytosis (10–50 cells/uL), high protein EMG/NCV: demyelination	Immunomodulating therapy, consider anti-CMV therapy in late onset IDP
MM Early: CD4 >200 Late: CD4 <100	Foot or wrist drop, facial weakness, focal pain	Multifocal cranial and peripheral neuropathy	EMG/NCV: multifocal axonal neuropathy	Immunomodulating therapy, consider anti-CMV therapy in late onset MM
PP Early: CD4 >200 Late: CD4 <100	Lower extremity weakness, paresthesias, sphincter dysfunction,	Flaccid paraparesis, saddle distribution anesthesia, depressed reflexes	CSF: polymorphonuclear pleocytosis (in CMV infection); lymphocytic pleocytosis (in lymphoma, syphilis, herpes); EMG/NCV: polyradiculopathy	Anti-CMV therapy (if CSF CMV PCR+); acyclovir for herpes radiculitis; PCN for neurosyphilitic radiculopathy; chemotherapy w/ or w/o RT for lymphomatous radiculopathy

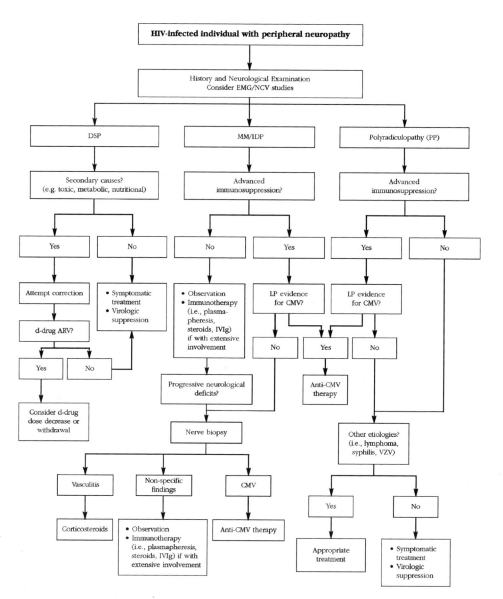

Figure 16.1   Algorithm for management of peripheral neuropathy in HIV-infected individuals.

7.   CONCLUSION

Peripheral neuropathies are the most common neurologic complications in HIV infection. They may result from the HIV infection itself, (directly or indirectly), from neurotoxic properties of HIV drugs, from opportunistic or other superimposed infections, or from a combination. DSP is the most common form and is the most disabling. Other neuropathies are much less common. A summary of the different forms of peripheral neuropathy that occur in HIV infection is given in Table 16.2. An algorithm summarizing the appropriate approach to an HIV-infected individual with neuropathy is shown in Fig. 16.1.

REFERENCES

1. Brinley F, Pardo C, Verma A. Human immunodeficiency virus and the peripheral nervous system workshop. Arch Neurol 2001; 58:1561–1566.
2. Pardo CA, McArthur JC, Griffin JW. HIV neuropathy: insights in the pathology of HIV peripheral nerve disease. J Peripher Nerv Syst 2001; 6(1):21–27.
3. So YT, Holtzman DM, Abrams DI, Olney RK. Peripheral neuropathy associated with acquired immunodeficiency syndrome. Prevalence and clinical features from a population-based survey. Arch Neurol 1988; 45(9):945–948.
4. Simpson D, Olney R. Peripheral neuropathies associated with human immunodeficiency virus infection. Peripheral Neuropathies: New Concepts Treat 1992; 685–711.
5. Schifitto G, McDermott M, McArthur J, Marder K, Sacktor N, Epstein L. Incidence of and risk factors for HIV-associated distal sensory polyneuropathy. Neurology 2002; 58(12):1764–1768.
6. Barohn RJ, Gronseth GS, LeForce BR, McVey AL, McGuire SA, Butzin CA. Peripheral nervous system involvement in a large cohort of human immunodeficiency virus-infected individuals [published erratum appears in Arch Neurol 1993 Apr; 50(4):388]. Arch Neurol 1993; 50(2):167–171.
7. Tagliati M, Grinnell J, Godbold J, Simpson DM. Peripheral nerve function in HIV infection: clinical, electrophysiologic, and laboratory findings. Arch Neurol 1999; 56(1):84–89.
8. Childs EA, Lyles RH, Selnes OA, Chen B, Miller EN, Cohen BA. Plasma viral load and CD4 lymphocytes predict HIV-associated dementia and sensory neuropathy. Neurology 1999; 52(3):607–613.
9. Simpson DM, Haidich AB, Schifitto G, Yiannoutsos CT, Geraci AP, McArthur JC. Severity of HIV-associated neuropathy is associated with plasma HIV-1 RNA levels. Aids 2002; 16(3):407–412.
10. Wulff EA, Wang AK, Simpson DM. HIV-associated peripheral neuropathy: epidemiology, pathophysiology and treatment. Drugs 2000; 59(6):1251–1260.
11. Herrmann DN, Griffin JW, Hauer P, Cornblath DR, McArthur JC. Epidermal nerve fiber density and sural nerve morphometry in peripheral neuropathies. Neurology 1999; 53(8):1634–1640.
12. Snider W, Simpson D, Nielsen S et al. Neurologic complications of acquired immunodeficiency syndrome; Analysis of 50 patients. Ann Neurol 1983; 14:403–418.
13. Simpson D, Cohen J, Sivak M et al. Neuromuscular complications in association with acquired immunodeficiency syndrome. Ann Neurol 1985; 18:160.
14. Cornblath DR, McArthur JC. Predominantly sensory neuropathy in patients with AIDS and AIDS-related complex. Neurology 1988; 38(5):794–796.
15. Lange DJ, Britton CB, Younger DS, Hays AP. The neuromuscular manifestations of human immunodeficiency virus infections. Arch Neurol 1988; 45(10):1084–1088.
16. Leger JM, Bouche P, Bolgert F, Chaunu MP, Rosenheim M, Cathala HP. The spectrum of polyneuropathies in patients infected with HIV. J Neurol Neurosurg Psychiatry 1989; 52(12):1369–1374.
17. Rance NE, McArthur JC, Cornblath DR, Landstrom DL, Griffin JW, Price DL. Gracile tract degeneration in patients with sensory neuropathy and AIDS. Neurology 1988; 38(2):265–271.
18. de la Monte SM, Gabuzda DH, Ho DD, Brown RH Jr, Hedley-Whyte ET, Schooley RT. Peripheral neuropathy in the acquired immunodeficiency syndrome. Ann Neurol 1988; 23(5):485–492.
19. Mah V, Vartavarian LM, Akers MA, Vinters HV. Abnormalities of peripheral nerve in patients with human immunodeficiency virus infection. Ann Neurol 1988; 24(6):713–717.
20. Lipkin WI, Parry G, Kiprov D, Abrams D. Inflammatory neuropathy in homosexual men with lymphadenopathy. Neurology 1985; 35(10):1479–1483.
21. Bailey RO, Baltch AL, Venkatesh R, Singh JK, Bishop MB. Sensory motor neuropathy associated with AIDS. Neurology 1988; 38(6):886–891.

22. Bradley WG, Shapshak P, Delgado S, Nagano I, Stewart R, Rocha B. Morphometric analysis of the peripheral neuropathy of AIDS. Muscle Nerve 1998; 21(9):1188–1195.

23. Martin C, Solders G, Sonnerborg A, Hansson P. Antiretroviral therapy may improve sensory function in HIV-infected patients: a pilot study [see comments]. Neurology 2000; 54(11):2120–2127.

24. Grafe M, Wiley C. Spinal cord and peripheral nerve pathology in AIDS: the roles of cytomegalovirus and human immunodeficiency virus. Ann Neurol 1989; 25:561–566.

25. Wesselingh S, Glass J, McArthur J, Griffin J, Griffin D. Cytokine Dysregulation in HIV-Associated Neurological Disease. Adv Neuroimmunol 1994; 4(3):199–206.

26. Tyor WR, Glass JD, Griffin JW, Becker PS, McArthur JC, Bezman L, Griffin DE. Cytokine expression in the brain during the acquired immunodeficiency syndrome. Ann Neurol 1992; 31:349–360.

27. Yoshioka M, Shapshak P, Srivastava AK, Stewart RV, Nelson SJ, Bradley WG. Expression of HIV-1 and interleukin-6 in lumbosacral dorsal root ganglia of patients with AIDS. Neurology 1994; 44(6):1120–1130.

28. Petratos S, Turnbull V, Papadopoulos R et al. Antibodies against peripheral myelin glycolipids in people with HIV infection. Immunol Cell Biol 1998; 76:535–541.

29. Petratos S, Turnbull V, Papadopoulos R. High titer anti-sulfatide antibodies in HIV-infected individuals. Neuroreport 1999; 10:2557–2562.

30. Petratos S, Turnbull V, Papadopoulos R et al. Peripheral nerve binding patterns of anti-sulphatide antibodies in HIV-infected individuals. Neuroreport 1999; 10:1659–1664.

31. Fuller GN, Jacobs JM, Guiloff RJ. Association of painful peripheral neuropathy in AIDS with cytomegalovirus infection [see comments]. Lancet 1989; 2(8669):937–941.

32. Breitbart W, Rosenfeld BD, Passik SD, McDonald MV, Thaler H, Portenoy RK. The undertreatment of pain in ambulatory AIDS patients. Pain 1996; 65(2–3):243–249.

33. Grond S, Zech D, Schug S, Lynch J, Lehmann K. Validation of World Health Organization guidelines for cancer pain relief during the last days and hours of life. J Pain Symptom Manage 1991; 6(7):411–422.

34. Simpson D, Olney R, McArthur J et al. A placebo-controlled trial of lamotrigine for painful HIV-associated neuropathy. Neurology 2000; 54:2115–2119.

35. McArthur JC, Yiannoutsos C, Simpson DM, Adornato BT, Singer EJ, Hollander H. A phase II trial of nerve growth factor for sensory neuropathy associated with HIV infection. AIDS Clinical Trials Group Team 291 [see comments]. Neurology 2000; 54(5):1080–1088.

36. Simpson DM, McArthur JC, Olney R, et al. Lamotrigine for HIV-associated painful sensory neuropathies: a placebo-controlled trial. Neurology 2003; 60:1508–1514.

37. Simpson D, Dorfman D, Olney R, McKinley G, Dobkin J, So Y. Peptide T in the treatment of painful distal neuropathy associated with AIDS; Results of a placebo-controlled trial. The Peptide T Neuropathy Study Group. Neurology 1996; 47:1254–1259.

38. Kieburtz K, Simpson D, Yiannoutsos C, Max MB, Hall CD, Ellis RJ. A randomized trial of amitriptyline and mexiletine for painful neuropathy in HIV infection. AIDS Clinical Trial Group 242 Protocol Team. Neurology 1998; 51(6):1682–1688.

39. Kemper CA, Kent G, Burton S, Deresinski SC. Mexiletine for HIV-infected patients with painful peripheral neuropathy: a double-blind, placebo-controlled, crossover treatment trial. J Acquir Immune Defic Syndr Hum Retrovirol 1998; 19(4):367–372.

40. Shlay JC, Chaloner K, Max MB, Flaws B, Reichelderfer P, Wentworth D. Acupuncture and amitriptyline for pain due to HIV-related peripheral neuropathy: a randomized controlled trial. Terry Beirn Community Programs for Clinical Research on AIDS [see comments]. J Am Med Assoc 1998; 280(18):1590–1595.

41. Yarchoan R, Perno C, Thomas R, Klecker R, Allain J, Wills R. Phase I studies of 2′3′-deoxycytidinein severe human immuno-deficiency virus infection as a single agent and alternating with zidovudine. Lancet 1988; 1:76–81.

42. Merigan T, Skowron G, Bozzette S, Richman D, Uttamchandani R, Fischl M. Circulating p24 antigen levels and responses to dideoxycytidine in human immunodeficiency virus (HIV) infections. Ann Intern Med 1989; 110:189–194.

43. Cooley T, Kunches L, Saunders C, Ritter J, Perkins C, Mclaren C. Once-daily administration of 2'3' didexyinosine (ddI) in patients with the acquired immunodeficiency syndrome or AIDS-related complex. N Engl J Med 1990; 322:1340–1345.

44. Lambert J, Seidlin M, Reichman R, Plank C, Laverty M, Morse G. Dideoxyinosine (ddI) in patients with the acquired immunodeficiency syndrome or AIDS-related complex: results of phase I trial. N Engl J Med 1990; 322:1333–1340.

45. Browne MJ, Mayer KH, Chafee SB, Dudley MN, Posner MR, Steinberg SM. 2',3'-didehydro-3'-deoxythymidine (d4T) in patients with AIDS or AIDS- related complex: a phase I trial. J Infect Dis 1993; 167(1):21–29.

46. Cooney D, Dalal M, Mitsuya H, McMahon J et al. Initial studies on the cellular pharmacology of 2'3'-dideoxycytidine, an inhibitor of HTLV-III infectivity. Biochem Pharmacol 1986; 35:2065–2068.

47. Pezeshkpour G, Krarup C, Buchthal F, Dimauro S, Bresolin N, McBurney J. Peripheral neuropathy in mitochondrial disease. J Neurol Sci 1987; 77:285–304.

48. Balzarini J, Herdewlin P, De Clercq E. Differential patterns of intracellular metabolism of 2'3'-dideoxythymidine and 3'-azido-2'3'-dideoxythymidine, two potent anti-human immuno-deficiency virus compounds. J Biol Chem 1989; 264:6127–6133.

49. Chen CH, Cheng YC. Delayed cytotoxicity and selective loss of mitochondrial DNA in cells treated with the anti-human immunodeficiency virus compound 2'3'-dideoxycytidine. J Biol Chem 1989; 264:11934–11937.

50. Martin J, Brown C, Davis N, Reardon J. Effects of antiviral nucleoside analogs on human DNA polymerases and mitchondrial DNA synthesis. Antimicrob Agents Chemother 1994; 38:2743–2749.

51. Cui L, Locatelli L, Xie M, Sommadossi J. Effect of nucleoside analogs on neurite regeneration and mitochondrial DNA synthesis in PC-12 cells. The Journal of Pharmacology and Experimental Therapeutics 1997; 280(3):1228–1234.

52. Gasnault J, Pinganaud C, Kousignian P et al. Subacute ascendant polyneuropathy revealing a nucleoside-induced mitochondrial cytopathy. Presented at The Seventh European Conference on Clinical Aspects and Treatment of HIV Infection. Lisbon, Portugal, Oct 23–27, 1999.

53. Moyle G, Sadler M. Peripheral neuropathy with nucleoside antiretrovirals. Drug Saf 1998; 19(6):481–494.

54. Angelucci L, Ramacci M, Taglialatela G et al. Nerve growth factor binding in aged rat central nervous system: effect of acetyl-L-carnitine. J Neurosci Res 1988; 20:491–496.

55. Colucci W, Gandour R. Carnitine acetyltransferase: a review of its biology, enzymology and bioorganic chemistry. Bioorg Chem 1988; 16:307–334.

56. Famularo G, Moretti S, Marcellini S, Trinchieri V, Tzantzoglou S, Santini G. Acetyl-carnitine deficiency in AIDS patients with neurotoxicity on treatment with antiretroviral nucleoside analogues. Aids 1997; 11(2):185–190.

57. Simpson DM, Katzenstein D, Haidich B, Millington D, Yiannoutsos C, Schifitto G. Plasma carnitine in HIV-associated neuropathy. Aids 2001; 15(16):2207–2208.

58. Tseng S, Pak G, Washenick K et al. Rediscovering thalidomide: a review of its mechanism of action, side effects, and potential uses. J Am Acad Dermatol 1996; 35:969–979.

59. Jacobson J, Greenspan J, Spritzler J et al. Thalidomide for the treatment of oral aphthous ulcers in patients with human immunodeficiency virus infection. N Eng J Med 1997; 336:1487–1493.

60. Biehl J, Skavlem J. Toxicity of isoniazid. Am Rev Tuberc 1953; 68:296–297.

61. Gammon G, Burge F, King G. Neural toxicity in tuberculous patients treated with isoniazid (isonicotinic acid hydrazide). AMA Archs Neurol Psychiatry 1953; 70:64–69.

62. Jones W, Jones G. Peripheral neuropathy due to isoniazid. Report of two cases. Lancet 1953; 1:1073–1074.

63. Biehl J, Vilter R. Effect of isonazid on vitamin B12 metabolism, its possible significance in producing isoniazid neuritis. Proc Soc Exp Biol Med 1954; 85:389–395.

64. Wiegand R. The formation of pyridoxal and pyridoxal 5-phosphate hydrazones. J Am Chem Soc 1956; 78:5307.

65. Price J, Brown R, Larson F. Quantitative studies on human urinary metabolites of tryptophan as affected by isoniazid and deoxypyridoxine. J Clin Invest 1957; 36:1600.

66. Girling D. Adverse effects of antituberculosis drugs. Drugs 1982; 23:56–74.

67. Snider D. Pyridoxine supplementation during isoniazid therapy. Tubercle 1980; 61:191–196.

68. Schaumburg H, Kaplan J, Windebank A. Sensory neuropathy from pyridoxine abuse. N Engl J Med 1983; 309:445–448.

69. Nisar M, Watkin SW, Bucknall RC, Agnew RA. Exacerbation of isoniazid induced peripheral neuropathy by pyridoxine. Thorax 1990; 45(5):419–420.

70. Berger A, Schaumburg H, Schroeder C, Appel S, Reynolds R. Dose response, coasting, and differential fiber vulnerability in human toxic neuropathy: a prospective study of pyridoxine neurotoxicity. Neurology 1992; 42:1367–1370.

71. Tugwell P, James S. Peripheral neuropathy with ethambutol. Postgrad Med J 1972; 48(565):667–670.

72. Nair V, LeBrun M, Kass I. Peripheral neuropathy associated with ethambutol. Chest 1980; 77(1):98–100.

73. Duffy L, Daum F, Fisher S, Selman J, Vishnubhakat S, Aiges H. Peripheral neuropathy in Crohn's disease. Patients treated with metronidazole. Gastroenterology 1985; 88:681–684.

74. Boyce E, Cookson E, Bond W. Persistent metronidazole-induced peripheral neuropathy. Ann of Pharmacotherapy 1990; 24:19–21.

75. Learned-Coughlin S. Peripheral neuropathy induced by metronidazole (letter). Ann Pharmacother 1994; 28:536.

76. Bradley W, Karlsson I, Rassol C. Metronidazole neuropathy. Br Med J 1977; 2(6087):610–611.

77. Coxon A, Pallis C. Metronidazole neuropathy. J Neuro Neurosurg and Psych 1976; 39:403–405.

78. Medina I, Mills J, Leoung G. Oral therapy for Pneumocystis carinii pneumonia in the acquired immunodeficiency syndrome: a controlled trial of trimethoprim-sulfamethoxazole versus trimethoprim-dapsone. N Engl J Med 1990; 323:776–782.

79. Saqueton A, Lorinez A, Vick N, Hamer R. Dapsone and peripheral motor neuropathy. Arch Dermatol 1969; 100:214–217.

80. Rapoport A, Guss S. Dapsone-induced peripheral neuropathy. Arch Neurol 1972; 27:184–185.

81. Epstein F, Bohm M. Dapsone-induced peripheral neuropathy. Arch Dermatol 1976; 112:1761–1762.

82. Fredericks E, Kugelman R, Kirsch N. Dapsone-induced motor polyneuropathy. Arch Dermatol 1976; 112:1158–1160.

83. Guttman L, Martin J, Welton W. Dapsone motor neuropathy—an axonal disease. Neurology 1976; 26:514–516.

84. Koller W, Gehlmann L, Malkinson F, Davis F. Dapsone-induced peripheral neuropathy. Arch Neurol 1977; 34:644–646.

85. Navarro S, Rosales R, Ordinario A, Izumo S, Osame M. Acute dapsone-induced peripheral neuropathy. Muscle Nerve 1989; 12:604–606.

86. Tuxen M, Hansen S. Neurotoxicity secondary to antineoplastic drugs. Cancer Treat Rev 1994; 20:191–214.

87. Legha S. Vincristine neurotoxicity: pathophysiology and management. Med Toxicol 1986; 1:421–427.

88. Macdonald D. Neurologic complications of chemotherapy. Neurol Clin 1991; 9:955–967.

89. Moore RD, Wong WM, Keruly JC, McArthur JC. Incidence of neuropathy in HIV-infected patients on monotherapy versus those on combination therapy with didanosine, stavudine and hydroxyurea. Aids 2000; 14(3):273–278.

90. Cornblath DR, McArthur JC, Kennedy PG, Witte AS, Griffin JW. Inflammatory demyelinating peripheral neuropathies associated with human T-cell lymphotropic virus type III infection. Ann Neurol 1987; 21(1):32–40.

91. Misha B, Sommers W, Koski C et al. Acute inflammatory demyelinating polyneuropathy in the acquired immunodeficiency syndrome. Ann Neurol 1985; 18:131–132.

92. Visser L, Van der Meché F, Meulstee J et al. Cytomegalovirus infection and Guillain–Barré syndrome: the clinical, electrophysiologic, and prognostic features. Neurology 1996; 47:668–673.

93. Griffin D, McArthur J, D C. Soluble interleukin-2 receptor and soluble CD8 in serum and cerebrospinal fluid during human immunodeficiency virus-associated neurologic disease. J Neuroimmunol 1990; 28:97–109.

94. Eidelberg D, Sotrel A, Vogel H, Walker P, Kleefield J, Crumpacker CSd. Progressive polyradiculopathy in acquired immune deficiency syndrome. Neurology 1986; 36(7):912–916.

95. Gozlan J, El Amrani M, Baudrimont M et al. A prospective evaluation of clinical criteria and polymerase chain reaction assay of cerebrospinal fluid for the diagnosis of cytomegalovirus-related neurological diseases during AIDS. AIDS 1995; 9:253–260.

96. Shinkai M, Spector S. Quantitation of human cytomegalovirus (HCMV) DNA in cerebrospinal fluid by competitive PCR in AIDS patients with different HCMV central nervous system diseases. Scand J Infect Dis 1995; 27:559–561.

97. Vogel J, Cinatl J, Lux A et al. New PCR assay for rapid and quantitative detection of human cytomegalovirus in cerebrospinal fluid. J Clin Microbiol 1996; 34:482–483.

98. The studies of ocular complication of AIDS Research Group in collaboration with the AIDS Clinical Trials Group. Combination foscarnet and ganciclovir therapy versus monotherapy for the treatment of relapsed cytomegalovirus retinitis in patients with AIDS. Arch Ophthalmol 1996; 114:23–32.

99. Simpson D, Olney RK. Peripheral neuropathies associated with human immunodeficiency virus infection. Neurol Clin 1992; 10(3):685–711.

100. Said G, Lacroix C, Chemouilli P, Goulon-Goeau C, Roullet E, Penaud D. Cytomegalovirus neuropathy in acquired immunodeficiency syndrome: a clinical and pathological study. Ann Neurol 1991; 29(2):139–146.

101. Gherardi RK, Chretien F, Delfau-Larue MH, Authier FJ, Moulignier A, Roulland-Dussoix D. Neuropathy in diffuse infiltrative lymphocytosis syndrome: an HIV neuropathy, not a lymphoma [see comments]. Neurology 1998; 50(4):1041–1044.

102. Miller RG, Parry GJ, Pfaeffl W, Lang W, Lippert R, Kiprov D. The spectrum of peripheral neuropathy associated with ARC and AIDS. Muscle Nerve 1988; 11(8):857–863.

103. Bradley WG, Verma A. Painful vasculitic neuropathy in HIV-1 infection: relief of pain with prednisone therapy. Neurology 1996; 47(6):1446–1451.

104. So Y, Olney R. The natural history of mononeuritis multiplex and simplex in HIV infection. Neurology 1991; 41(suppl 1):375.

105. Roullet E, Asseurus J, Gozlan J et al. Cytomegalovirus multifocal neuropathy in AIDS: analysis of 15 consecutive patients. Neurology 1994; 44:2174–2182.

17

Infectious and Granulomatous Neuropathies

Sharon P. Nations, Jaya R. Trivedi, and Gil I. Wolfe
University of Texas Southwestern Medical Center, Dallas, Texas, USA

ABSTRACT

Infectious and granulomatous neuropathies, including those associated with leprosy, Lyme disease, and sarcoidosis, share a number of clinical features. Asymmetric sensory and motor nerve involvement are typical, and cranial neuropathies are common, and help to distinguish infectious and granulomatous neuropathies from more common etiologies of peripheral nerve injury. Herpes zoster represents a re-activation of latent varicella zoster infection, and also results in asymmetric sensory loss, and less commonly weakness, in a radicular pattern. The diagnosis of infectious and granulomatous neuropathies rests on recognition of typical systemic involvement, serologic testing, and appropriate biopsy material. The diagnosis of herpetic neuropathies is made from the clinical features. Polymerase chain reaction techniques have an increasingly important role in diagnosis. Specific treatments are available for most infectious and granulomatous neuropathies and are generally effective in either reversing nerve damage or preventing further impairment. The prognosis is favorable when the cause is identified early in the disease course, but if treatment is delayed, permanent axonal damage is common in later stages. Herpetic neuropathies can be treated and post-herpetic pain successfully managed.

1. LEPROSY

1.1. Introduction

Leprosy or Hansen's disease is probably the earliest recorded form of infectious neuropathy, and remains a significant cause of morbidity worldwide, especially in developing countries. The causative organism, *Mycobacterium leprae*, is an acid-fast bacillus (AFB) with an affinity for skin and nerves. The organism enters its host via nasal droplet (1) or perhaps through abraded skin (2). It is carried hematogenously to cooler regions of the body including skin, superficial nerves, anterior portion of the eye, and testes. After an incubation period of years, patients develop symptoms of the disease.

1.2. Clinical Features

The initial manifestation, particularly in children, is often a single hypopigmented skin lesion with indistinct margins. Sensation loss within the lesion may be difficult to demonstrate. This stage, known as "indeterminate" leprosy, usually heals spontaneously but may progress to more extensive disease (3). The manifestations of the disease are determined by the host's T-cell-mediated immune response to the organism and range on a spectrum from tuberculoid to lepromatous (4).

In tuberculoid leprosy, the patient's strong immune response limits disease to a few hypopigmented, anesthetic skin lesions. If there is involvement of a nearby nerve trunk, a mononeuropathy develops. Biopsy of the skin lesion reveals well-formed epithelioid granulomas from subcutaneous tissue through the dermis (5). AFB are absent or only rarely detected in biopsy specimens and are not detected in slit-skin (tissue fluid) smears of the lesion or of earlobes, knees or elbows, which are typical sites of infection. Granulomas involving nerves may caseate and abscesses occasionally form.

In lepromatous leprosy, the patient fails to mount a cell-mediated immune response to the organism, and widespread infection occurs. Numerous erythematous macules, plaques, and nodules may spread over the face, trunk, and extensor surfaces of the extremities, sparing the scalp, crurae, and axillae. Loss of eyelashes and eyebrows (madarosis) and infiltration of nose and earlobes lead to the characteristic facial deformity (Fig. 17.1). Nasal congestion is a frequent complaint, and nasal mucus smears stain positive for AFB (6). Nasal septal perforation is seen in severe cases. A symmetric distal sensory polyneuropathy involving primarily pain, temperature, and autonomic modalities progresses proximally. A mononeuritis multiplex may become superimposed as larger superficial nerve trunks become involved. Skin biopsy reveals histiocytic infiltration of the dermis, with scant lymphocytes (5). Histiocytes are filled with clumps of bacilli ("globi").

Borderline leprosy patients fall in between these two extremes. These individuals have more widespread infection than tuberculoid patients, but are able to mount a somewhat greater immune response to the organism than patients at the lepromatous end of the spectrum. They may be further categorized into borderline tuberculoid, mid-borderline, or borderline lepromatous, depending on the range of their clinical and histopathological features within the spectrum. Skin biopsy shows numerous lymphocytes and macrophages. Biopsies from borderline tuberculoid patients may contain Langhans and undifferentiated giant cells, but those of mid-borderline and borderline lepromatous patients do not (5). Patients in borderline categories are at increased risk of immune-mediated "Type 1"

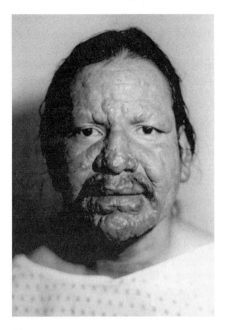

Figure 17.1 Patient with lepromatous leprosy.

reactions (discussed subsequently). A small minority of leprosy patients present with pure neuropathy symptoms, usually a mononeuritis or mononeuritis multiplex, without skin changes. This form of the disease is termed "neuritic" leprosy.

Complications of leprosy result from the loss of protective sensation and include bone resorption of phalanges (Fig. 17.2), repeated trauma and ulceration of distal limbs, and infection leading to osteomyelitis. Weakness of orbicularis oculi muscles and desensitization of the cornea due to infiltration of the ophthalmic division of the trigeminal nerve lead to repeated corneal abrasions and opacification. Glaucoma may result from iridocyclitis, usually occurring as a chronic, low-grade inflammation more common in patients with a high bacillary load (7). Up to 27% of all leprosy patients present with functional impairment secondary to neuropathy, and as many as half of multibacillary patients have neuropathic complications (8).

1.3. Laboratory Evaluation

Biopsy of a skin lesion is usually required for diagnosis. Even in cases of pure neuritic leprosy, skin biopsy from an anesthetic area may demonstrate inflammation and AFB, especially if the specimen is thick enough to include dermal nerves (9). However, a nerve biopsy is often necessary, preferably of an involved sensory nerve such as the sural, the superficial radial, or the superficial peroneal (Figs. 17.3 and 17.4). When the biopsy confirms the diagnosis, slit-skin smears are obtained to look for bacteria and aid in classification of the patient as either "paucibacillary" or "multibacillary" (see Section 1.5.). These require availability of personnel trained in the technique. A small incision is made in the skin of earlobes, elbows, and knees bilaterally with a scalpel blade. The inner edges of the incision are scraped to collect tissue fluid, which is then applied to a microscope slide. Samples of nasal mucus may also be collected via swab. Specimens are stained for AFB. The number of organisms per high power (oil immersion) field may be quantitated in log units on a scale from 0 to 6+ (the bacillary index or BI). The BI includes both viable and nonviable organisms. Smears should be negative in tuberculoid patients, but are strongly positive in lepromatous patients. Skin smears may be performed yearly for monitoring response to treatment or may be repeated in cases of suspected relapse. A decline in the BI of ∼1 log unit per year is expected with treatment (10).

The morphological index (MI) is the number of viable (solid-staining) organisms compared to nonviable (granular staining) organisms and can also be determined from

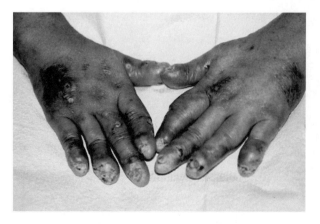

Figure 17.2 Hands of patient with lepromatous leprosy.

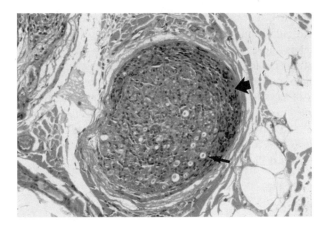

Figure 17.3 Cross-section of superficial radial nerve in neuritic leprosy demonstrating lymphocytic infiltration of the periphery (small arrow) and a few scattered remaining nerve axons (large arrow).

slit-skin smears. Interpretation of biopsy and slit-skin smear specimens is available through the National Hansen's Disease Center in Baton Rouge, LA, USA (1-800-642-2477). Polymerase chain reaction (PCR) for *M. leprae* may be obtained using nasal mucus or tissue specimens (11).

Nerve conduction studies (NCS) may be normal in patients with clinical involvement of only superficial dermal nerves. In patients with more extensive nerve involvement, NCS reveal slowed conduction velocities, particularly in the ulnar nerve across the elbow (12,13), the median nerve in the forearm, and the peroneal nerve in the popliteal fossa (14).

1.4. Differential Diagnosis

Leprosy should be readily recognized when a patient from an endemic area, which includes Texas and Louisiana in the United States, presents with a typical skin rash and

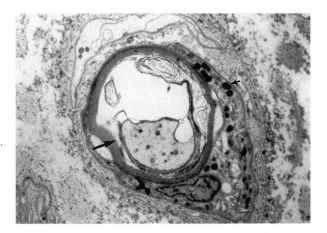

Figure 17.4 Electron microscopy demonstrating *M. leprae* (small arrow) within Schwann cell surrounding a degenerating nerve axon (large arrow).

a neuropathy. The diagnosis should also be considered in any patient from an endemic area who presents with neuropathy, particularly mononeuropathy or mononeuritis multiplex, without skin lesions. Recognition is more challenging in patients with pure neuritic forms. Preservation of proprioception and deep tendon reflexes are features characteristic of leprous neuropathy that may help to differentiate it from other causes of neuropathy. Although the skin manifestations of sarcoidosis, granuloma multiforme, and granuloma annulare include erythematous raised macules and plaques, they are not anesthetic. Histologically, the granulomas of these other diseases do not typically extend to the epidermal margin, whereas tuberculoid leprosy does. Conversely, epitheliod granulomas associated with normal nerve bundles argue against the presence of leprosy (5).

1.5. Management and Prognosis

The number of leprosy cases registered in treatment programs in 82 reporting countries in 1999 was about 730,000 (15), down from 5.4 million in 1991, due primarily to introduction of multidrug therapy (MDT) by the World Health Organization (WHO) in 1982. To facilitate the determination of the appropriate treatment regimen by healthcare workers in leprosy control programs, the classification of patients was simplified. The term "paucibacillary" refers to patients with five or fewer skin lesions. Neuropathy in the paucibacillary classification is limited to involvement of a single nerve trunk and/or anesthesia within skin lesions. No bacilli may be detected in biopsy of skin lesions or on slit-skin smears. All other patients are classified as multibacillary.

WHO treatment recommendations are presented in Table 17.1. Prior to initiating treatment, a glucose-6-phosphate dehydrogenase (G6PD) level should be obtained. Patients with G6PD deficiency cannot be treated with dapsone due to the risk of hemolysis. Other drugs such as minocycline, ofloxacin, or clarithromycin, are substituted.

The course of the disease is frequently complicated by immune-mediated reactions which can produce further nerve damage. These may occur prior to initiation of treatment, during treatment, or months to years after completing treatment. In Type 1 reactions, an increase in the immune response within skin and nerve lesions causes swelling and erythema of skin lesions, increased nerve tenderness, and new numbness or weakness (Fig. 17.5). Pain is often present but not invariably so. Prompt treatment with corticosteroids can reverse the symptoms. The corticosteroid dose is slowly tapered over several weeks. Some patients require the addition of other immunosuppressants, such as cyclosporine, for management of recurrent reactions or failure to tolerate a steroid taper.

Table 17.1 World Health Organization Recommendations for Treatment of Hansen's Disease

Disease classification	Antibiotics	Duration of treatment (months)
Paucibacillary	Dapsone 100 mg/day	6
	Rifampin 600 mg/month	6
Multibacillary	Dapsone 100 mg/day	12
	Rifampin 600 mg/month	12
	Clofazimine 50 mg/day plus 300 mg/month	12

Note: Antibiotic regimen modifications in US: rifampin 600 mg/day rather than monthly for paucibacillary and multibacillary; clofazimine 50–100 mg/day and omit monthly dose for multibacillary patients; duration of treatment 12 months for paucibacillary patients and 24 months for multibacillary patients.

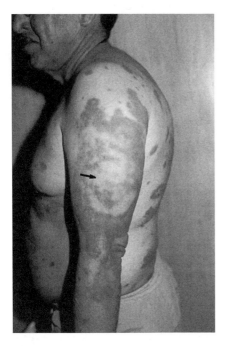

Figure 17.5   Reversal reaction. Patient denied sensory loss on examination until skin lesions became inflamed, with central anesthesia and hypopigmentation (arrow).

In the majority of cases, reversal reactions occur within the first 6 months of treatment (16). The presence of swollen, inflamed skin lesions or new neuropathy symptoms in the 6 months prior to diagnosis also suggests a possible reversal reaction at the time of diagnosis. Consideration should be given to starting prednisone therapy when initiating antibiotic treatment in these cases. As mentioned earlier, borderline leprosy patients are at greater risk for development of Type 1 reactions.

Type 2 reactions, or erythema nodosum leprosum (ENL), are the result of deposition of antigen–antibody complexes in various tissues. Patients at the lepromatous end of the spectrum are at greatest risk. Symptoms include fever, erythematous and tender skin nodules, neuritis, arthritis, orchitis, iridocyclitis, and nephritis. Biopsy of skin nodules reveals polymorphonuclear cells, differentiating this lesion from skin lesions of reversal reaction (17). Thalidomide 100–300 mg/day in nonpregnant patients is the treatment of choice. Thalidomide has well-known teratogenic effects, and male as well as female patients must use adequate contraception, as the drug is present in seminal fluid. Corticosteroids are also used in the treatment of ENL, especially if neuritis is present.

With MDT, recurrence rates in leprosy are extremely low. New skin lesions or neuropathy symptoms associated with a twofold or greater increase in the BI of slit-skin smears suggest relapse. The presence of AFB in skin or nerve biopsy specimens in treated patients cannot be used as evidence for recurrent infection, as nonviable bacilli may persist for years before being cleared by the immune system (18,19).

To avoid repeated trauma to insensitive hands and feet, patients must be instructed in proper foot care and in coping behaviors to prevent burns. Physical therapy and occupational therapy are important, particularly to prevent deformity and contractures. Regular ophthalmologic examinations are essential for early detection and management of ocular complications. After completing treatment, patients with "claw-hand" as a result of ulnar neuropathy may be candidates for tendon transfer. In the United States, these services may be obtained through the National Hansen's Disease Center (see Section 1.3. for contact information).

If the diagnosis of leprosy is made early before development of significant neurologic disability, prognosis is excellent for recovery with minimal or no sequelae. Nerve deficits present prior to initiation of treatment are usually not reversible, unless they have developed recently or are associated with reversal reaction. In cases of reaction, treatment with corticosteroids may reverse the neuropathy symptoms. Patient compliance with antibiotic treatment, as well as prompt recognition and treatment of immune-mediated reactions, can minimize disability.

1.6. Pathophysiology

The neurotropism of *M. leprae* is well known. Recent work suggests that this is due in part to the organism's affinity for laminin-2, a protein present in the basal lamina of Schwann cells (20). Laminin-2 complexes with α/β-dystroglycan on the surface of Schwann cells, and the interaction may provide the means of entry for *M. leprae* into the cells (21). However, other receptors are probably involved as blocking dystroglycan complex does not completely inhibit adhesion of the bacillus to Schwann cells (21). It is unclear whether the organism has a direct pathogenic effect on Schwann cells, but the mycobacterium most certainly is involved in inducing damage via both *M. leprae*-specific and autoreactive T-cells (22).

The earliest pathological change seen in the nerves of patients with lepromatous leprosy is edema, with proliferation of Schwann cells and perineurial cells forming an "onion peel" appearance (23). Infiltration of the perineurium and axons by macrophages ensues. As Schwann cells degenerate, myelin disruption may occur followed by axonal degeneration (23). In tuberculoid leprosy, nerve fibers are often completely destroyed by the prominent inflammatory response.

2. LYME DISEASE

2.1. Introduction

Lyme disease is the most common vector-borne disease in the United States (24). It is a systemic bacterial infection caused by the spirochete *Borrelia burgdorferi* and is transmitted to humans by infected *Ixodes scapularis* and *I. pacificus* ticks. Deer are the preferred host of this tick family. The majority of the cases begin in the spring and summer. Children aged 5–9 and adults aged 45–54 have the highest reported incidence (25). Annual incidence is 0.5% in endemic areas, which include the Northeast and upper Midwest of the United States (26).

2.2. Clinical Features

Lyme disease is classified into three stages. Stage 1 consists of erythema migrans (EM), which occurs at the site of the tick bite. The rash erupts 1–30 days after the tick bite and is almost pathognomonic for Lyme disease. EM classically appears as a nonpruritic bull's-eye lesion with central clearing, although it can also be raised, irregular, vesicular, or pruritic (27). EM is usually accompanied by malaise, fatigue, headache, arthralgias, myalgias, fever, and regional lymphadenopathy. Stage 2 follows days to weeks later in a disseminated form affecting the nervous system, heart, or joints. Stage 3 follows weeks to months later and consists of arthritis and/or neurologic features (26,28).

In the early stages of Lyme disease, cranial neuropathy, radiculopathy, or lymphocytic meningitis may occur independently or in combination, a disease complex known as the Garin–Bujadoux–Bannwarth syndrome. A wide variety of cranial neuropathies are associated with Lyme disease, either as a mononeuropathy or in combination. Facial nerve palsy occurs most commonly and may be unilateral or bilateral (26,29,30).

The radiculoneuritis seen in early stages of infection is relatively severe, predominantly axonal, and tends to resolve spontaneously. The interval between the appearance of cutaneous symptoms and the neurological presentation ranges from 18 days to 2 months (31). Symptoms consist of asymmetric pain, often in a radicular distribution, followed by weakness in proximal leg muscles. Reflexes are decreased to absent and sensory loss is limited to affected nerve roots. Electrophysiologic testing is remarkable for markedly reduced compound motor action potentials, some prolongation of distal and F-wave latencies, and reduced amplitudes of sensory responses. Needle EMG reveals rare fibrillation potentials. Sural nerve biopsies demonstrate loss of myelinated and unmyelinated fibers and myelin ovoids, consistent with axonal degeneration (31). About one-third of patients with early Lyme disease have peripheral neuritis. Patterns include thoracic sensory radiculitis, motor radiculitis, mononeuritis multiplex, mononeuritis, and brachial plexitis (30). Occasional patients in this early stage may present with acute inflammatory demyelinating polyneuropathy (32). Other rare neurological complications are phrenic nerve palsy (33) and autonomic neuropathy (34).

In later stages of Lyme disease, chronic peripheral nerve disorders are common. Chronic neuropathy occurs in ~5% of untreated patients, sometimes after long periods of latent infection. These neuropathies may affect any limb or an body segment in either a symmetrical or an asymmetrical pattern. Symptoms usually are reported as paresthesias or radicular pain. In one study of patients with Lyme disease and chronic peripheral neuropathy, about half presented with distal paresthesias and the other half with painful radiculopathy. Asymptomatic sensory loss was rarely observed, and some patients reported only numbness. Radicular pain occurred in cervical, thoracic, or lumbosacral distributions. For many patients, paresthesias and radicular symptoms were intermittent. Physical examination revealed sensory loss for both small- and large-fiber modalities. Weakness and hyporeflexia were less common. Most patients with either radicular pain or distal paresthesias had needle EMG evidence of proximal nerve segment involvement with denervation in paraspinal musculature as well as proximal and distal limb muscles. Isolated conduction block of the peroneal nerve between the ankle and the fibular head was noted in one patient (29).

Associated central nervous system (CNS) features in late stages of *B. burgdorferi* infection include progressive encephalopathy and neuropsychiatric disorders. Acrodermatitis chronica atrophicans (ACA) is a late manifestation of Lyme disease, occurring in up to two-thirds (35). It is a cutaneous eruption localized to acral parts of the extremities and appears as bluish-red skin lesions. In one series, an associated distal sensory polyneuropathy was found in 64% of subjects with ACA (35).

2.3. Laboratory Evaluation

The diagnosis of Lyme disease is usually based on the recognition of the characteristic clinical findings such as EM, a history of exposure in an endemic area, and antibody response to *B. burgdorferi* by enzyme-linked immunosorbent assay (ELISA) and western blot. Cultivation of *B. burdorferi* from skin or blood is the gold standard for demonstration of active infection, but it is expensive and lacks clinical sensitivity (36). The urine antigen test is unreliable and not commonly used (26).

There may be little or no detectable serum antibody in many patients during the first 4–6 weeks of the illness. IgM antibodies are first to appear and suggest recent infection. This is followed 6 weeks later by the detection of IgG antibodies. If antibiotics are given early in the course of Lyme disease, seroconversion may not occur. Positive IgM serology alone is not helpful in diagnosing active disease, when the illness has been present longer than a month due to the high frequency of false-positive results. If serology is negative in suspected early Lyme disease, paired acute- and convalescent-phase serum samples should be tested for evidence of seroconversion. False-positive serologies may occur in patients with other infectious and autoimmune disorders such as syphilis, leptospirosis, yaws, bejel, malaria, subacute bacterial endocarditis, rheumatoid arthritis, and systemic lupus erythematosus (26).

IgM or IgG antibody responses to *B. burgdorferi* may persist for 10–20 years without indicating the presence of active infection (37). The recombinant OspA Lyme disease vaccine may give positive IgG results by ELISA, as OspA is the major outer surface protein expressed in cultured *B. burgdorferi*. Thus, any seroassay that uses the whole organism as its antigen source cannot differentiate between vaccinated subjects and those who are naturally infected. A new sensitive and specific ELISA technique that utilizes recombinant chimeric *borrelia* proteins devoid of OspA (rNon-OspA) has been developed and can differentiate between patients who have been vaccinated and those with active or prior infection (38).

Cerebrospinal fluid (CSF) can also be tested for the presence of *B. burgdorferi* antibodies. Nonspecific CSF abnormalities include mononuclear pleocytosis, elevated protein, and normal glucose.

PCR is a highly sensitive means of detecting microbial DNA or RNA. However, *borrelia* DNA or RNA has not been detected reliably in blood, urine, or CSF of patients with early or late forms of Lyme disease (39). PCR has been found to be the most sensitive and specific test for detection of *B. burgdorferi* in skin biopsies from patients with dermatoborreliosis. For patients with neuroborreliosis, *B. burgdorferi* DNA was detectable in only 17–21% of CSF samples (40). There was a tendency for the PCR positive rate to be higher in patients with early neuroborreliosis (<2 weeks) when compared with those with longer disease duration. Thus, PCR can be helpful in early neuroborreliosis. However, PCR does not differentiate between the DNA of dead or live spirochetes (36) and will, therefore, not verify the presence of active infection. False-positive results from poor specimen handling and contamination must also be considered at the time of interpretation.

2.4. Differential Diagnosis

The differential diagnosis includes other disorders that can present with cranial and peripheral neuropathies. These include a number of other infectious diseases including human immunodeficiency virus (HIV), syphilis, mycobacteria including leprosy, and fungal infections. Connective tissue disorders and malignancy, such as lymphoma, should also be considered.

2.5. Management

Treatment of early Lyme disease usually prevents progression. Most patients with neuroborreliosis require parenteral antibiotics. Exceptions are patients with isolated facial nerve palsy and normal CSF examinations (30,41). These patients can be treated with a number of oral agents including doxycycline 100 mg p.o. bid, amoxicillin 500 mg p.o. tid, or tetracycline 500 mg p.o. tid for 2–4 weeks. Doxycycline is contraindicated during pregnancy and in children under the age of 8.

In other clinical scenarios, patients are treated with 2–4 weeks of intravenous ceftriaxone 2 g/day. Other parenteral antibiotics that may be used are intravenous cefotaxime 2 g every 8 h or penicillin G 3.3 million units every 4 h (27). Some authors advocate a combination of macrolide and hydroxychloroquine to treat late Lyme disease symptoms (39). Clinical features of acute neuroborreliosis usually resolve within weeks of antibiotic therapy, but those of chronic neuroborreliosis improve more slowly, over periods of several months (28). Complete recovery is rare in patients with longstanding disease (42).

2.6. Prevention

Patient education regarding proper clothing, careful inspection for ticks, and avoidance of infested habitats plays a key role in disease prevention. Chemoprophylaxis with a single dose of 200 mg doxycycline may be provided within 72 h of exposure to a tick bite (28,43). For immunoprophylaxis of high-risk individuals in endemic areas, a recombinant outer-surface protein (rOspA) Lyme disease vaccine (LYMErix) is available. The vaccine is given intramuscularly at a dose of 30 μg at 0, 1, and 12 months. A 76% efficacy in preventing infection has been demonstrated after the third dose (44). Booster doses may be needed every 1–3 years. Only transient mild-to-moderate vaccine-associated adverse events have been reported. The vaccine is not approved for use in children under the age of 15 or in pregnant women (45) and is licensed only for persons between 15 and 70 years of age.

2.7. Prognosis

Patients usually do well if diagnosed in early stages of infection after receiving appropriate antibiotic therapy (27). Response to therapy is less favorable in those with longer disease duration. Opinions differ on the outcome of chronic neuroborreliosis (42,46). Some have reported reversal of peripheral nerve manifestations with appropriate antibiotics (46), whereas others have reported more than a third of patients with chronic neurological manifestations that do not improve and about half who have a chronic progressive course (42). Poor outcomes were attributed to failure to eradicate the spirochete completely despite a 2 week course of intravenous antibiotics or to irreversible nervous system damage.

2.8. Pathophysiology

The pathogenesis of the nerve injury in Lyme disease remains unclear. Although injury directly related to the spirochete is a possibility, parainfectious immunologic mechanisms have also been proposed (41,47). Nerve biopsies show meningoradiculitis, lymphocytes, and plasma cells surrounding many epineurial, perineurial, and endoneurial vessels, without evidence of vessel wall necrosis. There is loss of both myelinated and unmyelinated fibers. Myelin ovoids consistent with axonal degeneration are seen (31). Sural nerve biopsy from a patient with chronic neuroborreliosis revealed complement membrane attack complexes and macrophages surrounding epineurial vessels and within the endoneurium. PCR demonstrated *B. burgdorferi* DNA from the nerve tissue (48).

3. SARCOIDOSIS

3.1. Introduction

Sarcoidosis is an immune-mediated, multisystem granulomatous disorder that presents with hilar adenopathy, pulmonary infiltration, and ocular and skin lesions. Sarcoidoisis was first recognized in 1869, but the cause remains unknown. No infectious agent has been identified. Immunoreactivity is enhanced in sarcoidosis with activated T-cells and macrophages producing a variety of proinflammatory mediators at sites of granuloma formation (49). Environmental exposures are believed to interact with genetic factors in determining the pattern of presentation, progression, and prognosis (50). Sarcoidosis commonly affects young and middle-age adults (51) with a slight female predominance in symptomatic cases. In the United States, the prevalence rate in African-Americans is roughly 10 times higher than that in Caucasians (51).

3.2. Clinical Features

The frequency of neurological involvement in sarcoidosis is ~5% (52). Most of these patients have other systemic manifestations of the disease. In two series of neurosarcoidosis, 48–65% of patients had neurologic dysfunction as their presenting manifestation (52,53). Neurologic manifestations are protean and may involve the central or peripheral nervous system. CNS involvement usually occurs in the early phase of the disease, whereas peripheral neuromuscular involvement is characteristically seen in the chronic stages (53).

Neurosarcoid patients may have single or multiple cranial nerve palsies (52), basilar meningitis, hydrocephalus, parenchymal disease of the nervous system, peripheral neuropathy, or myopathy (Table 17.2). Cranial nerve palsies occur in >50% of patients (54), with the facial nerve being most commonly affected (55). Most other cranial nerves may also be involved including I, II, III, IV, V, VI, VIII, IX, and X. The incidence of non-cranial peripheral neuropathy in sarcoidosis varies from 24% to 40% (54,55). The various patterns of peripheral neuropathy in sarcoidosis are listed in Table 17.3.

3.3. Polyneuropathy

Chronic sensorimotor polyneuropathy is the most common pattern of peripheral neuropathy in sarcoidosis. The polyneuropathy usually starts months to years after systemic features first appear (56). Patients typically present with a subacute to chronic progressive course of paresthesias, burning or shooting pain, and numbness distally in the hands and feet. Occasional patients develop respiratory failure secondary to diaphragmatic weakness (56,57). On examination, distal pan-sensory loss consistent with a length-dependent process, areflexia, and mild distal weakness are seen.

Table 17.2 Comparison of Clinical Manifestations in Neurosarcoidosis

	Chapelon et al. (55) (n = 35) (%)	Stern et al. (52) (n = 33) (%)	Sharma (54) (n = 37) (%)
Cranial nerve palsies	37	73	52
Meningitis	40	18	24
Peripheral involvement	40	6	24
Myopathy	26	12	8

Table 17.3 Patterns of Peripheral Neuropathy in Neurosarcoidosis

- Symmetric polyneuropathy
  - Sensorimotor (49,50)
  - Pure sensory (49,51)
  - Pure motor (55)
- Mononeuritis multiplex
- Mononeuropathy
- Polyradiculopathy (50,52,55)
- Guillain–Barré syndrome (49)
- Lumbosacral plexopathy (49)
- Phrenic neuropathy (53)
- Multifocal sensorimotor neuropathy with conduction block (51)

NCS reveal an axonal neuropathy with low-amplitude compound muscle action potentials and reduced to absent sensory nerve action potentials. Needle EMG may show active denervation in distal muscles.

3.4. Mononeuropathy and Mononeuritis Multiplex

This type of presentation is more often associated with cranial neuropathies as opposed to a neuropathy involving the limbs (58). Patients with mononeuropathy present with focal sensory and motor or sensorimotor symptoms that may include patchy sensory loss over the trunk (56). Onset is typically subacute with progressive involvement (59).

Electrophysiologic studies typically reveal an axonal pattern of injury. A multifocal demyelinating pattern has also been reported with asymmetric onset of weakness and numbness in the distal extremities that was responsive to corticosteroid therapy (59). Electrophysiologic studies in this report revealed conduction block in the median, ulnar, and peroneal nerves and a reduced sural amplitude.

3.5. Polyradiculopathy

This pattern is rarely seen in sarcoidosis. Presentation is usually in the fourth decade with back pain, lower extremity weakness most prominent proximally, sphincter dysfunction, and areflexia in the lower limbs (60). Thoracic, lumbar, and sacral roots are involved more frequently than the cervical distribution (55). A concurrent myelopathy may be present. Radicular involvement may arise from contiguous, hematogenous, or gravitational seeding of nerve root sleeves. Active denervation consistent with a nerve root localization can be demonstrated on needle EMG.

3.6. Guillain–Barré Syndrome

There have been rare cases of a Guillain–Barré syndrome (GBs)-like presentation in the setting of sarcoidosis (56). One case describes a young man with sarcoidosis who had subacute onset of facial and bulbar weakness accompanied by leg weakness. Electrophysiologic testing revealed prolonged distal latencies, low-amplitude motor amplitudes, prolonged late responses in the legs, absent sensory potentials, and prolonged blink reflexes. He improved with steroids, but had a mild relapse 3 years later. Other cases can present acutely leading to fulminant respiratory failure (59). Chronic inflammatory demyelinating polyradiculoneuropathy (CIDP) may also occur in association with sarcoidosis (58).

3.7. Lumbosacral Plexopathy with Chronic Sensorimotor Polyneuropathy

Proximal involvement is rare. A case report describes a patient with foot drop, ipsilateral absence of patellar reflex, bilaterally absent achilles reflexes, and vibratory loss in feet. Electrophysiologic studies demonstrated a left lumbosacral plexopathy superimposed on a sensorimotor polyneuropathy (56).

3.8. Subclinical Neuropathy

Subclinical mononeuritis multiplex appears to be common in sarcoidosis. In a comparison study of asymptomatic sarcoid patients to a similar number of age-matched control subjects, abnormal sensory amplitudes in one or more nerves were found in two-thirds of sarcoid patients when compared with few controls. Mean sensory amplitudes for the median, ulnar, and sural nerves were lower in patients than in controls. Asymptomatic compression of nerves by granulomata is the proposed mechanism (61).

3.9. Laboratory Evaluation

The diagnosis of sarcoidosis may be challenging when patients present with neurologic symptoms in the absence of systemic features. As the incidence of systemic involvement is high, routine chest radiography and ophthalmologic evaluation must be done to assess for hilar adenopathy, uveitis, or fundus granulomas (53). Chest radiographs are abnormal in 78–90% cases (54). Routine chemistry must be performed to exclude involvement of other organ systems. Hypercalcemia is seen in 17% of cases. Serum angiotensin converting enzyme (ACE) levels are elevated in 54–65% of cases, but are not highly sensitive or specific (54,55). Serum lysozyme is also used as a marker of sarcoidosis activity. It has a higher sensitivity, but lower specificity than ACE levels (62). CSF analysis may be normal (56) or may reveal an elevated protein (mean value, 326 mg/dL), lymphocytosis (mean value, 156 cells/mm^3), and hypoglycorrhachia (60). These findings, in the absence of positive cytology and cultures for bacteria, AFB, and fungi, are supportive of neurosarcoidosis. Myelography may demonstrate nerve root thickening and irregularity in patients with polyradiculopathy.

A definitive diagnosis of sarcoidosis requires histologic confirmation of noncaseating granulomas in the setting of a compatible clinical or radiologic picture. Muscle, nerve, skin, lymph node, conjunctival, or minor salivary gland biopsies can be performed for histologic confirmation. Because pulmonary involvement is very common with sarcoidosis, transbronchial biopsy or mediastinoscopy are options. Gallium scan or computed tomography of the chest may also be helpful in the evaluation.

3.10. Differential Diagnosis

Sarcoidosis is a multisystem disease and neurologic involvement may occur in isolation without the typical systemic features. Hence, when patients present with the various cranial and peripheral manifestations, etiologies such as HIV infection, mycobacterial and fungal infections including leprosy, lymphoma, syphilis, and Lyme disease must be kept in mind. Vasculitides in isolation or in association with connective tissue disorders should also be considered. Common causes of polyradiculopathy and sensorimotor polyneuropathy, such as diabetes mellitus, must also be excluded.

3.11. Management and Prognosis

Treatment is not indicated for asymptomatic or minimally symptomatic disease (63), and these patients may improve spontaneously (53). In patients with more significant disease, corticosteroids remain the mainstay of treatment. Prednisone is usually sufficient in controlling the underlying inflammatory process (52). Prednisone doses range from 0.5 to 1 mg/kg daily, depending on the clinical scenario. Treatment at this higher dosage should continue for at least 2 months, with lower doses continued for longer periods to maintain functional improvement (55,63). In patients with relapses, intravenous corticosteroids (solumedrol 1 g/day × 3 days) should be considered. If patients fail to respond to this regimen, azathioprine, chlorambucil, methotrexate, cyclosporine, or cyclophosphamide are options. Decompressive laminectory may be appropriate when there is mass effect and it also provides tissue for diagnosis (60). Patients presenting with a clinical picture consistent with GBS or CIDP should be treated with plasma exchange or intravenous gammaglobulin (58), as one would in cases not associated with sarcoidosis.

The overall prognosis of neurosarcoidosis is relatively favorable. A positive outcome has been observed in two-thirds of well-documented episodes of neurologic dysfunction (52). However, outcomes for patients with peripheral nerve involvement are somewhat less favorable than for neurosarcoidosis of the CNS, two-thirds of patients with CNS manifestations recovered compared with 42% with peripheral neuropathy (55). In patients with chronic neurosarcoidosis, the prognosis is relatively poor, with death occurring in 20% from complications related to sarcoidosis (54).

3.12. Pathophysiology

Nerve biopsy specimens show noncaseating granulomas in the epineurial and perineurial spaces, periangiitis, panangiitis, and axonal degeneration (64). Axonal degeneration is probably a result of involvement of the vasa nervorum and direct compression by the granulomas. Immune dysfunction may also play a role in the pathogenesis as a number of autoimmune disorders are associated with sarcoidosis.

4. HERPES ZOSTER

4.1. Introduction

Radiculitis or cranial neuritis due to herpes zoster, commonly referred to as "shingles," is the result of re-activation of latent varicella zoster virus (VZV) in sensory ganglia. Decreased immune responsiveness associated with advancing age, malignancy, use of cytotoxic agents, or infection with HIV increases the risk of developing herpes zoster.

4.2. Clinical Features

A vesicular rash appears in a trigeminal or dermatomal distribution, associated with radicular pain and paresthesias that usually conform to the same body region. Loss of pain and temperature sensation is typically patchy within the dermatome. Pain may precede the rash by a week or more. Fever, malaise, and headache may also occur.

In nonimmunocompromised patients, the vesicles resolve in 2–3 weeks, usually with no sequelae.

Patients may develop focal weakness in a radicular distribution. Ramsay–Hunt syndrome, the development of facial paresis after herpes zoster oticus, is the most common example. In general, myotomal involvement correlates to the dermatome(s) affected by rash, although rarely weakness may not coincide anatomically with the cutaneous eruption (65–68). Weakness progresses over hours or days, then plateaus. Most of the time, the rash precedes the weakness but rarely, weakness may antedate the rash.

Focal weakness in a spinal nerve root or cranial nerve distribution is rare (5%), with a latency varying from 1 day to 5 weeks after eruption of the rash (65). Motor involvement ranges from mild weakness in a single myotome to nearly complete paralysis of an extremity. Deep tendon reflexes are reduced, often out of proportion to the degree of muscle weakness, consistent with involvement of the afferent arc of the spinal reflex. Oculomotor paresis, both with and without pupillary involvement, may occur in association with rash in the distribution of the ophthalmic division of the trigeminal nerve.

Rarely, in both immunocompetent and immunocompromised individuals, focal sensory and motor symptoms may occur in the absence of the vesicular rash, the so-called zoster sine herpete (69–71). In the absence of rash, diagnosis is challenging. PCR for VZV in CSF or detection of VZV antibody in CSF can be helpful in establishing the diagnosis (70,72). Recurrent polyneuropathies without cutaneous manifestations of herpes zoster have been diagnosed in the setting of presumed chronic VZV infection that was based on the presence of VZV antibodies in the CSF (73). Other uncommon neurological complications of VZV are aseptic meningitis, encephalitis, transverse myelitis, and urinary retention. These complications occur in <1% of immunocompetent patients, but in as many as 35% of immunocompromised hosts (74).

Post-herpetic neuralgia (PHN) is a chronic pain syndrome that is seen in greater frequency in older patients. The number of patients reporting persistent pain ≥3 months after resolution of the rash ranges from 11% in patients <30 years (75) to 39% in patients >50 years (76,77).

4.3. Laboratory Evaluation

In the setting of the trademark vesicular rash and uncomplicated sensory symptoms, the diagnosis is straightforward and requires no specific laboratory testing. In cases without rash or when severe complications arise, further investigation is indicated. Magnetic resonance imaging (MRI), T1-weighted sequences before and after infusion of gadolinium may show enhancement of spinal nerve roots or cranial nerves (68,78). T2 and proton density sequences may show high-signal intensity in the spinal cord in cases of myelitis (79) and in subcortical white matter or brainstem in cases of encephalitis (79–83). However, MRI may be normal even in cases of encephalitis (81). CSF analysis often shows mild-to-moderate elevation of protein and a variable lymphocytic pleocytosis with normal glucose. PCR for VZV in CSF is an important and specific method of detecting infection, as are immunosorbent assays for IgG and IgM antibodies to VZV in the CSF (84).

In the cases of segmental paresis, NCS reveal normal sensory and motor responses in most patients (65). However, other studies have shown reduced sensory nerve action potentials in as many as 52% (85). Motor nerve responses may be normal or have low-amplitudes (65,85). Needle EMG performed ≥2 weeks after onset of weakness usually demonstrates active denervation potentials in clinically weak muscles, but have also been reported in a myotomal distribution corresponding to the affected dermatomes even when no clinical weakness is apparent (86).

4.4. Differential Diagnosis

In cases of zoster sine herpete, the differential diagnosis includes other structural, inflammatory, or infectious causes of radiculopathy or cranial neuropathy, including herniated vertebral disc, diabetes, or Lyme disease. In the setting of myelitis or encephalitis, viral infection including HIV or lupus or other inflammatory processes should be considered.

4.5. Management and Prognosis

To reduce the time for healing of cutaneous lesions and possibly to reduce the incidence of segmental paresis (85), immunocompetent patients should be treated with valacyclovir 1000 mg p.o. three times daily for 7 days, famciclovir 500 mg p.o. three times daily for 7 days, or acyclovir 800 mg p.o. five times daily for 7–10 days. Treatment started within 72 h of onset of the rash is the most advantageous. The incidence of PHN is not reduced by antiviral therapy, but the duration of pain may be shortened (85,87). Intravenous acyclovir is effective in preventing dissemination of herpes zoster in immunocompromised individuals. The use of steroids is probably not indicated and should be avoided in immunocompromised patients.

For PHN, amitriptyline and other tricyclic antidepressants and gabapentin are effective. Carbamazepine may be especially useful for treating lancinating pain. Short-term use of narcotics should be considered, especially in refractory patients.

The prognosis for full recovery is good. Even patients who develop focal weakness usually regain normal strength or have only slight residual numbness or weakness.

4.6. Pathophysiology

With re-activation of VZV, replication and release of the virus occur in dorsal root ganglia and spread to the entire ganglion. Involved dorsal root ganglia on autopsy show inflammation and necrosis (88). Destruction of sensory neurons leads to temporary or permanent sensory loss in the corresponding dermatome, but also removes reservoirs for the virus (89). The active infection explains the pleocytosis seen in CSF. VZV spreads along the nerve to the skin. Light microscopy demonstrates perivascular lymphocytic infiltration in the early erythematous cutaneous stage. During the vesicular stage, viral antigens may be detected in epidermis and in capillary and venule endothelial cells and the perineurium of dermal nerves (90).

The pathogenesis of PHN is not well understood. PHN may arise from structural or physiologic changes in the DRG (89). Alternatively, C-fiber nociceptors may become sensitized, with development of spontaneous or stimulus-evoked pain. Further, continuous nociceptor discharge may lead to central hyperexcitability of spinal DRG. These neurons may have exaggerated responses to input and may contribute to development of allodynia (91). Skin biopsies of patients with pain 3 months after resolution of HZV rash show significantly fewer epidermal nerve endings than do biopsies of patients without pain (92).

REFERENCES

1. Rees RJW, McDougall AC. Airborne infection with *Mycobacterium leprae* in mice. Int J Lepr 1976; 44:99–103.
2. Abraham S, Mozhi NM, Joseph GA, Kurian N, Rao PSSS, Job CK. Epidemiological significance of first skin lesion in leprosy. Int J Lepr 1998; 66:131–139.

3. Lara CB, Nolasco JO. Self-healing, or abortive, and residual forms of childhood leprosy and their probable significance. Int J Lepr 1956; 24:245–263.

4. Ridley DS, Jopling WH. Classification of leprosy according to immunity. A five-group system. Int J Lepr 1966; 34:255–273.

5. Fields JP, Meyers WM. Mycobacterial infections. In: Farmer ER, Hood AF, eds. Pathology of the Skin. 2nd ed. McGraw-Hill: New York, 2000:553–578.

6. Davey TF, Rees RJW. The nasal discharge in leprosy: clinical and bacteriological aspects. Lepr Rev 1974; 45:121–134.

7. Lewallen S. Prevention of blindness in leprosy: an overview of the relevant clinical and pro-gramme-planning issues. Ann Trop Med Parasitol 1997; 91:341–348.

8. van Brakel WH. Peripheral neuropathy in leprosy and its consequences. Lepr Rev 2000; 71(suppl):S146–S153.

9. Rodriguez G, Sanchez W, Chatela JG, Soto J. Primary neuritic leprosy. J Am Acad Dermatol 1993; 29:1050–1052.

10. Amenu A, Saunderson P, Desta K, Byass P. The pattern of decline in bacillary index after 2 years of WHO recommended multiple drug therapy: the AMFES cohort. Lepr Rev 2000; 71:332–337.

11. De Wit MY, Douglas JT, McFadden J, Klaster PR. Polymerase chain reaction for detection of *Mycobacterium leprae* in nasal swab specimens. J Clin Microbiol 1993; 31:502–506.

12. Hackett ER, Shipley DE, Livengood R. Motor nerve conduction velocity studies of the ulnar nerve in patients with leprosy. Int J Lepr 1968; 36:282–287.

13. Antia NH, Pandya SS, Dastur DK. Nerves in the arm in leprosy: I. Clinical, electrodiagnostic and operative aspects. Int J Lepr 1970; 38:12–29.

14. Swift TR, Hackett ER, Shipley DE, Miner KM. The peroneal and tibial nerves in lepromatous leprosy: clinical and electrophysiologic observations. Int J Lepr 1973; 41:25–34.

15. Anonymous. Global leprosy situation, September, 1999. Wkly Epidemiol Rec 1999; 74:313–316.

16. Roche PW, Le Master J, Butlin CR. Risk factors for type 1 reactions in leprosy. Int J Lepr 1997; 65:450–455.

17. Naafs B. Current views on reactions in leprosy. Indian J Lepr 2000; 72:97–122.

18. Sharma A, Sharma VK, Rajwanshi A, Das A, Kaur I, Kumar B. Presence of *M. leprae* in tissues in slit skin smear negative multibacillary (MB) patients after WHO-MBR. Lepr Rev 1999; 70:281–286.

19. Ebenezer GJ, Job A, Abraham S, Arunthathi S, Rao PSSS, Job CK. Nasal mucosa and skin of smear-positive leprosy patients after 24 months of fixed duration MDT: histopathological and microbiological study. Int J Lepr 1999; 67:292–297.

20. Rambukkana A, Salzer JL, Yurchenco PD, Tuomanen EI. Neural targeting of *Mycobacterium leprae* mediated by the G domain of the laminin-*a*2 chain. Cell 1997; 88:811–821.

21. Rambukkana A, Yamada H, Zanazzi G, Mathus T, Salzer JL, Yurchenco PD, Campbell KP, Fischetti VA. Role of *a*-dystroglycan as a Schwann cell receptor for *Mycobacterium leprae*. Science 1998; 282:2076–2079.

22. Spierings E, de Boer T, Zulianello L, Ottenhoff THM. The role of Schwann cells, T cells and *Mycobacterium leprae* in the immunopathogenesis of nerve damage in leprosy. Lepr Rev 2000; 71(suppl):S121–S129.

23. Job CK. Pathology of peripheral nerve lesions in lepromatous leprosy—a light and electron microscopic study. Int J Lepr 1971; 39:251–268.

24. Piacentino JD, Schwartz BS. Occupational risk of Lyme disease: an epidemiological review. Occup Environ Med 2002; 59:75–84.

25. Orloski KA, Hayes EB, Campbell GL, Dennis DT. Surveillance for Lyme disease-United States, 1992–1998. MMWR CDC Surveill Summ 2000; 49:1–11.

26. Verdon ME, Sigal LH. Recognition and management of Lyme disease. Am Fam Physician 1997; 56:427–436.

27. Coyle PK, Schutzer SE. Neurologic aspects of Lyme disease. Med Clin North Am 2002; 86:261–284.

28. Steere AC. Lyme disease. N Engl J Med 2001; 345:115–125.
29. Logigian EL, Steere AC. Clinical and electrophysiologic findings in chronic neuropathy of Lyme disease. Neurology 1992; 42:303–311.
30. Pachner AR, Steere AC. The triad of neurologic manifestations of Lyme disease: meningitis, cranial neuritis, and radiculoneuritis. Neurology 1985; 35:47–53.
31. Vallat JM, Hugon J, Lubeau M, Leboutet MJ, Dumas M, Desproges-Gotteron R. Tick-bite meningoradiculoneuritis: clinical, electrophysiologic, and histologic findings in 10 cases. Neurology 1987; 37:749–753.
32. Crisp D, Ashby P. Lyme radiculoneuritis treated with intravenous immunoglobulin. Neurology 1996; 46:1174–1175.
33. Faul JL, Ruoss S, Doyle RL, Kao PN. Diaphragmatic paralysis due to Lyme disease. Eur Respir J 1999; 13:700–702.
34. Chatila R, Kapadia CR. Intestinal pseudoobstruction in acute Lyme disease: a case report. Am J Gastroenterol 1998; 93:1179–1180.
35. Kindstrand E, Nilsson BY, Hovmark A, Pirskanen R, Asbrink E. Peripheral neuropathy in acrodermatitis chronica atrophicans—a late Borrelia manifestation. Acta Neurol Scand 1997; 95:338–345.
36. Bunikis J, Barbour AG. Laboratory testing for suspected Lyme disease. Med Clin North Am 2002; 86:311–340.
37. Kalish RA, McHugh G, Granquist J, Shea B, Ruthazer R, Steere AC. Persistence of immunoglobulin M or immunoglobulin G antibody responses to *Borrelia burgdorferi* 10–20 years after active Lyme. Clin Infect Dis 2001; 33:780–785.
38. Gomes-Solecki MJ, Wormser GP, Schreifer M, Neuman G, Hannafey L, Glass JD, Dattwyle RJ. Recombinant assay for serodiagnosis of lyme disease regardless of OspA vaccination status. J Clin Microbiol 2002; 40:193–197.
39. Donta ST. Late and chronic Lyme disease. Med Clin North Am 2002; 86:341–349.
40. Lebech AM. Polymerase chain reaction in diagnosis of *Borrelia burgdorferi* infections and studies on taxonomic classification. APMIS 2002; 105(suppl):1–40.
41. Logigian EL. Peripheral nervous system Lyme borreliosis. Semin Neurol 1997; 17:25–30.
42. Logigian EL, Kaplan RF, Steere AC. Chronic neurologic manifestations of Lyme disease. N Engl J Med 1990; 323:1438–1444.
43. Nadelman RB, Nowakowski J, Fish D, Falco RC, Freeman K, McKenna D, Welch P, Marcus R, Aguero-Rosenfeld ME, Dennis DT, Wormser GP. Tick Bite Study Group. Prophylaxis with single-dose doxycycline for the prevention of Lyme disease after an *Ixodes scapularis* tick bite. N Engl J Med 2001; 345:79–84.
44. Poland GA, Jacobson RM. The prevention of Lyme disease with vaccine. Vaccine 2001; 19:2303–2308.
45. Rahn DW. Lyme vaccine: issues and controversies. Infect Dis Clin North Am 2001; 15:171–187.
46. Halperin J, Luft BJ, Volkman DJ, Dattwyler RJ. Lyme neuroborreliosis. Peripheral nervous system manifestations. Brain 1990; 113:1207–1221.
47. Sigal LH. Immunologic mechanisms in Lyme neuroborreliosis: the potential role of autoimmunity and molecular mimicry. Semin Neurol 1997; 17:63–68.
48. Maimone D, Villanova M, Stanta G, Bonin S, Malandrini A, Guazzi GC, Annunziata P. Detection of *Borrelia burgdorferi* DNA and complement membrane attack complex deposits in the sural nerve of a patient with chronic polyneuropathy and tertiary Lyme disease. Muscle Nerve 1997; 20:969–975.
49. Moller DR. Etiology of sarcoidosis. Clin Chest Med 1997; 18:695–706.
50. Martinetti M, Dugoujon JM, Tinelli C, Cipriani A, Cortelazzo A, Salvaneschi L, Casali L, Semenzato G, Cuccia M, Luisetti M. HLA-Gm/kappam interaction in sarcoidosis. Suggestions for a complex genetic structure. Eur Respir J 2000; 16(1):74–80.
51. Hosoda Y, Yamaguchi M, Hiraga Y. Global epidemiology of sarcoidosis. What story do prevalence and incidence tell us? Clin Chest Med 1997; 18:681–694
52. Stern BJ, Krumholz A, Johns C, Scott P, Nissim J. Sarcoidosis and its neurological manisfestations. Arch Neurol 1985; 42:909–917.

53. Delaney P. Neurological manifestations in sarcoidosis. Review of the literature, with a report of 23 cases. Ann Intern Med 1977; 87:336–345.

54. Sharma OP. Neurosarcoidosis. A personal perspective based on the study of 37 patients. Chest 1997; 112:220–228.

55. Chapelon C, Ziza JM, Piette JC, Levy Y, Raguin G, Wechsler B, Bitker MC, Bletry O, Laplane D, Bousser MG, Godeau P. Neurosarcoidosis: signs, course and treatment in 35 confirmed cases. Medicine 1990; 69:261–276.

56. Zuniga G, Ropper AH, Frank J. Sarcoid peripheral neuropathy. Neurology 1991; 41:1558–1561.

57. Robinson LR, Brownsberger R, Raghu G. Respiratory failure and hypoventilation secondary to neurosarcoidosis. Am J Respir Crit Care Med 1998; 157:1316–1318.

58. Mendell JR, Kissel JT, Cornblath DR. Diagnosis and Management of Peripheral Nerve Disorders. Oxford University Press, Inc., 2001.

59. Said G, Lacroix C, Plante-Bordeneuve V, Page LL, Pico F, Presles O, Senant J, Remy P, Rondepierre P, Mallecourt J. Nerve granulomas and vasculitis in sarcoid peripheral neuropathy. A clinicopathological study of 11 patients. Brain 2002; 125:264–275.

60. Koffman B, Junck L, Elias SB, Feit HW, Levine SR. Polyradiculopathy in sarcoidosis. Muscle Nerve 1999; 22:608–613.

61. Challenor YB, Felton CP, Brust JC. Peripheral nerve involvement in sarcoidosis: an electrodiagnostic study. J Neurol Neurosurg Psychiatry 1984; 47:1219–1222.

62. Tomita H, Sato S, Matsuda R, Sugiura Y, Kawaguchi H, Niimi T, Yoshida S, Morishita M. Serum lysozyme levels and clinical features of sarcoidosis. Lung 1999; 177:161–167

63. Johns CJ, Michele TM. The clinical management of sarcoidosis. A 50-year experience at the Johns Hopkins hospital. Medicine 1999; 78:65–111.

64. Oh SJ. Sarcoid polyneuropathy: a histologocally proved case. Ann Neurol 1980; 7:178–181.

65. Thomas JE, Howard FM. Segmental zoster paresis—a disease profile. Neurology 1972; 22:459–466.

66. Taterka JH, O'Sullivan ME. The motor complications of herpes zoster. J Am Med Assoc 1943; 122:737–739.

67. Kendall D. Motor complications of herpes zoster. Br Med J 1957; 2:616–618.

68. Hanakawa T, Hashimoto S, Kawamura J, Nakamura M, Suenago T, Matsuo M. Magnetic resonance imaging in a patient with segmental zoster paresis. Neurology 1997; 49:631–632.

69. Osaki Y, Mutsubayashi K, Okumiya K, Wada T, Doi Y. Polyneuritis cranialis due to varicella-zoster virus in the absence of rash. Neurology 1995; 45:2293.

70. Gilden DH, Wright RR, Schneck SA, Gwaltney JM, Mahalingam R. Zoster sine herpete, a clinical variant. Ann Neurol 1994; 35:530–533.

71. Elliott KD. Other neurological complications of herpes zoster and their management. Ann Neurol 1994; 35(suppl):S57–S61.

72. Gilden DH, Dueland AN, Devlin ME. Varicella-zoster reactivation without rash. J Infect Dis 1992; 166(suppl 1):S30–S34.

73. Fox RJ, Galetta SL, Mahalingamm R, Wellish M, Forghani B, Gilden DH. Acute, chronic, and recurrent varicella zoster virus neuropathy without zoster rash. Neurology 2001; 57:351–354.

74. Weller TH. Varicella and herpes zoster: changing concepts of the natural history, control and importance of a not-so-benign virus (part two). N Engl J Med 1983; 309:1434–1440.

75. Goh CL, Khoo L. A retrospective study of the clinical presentation and outcome of herpes zoster in a tertiary dermatology outpatient referral clinic. Int J Dermatol 1997; 36:667–672.

76. Ragozzino MW, Melton IJ, Kurland LT. Population based study of herpes zoster and its sequelae. Medicine 1982; 21:310–316.

77. de Moragas JM, Kierland RR. The outcome of patients with herpes zoster. Arch Dermatol 1957; 75:193–196.

78. Osumi A, Tien RD. MR findings in a patient with Ransay–Hunt syndrome. J Comput Assist Tomogr 1990; 14:991–993.

79. Haanpaa M, Dastidar P, Weinberg A, Levin M, Miettinen A, Lapinlampi A. CSF and MRI finding in patients with acute herpes zoster. Neurology 1998; 51:1405–1411.

80. Tien RD, Felsberg GJ, Osumi AK. Herpes virus infections in the CNS: MR findings. Am J Roentgenol 1993; 161:167–176.

81. De la Blanchardiere A, Rozenberg F, Caumes E, Picard O, Lionnet F, Livartowski J, Coste J, Sicard D, Lebon P, Salmon-Ceron D. Neurological complications of varicella-zoster virus infection in adults with human immunodeficiency virus infection. Scand J Infect Dis 2000; 32:263–269.

82. Kidd D, Duncan JS, Tompson EJ. Pontine inflammatory lesion due to shingles. J Neurol Neurosurg Psychiatry 1998; 65:208.

83. Weaver S, Rosenblum MK, DeAngelis LM. Herpes varicella zoster encephalitis in immuno-compromised patients. Neurology 1999; 52:193–197.

84. Kleinschmidt-DeMasters, Gilden DH. Varicella-zoster virus infections of the nervous system. Arch Pathol Lab Med 2001; 125:770–780.

85. Mondelli M, Romano C, Passero S, Della Porta P, Rossi A. Effects of acyclovir on sensory axonal neuropathy, segmental motor paresis and postherpetic neuralgia in herpes zoster patients. Eur Neurol 1996; 36:288–292.

86. Greenberg MK, McVey AL, Hayes T. Segmental motor involvement in herpes zoster: an EMG study. Neurology 1992; 42:1122–1123.

87. Alper BS, Lewis PR. Does treatment of acute herpes zoster prevent or shorten postherpetic neualgia? A systematic review of the literature. J Fam Pract 2000; 49:256–264.

88. Lungo O, Ammunziato PW, Gershon A, Staugaitis SM, Josephson D, LaRussa P, Silverstein SJ. Reactivated and latent varicella-zoster virus in human dorsal root ganglia. Proc Natl Acad Sci USA 1995; 92:10980–10984

89. Steiner I. Human herpes viruses latent infection in the nervous system. Immunol Rev 1996; 152:158–173.

90. Muraki R, Baba T, Iwasaki T, Sata T, Kurata T. Immunohistochemical study of skin lesions in herpes zoster. Pathol Anat Histopathol 1992; 420:71–76.

91. Bennett GJ. Hypotheses on the pathogenesis of herpes zoster—associated pain. Ann Neurol 1994; 35(suppl):S38–S40.

92. Oaklander AL. The density of remaining nerve endings in human skin with and without postherpetic neuralgia after shingles. Pain 2001; 92:139–145.

18
Critical Illness Polyneuropathy and Myopathy

J. Robinson Singleton and Estelle S. Harris
University of Utah, Salt Lake City, Utah, USA

ABSTRACT

Weakness is common in patients requiring intensive care and is often attributable to injury to either peripheral nerves or muscle. Critical illness polyneuropathy (CIP) is a distal axonal neuropathy observed in severely ill patients with sepsis and multiple organ system failures. Critical illness myopathy (CIM) is a catabolic injury to skeletal muscle that occurs in the same setting. There is controversy over the relative contribution of these two entities to the spectrum of clinical weakness observed in critically ill patients. Up to 70% of patients receiving intensive care develop weakness associated due to CIP, CIM, or both. Diagnosis of either entity may be delayed because superimposed medical problems can obscure clinical weakness. This chapter will review the differential diagnosis, clinical and electrodiagnostic features of CIP, and describe the common pathogenesis shared by CIP and the closely related CIM.

1. INTRODUCTION

Weakness is common in critically ill patients. In 1984, Bolton et al. (1) formulated the concept that the attendant metabolic and immune stressors of sepsis and critical illness cause reversible injury to peripheral nerve and muscle (2). Since that time, there has been an apparent increased prevalence of critical illness polyneuropathy (CIP) as neurologists and intensive care specialists became familiar with these disorders. Prevalence figures also depend on diagnostic criteria, with older studies identifying few patients with severe and protracted weakness, to identification of 70% of patients with electrodiagnostic abnormalities consistent with motor-predominant axonal injury (3,4). Recent studies question whether these patients may in fact have a critical illness myopathy (CIM) instead of or in addition to, CIP.

It is challenging to detect and diagnose weakness in critically ill patients. They are usually intubated, often sedated and sometimes paralyzed. Many have altered consciousness or mental status, and questions about weakness or sensory symptoms are limited or impossible. Physical examination may be restricted by the paraphernalia of critical illness, including intravenous and arterial lines, endotracheal tubes, splints, and alternating compression devices. Weakness is often undetected until transfer to convalescent care or until weakness leads to difficulty weaning from assisted ventilation. Accordingly, ICU care providers should be attentive to evidence of weakness in critically ill patients and not mistakenly ascribe weakness to drugs or sedation. It is important to request that neuromuscular blocking agents and sedation be held, if possible, before the neurological examination. Simple resistive strength testing can establish the degree of weakness and help to distinguish symmetric weakness associated with CIP or CIM from other causes of weakness.

2. DIFFERENTIAL DIAGNOSIS

The broad differential diagnosis of weakness in this setting includes metabolic abnormalities, disorders of the central nervous system, and disorders of the peripheral nervous system. Stroke or diffuse anoxic brain injury frequently accompany acute myocardial infarction or respiratory arrest. Vertebral dissection or traumatic myelopathy can be late or unrecognized consequences of head and neck trauma (5). Ischemic myelopathy can be an initially unnoticed complication following major thoracic or abdominal surgical procedures. Psychomotor retardation from advanced dementia, severe bradykinesia in parkinsonism, catatonia, and a variety of metabolic abnormalities can mimic neuromuscular weakness.

The differential diagnosis of neuromuscular causes of weakness includes diseases that can occur in conjunction with critical illness or are caused by critical illness. Among, the former is Guillain–Barré Syndrome (GBS) which causes rapidly progressive ascending limb weakness accompanied by sensory complaints and diffuse back and body pain. Diaphragmatic weakness impairs ventilation in 20% and requires intubation in 5–10%, leading to ICU admission. Patients with limb weakness that precedes respiratory compromise usually do not present a diagnostic challenge. However, GBS can also be precipitated by a critical illness. Although the most common form of GBS, acute inflammatory demyelinating polyradiculoneuropathy (AIDP), typically causes primary multisegmental demyelination, axonal forms of GBS are also described. Acute motor and sensory axonal neuropathy (AMSAN) is recognized as a severe form of GBS with prolonged weakness and poor prognosis. These AIDP variants are frequently associated with specific anti-ganglioside antibodies (anti-GM1 and anti-GD1A) (6,7), but are likely to be difficult to distinguish from CIP clinically or electrodiagnostically (8).

Exacerbations of myasthenia gravis can lead to respiratory compromise or pneumonia during an exacerbation. Although rare, sepsis, organ failure, or surgery can precipitate a myasthenic crisis in a patient not known to have the disease. Botulism, acetylcholinesterase inhibitors, and a variety of toxins cause precipitous weakness, respiratory failure, and autonomic dysfunction. Prolonged neuromuscular blockade without evidence of myopathy has been described after withdrawal of neuromuscular blocking agents (especially vecuronium) and in association with aminoglycosides (9,10). Acute heavy metal intoxications (thallium and arsenic) and porphyria can precipitate metabolic dysequilibrium and diffuse neuropathy that occur simultaneously.

CIP and CIM are unique as neuromuscular diseases because they appear to be directly caused by critical illness. CIP is more common in patients with sepsis and multiorgan failure, whereas glucocorticoids and neuromuscular blocking agents predispose to CIM. Distinguishing CIM from CIP can be difficult both clinically and electrodiagnostically. Because of overlap between the two syndromes in terms of setting, clinical presentation, electrodiagnostic findings, and pathogenesis, they may be best regarded as poles in a spectrum of neuromuscular disease associated with critical illness.

3. CLINICAL PRESENTATION OF CIP

CIP is an acute or subacute, axonal, length-dependent neuropathy that occurs in severely ill patients in proportion to the acuity of systemic disease. The neuropathy is monophasic and self-limited and generally gradually resolves if the patient survives. Confusion exists about the clinical boundaries of CIP. The prototypical presentation is rapid development of profound weakness affecting limbs in a distal to proximal gradient days to weeks after acquiring a severe illness. Acute axonal injury has been reported to occur within 72 h after ICU admission (11–13). In severe cases, muscles of respiration are also involved, resulting in respiratory failure, but more commonly as failure to wean from ventilatory support. Weakness is accompanied by muscle atrophy and hyporeflexia. Complete areflexia is rare, even in severely affected patients, distinguishing CIP from AIDP clinically.

Sensory symptoms should be a key feature in distinguishing CIP from CIM, but sensory involvement is variable (14). It is often difficult or impossible to clinically evaluate sensory loss in the acute care setting. A forced choice technique, such as joint position sense testing, has the greatest chance of providing objective data. However, CIP is viewed as a motor predominant or exclusive disease by most authors (15–18), and this view is generally borne out by electrodiagnostic testing.

Ancillary laboratory tests are rarely instructive. Creatine phosphokinase (CPK) is normal or minimally elevated. CPK elevations greater than twice the upper limit of normal suggest CIM, whereas CPK values >2000 IU/dL more likely reflect myonecrosis. Cerebral spinal fluid protein is normal (in contrast to findings in GBS) with no elevation of white blood cells.

Little pathological data are available. A review of autopsy specimens for nine patients with clinical CIP who died of their critical illness (19) showed primary axonal degeneration of both motor and sensory nerve fibers, but little or no evidence of inflammation, vascular injury, or demyelination. Skeletal muscle showed extensive atrophy described as being due to denervation.

4. ELECTRODIAGNOSIS OF CIP

Electrodiagnostic testing in the ICU has special challenges. Sedation may preclude voluntary muscle activation. Bedside instruments and equipment, peripheral edema, and skin breakdown can limit placement of recording electrodes. Electrical interference can obscure the detection of low amplitude responses. Interference can be minimized by plugging the EMG machine into the same bank of outlets used for the ventilator, intravenous pumps, and other patient care machines. This also minimizes the risk of electrical shock to the patient by eliminating possible differences in ground potentials. If 60 cycle/s interference significantly obscures the recording, all nonessential equipment should be turned off during sensory nerve conduction and assessment for abnormal spontaneous activity during EMG recording. Sensory nerve action potentials (SNAPs) are of low amplitude ($5-30\ \mu V$) and can easily be obscured by 60-cycle electrical interference or blunted by distal limb edema. Assessing the radial sensory response is useful because it is rarely absent in CIP or other severe axonopathies and serves as a check that a sensory response can be discerned. Averaging sensory responses is also helpful.

The electrodiagnostic features of CIP are consistent with a distal, motor-predominant axonal polyneuropathy. Compound motor action potentials (CMAPs) are reduced in amplitude or entirely absent in severe cases. CMAP amplitude reduction is not specific, for CIP, and can be due to pre-existing polyneuropathy, CIM, AIDP or AMSAN. Features of demyelination, such as prolongation of distal latency, proximal nerve conduction slowing, or F-wave latency prolongation are typically not present or mild. Prominent conduction slowing or block suggests AIDP. Repetitive stimulation should be performed to exclude unrecognized neuromuscular junction disorders.

Assessment of distal SNAP amplitudes is helpful to distinguish CIM from CIP, because SNAP amplitude is normal in CIM. However, the degree of sensory nerve involvement in CIP is variable, and mean SNAP amplitudes tend to be normal, whereas mean CMAP amplitudes are 60% of the lower limit of normal (16,20).

Abnormal spontaneous activity on needle EMG examination develops within $1-3$ weeks of the onset of weakness, consistent with an acute axonal injury. If the patient is able to voluntarily activate muscles, decreased recruitment of normal appearing motor units is typical early in the disease course. During convalescence, increased motor unit complexity or size supports re-innervation. A mixture of myopathic and neuropathic electromyographic features is common and consistent with the frequent coexistence of CIM in these patients. Data from quantitative motor unit analysis techniques indicate that myopathic features are more common and prominent than neuropathic features (18).

5. CRITICAL ILLNESS MYOPATHY

Myopathy is a recognized complication of critical illness. The term "acute quadriplegic myopathy" is applied to severely affected patients, but we prefer the more inclusive term CIM to emphasize the close association with CIP, because most patients probably have relatively mild weakness ($21-24$). CIM is recognized clinically in $1-5\%$ of critically ill patients as rapidly progressive weakness of limbs and diaphragm. Patients are typically septic, intubated, and receiving nondepolarizing neuromuscular junction blocking agents to aid ventilation (24). High dose glucocorticoids predispose patients to CIM. As with CIP, the incidence of CIM diagnosed by clinical observation is an underestimate. CIM was first recognized as a failure to wean from ventilation in young asthmatics receiving high dose steroids, and the diagnosis is still often overlooked unless the patient is very weak.

Biopsy of affected muscle shows severe atrophy of myofibers, especially in type II fibers, and sarcomeric disruption with profound loss of myosin thick filaments, a condition often referred to as "sarcomeric disarray" (25). As a result, a low myosin/actin ratio after electrophoretic separation of muscle proteins has been suggested as a reliable and rapid method to establish the diagnosis of CIM (26). These changes in sacromeric protein are similar in form, but more severe, than those recognized in myopathy produced by chronic glucocorticoid use and underscore the central role of steroid administration to the pathogenesis of this myopathy (27). In contrast to myopathy associated with chronic steroid use, myotubular fragmentation and lysis often occur in CIM and results in elevated serum CPK, abnormal spontaneous activity on electromyography, and evidence of scattered myotubular necrosis on muscle biopsy (24,28). Finally, there is disruption of electrical signaling in affected myotubes. Murine models of CIM combining high dose intravenous steroids with acute focal denervation confirm the observation in human patients of electrical inexcitability of many myofibers in CIM (29). These findings suggest that weakness in CIM results, in part, from reversible changes in sodium and chloride channels causing inhibition of muscle depolarization (30).

6. DISTINGUISHING CIP AND CIM

The overlap in clinical and electrodiagnostic features, and the common pathogenetic factors, supports abandoning the polar terms of CIP and CIM in favor of more global and descriptive terms of "critical illness weakness" or "critical illness polyneuropathy and myopathy" (31). However, one reason to distinguish between the two polar terms is that the prognosis for patients with clear CIP appears to be worse than for those with CIM alone. Routine electromyography is of little value in distinguishing CIP from CIM in the acute time period, as both diseases feature reduced CMAP amplitudes and abnormal spontaneous activity on needle EMG, and patients usually cannot voluntarily recruit motor units to distinguish between neurogenic and myopathic recruitment patterns. Howerver, special electrodiagnostic testing may help to distinguish between the two (Table 18.1). In severe CIM, muscle is inexcitable to direct electrical stimulation (29). Conversely, in CIP, axonal injury prevents neuromuscular junction transmission, but leaves individual muscle fibers able to be depolarized in response to direct electrical stimulation. Motor unit number estimation (MUNE) estimates the number of motor units participating in

Table 18.1 Features of CIP and CIM

Parameter	CIP	CIM
Weakness	Rapidly progressive, distal predominant	Rapidly progressive, distal and proximal
Diaphragm involvement	Occasionally	Frequently
Sensory loss	Frequently	No
Nerve conduction studies	Low amplitude or absent CMAPs Low amplitude SNAPs Normal conduction velocities	Low amplitude or absent CMAPs Preserved SNAPs Normal conduction velocities
Electromyography	Abundant ASP Excitable muscle	ASP Inexcitable muscle
CPK	Normal to 2× normal	Normal to 20× normal

Note: ASP, abnormal spontaneous potentials.

the CMAP. When weakness is due to a neuropathy MUNE values should be reduced, whereas when it is due to a myopathy MUNE values will be normal, if a CMAP can be obtained. Using these special techniques, the prevalence of CIM exceeds that of CIP, or put another way, myopathic injury is a more common component of critical illness weakness than axonal injury (18,29,32,33).

7. RISK FACTORS AND PATHOGENESIS

CIP occurs in patients with the systemic inflammatory response syndrome (SIRS), which includes sepsis and multiple organ dysfunction syndrome (MODS, i.e., renal failure). Sepsis results in more than 200,000 deaths in the United States each year, more than from breast, colon/rectal, pancreatic, and prostate cancer combined. Severe sepsis, defined as sepsis accompanied by acute dysfunction of one or more organs (i.e., renal failure), has a mortality rate of 40% with a high rate of morbidity in the surviours.

SIRS is the generalized inflammatory host response that occurs as a consequence of severe illness. Clinically, SIRS is heralded by increased heart rate, elevated respiratory rate, and increased or decreased temperature or leukocyte count (Table 18.2). The SIRS response is often characterized by uncontrolled inflammation via a variety of "proinflammatory" mediators including IL-1, TNF-α, and IL-6 that lead to widespread tissue injury. Extension of this pathologic inflammatory process to normal organs causes MODS. Common examples include altered consciousness or depressed mental status, acute respiratory failure or distress syndrome (ARDS), and acute liver or renal failure. CIP has been considered to be organ dysfunction or failure of peripheral nerves.

Up to 70% of patients with sepsis have a length-dependent motor and sensory axonal neuropathy (4,14,34). Explanations for the development of nerve damage in CIP include direct physical injury, exposure to toxins, circulating serum factors (IL-1 and IL-6), electrolyte abnormalities, hyperosmolar states, and vascular insufficiency. Inflammation has been demonstrated in muscle biopsies from patients with CIP or CIM. Evidence of inflammation in nerve biopsies includes perivascular lymphocytic infiltrates, perimysial lymphocytes, macrophages, and cytokine expression (IL-1β, INFγ, and IL-12) (35). These changes are consistent with a destructive immune response as a contributor to CIP or CIM pathogenesis. A single small and uncontrolled clinical study reported that early treatment with intravenous immunoglobulin (IVIG) reduced or prevented the development of CIP in patients with gram negative sepsis and MODS (36). Unfortunately, no subsequent prospective trials have evaluated IVIG treatment in the prevention or attenuation of CIP.

Another pathogenic factor for both CIP and CIM is sepsis-induced maldistribution of microvascular blood flow leading to decreased capillary oxygen extraction and local ischemia to nerves and muscle. A rat model of sepsis demonstrated a maldistribution of oxygen transport from two principal mechanisms: stopped or "clogged" blood flow in low flow capillaries and a twofold increase in diffusion distances across swollen membranes in regions of tissues containing normal or high flow capillaries (37).

Table 18.2 Diagnostic Criteria for SIRS

Two or more of the following must be present:
  Temperature >38°C or <36°C
  Heart rate >90 beats/min
  Respiratory rate >20 breaths/min or PaCo$_2$ <32 mmHg
  Abnormal white blood cell count [>12,000 cells/mm^3,
    <4000 cells/mm^3, or >10% immature (band) forms]

The maldistribution of microvascular blood flow in tissues is felt to be similar to the ventilation and perfusion mismatch in the lung observed in many respiratory diseases including ARDS.

Nutritional status and hyperglycemia likely contribute to the development of CIP. Serum albumin levels were significantly lower in critically ill patients who developed CIP (34). Hyperalimentation formulas lacking essential nutrients may lead to a "nutritional neuropathy" in critically ill patients who receive prolonged total parenteral nutrition (1). CIP has also been associated with "hyperosmolar" states, including hyperalimentation, hypernatremia, and hyperglycemia (38). Hyperglycemia is common in sepsis and trauma and has been identified as an independent risk factor for the development of CIP (34,39). The concept of acute hyperglycemia-induced neurotoxicity is strengthened by prospective evidence that tight glycemic control using an insulin infusion reduced the incidence of CIP in surgical intensive care unit patients by 44% (incidence of 20.5% vs. 26.3%) (39).

8. PROGNOSIS IN CIP AND CIM

CIP occurs in critically ill patients with multiorgan involvement, and thus is a marker for severe illness. As a consequence, the short-term prognosis is poor due to the underlying illness. In-hospital mortality for electrodiagnostically confirmed CIP is 84% when compared with 56% mortality for patients matched for age and APACHE score who did not have axonal injury (40). It is not known whether CIP itself increases mortality, but the length of mechanical ventilation and hospitalization is significantly longer among patients with CIP who are discharged alive from the ICU (40).

There are little data on the long-term functional recovery of patients with CIP or CIM. Approximately 10% have persistent severe limb weakness and ventilator dependency (34). Most, if not all, patients have electrodiagnostic evidence of persistent axonal injury, and most clinical evidence of persistent weakness 1–2 years after discharge. However, evidence of any residual myopathy has not been found, and CIM may be associated with a much better long-term recovery than CIP (41).

9. TREATMENT

No specific treatment has been effective for CIP or CIM. At this stage, the focus must be on prevention including early and aggressive physical therapy. Recognition and treatment of risk factors may decrease the incidence of CIP. The use of glucocorticoids and neuromuscular blocking agents should be minimized. Rigorous control of hyperglycemia may also be practical CIP prophylaxis. Maintenance of serum glucose between 80 and 110 mg/dL reduced incidence of CIP by 44% in a large prospective study of surgical intensive care patients (39). Early and aggressive treatment of sepsis, including surgical drainage of infectious foci, can limit the severity of severe sepsis and posibly attenuate CIP. Additional recommendations about prevention and/or treatment of critical illness weakness are lacking until further work in this area is forthcoming.

REFERENCES

1. Bolton CF, Lavert DA, Brown JD. Polyneuropathy in critically ill patients. J Neurol Neurosurg Psychiatry 1984; 45:1223–1231.
2. Bolton CF. Sepsis and the systemic inflammatory response syndrome: neuromuscular manifestations. Crit Care Med 1996; 24:1408–1416.

3. Wijdicks EF, Litchy WJ, Harrison BA, Gracey DR. The clinical spectrum of critical illness polyneuropathy. Mayo Clin Proc 1994; 69:955–959.

4. Berek K, Margreiter J, Willeit J, Berek A, Schmutzhard E, Mutz NJ. Polyneuropathies in critically ill patients: a prospective evaluation. Intensive Care Med 1996; 22:849–855.

5. Schellinger P, Schwab S, Krieger D, Fiebach J, Steiner T, Hund E, Hacke W, Meinck H. Masking of vertebral artery dissection by severe trauma to the cervical spine. Spine 2001; 26:314–319.

6. Yuki N, Kuwabara S, Koga M, Hirata K. Acute motor axonal neuropathy and acute motor-sensory axonal neuropathy share a common immunological profile. J Neurol Sci 1999; 168:121–126.

7. Ho TW, Willison HJ, Nachamkin I, Li CY, Veitch J, Ung H, Wang GR, Liu RC, Cornblath DR, Asbury AK, Griffin JW, McKhann GM. Anti-GD1a antibody is associated with axonal but not demyelinating forms of Guillain–Barre syndrome. Ann Neurol 1999; 45:168–173.

8. de Letter MA, Visser LH, van der Meche FG, Ang W, Savelkoul HF. Distinctions between critical illness polyneuropathy and axonal Guillain–Barre syndrome. J Neurol Neurosurg Psychiatry 2000; 68:397–398.

9. Segredo V, Caldwell JE, Matthay MA, Sharma ML, Gruenke LD, Miller RD. Persistent paralysis in critically ill patients after long-term administration of vecuronium. N Engl J Med 1992; 327:524–528.

10. Gooch J. AAEM case report #29: prolonged paralysis after neuromuscular blockade. Muscle Nerve 1995; 18:937–942.

11. Tennila A, Salmi T, Pettila V, Roine RO, Varpula T, Takkunen O. Early signs of critical illness polyneuropathy in ICU patients with systemic inflammatory response syndrome or sepsis. Intensive Care Med 2000; 26:1360–1363.

12. Woittiez AJ, Veneman TF, Rakic S. Critical illness polyneuropathy in patients with systemic inflammatory response syndrome or septic shock. Intensive Care Med 2001; 27:613.

13. Tepper M, Rakic S, Haas JA, Woittiez AJ. Incidence and onset of critical illness polyneuropathy in patients with septic shock. Neth J Med 2000; 56:211–214.

14. Latronico A, Fenzi F, Recupero D, Guarneri B, Tomelleri G, Tonin P, De Maria G, Antonini, Rizzuto N, Candiani A. Critical illness myopathy and neuropathy. Lancet 1996; 347:1579–1582.

15. Gorson KC, Ropper AH. Acute respiratory failure neuropathy: a variant of critical illness polyneuropathy. Crit Care Med 1993; 21:267–271.

16. Hund E, Genzwurker H, Bohrer H, Jakob H, Thiele R, Hackle W. Predominant involvement of motor fibres in patients with critical illness polyneuropathy. Br J Anaesth 1997; 78:274–278.

17. Zifko U, Zipko H, Bolton C. Clinical and electrophysiological findings in critical illness polyneuropathy. J Neurol Sci 1998; 19:186–193.

18. Trojaborg W, Weimer L, Hays A. Electrophysiologic studies in critical illness weakness: myopathy or neuropathy—a reappraisal. Clin Neurophysiol Col 2001; 112:1586–1593.

19. Zochodne DW, Bolton CF, Wells GA, Gilbert JJ, Hahn AF, Brown JD, Sibbald WA. Critical illness polyneuropathy. A complication of sepsis and multiple organ failure. Brain 1987; 110:819–841.

20. Hinds C, Yarwood G, Coakley J. Acquired neuromuscular abnormalities in intensive care patients. In: Vincent J ed. Yearbook of Intensive Care and Emergency Medicine. Berlin: Springer-Verlag, 1994:655–667.

21. Kaminski HJ, Ruff RL. Endocrine myopathies (hyper- and hypofunction of adrenal, thyroid, pituitary and parathyroid glands and iatrogenic corticosteroid myopathy). In: Engel AG, Franzini-Armstrong C, eds. Myology. New York: McGraw Hill, 1995:1726–1747.

22. MacFarlane IA, Rosenthal FD. Severe myopathy after status asthmaticus. Lancet 1977; 2:615.

23. Kaplan KH, Rocha W, Sanders DB, D'Souza B, Spock A. Acute steroid-induced tetraplegia following status asthmaticus. Pediatrics 1986; 78:121–123.

24. Danon MJ, Carpenter S. Myopathy with thick filament (myosin) loss following prolonged paralysis with vecuronium during steroid treatment. Muscle Nerve 1991; 14:1131–1139.

25. Al-Lozi MT, Pestronk A, Yee WC, Flaris N, Cooper J. Rapidly evolving myopathy with myosin-deficient muscle fibers. Ann Neurol 1994; 5:273–279.
26. Stibler H, Edstrom L, Ahlbeck K, Remahl S, Ansved T. Electrophoretic determination of the myosin/actin ratio in the diagnosis of critical illness myopathy. Intensive Care Med 2003; 29:1515–1527.
27. Gutmann L, Blumenthal D, Gutmann L, Schochet SS. Acute type II myofiber atrophy in critical illness. Neurology 1996; 46:600–601.
28. Zochodne DW, Ramsay DA, Saly V, Shelley S, Moffatt S. Acute necrotizing myopathy of intensive care: electrophysiologic studies. Muscle Nerve 1994; 17:285–292.
29. Rich MM, Teener JW, Raps EC, Schotland DL, Bird SJ. Muscle is electrically inexcitable in acute quadriplegic myopathy. Neurology 1996; 46:731–736.
30. Rich MM, Pinter MJ, Kraner SD, Barchi RL. Loss of electrical excitability in an animal model of acute quadriplegic myopathy. Ann Neurol 1998; 43:171–179.
31. De Letter MA, Schmitz PI, Visser LH, Verheul FA, Schellens RL, Op de Coul DA, van der Meche FG. Risk factors for the development of polyneuropathy and myopathy in critically ill patients. Crit Care Med 2001; 29:2281–2286.
32. Lacomis D, Petrella JT, Giuliani MJ. Cause of neuromuscular weakness in the intensive care unit: a study of ninety-two patients. Muscle Nerve 1998; 21:610–617.
33. Bednarik J, Lukas Z, Vondracek P. Critical illness polyneuromyopathy: the electrophysiological components of a complex entity. Intensive Care Med 2003; 29:1505–1514.
34. Witt NJ, Zochodne DW, Bolton CF, Grand'Maison F, Wells G, Young B, Sibbald WJ. Peripheral nerve function in sepsis and multiple organ failure. Chest 1991; 99:176–184.
35. De Letter MA, van Doorn PA, Savelkoul HF, Laman JD, Schmitz PI, Op de Coul AA, Visser LH, Kros JM, Teepen JL, van der Meche FG. Critical illness polyneuropathy and myopathy (CIPNM): evidence for local immune activation by cytokine-expression in the muscle tissue. PG-206-13. J Neuroimmunol 2000; 106:206–213.
36. Mohr M, Englisch L, Roth A, Burchardi H, Zielmann S. Effects of early treatment with immunoglobulin on critical illness polyneuropathy following multiple organ failure and gram-negative sepsis. Intensive Care Med 1997; 23:1144–1149.
37. Ellis CG, Bateman RM, Sharpe MD, Sibbald WJ, Gill R. Effect of a maldistribution of microvascular blood flow on capillary O(2) extraction in sepsis. Am J Physiol Heart Circ Physiol 2002; 282:H156–H164.
38. Bolton CF, Young GB. Critical illness polyneuropathy due to parenteral nutrition (letter). Intensive Care Med 1997; 23:924–925.
39. van den Berghe G, Wouters P, Weekers F, Verwaest C, Bruyninckx F, Schetz M, Vlasselaers D, Ferdinande P, Lauwers P, Bouillon R. Intensive insulin therapy in the critically ill patients. N Engl J Med 2001; 345:1359–1367.
40. Garnacho-Montero J, Madrazo-Osuna J, Garcia-Garmendia JL, Ortiz-Leyba C, Jimenez-Jimenez FJ, Barrero-Almodovar A, Garnacho-Montero MC, Moyano-Del-Estad MR. Critical illness polyneuropathy: risk factors and clinical consequences. A cohort study in septic patients. Intensive Care Med 2001; 27:1288–1296.
41. Fletcher SN, Kennedy DD, Ghosh IR, Misra VP, Kiff K, Coakley JH, Hinds CJ. Persistent neuromuscular and neurophysiologic abnormalities in long-term survivors of prolonged critical illness. Crit Care Med 2003; 31:1012–1016.

19

Nutritional Neuropathies

Patrick C. Nolan and James W. Albers
University of Michigan, Ann Arbor, Michigan, USA

ABSTRACT

Nutritional neuropathies occur in many settings, including alcohol abuse, malnutrition, fad diets, parenteral nutrition, and gastric surgeries. The challenge for the clinician is to recognize the historical clues and clinical features associated with the patient's neuropathy in order to focus the evaluation. Treatment of nutritional neuropathies involves supplementation for specific deficiencies or abstinence from toxic compounds. Therapy for individual deficiencies is variably effective ranging from full resolution of symptoms and signs to arrest of progression. This chapter defines several neuropathy syndromes associated with individual nutritional deficiencies. The neuropathies related to chronic alcoholism and pyridoxine toxicity are included in this chapter. The former is closely tied with malnutrition and specific vitamin deficits, whereas the latter is an essential vitamin whose toxicity and deficiency result in phenotypically different neuropathies. Neuropathies that develop in the setting of gastric surgery also will be discussed in the context of nutritional deficiency.

1. INTRODUCTION

Nutritional neuropathies continue to be diagnostically challenging and demand a high clinical suspicion for initial recognition. These neuropathies are preventable and generally respond best to therapy when diagnosed and treated in the early stages. Neuropathies arising from nutritional deficiencies were historically recognized among patients suffering from prolonged caloric restriction or chronic alcoholism. Although malnutrition is now less common in Western medicine, recent research has identified multiple patient populations at high risk for specific nutritional neuropathies. Gastric resection, malabsorption syndromes, fad diets, prolonged parenteral nutrition, genetic disorders, and parasitic infection can result in neuropathies associated with specific nutritional deficits. Understanding the neuropathies arising from individual nutritional deficiencies and toxicities provides a starting point to understand the epidemic neuropathic syndromes that continue to arise throughout the world.

Neuropathy associated with a specific nutritional deficit commonly presents as a constellation of neurological and systemic symptoms and signs that can help differentiate individual nutritional neuropathies from other etiologies. As in all facets of medicine, a careful history and detailed physical examination can establish the presence of neuropathy and focus the evaluation that may require serological, electrophysiologic, or histologic evaluation to identify the underlying etiology. However, many patients who present with complaints suspicious of a nutritional neuropathy have complex medical conditions or complicated nutritional histories. A lack of definitive research continues to fuel debate in many areas discussed in this chapter. Areas of debate include the etiology of alcohol-associated neuropathy, the existence of neuropathy in the setting of single vitamin deficiencies, and the biochemical mechanism responsible for many of the neuropathies discussed. In the text that follows, "neuropathy" is used synonymously with the terms peripheral neuropathy or polyneuropathy to indicate a peripheral disorder generally showing a symmetric stocking-glove distribution of sensory loss or weakness.

2. ALCOHOL-ASSOCIATED NEUROPATHY

Neuropathy is commonly associated with evidence of chronic alcoholism, yet the etiology of the neuropathy is surrounded with controversy. Alcohol-associated neuropathy has been well described among patients with chronic alcohol exposure who also have poor nutritional status (68,70). Although the alcoholic population does not often present for medical evaluation, estimates of neuropathy among patients with alcoholism range from 9% (68) to 67% (7). The higher estimates include evidence of subclinical neuropathy based on use of electrophysiological tests to evaluate peripheral nerve function. There may be gender differences, with females more frequently and more severely affected by the neuropathy associated with alcoholism than males (7,10,44). Because the caloric content of alcohol can replace food, many patients who abuse alcohol develop multiple nutrient deficiencies. Alcohol is known to inhibit the absorption and metabolism of thiamine, and alcohol-associated neuropathy has many similarities to thiamine deficiency neuropathy. Some argue that alcohol-associated neuropathy is indistinguishable from thiamine neuropathy (68,70,76). Support for a nutritional cause includes evidence that individuals who consume excessive amounts of alcohol but also receive nutritional supplements do not develop neuropathy (70). This view contrasts to the observations of others who report that a typical alcohol-associated neuropathy may occur in the setting of normal nutrition (10,44). Extensive research involving humans and laboratory animals has investigated whether alcohol has direct toxic effects on peripheral nerves. Although this question remains unanswered, clinical treatment of alcohol-associated neuropathy should address both alcohol abstinence and thiamine (vitamin B_1) supplementation.

2.1. Clinical Features

The initial symptoms of alcohol-associated neuropathy include painful, burning dysesthesias and lancinating leg pains historically described as "pseudotabes" (68). The pain is accompanied by subjective numbness that progresses in a stocking-glove pattern. Clinical signs include distal, symmetric loss of fine touch, pain, temperature, and vibration sensations (19,44,53,76). Reflexes are diminished or absent at the ankles. Weakness of the distal lower extremities develops late in the course of the neuropathy but can be severe. Progression of the neuropathy is generally gradual, over months to years, but can also occur subacutely over months.

Autonomic abnormalities are prominent in alcohol-associated neuropathy. Hyperhydrosis, hair loss, and thinning of the skin go along with the distal distribution of sensory loss. Sympathetic-mediated orthostasis, parasympathetic-mediated cardiac irregularities, and esophageal dysmotility can be demonstrated in up to one-quarter of patients known to abuse alcohol (44,53).

Alcohol-associated neuropathy usually is accompanied by other stigmata of chronic alcoholism that reflect direct alcohol toxicity or concomitant thiamine deficiency. Myopathy is common and presents chronically as diffuse cramps, local pain, and selective loss of proximal type II muscle fibers. A rare form of acute myopathy also can occur after alcohol binges (19). Other neurological findings include truncal ataxia with wide-based gait related to vermal cerebellar degeneration, amblyopia, and the Wernicke–Korsakoff syndrome. Systemic abnormalities found with chronic alcoholism include evidence of liver damage that can progress to cirrhosis, anemia, and hypoglycemia with ketoacidosis (Table 19.1).

2.2. Laboratory Evaluation

2.2.1. Serology

Evaluation of serum alcohol levels can be helpful to establish acute intoxication. Chronic excessive alcohol use can result in elevated transaminases and γ glutamyltransferase with a relative red cell macrocytosis. If liver toxicity has progressed to cirrhosis, transaminases can be low or normal but liver synthetic activity, evaluated by serum albumin and clotting factors, will be diminished (19,68,76).

2.2.2. Electrodiagnostic Testing

Nerve conduction studies reveal low amplitude sensory responses, especially in the lower extremities; motor responses are usually normal early in the course of neuropathy, but may be of very reduced amplitude, particularly when recorded from weak distal leg muscles (7,10,44,53). Motor and sensory conduction velocities recorded from the upper and lower extremities show only mild slowing with prolonged distal latency without conduction block (7,10,44). The combined findings are those of a sensory or sensorimotor neuropathy of the axonal type. Axonal loss is confirmed by evidence of denervation and reinnervation on needle EMG examination (10).

2.2.3. Pathologic Features

Recent studies by Koike et al. (44) found reduced myelinated fiber density, especially in small myelinated and unmyelinated fibers, whereas Behse and Buchthal (10) found a

Table 19.1 Additional Signs and Symptoms
Associated with Vitamin Deficiencies

Alcohol toxicity
   Wernicke's encephalopathy/Korsakoff syndrome
   Cerebellar ataxia/gait disturbances
   Myopathy (chronic and acute)
   Amblyopia
   Liver cirrhosis
   Anemia
Thiamine (vitamin B_1) deficiency
   Wernicke's encephalopathy/Korsakoff syndrome
   Dilated cardiac hypertrophy (acute)
   Peripheral edema (acute)
   Chorea/myoclonus
Pyridoxine (vitamin B_6) deficiency
   Lethargy/anorexia/nausea
   Dermatological changes
     Facial seborrheic dermatitis/cheliosis
   Conjunctivitis/glossitis/oral ulcers
   Seizures in congenital deficiency state
Cyanocobalamin (vitamin B_{12}) deficiency
   Myelopathy (dorsal columns)
   Encephalopathy (dementia, memory loss, psychosis)
   Altered smell and taste/anosmia
   Visual impairment/optic atrophy
   Megaloblastic anemia
   Glossitis/diarrhea/yellow-pigmented skin and nails
   Hypospermia
α-Tocopherol (vitamin E) deficiency
   Myelopathy (dorsal columns)
   Ataxia
   Dysarthria
   Tongue fasciculations
   Pes cavus and kyphoscoliosis
Phosphate deficiency
   Dysarthria
   Confusion/obtundation/coma
   Seizures
   Rhabdomyolysis

substantial loss of large myelinated fibers among patients with excessive alcohol consumption but normal serum thiamine levels. Unmyelinated fibers also showed evidence of degeneration. Axonal sprouting was noted to be abundant only among patients with a prolonged (>2 years) course of neuropathy (44). Teased fiber preparations showed axonal degeneration with rare segmental demyelination (10,44).

2.3. Differential Diagnosis

The differential diagnosis for primary sensory greater than motor neuropathies of the axonal type is broad and included in Table 19.3. Multiple nutritional neuropathies also show an axonal predominance with painful dysesthesias. A careful history and accompanying clinical abnormalities should help to focus the neuropathy evaluation. Prescription drugs and hereditary causes for neuropathy are often overlooked. Diabetic neuropathy, amyloidosis, and Fabry's disease can produce neuropathy with painful dysesthesias and autonomic symptoms, although Fabry's disease usually presents in early adulthood.

2.4. Management and Prognosis

Abstinence of alcohol is the primary treatment for alcohol-associated neuropathy. As most clinical presentations of alcoholic neuropathy are associated with malnutrition, vitamin supplementation with B complex vitamins is also recommended. Noticeable improvement in dysesthesias and sensory deficits often requires months to years of abstinence and is often incomplete (10,44,68,76).

2.5. Pathogenesis

Determination of a patient's alcohol intake is highly unreliable, but careful retrospective studies of patients diagnosed with alcoholism demonstrate a good correlation between the lifetime dose of alcohol and the presence of neuropathy (7,53). These studies suggest that a cumulative dose >15 kg of alcohol per kilogram of body weight is an independent risk factor for peripheral and autonomic neuropathies. In practical terms, this equates to 300 mL of distilled spirits daily for 25 years. However, Behse and Buchthal (10) found neuropathic evidence among patients imbibing $\sim$100 mL of alcohol per day for at least 3 years.

   The pathogenesis of alcoholic neuropathy is still debated and may relate to a combination of malnutrition with thiamine (vitamin B_1) deficiency, direct toxic effects of alcohol and its metabolites on peripheral nerves, as well as genetic predisposition. Recent comprehensive reviews and new human data suggest alcohol may play a direct role in neurotoxicity (10,28,44,68,70,76). However, in the clinical setting where most patients presenting with alcoholic neuropathy are malnourished, both alcohol abstinence and thiamine (vitamin B_1) supplementation should be stressed.

3. THIAMINE (VITAMIN B_1) DEFICIENCY NEUROPATHY

The neuropathy associated with thiamine deficiency was termed beriberi by Western medicine in 1611 (68). This term translates to extreme weakness, which is a prominent feature of thiamine deficiency. After multiple epidemics of neuropathy in the next 300 years, it was determined that a diet of white rice stripped of the thiamine-containing pericarp resulted in what was, by then, a well-described disease in both humans and domestic fowl. Research in the early 1900s defined thiamine as the essential agent in this neuropathy and introduced the concept of the vitamin to medicine (35,68).

   Although pure thiamine deficiency is relatively rare, some countries continue to have endemic beriberi resulting from a diet high in polished rice (21). In the West, faddiets, chronic dialysis, and surgical gastrectomy have resulted in patients with signs of both acute or "wet" beriberi and the more chronic or "dry" beriberi, although some of these syndromes may be related to multiple deficiencies (33,34,43,57,66). Other causes of thiamine deficiency are listed in Table 19.2 and include diets rich in thiaminase found in raw fish (72). The acute presentation of thiamine deficiency (wet beriberi) is associated with dilated cardiomyopathy causing congestive heart failure and resultant edema in association with neuropathy and other CNS findings. Dry beriberi refers to a

Table 19.2 Clinical Conditions Associated with Metabolic Neuropathies

Thiamine (vitamin B_1) deficiency
  Alcoholism
  Malnutrition
    Fad diets
    HIV
    Cachexia
    Malabsorption
  Peritoneal dialysis and hemodialysis
  Raw fish diet (thiaminases)
Pyridoxine (vitamin B_6) deficiency
  Isolated deficiency in neonatal formula
  Prescription drug inactivation of vitamin
    Cycloserine
    Hydralazine
    Isoniazid
    Penicillamine
    Phenelzine
Cyanocobalamin (vitamin B_{12}) deficiency
  Genetic mutations affecting B_{12} metabolism
  Malabsorption
    Intrinsic factor deficiency
      Pernicious anemia
      Celiac and tropical sprue
      Gastric resection
      Genetic disorders affecting absorption
    Pancreatic insufficiency
    Achlorhydria [common in elderly (16–40%)]
    Absent terminal ileum (resection or disease)
  Consumption of cobalamin
    Blind loop syndrome (bacterial overgrowth)
    Fish tapeworm infection (*D. latum*)
  Vegetarianism–Veganism
  Nitrous oxide exposure (inactivates cobalamin)
α-Tocopherol (vitamin E) deficiency
  Genetic mutations affecting vitamin E metabolism
    Abetalipoproteinemia (Bassen–Kornzweig syndrome)
    Vitamin E transporter deficiency
  Malabsorption
    Chronic cholestasis/liver disease
    Cystic fibrosis
    Bowel disease with steatorrhea
      Celiac/tropical sprue
      Whipple's disease
      Pancreatitis
      Inflammatory bowel disease
      Parenteral nutrition (chronic)
    Postgastrectomy/short bowel syndrome

(*continued*)

Table 19.2 *Continued*

Phosphate deficiency
   Carbohydrate infusions
   Hyperparathyroidism
   Respiratory alkalosis
   Phosphate-binding antacids
   Extensive burns
   Pancreatitis

more gradual development of thiamine deficiency resulting in the same neurological symptoms without cardiomyopathy and edema.

3.1. Clinical Features

Acute thiamine deficiency in the absence of excessive alcohol use presents with edema, sensory loss, and extremity weakness. Symptoms related to neuropathy include distal sensory loss and weakness. In classic thiamine deficiency associated with a diet exclusively of polished white rice, the numbness is associated with tingling paresthesias but without the lancinating or dysesthetic pain described in alcohol-associated neuropathy (57,66). Examination reveals diminished lower extremity sensation for all sensory modalities, weakness of foot dorsiflexors and wrist extensors, and depressed or absent patellar and ankle reflexes.

Distal weakness and sensory loss with or without peripheral edema can appear within 2–12 months of beginning a thiamine-restricted diet or may develop insidiously over years without any signs of cardiac abnormalities (33,57,66). Cranial nerve involvement was reported in early accounts of thiamine deficiency neuropathy, characterized by weakness of laryngeal, facial, and tongue muscles (76). More recent studies of patients developing neuropathy after consuming exclusive rice diets have not reported cranial nerve involvement (57,66).

Acute thiamine deficiency can occur in the setting of malnutrition and alcoholism. An acute alcoholic binge followed by increased metabolic stress can result in Wernicke's encephalopathy described as a triad of confusion, impaired extraocular movements with nystagmus, and truncal ataxia (68). Wernicke's encephalopathy can develop within hours or evolve over days. The mental status changes include apathy, confusion, and poor concentration. Eye movement abnormalities are most often associated with nystagmus and lateral rectus paresis. Rapid thiamine supplementation is crucial to prevent brainstem and hypothalamic damage. In 80% of patients presenting with this acute encephalopathy, retrograde and anterograde amnesia persists. The more chronic mental status abnormality associated with thiamine deficiency is termed Korsakoff syndrome and consists of an amnesia that is primarily retrograde. Although confabulation has been included in the classic description of Korsakoff syndrome, it is not a requisite component.

Recently, patients who were undergoing peritoneal dialysis or hemodialysis were found to have poor nutritional status, reduced thiamine levels, and many clinical characteristics of thiamine deficiency. Neuropathy and cardiac abnormalities due to other causes may confuse the presentation among patients undergoing dialysis, but subacute onset of chorea, confusion, and myoclonus have shown remarkable improvement in association with thiamine supplementation (33,34). Many of these patients did not show the typical ataxia and eye movement abnormalities found in classic Wernicke's encephalopathy.

Systemic abnormalities associated with thiamine deficiency include congestive heart failure in the acute syndrome with secondary tachycardia and lower extremity edema. Heart failure is associated with dilated cardiomyopathy (66) (Table 19.1).

3.2. Laboratory Evaluation

3.2.1. Serology

Modern evaluation of serum thiamine employs whole-blood high performance liquid chromatography (HPLC) for thiamine level evaluation (43). Thiamine stores can also be evaluated by assays of blood cell transketolase activity. The response can then be compared with the activity after addition of thiamine pyrophosphate (TPP) (35,72,76). If clinical suspicion for thiamine deficiency is high, prompt supplementation is warranted before evaluation of vitamin levels.

3.2.2. Electrodiagnostic Testing

Most reports of electrodiagnostic evaluation of patients who have thiamine deficiency are complicated by secondary vitamin deficiencies or only limited evaluations. Koike et al. (43) described 17 patients who developed thiamine deficiency and occasional other vitamin B deficiencies postgastrectomy. In this population, most patients showed marked reduction of lower limb sensory and motor responses. They also showed only mild slowing of sensory and motor conduction velocities and distal latencies. These findings are similar to reports of studies in humans with restricted diets of polished rice (21,66). Further evaluation revealed prolonged H-reflex latencies with only mildly slowed F-wave latencies (21). Needle EMG evaluation of distal limbs in all studies reflected neurogenic changes with some evidence of denervation and reinnervation.

3.2.3. Pathologic Features

Sural nerve pathology among patients eating diets of only polished rice demonstrates a preferential degeneration of large myelinated axons (57,66). Teased fiber preparations demonstrate rare to absent segmental demyelination and onion bulbs, although one study in two patients found some segmental demyelination that was attributed to axonal regeneration (57,66). Studies of patients with thiamine deficiency and occasional other vitamin deficiencies or alcohol abuse associated with thiamine deficiency show a more global axonal loss with less preference for large fibers (43,73). These pathological findings are consistent with the clinical observations of sensory and autonomic symptoms in the patients studied. Endoneural edema was noted in all nerve biopsy studies performed before thiamine replacement therapy (43,57,66).

3.3. Differential Diagnosis

As with alcohol-associated neuropathy, the preferential loss of small axons can be seen in many neuropathies, including multiple vitamin deficiencies (Table 19.3). Microscopic evaluation of distal innervation in experimental animals deprived of dietary thiamine shows a "dying back" neuropathy also seen in numerous toxic neuropathies, including those associated with vincristine and acrylamide. As with all metabolic neuropathies, the accompanying clinical syndrome (Table 19.1) and a detailed history about diet and alcohol intake should help to limit the diagnostic evaluation before serological tests are required.

Table 19.3 Axonal Neuropathies with Sensory Greater than Motor Loss

Acromegaly	Thiamine (vitamin B_1)
Amyloidosis	Pyridoxine (vitamin B_6)
Chronic illness neuropathy	Postgastrectomy
Connective tissue disease	Pharmaceuticals
Rheumatoid arthritis	Amitriptyline
Periarteritis nodosa	Colchicine
Churg–Strauss vasculitis	Ethambutol
Degenerative disorders	Isonicotine hydrazine
Friedreich's ataxia	Metronidazole
Olivopontocerebellar	Nitrous oxide
atrophy	Phenytoin
Gout	Thallium
Hypothyroidism	Vincristine
Metals	Polycythemia vera
Arsenic	Sarcoidosis
Gold	Toxic
Lithium	Acrylamide
Mercury	Carbon disulfide
Multiple myeloma	Ethyl alcohol
Myotonic dystrophy	Hexacarbons
Nutritional deficiencies	Organophosphorus esters
Chromium	
Cobalamin (vitamin B_{12})	

Source: Adapted from Donofrio and Albers (1990).

3.4. Management and Prognosis

In the acute presentation of Wernicke's encephalopathy among chronically malnourished patients who abuse alcohol, rapid administration of 100 mg of thiamine intravenously usually results in improvement of ataxia, confusion, and eye movement abnormalities over hours. Thiamine should be administered before glucose, which can increase metabolic stress and produce subsequent metabolic lactic acidosis. If left untreated, these abnormalities can become irreversible. A dose of 100 mg of thiamine should be continued intramuscularly for 3–5 days and then continued orally. Oral supplements are then recommended at doses of 50–100 mg daily thereafter.

The same oral dose also is beneficial for chronic thiamine deficiency and should probably be continued indefinitely. Parenteral supplementation may be preferred for patients who have evidence of malabsorption or who are undergoing dialysis. The response to thiamine supplementation can result in improvement of neuropathy symptoms in a few weeks and in some cases show complete resolution (57,66). Pathologic studies of sural nerve show active regeneration in patients with thiamine supplementation (66). Edema and presumed cardiac pathology can also respond dramatically in acute thiamine deficiency within weeks (43,57).

3.5. Pathogenesis

Thiamine is a ubiquitous water-soluble vitamin found in many foods, including cereal grains, meat, yeast, and rice husks. It is converted to TPP and is required for the oxidative decarboxylation of pyruvate into acetyl CoA. Under conditions of extreme metabolic activity, TPP is also required in the pentose phosphate shunt. In the absence of TPP, pyruvate can accumulate and result in an increase of lactate in metabolically active tissues (35). Tissues of the central nervous system, especially brain stem structures, are most sensitive to acute changes in lactate concentrations (45).

The primary pathology associated with thiamine deficiency neuropathy involves a preferential loss of the largest myelinated axons. The distal distribution is that of a dying-back process, consistent with defective axonal transport. As fast axoplasmic transport requires oxidative metabolism for nerve health, a proposed mechanism for thiamine-induced neuropathy may be related directly to its role in energy metabolism (18,60,66).

4. PYRIDOXINE (VITAMIN B₆) DEFICIENCY NEUROPATHY

Pyridoxine is an essential vitamin necessary for the metabolism of many substances, including proteins, carbohydrates, and fatty acids. The neuropathy associated with pyridoxine deficiency is rarely encountered in isolation, although it may play an important role in the neuropathy observed with combined deficiency of the B vitamins in malnutrition. Because pyridoxine is an essential vitamin, both the deficiency and toxicity state, which can result in phenotypically distinct neuropathies, are considered in this chapter. Because of the ubiquitous nature of pyridoxine in most foods, isolated pyridoxine deficiency rarely results from dietary restriction. Rather, it is usually encountered in the setting of pharmacologic therapy. For example, isoniazid competitively inhibits the action of pyridoxine, and pyridoxine supplementation during isoniazid therapy is necessary to prevent development of a pyridoxine deficiency neuropathy (64).

Since the description of pyridoxine deficiency neuropathy after the introduction of isoniazid for tuberculosis therapy, it has been related to therapy with cycloserine, hydralazine, penicillamine, and phenelzine.

4.1. Clinical Features

Pyridoxine deficiency neuropathy is a distal, symmetric, sensorimotor neuropathy. Symptoms of lower extremity numbness, tingling, and painful paresthesias dominate the clinical presentation. Examination reveals decreased lower extremity sensation, mild distal weakness, and depressed ankle, and occasionally patellar, reflexes (2,30,55). Clinically evident pyridoxine neuropathy can appear within 4–6 months of initiating isoniazid at dosages of 200–500 mg/day (2). The rate of progression is related to the dose of isoniazid, the patient's nutritional status, and the rate at which the patient inactivates isoniazid (2). Other medications show a variable rate of presentation of neuropathic symptoms (30,61). Additional systemic symptoms sometimes attributed to pyridoxine deficiency include cognitive changes, muscle cramps, skin changes, and glossitis (Table 19.4) (55,71).

4.2. Laboratory Evaluation

4.2.1. Serology

Pyridoxine levels may be directly measured in the clinical setting with HPLC.

4.2.2. Electrodiagnostic Testing

The electrophysiological findings depend on the severity of the neuropathy, and some patients thought to have a mild pyridoxine deficiency neuropathy may demonstrate no

Table 19.4   Clinical Characteristics of Metabolic Neuropathies

Alcohol toxicity
   Poorly defined, distal symmetric sensory loss (pain/temperature > vibration/proprioception)
   Severe paresthesias with shooting pains in lower legs ("pseudotabes")
   Calf tenderness on palpation
   Autonomic involvement
      Hyperhydrosis, hair loss, and thinning skin over affected areas
      Orthostasis
      Incontinence
      Esophageal dysmotility
Thiamine (vitamin B_1) deficiency
   Distal, symmetric sensory loss (all modalities)
   Mild lower extremity paresthesias or burning feet (variable)
   Early weakness of foot and wrist extensors with muscle wasting
   Cranial nerve involvement (disputed)
Pyridoxine (vitamin B_6) deficiency
   Distal, symmetric sensory loss (all modalities)
   Burning distal paresthesias
Pyridoxine (vitamin B_6) toxicity
   Rapidly progressive, symmetric sensory loss (all modalities)
   Painless
   Autonomic involvement in severe cases
      Ileus
      Urinary retention
Cyanocobalamin (vitamin B_{12}) deficiency
   Distal, symmetric sensory loss (vibration/proprioception > pain/temperature)
   Tingling paresthesias both upper and lower extremities early
   Variable distal deep tendon reflexes (often with plantar extensor reflex)
   Autonomic involvement
      Orthostasis
      Impotence
      Incontinence
α-Tocopherol (vitamin E) deficiency
   Distal, profound, symmetric sensory loss (vibration/proprioception > pain/temperature)
   Painless
   Variable distal deep tendon reflexes (often with plantar extensor reflex)
Phosphate deficiency
   Mild, distal, symmetric sensory loss (all modalities)
   Mild lower extremity and perioral paresthesias
   Early, profound, ascending weakness
   Ataxia out of proportion to sensory loss

nerve conduction study abnormalities. The limited published descriptions of abnormal electrodiagnostic results attributed to pyridoxine deficiency show evidence suggestive of a general sensorimotor neuropathy (2,30).

4.2.3. Pathologic Features

Microscopic studies of human nerve taken from isoniazid-treated patients with clinically evident neuropathy reveal axonal degeneration of medium-sized nerve fibers and sparing of large myelinated fibers (55). Animal studies show similar changes in peripheral nerves and suggest more severe changes distally in the nerve (2,69).

4.3. Differential Diagnosis

A careful exposure history, including prescription and nonprescription medications and drug exposure, is required to distinguish this neuropathy from the many other causes of sensorimotor axonal neuropathies (Table 19.3). The presence of painful paresthesias may be helpful to differentiate this neuropathy, but the evidence in the literature for the aforementioned cognitive and dermatological changes is scant. A high degree of suspicion and confirmatory serum levels of pyridoxine may be helpful at the time of treatment.

4.4. Management and Prognosis

The recommended daily allowance for a normal adult diet is ∼2.0 mg/day. During isoniazid therapy, oral supplementation should be between 50 and 100 mg daily (2). However, adult supplementation should not exceed 150 mg daily. Response to pyridoxine supplementation can reverse symptoms in early stages but usually only halts progression in cases showing electromyographic changes (30,61,71).

4.5. Pathogenesis

Pyridoxine is a common water-soluble vitamin found in grains, meats, and vegetables and fruits. It is especially plentiful in oranges, bananas, and avocados. It is converted by pyridoxal kinase or pyridoxine phosphate oxidase to pyridoxal phosphate, an essential coenzyme in both decarboxylation and transamination reactions. Proposed essential reactions associated with neuropathy may relate to the essential role of pyridoxal phosphate in synthesizing sphingomyelin with serine palmityl transferase (2,59,61). The aldehyde group on pyridoxal phosphate is available to bond the carbonyl group on isoniazid and hydralazine as well as the other drugs noted earlier. Formation of a bond forms a hydrozone compound that inactivates the coenzyme function of pyridoxal phosphate (30,61,71). Why a perturbation in the availability of pyridoxal phosphate results in a sensorimotor axonal neuropathy has not been fully explored.

5. PYRIDOXINE (VITAMIN B$_6$) INTOXICATION NEUROPATHY

Unlike most water-soluble vitamins, pyridoxine is neurotoxic at doses higher than provided in a normal diet. Following excessive exposure, pyridoxine produces a pure sensory axonal neuropathy. At relatively low, yet still excessive, exposures to this essential vitamin, sensory axons degenerate in a length-dependent distribution. At higher excessive doses, the neuronal cell bodies of the dorsal root ganglion (DRG) degenerate, resulting in a severe sensory neuronopathy.

Pyridoxine intoxication requires ingestion far beyond what can be obtained in a normal diet; however, modern vitamin supplements allow easy access to toxic levels. Most patients who present with pyridoxine-induced neuropathy do so in the setting of self-treatment for water retention, bodybuilding, or fad diets. Occasionally, misinterpretation of symptoms of pyridoxine intoxication has been confused with the indication for additional treatment (as in the treatment of some types of mushroom poisoning), prompting the use of supratherapeutic doses and a resultant poorly reversible sensory neuronopathy (5). Medical trials for schizophrenia and autism have also employed neurotoxic doses of pyridoxine (62).

5.1. Clinical Features

The initial symptoms of a pyridoxine-induced neuropathy are lower extremity numbness and paresthesias. Gait unsteadiness is often the presenting complaint. Occasional patients describe symptoms consistent with Lhermitte's sign (12,58). Symptoms can progress to involve the upper extremities, depending on cumulative dose. Examination reveals reduced touch, vibratory, and joint position sensations. Sensory ataxia and choreoathetoid movements (pseudoathetosis) develop in association with decreased proprioceptive sensation. At this level of sensory impairment, marked functional impairment develops, and patients are sometimes thought to show motor involvement. Close evaluation reveals normal strength but with activation limited by poor proprioception. With mild neuropathy, reflexes may be globally hypoactive or absent only at the ankles. With increasing severity, areflexia develops, sparing only the masseter reflex. Autonomic dysfunction has been described in the setting of large, acute doses of pyridoxine (2 g/kg) (5). Evidence of dysautonomia includes ileus and urinary retention. The severity and rate of symptom onset are related to the total dosage. Symptoms can occur subacutely with massive doses extending to gradual onset of symptoms in 36 months at doses of 200 mg/day (5,16,58).

5.2. Laboratory Evaluation

5.2.1. Electrodiagnostic Testing

In early stages, electrodiagnostic testing may give normal results (12). As severity increases, nerve conduction studies reveal reduced sensory amplitudes progressing to absent sensory responses in all nerves tested; motor responses remain normal (12,58). In case reports of profound toxicity, mild motor abnormalities consisting of mildly reduced amplitude and conduction, presumably attributable to limb disuse have been described (5). Needle electromyography reveals no abnormalities, even among patients with severe pyridoxine intoxication.

5.2.2. Pathologic Features

Pyridoxine toxicity results in a sensory neuronopathy at the level of the dorsal root and trigeminal ganglion. Dose dependence has been demonstrated with careful histological studies in animals (77). Chronic low-level exposure results in proximal axonal atrophy in the presence of normal appearing neurons; higher-level exposure results in death of sensory neurons in the DRG. Humans appear to be the most sensitive to the neurotoxic effects of pyridoxine on a weight per dose basis of all animals studied (77). The results of human sural nerve biopsy in pyridoxine intoxication are consistent with pathological investigations in animals and show moderate reduction in myelinated fiber density without evidence of segmental demyelination or regeneration (58).

5.3. Differential Diagnosis

The sensory neuronopathy of pyridoxine deficiency has a limited differential diagnosis. The most common systemic disorders causing a sensory neuronopathy include paraneoplastic antineuronal antibodies (Hu or ANNA-1) most often related to small-cell lung cancer, Sjögren's syndrome, and idiopathic sensory ganglionopathy. Medications that produce sensory neuropathy with or without loss of DRG cells include cisplatin, metronidazole, and thalidomide.

5.4. Management and Prognosis

Therapy involves prompt discontinuation of pyridoxine supplementation. Upon discontinuation of pyridoxine, paresthesias and sensory loss may continue to progress for many weeks. This phenomenon is termed "coasting" and is observed in many other toxic neuropathies (12,16). Recovery can be complete if the presenting symptoms are mild. In the setting of high doses and severe presentation, recovery may only be partial after pyridoxine discontinuation (4,58).

5.5. Pathogenesis

The dose of pyridoxine required to produce neuropathy in humans has been suggested to be as low as 200 mg daily. This dose results in an insidious presentation after prolonged exposure. In contrast, much higher doses of pyridoxine (many grams over a short period of time) can result in rapid onset of severe neuropathic symptoms. The present theory of pathogenesis suggests that an overabundance of pyridoxine is directly toxic to neurons. Support for this theory is the observation that dosage strength results in a differential toxicity to DRG neurons (58,77). Further, in the case of extreme doses (2 g/kg), autonomic abnormalities were noted with profound sensory loss (5). Selective toxicity of the DRG neurons and, in higher doses, autonomic neurons may be due to reduced permeability of the blood–nerve barrier at these locations. Pathologic changes occur in the largest diameter DRG neurons and axons, preferentially. These neurons are purported to have higher metabolic requirements and may reflect impaired energy metabolism (18,77).

6. COBALAMIN (VITAMIN B$_{12}$) DEFICIENCY NEUROPATHY

In the early part of the 20th century, the distal sensory loss associated with cobalamin deficiency was attributed to myelopathy (68). The clinical findings were named subacute combined degeneration in reference to the degeneration of the dorsal and lateral columns of the spinal cord. However, the clinical findings of variably depressed reflexes and electromyographic studies demonstrating peripheral nerve abnormalities suggested a concurrent neuropathy. Neuropathological studies of peripheral nerves later confirmed the presence of peripheral axonal loss and occasional demyelination (51,76). The frequency and clinical relevance of myelopathy in relation to the neuropathy associated with cobalamin deficiency have not been conclusively settled (6,68,76). Most studies have been limited by sample size (20,68) or limited electrophysiological or histological investigation of peripheral nerve (29).

Unlike most nutritional neuropathies, cobalamin deficiency typically occurs in patients with normal caloric intake and no signs of malnutrition. Most causes are related to gastric malabsorption. The majority of cases (80%) occur in the setting of pernicious anemia, although as many as 25% of patients with cobalamin deficiency do not have the expected megaloblastic anemia (29,31,41). Patients with chronic atrophic gastritis and subsequent achlorhydria also are at great risk for cobalamin deficiency (6,29). Other causes of cobalamin deficiency include genetic defects affecting cobalamin metabolism and competition for cobalamin stores with intestinal flora and occasional parasites (Table 19.2).

6.1. Clinical Features

Early clinical findings of cobalamin deficiency neuropathy include ill-defined paresthesias of the extremities. In contrast to typical distal neuropathies that first involve the feet, the hands are reported to be affected equally or more severely than the feet in cobalamin deficiency neuropathy (31,68,70). Painful, tingling paresthesias can be disabling. Vibration and position sensations are variably impaired out of proportion to decreased pain and temperature sensations. Distal leg weakness and gait ataxia typically develop within 4 months of the initial sensory complaints (29). Reflexes are variable, but may be depressed from the neuropathy early in the course of disease or brisk with extensor planter responses reflecting a simultaneous myelopathy (29,31).

The onset of cobalamin deficiency neuropathy is insidious and the clinical signs of neuropathy exist in the setting of confounding myelopathic findings. In a retrospective study of patients with cobalamin deficiency, Healton et al. (29) found that 114 of 153 patients had neurologic symptoms at the time of the laboratory diagnosis. Coexisting signs of neuropathy and myelopathy were present in 41% of these patients, whereas neuropathy alone was present in 25% and myelopathic changes alone were present in 12% of the patients. A recent large retrospective study of patients with cobalamin deficiency found that the laboratory diagnosis normally resulted in prompt treatment without electrophysiologic testing (29). This common clinical practice may explain the under-representation of neuropathy in the classic descriptions of cobalamin deficiency.

Symptoms of cobalamin deficiency normally develop gradually. However, patients with borderline-low cobalamin stores may develop symptoms acutely after exposure to nitrous oxide (48). Nitrous oxide oxidizes the cobalt in cobalamin, inactivating gastrointestinal stores of methylcobalamin. Nitrous oxide is commonly used in surgical and dental procedures, and it also has illicit recreational usage. Historically, even single exposures can result in symptoms and should be considered in any postoperative patient with new extremity paresthesias (40).

Other neurologic manifestations of cobalamin deficiency include autonomic neuropathy with orthostasis, impotence, and bladder dysfunction (29,31,51). Evidence of orthostatic hypotension may suggest involvement of small unmyelinated axons (51). Cognitive symptoms and signs, as well as dysgeusia, dysosmia, and visual disturbances occasionally occur (29,31). Impaired central vision may reflect a bilateral optic neuropathy. Cognitive abnormalities range from mild short-term memory deficits to clinically evident dementia with psychomotor slowing. Occasionally, depression and psychosis develop (49). Non-neurological manifestations include glossitis, diarrhea, and yellow-pigmented skin and fingernails (26) (Table 19.1).

6.2. Laboratory Evaluation

6.2.1. Serology

The characteristic blood abnormality associated with cobalamin deficiency is a megaloblastic anemia. Serum levels of cobalamin can be measured, and levels <200 pg/mL should arouse suspicion of a cobalamin deficit. As described subsequently, folate levels should be measured at the same time. Deficiency of cobalamin is confirmed by demonstrating elevated serum methylmalonic acid and homocysteine levels, and both should be evaluated even when cobalamin levels are in the low-normal range (29,41). The cause of cobalamin deficiency should be first addressed by testing for intrinsic factor-blocking antibody, although elevated antibody levels are identified only in ~50% of cases of pernicious anemia (41). When intrinsic factor-blocking antibodies are not found, but there remains a high suspicion for pernicious anemia, a Schilling test can further differentiate between pernicious anemia and defects involving absorption (terminal ileum damage) or digestive competition for cobalamin (blind loop or infection with the fish tapeworm *Diphyllobothrium latum*). In pernicious anemia, the Schilling test will be abnormal after the first administration of radiolabeled cobalamin (Part I). Vegetarians and patients who have achlorhydria demonstrate a normal response to Part I of the test because of the purified supply of cobalamin provided in the test. When combined with intrinsic factor (Part II), absorption is corrected in pernicious anemia. Complications of intestinal absorption, such as blind loop syndrome, parasite infection, pancreatic disease, or ileal malabsorption, produce abnormal results of Part II.

6.2.2. Electrodiagnostic Testing

Depending on the severity and duration of symptoms, patients with cobalamin deficiency may demonstrate no nerve conduction or electromyographic abnormalities (31). Electrophysiologic evaluation of 20 patients with pernicious anemia identified 13 (65%) who showed evidence of neuropathy (20). When abnormalities are present, they are consistent with an axonal neuropathy, although occasional patients have findings suggestive of demyelination. Most reports include evidence of low amplitude sensory and motor responses (25,29,31). In contrast, conduction velocities, including F response latencies, are only mildly slowed, consistent with an axonal neuropathy (20,25,29,31). Severely slowed nerve conduction and coexisting partial conduction block have been described as reversible with cobalamin replacement in two individual patients (3,31). Needle EMG studies show evidence of distal denervation and reinnervation of distal muscles of patients with severe neuropathy (29).

6.2.3. Pathologic Features

Sural nerve pathology in cobalamin deficiency neuropathy shows predominant axonal loss of large myelinated fibers (51). McCombe and McLeod found no evidence of primary demyelination in the three sural nerves evaluated in their study but did note axonal degeneration, which was severe in two of the three cases. Neuropathological studies of spinal cord demonstrate multifocal axonal loss and demyelination, predominantly in the dorsal and lateral columns. Similar lesions are found in the cerebrum in late stages of the disease (76).

6.3. Differential Diagnosis

The clinical presentation of cobalamin deficiency is highly variable, and the neuropathy may be present without evidence of myelopathy or cognitive impairment. The differential diagnosis for distal paresthesias in the setting of a mild, nonspecific axonal neuropathy is broad (Table 19.3). In the more classic combined syndrome of myelopathy and neuropathy, with or without cognitive changes, the differential diagnosis includes Friedreich's ataxia, α-tocopherol (vitamin E) deficiency, and adrenoleukodystrophy. These disorders also have neurophysiological and neuropathological findings similar to those of cobalamin deficiency (25).

6.4. Management and Prognosis

Before cobalamin was purified, Nobel Prize research performed in 1926 demonstrated that feeding animal liver to patients with subacute combined system disease resulted in clinical improvement (52). The response to treatment of cobalamin deficiency can be dramatic if replacement is initiated before significant myelopathy occurs. In the setting of pernicious anemia, typical therapy consists of prompt administration of subcutaneous or intramuscular cobalamin at a dose of 100–1000 µg daily for 5 days, followed by

100–1000 μg monthly (26). There is also evidence that oral supplementation of coba-lamin at doses of 2 mg daily in patients with pernicious anemia is as effective as the intra-muscular 1 mg administered monthly (46). The normalization of serum methylmalonic acid can be monitored as a therapeutic marker in the setting of normal hematological parameters. Maximal improvement of neurological symptoms and signs may require up to 18 months, although paresthesias usually improve rapidly. Clinical symptoms may respond much more than electrophysiologic parameters, although some studies suggest abnormal nerve conduction studies improve significantly (20). Autonomic symptoms, visual changes, and even cognitive changes have been reported to improve or resolve after cobalamin supplementation (29,49,51). Myelopathy deficits usually do not respond fully to replacement (29,31,51).

6.5. Pathogenesis

Because of the prevalence of cobalamin in animal-related proteins and a large capacitance of hepatic stores, cobalamin is present in most diets at adequate levels and deficiency syn-dromes usually develop slowly. Pernicious anemia is responsible for >70% of cases of coba-lamin deficiency (29). Other causes are presented in Table 19.2. Cobalamin has a complex mechanism for absorption. It is initially released from dietary animal proteins in the low-pH environment of the stomach and binds to salivary proteins. Pancreatic enzymes in the duo-denum and jejunum cleave the binding proteins and the cobalamin binds with intrinsic factor secreted from gastric parietal cells. The cobalamin–intrinsic factor complex is absorbed through a receptor-mediated mechanism in the terminal ileum where it is bound to serum proteins transcobalamin I and II. The cobalamin bound to transcobalamin II is biologically active and available for intracellular enzymatic reactions or is stored in the liver. Tissue stores of cobalamin usually last 3–4 years. Cobalamin acts as a coenzyme for two essential metabolic reactions. Although significant debate exists, it is unknown which reaction is the essential mechanism resulting in the neurological abnormalities (9).

7. FOLATE DEFICIENCY NEUROPATHY

The metabolic linkage between folate and cobalamin (vitamin B_{12}) metabolism results in an interdependence that can mask alternate deficiencies (41). Consequently, folate sup-plementation in the setting of a cobalamin deficiency can improve a megaloblastic anemia but may not improve and may even worsen the neurologic symptoms of cobalamin deficiency (29).

The presence of peripheral neuropathy in the setting of isolated folic acid deficiency continues to be debated in the literature. The clinical symptoms are reported to be similar to cobalamin deficiency, often including a myelopathy and neuropathy (6,13). Botez et al. (13) described two patients who displayed clinical and electrophysiologic evidence of both myelopathy and peripheral neuropathy and three patients who showed evidence of an iso-lated neuropathy. All had reduced serum folate levels and all improved or resolved after folate supplementation. All patients had longstanding gastrointestinal disease and normal serum cobalamin levels. Other published studies are often complicated by coexisting vitamin deficiencies or alcoholism limiting the understanding of an isolated deficiency.

8. α-TOCOPHEROL (VITAMIN E) DEFICIENCY NEUROPATHY

The tocopherols (α, β, γ, and δ) are a group of fat-soluble antioxidants thought to prevent peroxidation of fatty acids in cell membranes (39). Vitamin E or α-tocopherol is the most common and potent antioxidant in this group of compounds. The ubiquitous nature of the tocopherols makes dietary insufficiency nearly impossible. However, functional deficiencies related to vitamin metabolism and absorption have been described (Table 19.2). Malabsorption and steatorrhea comprise the most common cause of α-tocopherol deficiency as observed in celiac disease, Whipple's disease, and pancreatitis (36). Genetic defects associated with vitamin metabolism have also been described, including defects in lipid transport proteins (32).

A well-defined autosomal recessive disorder resulting in α-tocopherol deficiency is abetalipoproteinemia (Bassen–Kornzweig Syndrome). The congenital absence of apoprotein B results in deficits in vitamins E and A. The clinical characteristics of this disease are a progressive ataxia, areflexia, steatorrhea, and retinitis pigmentosa attributable to both vitamin E and A deficiencies (6,15). A second, autosomal recessive defect in the α-tocopherol transporter protein results in inadequate incorporation of α-tocopherol into very low-density lipoproteins in liver cells and in an isolated α-tocopherol deficiency (32). Patients exhibiting either of these disorders have normal gastrointestinal function.

8.1. Clinical Features

The neuropathy associated with α-tocopherol deficiency is relatively mild in early stages and usually not painful. Most often it is limited to the lower extremities. Similar to the presentation of cobalamin deficiency, it most often presents as a mixed syndrome of neuropathy and myelopathy. The presentation usually includes an unsteady gait and complaints of lower extremity numbness. The onset of symptoms is insidious and progression slow. In the setting of genetic defects in metabolism, impaired gait may develop between the ages of 5 and 10 years (27). When the defect is partial or acquired, abnormalities may present after intervals of 5–20 years (6,36,76). Examination reveals decreased proprioception and vibration sensation with preserved pinprick, temperature, and light-touch sensation. Diminished proprioception, when severe, results in pseudoathetosis. Reflexes are depressed or absent, and the response to plantar stimulation is variable. Truncal and extremity ataxia as well as tremor and dysarthria attributable to cerebellar dysfunction can also be observed. Opthalmoplegia, retinitis pigmentosa, and optic nerve abnormalities are common findings in combined fat-soluble vitamin disorders but have not been described in isolated α-tocopherol deficiency states (11,36,42). Over time, pes cavus and kyphoscoliosis often develop in the setting of the progressive neuropathy and myelopathy.

8.2. Laboratory Evaluation

8.2.1. Serology

Serum level of α-tocopherol is a reasonable measure of body stores, having a normal range of 5.5–17.0 mg/L. γ- and β-tocopherols also can be assayed. Although the ratio of α-tocopherol to total serum lipids may be a more accurate measure that corrects for hyperlipidemia, in most patients with α-tocopherol deficiency, levels are undetectable. A trial loading dose of 2–5 g of α-tocopherol can be followed over 5 days to establish the effectiveness of vitamin absorption (76).

8.2.2. Electrodiagnostic Testing

Occasionally, nerve conduction and electromyographic studies may be normal in symptomatic α-tocopherol deficiency neuropathy (36,39). As severity of the neuropathy increases, sensory responses decline in amplitude and may be unobtainable in the legs.

The accompanying reduction in sensory conduction velocity reflects the loss of sensory axons. Needle EMG is normal (14,75).

8.2.3. Pathologic Features

Dorsal root neurons appear most sensitive to α-tocopherol deficiency. The results of sural nerve biopsies can be normal or show retrograde degeneration of large-caliber myelinated axons (36,54,67). Most patients with abetalipoproteinemia show a marked loss of large-diameter fibers (75). The distal projection of the central afferents of the dorsal root neuron shows marked degeneration in the fasciculi gracilis and cuneatus (47,76).

8.3. Differential Diagnosis

As a neuropathy, α-tocopherol deficiency resembles a sensory ganglionopathy with its painless loss of large-fiber modalities. However, when considering the combined syndrome of neuropathy, myelopathy, and ataxia, the differential diagnosis should include Friedreich's ataxia, cobalamin (vitamin B_{12}) deficiency, and Refsum's disease.

8.4. Management and Prognosis

The normal recommended daily allowance of α-tocopherol is 10 mg/day for males and 8 mg/day for females. There have been no reported toxic effects of α-tocopherol, and doses of 200 mg to 2 g/day have been used for therapeutic replacement in the event of a demonstrated deficiency. Patients with malabsorption require 1–4 g/day or may require a water-soluble α-tocopherol preparation (36,39). In abetalipoproteinemia, the recommended dose of α-tocopherol is 100–200 mg/kg per day in addition to vitamin A and vitamin K supplementation (39). The goal of all therapy in α-tocopherol deficiency is to arrest neurologic progression. In the setting of early neuropathy, case reports have described substantial clinical and electrophysiological improvement after α-tocopherol supplementation (17,42,50). There is poor evidence for substantial recovery after progression includes prominent cerebellar dysfunction and other central signs.

8.5. Pathogenesis

Tocopherols are a component of vegetable products, and they are especially concentrated in vegetable oils and wheat germ. They are solubilized with bile acids and absorbed in the small intestine as mixed micelles and incorporated into chylomicrons. α-tocopherol is specifically transferred through a binding protein into LDL and VLDL particles for systemic use. The mechanism of uptake in neural tissues is unknown, but the loss of the antioxidant function is thought to result in the pathologic changes associated with α-tocopherol deficiency (36).

9. PHOSPHATE DEFICIENCY NEUROPATHY

Severe hypophosphatemia can result in a reversible neuropathy that resembles acute inflammatory demyelinating polyradiculoneuropathy (AIDP). The clinical presentation includes generalized weakness, perioral paresthesias, acral sensory loss, dysarthria, ataxia, and absent reflexes (63). Weakness can rapidly progress and result in respiratory failure and need for assisted ventilation. Electrodiagnostic evaluations have suggested the presence of a demyelinating neuropathy with partial conduction block and conduction slowing. However, the rapid resolution of clinical and electrodiagnostic abnormalities over days to weeks suggests a metabolic mechanism for the conduction abnormalities.

Hypophosphatemia is most often found in profoundly ill patients in the setting of poorly supplemented parenteral nutrition. Acute carbohydrate loads can cause a shift of phosphate to the intracellular space in a patient with already depleted stores resulting in severe weakness (65). Hypophosphatemia frequently is not recognized, and it can be caused or worsened by alcoholism, phosphate-binding antacids, severe burns, respiratory alkalosis, and hyperparathyroidism (65,78). Other manifestations of severe hypophosphatemia include rhabomyolysis, delirium, seizure, and coma (63,65).

Following intravenous replacement of phosphate, the neuropathy can be reversed within days to weeks. It is proposed to result from decreased phosphate metabolism and recruitment of ATP in the largest axons that have the highest metabolism (18,63,74,78).

10. CHROMIUM DEFICIENCY NEUROPATHY

A rare neuropathy related to chromium deficiency has been described in three patients in the setting of prolonged total parenteral nutrition (37). This syndrome consists of a sensorimotor neuropathy and impaired glucose tolerance, which both resolved following chromium replacement in the parenteral nutrition formulation (37,38).

11. CUBAN EPIDEMIC NEUROPATHY

Between 1991 and 1994, an epidemic of neuropathy and optic neuropathy occurred in Cuba, with over 50,000 reported cases (23). The "epidemic neuropathy" was initially thought to represent an exposure to some unrecognized neurotoxicant. However, the epidemic appeared in association with acute worsening of the economic situation, and the syndrome was eventually attributed to acute nutritional deficiencies caused by malnutrition, possibly in combination with alcohol consumption (tobacco–alcohol amblyopia) and exposure to other unidentified substances (56). Support for a deficiency syndrome hypothesis was provided by disappearance of additional cases after widespread vitamin supplementation (23).

12. POSTGASTRECTOMY NEUROPATHY

Clinically evident nutritional neuropathies often represent combined deficiencies related to dietary insufficiency or malabsorption. Because of the presence of overlapping deficiency syndromes, diagnosis can be challenging. One of the most common presentations of nutritional neuropathy occurs in the setting of remote gastric resection or diversion. A recent review suggests that ~5% of patients undergoing gastric restriction surgery for morbid obesity developed some neurologic complication (1). The resultant neuropathy reflects the type of gastric resection and the resultant malabsorption syndrome. In the setting of gastric resection for carcinoma or severe gastric ulcer disease, the neuropathy presents 5–15 years after the procedure.

The clinical symptoms associated with postgastrectomy neuropathy include distal dysesthesias and weakness, most severe in the lower limbs. Examination shows distal sensory loss, weakness, and hypoactive or absent reflexes without signs of corticospinal tract dysfunction (8,10,43). Most of the patients described in these studies demonstrated multiple vitamin deficiencies, including low serum levels of thiamine, pyridoxine, folate, and cobalamin (8,10,43). Histological evaluations in three sural nerves studied by Behse and Buchthal (10) showed reduced fiber density, perineural edema, and segmental demyelination in two nerves. The other study which evaluated sural nerve histology reported similarly reduced fiber density and perineural edema, but found that segmental demyelination occurred rarely among the 12 nerves examined (43).

In the setting of neuropathic symptoms and past gastric surgery, evaluation should include serum levels of the B vitamins and folate with therapy addressing any and all deficiencies. The index of suspicion for cobalamin deficiency should be high because of the high prevalence of unrecognized cobalamin deficiency in the general population. In the setting of steatorrhea, α-tocopherol (vitamin E) also should be included. When multiple vitamin deficiencies are present, historical reports suggest a mild and incomplete response to comprehensive vitamin supplementation.

A more severe neuropathy has been described in association with gastric diversion, banding, or plication in the obese compared with the combined deficiency sensorimotor neuropathy described earlier. This neuropathy presents acutely, 2–4 months after the surgical procedure, with sensory loss, distal weakness, and hypoactive or absent reflexes. The neuropathy usually develops in the presence of significant weight loss and frequent vomiting (1). Neuropathological investigation of a single patient who displayed this profile showed lipofuscin in dorsal root and anterior motor neurons with lipid accumulation in Schwann cells (24). The neuropathy resembled a form of AIDP but without an elevated CSF protein level. The coexisting confusional state suggested a diagnosis of Wernicke's encephalopathy, which also had been reported to occur within months of gastric restrictive surgery (1). Vitamin supplementation in this setting should probably include parenteral B complex vitamins in the high normal range, although the reported response to aggressive supplementation has been reported to be incomplete (1,24).

13. CONCLUSION

Although Western medicine has substantial experience with neuropathy developing in the setting of famine and nutritional deficiency, a lack of definitive research promotes confusion about the etiology and presenting characteristics of specific nutritional neuropathies. These neuropathies must be suspected by their clinical presentation and in the context of a carefully gathered history. Specific nutritional neuropathies can develop in the setting of malabsorption syndromes, gastric disorders, and some disease states that predispose to specific nutritional deficiencies. Prescription medications, dietary supplements, prolonged dialysis, or inadequate parenteral nutrition can also result in iatrogenic neuropathy. More infrequent are neuropathies due to select trace mineral deficiencies and specific genetic disorders. Therapy involves supportive care and nutrient replacement.

REFERENCES

1. Abarbanel JM, Berginer VM, Osimani A, Solomon H, Charuzi I. Neurologic complications after gastric restriction surgery for morbid obesity. Neurology 1987; 37:196–200.
2. Aita JF, Calame TR. Peripheral neuropathy secondary to isoniazid-induced pyridoxine deficiency. Md State Med J 1972; 21:68–70.

3. Al-Shubaili AF, Farah SA, Hussein JM, Trontelj JV, Khuraibet AJ. Axonal and demyelinating neuropathy with reversible proximal conduction block, an unusual feature of vitamin B12 deficiency. Muscle Nerve 1998; 21:1341–1343.

4. Albin RL, Albers JW. Long-term follow-up of pyridoxine-induced acute sensory neuropathy–neuronopathy. Neurology 1990; 40:1319.

5. Albin RL, Albers JW, Greenberg HS, Townsend JB, Lynn RB, Burke JM, Alessi AG. Acute sensory neuropathy–neuronopathy from pyridoxine overdose. Neurology 1987; 37:1729–1732.

6. Albers JW, Nostrant TT, Riggs JE. Neurologic manifestations of gastrointestinal disease. Neurol Clin 1989; 7:525–548.

7. Ammendola A, Tata MR, Aurilio C, Ciccone G, Gemini D, Ammendola E, Ugolini G, Argenzio F. Peripheral neuropathy in chronic alcoholism: a retrospective cross-sectional study in 76 subjects. Alcohol & Alcoholism 2001; 36:271–275.

8. Banerji NK, Hurwitz LJ. Nervous system manifestations after gastric surgery. Acta Neurol Scand 1971; 47:485–513.

9. Beck WS. Cobalamin and the nervous system. New Engl J Med 1988; 318(26):1752–1754.

10. Behse F, Buchthal F. Alcoholic neuropathy: clinical, electrophysiological, and biopsy findings. Ann Neurol 1977; 2:95–110.

11. Benomar A, Yahyaoui M, Marzouki N, Birouk N, Bouslam N, Belaidi H, Amarti A, Ouazzani R, Chkili T. Vitamin E deficiency ataxia associated with adenoma. J Neurol Sci 1999; 162:97–101.

12. Berger AR, Schaumburg HH, Schroeder C, Apfel S, Reynolds R. Dose response, coasting, and differential fiber vulnerability in human toxic neuropathy: a prospective study of pyridoxine neurotoxicity. Neurology 1992; 42:1367–1370.

13. Botez MI, Peyronnard J, Bachevalier J, Charron L. Polyneuropathy and folate deficiency. Arch Neurol 1978; 35:581–584.

14. Brin MF, Fetell MR, Green PHA, Kayden HJ, Hays AP, Behrens MM, Baker H. Blind loop syndrome, vitamin E malabsorption, and spinocerebellar degeneration. Neurology 1985; 35:338–342.

15. Brin MF, Pedley TA, Lovelace RE, Emerson RG, Gouras P, MacKay C, Kayden HJ, Levy J, Baker H. Electrophysiologic features of abetalipoproteinemia: functional consequences of vitamin E deficiency. Neurology 1986; 36:669–673.

16. Bromberg, MB. Peripheral neurotoxic disorders. Neurol Clin 2000; 18:681–694.

17. Burck U, Goebel HH, Kuhlendahl HD, Meier C, Goebel KM. Neuromyopathy and vitamin E deficiency in man. Neuropediatrics 1981; 12:267–278.

18. Cavanagh JB. The problems of neurons with long axons. Lancet 1984; 1:1284–1287.

19. Charness ME, Simon RP, Greenberg DA. Medical progress: ethanol and the nervous system. N Engl J Med 1989; 321:442–454.

20. Cox-Klazinga M, Endtz LJ. Peripheral nerve involvement in pernicious anemia. J Neurol Sci 1980; 45:367–371.

21. Djoenaidi W, Notermans SLH. Electrophysiologic evaluation of beri-beri neuropathy. Electromyogr Clin Neurophysiol 1990; 30:97–103.

22. Donofrio PD, Albers JW. Polyneuropathy: classification by nerve conduction studies and electromyography. Muscle Nerve 1990; 13:889–903.

23. Anonymous. Epidemic neuropathy—Cuba, 1991–1994. MMWR Morb Mortal Wkly Rep 1994; 43:189–192.

24. Feit H, Glasberg M, Ireton C, Rosenberg RN, Thal E. Peripheral neuropathy and starvation after gastric partitioning for morbid obesity. Ann Int Med 1982; 96:453–455.

25. Fine EJ, Hallett M. Neurophysiological study of subacute combined degeneration. J Neurol Sci 1980; 45:331–336.

26. Green R, Kinsella LJ. Current concepts in the diagnosis of cobalamin deficiency. Neurology 1995; 45:1435–1440.

27. Guggenheim MA, Jackson V, Lilly J, Silverman A, Grabert BE. Progressive neuromuscular disease in children with chronic cholestasis and vitamin E deficiency: diagnosis and treatment with alpha-tocopherol. J Pediatr 1982; 100:51–58.

28. Hallett M, Fox JG, Rogers AE, Nicolosi R, Schoene W, Goolsby HA, Landis DMD, Pezeshkpour G. Controlled studies on the effects of alcohol ingestion on peripheral nerves of macaque monkeys. J Neurol Sci 1987; 80:65–71.

29. Healton EB, Savage DG, Brust JC, Garrett TJ, Lindenbaum J. Neurologic aspects of cobalamin deficiency. Medicine 1991; 70(4):229–245.

30. Heller CA, Friedman PA. Pyridoxine deficiency and peripheral neuropathy associated with long-term phenelzine therapy. Am J Med 1983; 75:887–888.

31. Hemmer B, Glocker FX, Schumacher M, Deuschl G, Lucking CH. Subacute combined degeneration: clinical, electrophysiological, and magnetic resonance imaging findings. J Neurol Neurosurg Psychiatry 1998; 65(6): 822–827.

32. Hentati A, Deng HX, Hung WY, Nayer M, Ahmed MS, He X, Tim R, Stumpf DA, Siddique T. Human α-tocopherol transfer protein: gene structure and mutations in familial vitamin E deficiency. Ann Neurol 1996; 39(3):295–300.

33. Hung SC, Hung SH, Tarng DC, Yang WC, Chen TW, Huang TP. Thiamine deficiency and unexplained encephalopathy in hemodialysis and peritoneal dialysis patients. Am J Kidney Dis 2001; 38:941–947.

34. Ihara M, Ito T, Yanagihara C, Nishimura Y. Wernicke's encephalopathy associated with hemodialysis: a report of two cases and review of the literature. Clin Neurol Neurosurg 1999; 101:118–121.

35. Itokawa Y. Thiamine and nervous system function: an historical sketch. Metabol Brain Dis 1996; 11:1–7.

36. Jackson CE, Amato AA, Barohn RJ. Isolated vitamin E deficiency. Muscle Nerve 1996; 19:1161–1165.

37. Jeejeebhoy KN, Chu RC, Marliss EB, Greenburg GR, Bruce-Robertson A. Chromium deficiency, glucose intolerance, and neuropathy reversed by chromium supplementation, in a patient receiving long-term total parenteral nutrition. Am J Clin Nutr 1977; 30:531–538.

38. Jeejeebhoy KN. Chromium and parenteral nutrition. J Trace Elem Exp Med 1999; 12:85–89.

39. Kayden HK. The neurological syndrome of vitamin E deficiency: a significant cause of ataxia. Neurology 1993; 43:2167–2169.

40. Kinsella LJ, Green R. "Anesthetesia paresthetica": nitrous oxide-induced cobalamin deficiency. Neurology 1995; 45:1608–1610.

41. Klee GG. Cobalamin and folate evaluation: measurement of methylmalonic acid and homocysteine vs vitamin B_{12} and folate. Clin Chem 2000; 46:1277–1283.

42. Ko HY, Park-Ko I. Electrophysiologic recovery after vitamin E-deficient neuropathy. Arch Phys Med Rehabil 1999; 80:964–967.

43. Koike H, Misu K, Hattori N, Ito H, Hirayama M, Nagamatsu M, Sasaki I, Sobue G. Postgastrectomy polyneuropathy with thiamine deficiency. J Neurol Neurosurg Psychiatry 2001; 71:357–362.

44. Koike H, Mori K, Misu K, Hattori N, Ito H, Hirayama M, Sobue G. Painful alcoholic polyneuropathy with predominant small-fiber loss and normal thiamine status. Neurology 2001; 56:1727–1732.

45. Kril JJ. Neuropathology of thiamine deficiency disorders. Metabol Brain Dis 1996; 11:9–17.

46. Kuzminski AM, Del Giacco EJ, Allen RH, Stabler SP, Lindenbaum J. Effective treatment of cobalamin deficiency with oral cobalamin. Blood 1998; 94:1191–1198.

47. Landrieu, P. Peripheral nerve involvement in children with chronic cholestasis and vitamin E deficiency. Neuropediatrics 1985; 16:194–201.

48. Layzer RB, Fishman RA, Schafer JA. Neuropathy following abuse of nitrous oxide. Neurology 1978; 28:504–506.

49. Lindenbaum J, Healton EB, Savage DG, Brust JCM, Garrett TJ, Podell ER, Marcell PD, Stabler SP, Allen RH. Neuropsychiatric disorders caused by cobalamin deficiency in the absence of anemia or macrocytosis. New Engl J Med 1988; 318:1720–1728.

50. Martinello F, Fardin P, Ottina M, Ricchieri GL, Koenig M, Cavalier L, Trevisan CP. Supplemental therapy in isolated vitamin E deficiency improves the peripheral neuropathy and prevents the progression of ataxia. J Neurol Sci 1998; 156:177–179.

51. McCombe PA, McLeod JG. The peripheral neuropathy of vitamin B_{12} deficiency. J Neurol Sci 1984; 66:117–126.

52. Minot GR, Murphy WP. Treatment of pernicious anemia by a special diet. J Am Med Assoc 1926; 87:470–476.

53. Monforte R, Estruch R, Valls-Sole J, Nicolas J, Villalta J, Urbano-Marquez A. Autonomic and peripheral neuropathies in patients with chronic alcoholism: a dose-related toxic effect of alcohol. Arch Neurol 1995; 52:45–51.

54. Nelson JS. Neuropathological studies of chronic vitamin E deficiency in mammals including humans. Ciba Found Symp 1983; 101:92–105.

55. Ochoa J. Isoniazid neuropathy in man: quantitative electron microscope study. Brain 1970; 93:831–850.

56. Ordunez-Garcia PO, Nieto FJ, Espinosa-Brito AD, Caballero B. Cuban epidemic neuropathy, 1991–1994: history repeats itself a century after the "amblyopia of the blockade." Am J Public Health 1996; 86:738–743.

57. Ohnishi A, Tsuji S, Igisu H, Murai Y, Goto I, Kuriowa Y, Tsujihata M, Takamori M. Beriberi neuropathy: morphometric study of sural nerve. J Neurol Sci 1980; 45:177–190.

58. Parry GJ, Bredessen DE. Sensory neuropathy with low-dose pyridoxine. Neurology 1985; 35:1466–1468.

59. Pellock JM, Howell J, Kendig EL, Baker H. Pyridoxine deficiency in children treated with isoniazid. Chest 1985; 5:658–661.

60. Prineas J. Peripheral nerve changes in thiamine-deficient rats. Arch Neurol 1970; 23:541–548.

61. Raskin NH, Fishman RA. Pyridoxine-deficiency neuropathy due to hydralazine. New Engl J Med 1965; 25:1182–1185.

62. Schaumburg HH, Kaplan J, Windebank AJ, Vick N, Rasmus S, Pleasure D, Brown MJ. Sensory neuropathy from pyridoxine abuse: a new megavitamin syndrome. New Engl J Med 1983; 309:445–448.

63. Siddiqui MF, Bertorni TE. Hypophosphatemia-induced neuropathy: clinical and electro-physiologic findings. Muscle Nerve 1998; 21:650–652.

64. Snider DE Jr. Pyridoxine supplementation during isoniazid therapy. Tubercle 1980; 61:191–196.

65. Subramanian R, Khardori R. Severe hypophosphatemia: pathophysiologic implications, clinical presentations and treatment. Medicine 2000; 79:1–8.

66. Takahishi K, Nakamura H. Axonal degeneration in beriberi neuropathy. Arch Neurol 1976; 33:836–841.

67. Traber MG, Sokol RJ, Ringel SP, Neville HE, Thellman CA, Kayden HJ. Lack of tocopherol in peripheral nerves of vitamin E-deficient patients with peripheral neuropathy. New Engl J Med 1987; 317:262–265.

68. Victor M. Polyneuropathy due to nutritional deficiency and alcoholism. In: Dyck PJ, Thomas RK, Bunge RP, eds. Peripheral Neuropathy. Vol. 2. 2nd ed. Philadelphia: WB Saunders, 1984:1899–1940.

69. Victor M, Adams RD. The neuropathy of experimental vitamin B6 deficiency in monkeys. Am J Clin Nutr 1956; 4:346–353.

70. Victor M, Adams RD, Collins GH. The Wernicke–Korsakoff syndrome and related neurologic disorders due to alcoholism and malnutrition. Contemporary Neurology Series. Vol. 3. Philadelphia: FA Davis, 1989.

71. Vilter RW, Mueller JF, Glazer HS, Jarrold T, Abraham J, Thompson C, Hawkins VR. The effect of vitamin B6 deficiency induced by desoxypyridoxine in human beings. J Lab Clin Med 1953; 42:335–357.

72. Vimokesant SL, Hilker DM, Nakornchai S, Rungruangsak K, Dhanamitta S. Effects of betel nut and fermented fish on the thiamine status of northeastern Thais. Am J Clin Nutr 1975; 28:1458–1463.

73. Walsh JC, McLeod JG. Alcoholic neuropathy: an electrophysiological and histological study. J Neurol Sci 1970; 10:457–469.

74. Weintraub MI. Hypohphosphatemia mimicking acute Guillain–Barré–Strohl syndrome: a complication of hyperalimentation. J Am Med Assoc 1976; 235:1040–1041.

75. Wichman A, Buchthal F, Pezeshkpour GH, Gregg RE. Peripheral neuropathy in abetalipopro-
    teinemia. Neurology 1985; 35:1279–1289.
76. Windebank AJ. Polyneuropathy due to nutritional deficiency and alcoholism. In: Dyck PJ,
    Thomas RK, eds. Peripheral Neuropathy. Vol. 2. 3rd ed. WB Saunders, 1993:1310–1321.
77. Xu Y, Sladky JT, Brown MJ. Dose-dependent expression of neuronopathy after experimental
    pyridoxine intoxication. Neurology 1989; 39:1077–1083.
78. Yagnik P, Singh N, Burns R. Peripheral neuropathy with hypophosphatemia in a patient receiv-
    ing intravenous hyperalimentation. South Med J 1985; 78:1381–1384.

20
Toxic Neuropathy

Eric J. Sorenson and A. Gordon Smith
University of Utah, Salt Lake City, Utah, USA

ABSTRACT

Peripheral neuropathies caused by toxic agents are often misdiagnosed. To make the diagnosis of a toxic neuropathy, the physician must have a high index of clinical suspicion and pursue the history to identify the offending agent. In many cases, there is no specific diagnostic test, and diagnosis relies on the clinical and electrodiagnostic evaluation. Given the very large number of peripheral nerve toxins, it is not possible to review all of them, and this chapter focuses on the most common toxins that cause clinically relevant peripheral neuropathy. Characteristic features of each disorder as well as general principles of neurotoxicology are emphasized. The toxins are organized into three categories: occupational and environmental exposures, recreational substance abuse, and iatrogenic exposures. Historically, occupational and environmental exposures provided the greatest risk of toxic neuropathy. However, with improving work conditions and careful precautions, these have become less frequent. Currently, the principal source of toxic neuropathies is prescription medication. Because of the users' socio-economic status, neuropathies from recreational substances have been more difficult to study in a systematic fashion.

1. INTRODUCTION

There are several general principle of neurotoxicology that are important to consider when evaluating patients with possible toxic neuropathy. Patients frequently question if prior or ongoing exposure has caused their peripheral neuropathy. In many cases, the agents in question have not been systematically studied and it may be impossible to conclusively exclude a relationship. The Bradford Hill criteria define an organized approach to addressing the issue of causation (Table 20.1). Before an agent can be judged to cause neuropathy, there must be a strong association between the potential toxin and neuropathy, appropriate timing of exposure and signs, a dose response effect, improvement following removal from exposure, an animal model, a consistent clinical spectrum across studies, and biological plausibility (is an etiological link consistent with current knowledge) (1,2). Full consideration of these criteria is useful in the clinical setting. Although it is unlikely that an agent not yet known to cause neuropathy will fulfill all criteria in a single clinical setting or outbreak, if many are met, an association or causal relationship becomes more likely, justifying public health efforts to reduce risk while experimental and epidemiological studies are undertaken.

Recognition of toxic neuropathy depends on a high index of suspicion. In some cases, a patient's occupation or a history of using a particular medication or substance of abuse will suggest the diagnosis. In many instances, however, the exposure history may not be readily apparent. Furthermore, diagnosis may be complicated by continued progression of the neuropathy for weeks or even months following cessation of exposure (coasting). Although the term coasting is most often used to refer to *n*-hexane neuropathy, the phenomenon is observed with many other toxins (3–5). Useful clinical features that suggest a toxic etiology include features atypical for idiopathic or typical metabolic neuropathies (e.g., diabetes). A subacute time-course or prominent weakness or sensory loss should prompt a particularly careful search for a toxic etiology.

Table 20.1 The Bradford Hill Criteria Outline an Organized Approach to Determine a Causal Relationship Between a Potential Toxin and Neuropathy

Strength of association: The stronger the relationship between the neuropathy and the toxic agent, the less likely it is that the relationship is due to some other variable.

Temporality: The toxic exposure must precede development of neuropathy.

Consistency: Multiple independent observations of an association by different investigators, using multiple techniques increase the likelihood of a casual association.

Theoretical plausibility: The relationship between neuropathy and the toxic agent should make theoretical sense.

Coherence: A cause-and-effect relationship is most likely when there is no conflict with what is known about the toxic agent and exposure and when there are no plausible competing theories or rival hypotheses.

Specificity in the causes: Ideally, the outcome (the specific type of neuropathy) should have only one cause. This criterion is uncommonly met in toxic neuropathy. However, the more distinctive the clinical syndrome, the more likely there is an association.

Dose–response relationship: Larger doses (exposures) should cause more severe neuropathy. The larger the exposure (dose) the more severe the neuropathy should be.

Experimental evidence: Cell culture and animal models of the toxic neuropathy support a direct causal relationship.

Analogy: Sometimes a commonly accepted phenomenon in one area can be applied to another area (e.g., nucleoside analog reverse transcriptase inhibitors).

Note: The more of the criteria are fulfilled, the more likely the association is valid and causative.

The electrodiagnostic evaluation is an important part of the diagnostic evaluation of toxic neuropathy. Most neurotoxins cause an axonal sensory motor peripheral neuropathy. Sensory nerve action potential amplitudes are reduced or absent in a length dependent fashion. Compound muscle action potential amplitudes may be reduced if there is significant motor axonal loss. Fibrillations and reduced recruitment of large motor units may be observed in distal muscles. Rare toxic neuropathies may cause primary demyelination, and the finding of demyelination of nerve conduction studies is one of the useful diagnostic clues (Table 20.2).

Table 20.2 Demyelinating Toxic Neuropathies: Demyelinating Neuropathies are Uncommon

n-Hexane
Suramin
Amiodarone
Perhexiline
Chloroquine
Cytosine arabinoside
Arsenic (rarely in the acute stage)
Tacrolimus
Procainamide
Gold

Note: When encountered, exposure to these agents should be sought. Toxins in italics are discussed in further detail in the text.

Patients with pre-existing peripheral neuropathy may be at risk to develop significant worsening of their neuropathy following exposure to neurotoxic medication (6). The best example of this phenomenon is the development of a severe motor neuropathy in patients with unrecognized Charcot–Marie–Tooth disease who receive vincristine chemotherapy (7). Care should be exercised when prescribing potentially neurotoxic medication to patients with underlying peripheral neuropathy, and alternative treatments should be used whenever possible.

2. OCCUPATIONAL AND ENVIRONMENTAL EXPOSURES

Occupational and environmental peripheral nerve toxicity is relatively uncommon in developed countries. Care must be taken when counseling patients with a possible exposure given the significant medical legal implications. The Bradford Hill criteria should be carefully evaluated. A number of chemicals have been studied and their role in peripheral neuropathy have been established. These include heavy metals, organo-phosphates, and organic solvents.

2.1. Heavy Metals

Occupational exposure to heavy metals has become increasingly rare with improvements in worker safety. Currently, the most common source of heavy metal exposure leading to peripheral neuropathy is intentional poisoning. The diagnosis of heavy metal neuropathy requires a high degree of suspicion. Although the neuropathy may be non-specific, the associated systemic features of heavy metal toxicity should suggest the correct diagnosis.

2.1.1. Lead

Because of its ease of malleability lead has historically been a popular agent in metallurgy. This is despite recognition of its adverse health effects even in antiquity. Lead toxicity most commonly occurs following ingestion of lead containing paints and from the mining industry. Toxicity from lead paint occurs in children who ingest paint flakes. Low socio-economic status is a major risk factor due to inhabitation of older homes that have not been renovated. Childhood lead toxicity causes an encephalopathy rather than neuropathy. Lead neuropathy usually occurs following occupational exposure. Industries at risk include lead smelting and refining, steel and iron factories, gasoline stations, and battery manufacturing (8). Miners may be exposed via inhalation during the smelting of ore to extract silver (9). There are several reports of lead neuropathy due to retained bullet fragments many years after a gunshot wound (10). Fortunately as a result of increasing governmental regulations significant industrial exposure to lead has diminished considerably.

As with other heavy metals, the systemic manifestations often suggest the diagnosis. Abdominal pain, constipation, and anemia are prominent in acute lead poisoning (11). Abdominal pain and constipation may not be as prominent with chronic toxicity. Occasionally, a lead line may appear in the gingiva of the mouth suggesting chronic exposure. Lead inhibits δ-aminolevulinic acid dehydrase, the rate limiting enzyme in heme biosynthesis. This results in a microcytic, hypochromic anemia with basophilic stippling. δ-Aminolevulinic can be detected in the urine.

Lead neuropathy is classically motor-predominant with little sensory involvement. In adults, it has a predilection for the upper limbs, in particular the nerves innervating wrist and finger extensor muscles. When the legs are involved, the neuropathy affects ankle dorsiflexors resulting in foot drop. Involvement of the lower extremities is more likely to occur in children than in adults (12). More recent data have called into question this classic pattern of weakness and suggest chronic industrial exposure leads to a sensory-predominant neuropathy primarily involving the legs (13). It seems likely that two forms of lead neuropathy exist: an acute intoxication leading to the classically described pattern of wrist drop and a chronic intoxication leading to a length-dependent sensory greater than motor neuropathy.

Most of the clinical experience predates the development of electromyography, and the electrophysiological changes are not well described. Similarly, because of co-morbidities and misdiagnoses, the pathology of the condition also has not been firmly established in humans. In a rat model of lead neuropathy, segmental demyelination is prominent (14). In humans, however, the available evidence suggests that the primary process is axonal loss (15).

The diagnosis of lead neuropathy is usually suggested by a typical pattern of weakness in association with anemia. If exposure is ongoing, the diagnosis may be confirmed by demonstrating elevated lead levels in the blood or a 24 h urine specimen. δ-Aminolevulinic levels are elevated in the urine of all patients with lead toxicity. If the exposure is not ongoing, these tests may be normal. It has been suggested that chelation with ethylene-diaminetetra-acetic acid (EDTA) may mobilize tissue lead that can then be measured in the urine (16). This approach has not been well studied, however, and diagnosis of lead neuropathy months after the exposure usually rests on recognition of the typical neuropathy, a plausible route of exposure, and exclusion of other etiologies.

Treatment must first be directed at removing the patient from the exposure. While controlled studies are lacking, chelation therapy is generally recommended, particularly if the blood levels are >10 μg/dL (17). There are several chelating agents available: dimercaprol (BAL), penicillamine, succimer, and EDTA. Which agent and route of administration are most effective remains debated.

Lead is believed to have its clinical effects via inhibition of heme synthesis by blocking the activity of δ-aminolevulinic acid dehydratase (18,19). This enzyme converts δ-aminolevulinic acid to porphobilinogen (a pyrole ring). Synthesis of hemoglobin and heme containing enzymes (e.g., mitochondrial electron transport chain cytochrome P450 enzymes) is disturbed.

2.1.2. Arsenic

Arsenic has had many uses throughout history. In antiquity, it was used for medicinal purposes. As recently as the early 20th century arsenic was used to treat syphilis and other infections because of its antibacterial effects. In more recent years, it has been used in pesticides and in the lumber industry as a wood preservative. Inorganic forms of arsenic are far more toxic than the organic form. Most organic exposures to arsenic are the result of seafood ingestion. Fish and shellfish absorb arsenic from the water in which they live. Organic exposures are relatively non-toxic and the arsenic is quickly excreted in the urine. Industrial exposure to inorganic arsenic has been described in the smelting industry (20,21). Neuropathy may occur following inhalation of smoke emanating from burning wood preserved with arsenic or from contaminated dust or soil (22). Exposure to contaminated water via wading or oral consumption may also result in toxicity (23). However, intentional poisoning, often with a rodenticide, is currently the most common cause of arsenic intoxication in the developed world (Fig 20.1).

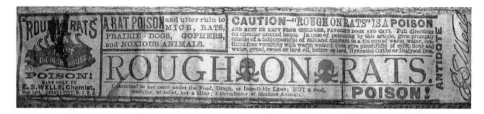

Figure 20.1   The most common source of arsenic is rodenticides. Rough on Rats was a late 19th century rat poison. A patient with acute arsenic neuropathy attempted suicide by ingesting this poison.

As with lead, acute arsenic intoxication commonly presents with systemic symptoms including severe abdominal pain, nausea, and diarrhea. Acute tubular necrosis may result in the need for hemodialysis (24). Acute arsenic poisoning often causes hematologic abnormalities including anemia and pancytopenia (25). In severe cases, vasomotor collapse and death occur within hours. Those that survive the cardiovascular insult develop a progressive neuropathy over weeks (26). The initial manifestations are distal pain and sensory loss. Weakness typically follows in a length dependent fashion. When severe, proximal muscles are also affected. Reflexes are preserved early on, suggesting a primary axonal rather than demyelinating insult. Given the prodrome of abdominal pain and diarrhea, acute arsenic poisoning may be confused with the Gullain–Barré syndrome (acute inflammatory demyelinating polyradiculoneuropathy). Diagnostic clues for arsenic toxicity include prominent sensory loss, pain, distal predominance, and hematologic abnormalities.

A variety of cutaneous manifestations of arsenic poisoning have been described. Acute dermatologic findings include facial edema and desquamation of the palms and soles (Fig. 20.2) (27). A pale transverse line in the finger and toe nails (Mee's lines) is the most commonly recognized finding (28). Mee's are visible several weeks following acute intoxication, and are only useful diagnostically later in the disease course, or in patients with repeated exposures.

Chronic arsenic exposure may also cause slowly progressive distal sensory loss, pain, and mild weakness. Abdominal pain and diarrhea are not characteristic. Other systemic features include chronic lung disease and hepatotoxicity due to liver fibrosis. Dermatologic features include hyperkeratosis and skin cancer (23,29).

The results of electrodiagnostic studies depend on the timing of the study. If performed within the first 1–2 weeks of the illness elements of partial motor conduction block may be observed (30). This finding is thought to be due to acute axonal injury rather than segmental demyelination. After several weeks of progression, axonal features predominate including prominent fibrillation potentials. Pathologic data support primary axonal loss. There is no specific nerve biopsy change associated with arsenic toxicity (26).

Diagnosis of arsenic intoxication rests on recognition of the systemic features in association with the characteristic neuropathy. A history of recognized exposure is usually absent, or difficult to establish, especially before the diagnosis is confirmed. The diagnosis is confirmed by measuring urinary arsenic in a 24 h sample. Because arsenic is deposited in hair and nails, it may be detected in these sites for many weeks or months following exposure. CSF examination reveals elevated protein without pleocytosis.

The mechanisms underlying arsenic toxicity to nerve are unclear. Arsenic binds to sulfhydryl groups, resulting in the disruption of over 200 enzymes. Cellular energy

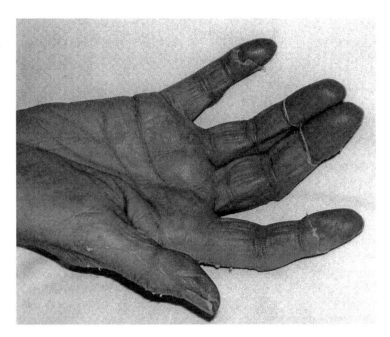

Figure 20.2 Arsenic toxicity may cause a variety of cutaneous manifestations, including peeling of the skin on the hands and feet. Acrylamide toxicity may also cause peeling palms.

systems, including respiratory chain enzymes, are affected and oxidative phosphorylation is uncoupled. Different mechanisms may underlie carcinogenesis (31).

Treatment is similar to that of lead intoxication. The principal therapy is removal from the exposure. Chelating agents have been utilized to both increase arsenic excretion and block its biological effects. Rigorous examination on the effects of chelating agents has failed to demonstrate clear benefit. In addition, it should be noted that the neuropathy of arsenic intoxication may continue to worsen for a few weeks after treatment is begun. The chelating agent of choice remains debated. Traditionally, intramuscular dimercaprol (BAL) has been used at a dose of 3–5 mg/kg of body weight administered intramuscularly every 4 h for 2 days, every 6 h for 1 day, and then every 12 h for 10 days (Hu, 2001). Because intramuscular BAL is painful and has a low therapeutic index, newer chelating agents have been suggested to replace BAL. These include 2,3-dimercaptopropanesulphonate sodium (DMPS) and meso-2,3-demercaptosuccinic acid (DMSA). It remains debated if these newer agents result in improved outcomes (32). In cases of renal failure, hemodialysis may be necessary to remove the chelator-arsenic compounds. Recovery of the neuropathy following arsenic intoxication is prolonged and often incomplete.

2.1.3. Thallium

Thallium was utilized in the 1800s as a treatment for tuberculosis and is currently used in commercial insecticides. As with arsenic, a majority of thallium intoxications today occur in the form of intentional poisoning. Exposure to thallium can be through skin, inhalation, or via oral ingestion.

The presentation is very similar to arsenic intoxication. Acute intoxication causes abdominal pain, nausea, and diarrhea followed by an ascending sensorimotor neuropathy.

Unlike arsenic neuropathy, cranial nerve involvement with severe thallium intoxication is not uncommon (33). The hallmark of thallium intoxication is alopecia, which typically begins ~2 weeks after the exposure and involves the scalp more than other areas of hair growth (34).

The diagnostic approach is the same as for the other metals: confirming increased level in blood, a 24 h urine sample, or hair and nails. Treatment is similar to the other metals, with elimination of the source of toxicity as the first step. There is no evidence that chelating agents are useful (35). Other treatments attempted have included forced diuresis, dialysis, and Prussian blue therapy, but none are of proven efficacy (35). Treatment at this point is largely supportive. Recovery is slow given the axonal nature to the neuropathy. If the neuropathy is severe, recovery is often incomplete.

2.1.4. Mercury

Mercury toxicity in the past has generally occurred as an occupational exposure. During the 19th century, inorganic mercury salts were used in felt hat industry, leading to the phrase "Mad as a Hatter." Mercury exposure can come in the form of elemental, inorganic, or organic mercury. Elemental mercury is poorly absorbed from the gastrointestinal tract, with nearly all being eliminated in feces. However, vaporized elemental mercury is readily absorbed by inhalation. Inorganic mercury is principally absorbed via the gastrointestinal tract or transdermally. Organic mercury can be absorbed via the gastrointestinal tract or via inhalation (36).

Mercury toxicity primarily affects the central nervous system, resulting in cognitive disturbance, tremor, and ataxia. Gingivitis may be observed (36). A sensory predominant peripheral neuropathy is common, although it is nearly always overshadowed by central nervous system disease. Dorsal root ganglia neurons may be particularly sensitive to mercury salts (37). The principal pathologic lesions are located within the visual cortex, cerebellar vermis, and the postcentral cortex (38).

Diagnosis is made by demonstrating increased mercury content in the 24 h urine sample and confirmed by quantitating mercury content in the blood. Treatment focuses on removal from the exposure and chelation. The chelation agent of choice depends on the temporal profile of the exposure. In acute intoxications with mercury salts dimercaprol (BAL) is preferred (39). N-Acetyl penicillamine was designed specifically as a mercury chelator and may ultimately be the preferred chelator in humans (40). It may have a superior side effect profile compared with D, L-penicillamine, and a similar side effect profile to D-penicillamine with stronger binding of mercury than either. N-Acetyl penicillamine remains experimental and is not widely available for human use (41).

2.2. Organophosphates

Organophosphates are potent inhibitors of acetylcholinesterase, the enzyme responsible for degrading acetylcholine. Because of this action, these agents have been utilized as pesticides in the agrochemical industry and as agents of chemical warfare. Organophosphates have industrial application as petroleum additives and softeners in the plastics industry. Exposure may occur transdermally, via the respiratory tree or from the gastrointestinal tract. The most common source of exposure is pesticide use in the agricultural industry, although cases of intentional poisoning may also occur.

Organophosphate intoxication occurs in two phases: an acute syndrome with prominent neuromuscular weakness and autonomic features and a delayed length-dependent peripheral neuropathy. The acute phase is due to blockade of both muscarinic and nicotinic acetylcholine receptors resulting in acute cholinergic overload. Abdominal cramping, diarrhea, excessive lacrimation and salivation occur within the first few hours following exposure. Weakness follows due to depolarizing blockade of the post-synaptic neuromuscular junction (42). Weakness is generalized, involving proximal, distal, and cranial nerve innervated muscles. With supportive therapy, weakness resolves in 1–2 weeks.

The acute phase may be followed by a length-dependent peripheral neuropathy. Onset is usually several weeks following exposure and it may be progressive and severe (42). Distal weakness and atrophy are prominent and overshadow sensory loss. Reflexes remain relatively preserved, suggesting that the neuropathy is predominately axonal.

Diagnosis requires the identification of an appropriate exposure. Quantitation of erythrocyte acetylcholinesterase or plasma cholinesterase can be used for the confirmation of acute toxicity. Autonomic symptoms begin at 40–50% enzymatic inhibition and neuromuscular blockage at 80% inhibition (43). Electrodiagnostic testing may reveal multiple afterpotentials following the compound muscle action potential due to depolarizing blockade of post-synaptic acetylcholine receptors. A decremental response to repetitive nerve stimulation may also be observed, reflecting the defect of neuromuscular transmission that accompanies the acute form of toxicity. These findings are similar to those seen in some congenital myasthenic syndromes.

Diagnosis of organophosphate-induced neuropathy rests on recognition of an appropriate exposure in a patient with a progressive motor greater than sensory neuropathy. Electrodiagnostic studies demonstrate an axonal neuropathy. There are no specific pathologic features and nerve biopsy reveals axonal loss without evidence of demyelination (44).

Organophosphates neuropathy is thought to be due to inhibition of the enzyme neurotoxic esterase (45). The organophosphate esters that cause permanent inhibition of neurotoxic esterase are the most toxic. Less potent agents require repeated or prolonged exposure before causing neuropathy. Occasionally, neuropathy may occur following a single large exposure of the more common but less potent agents. There is no known effective treatment of the organophosphate-induced delayed neuropathy. Only supportive and symptomatic care is available. Acute toxicity can be treated with atropine to block the muscarinic effects (symptoms of gastrointestinal distress, excessive lacrimation and salivation). Atropine does not prevent nicotinic mediated symptoms (neuromuscular blockade). Pralidoxime (PAM) may prevent weakness if given soon after the exposure. PAM reactivates acetylcholinesterase if the organophosphates have not yet irreversibly inactivated the enzyme (43). Randomized controlled clinical trials of PAM in acute organophosphate poisoning, however, have not performed (46).

2.3. Organic Solvents

Patients often question if their neuropathy could be due to occupational exposure to toxic chemicals. Concern is often highest among individuals who have a history of exposure to organic solvents. In considering the question of exposure, the clinician must carefully evaluate the Bradford Hill criteria. Often, the exposure occurred years before the onset of symptoms, and an association is doubtful. In other instances, the chemical in question has not been linked to peripheral neuropathy and examination of other exposed individuals may be informative. Several organic solvents have been shown to cause neuropathy, including acrylamide, carbon disulfide, ethylene oxide, and triorthocresylphosphate. Fortunately, neuropathy secondary to industrial solvent exposure is very rare in the developed world. N-Hexane is probably the most common neurotoxic solvent. Because exposure typically occurs in the setting of recreational drug abuse, this agent is considered in the following section.

2.3.1. Acrylamide

Acrylamide is used industrially as either a monomer or a polymer. The polymer is widely used as a flocculator (a substance used to separate suspended solids from liquids) and as a grouting agent. The polymer itself is generally considered to be nontoxic. However, acrylamide monomer, which serves as a precursor to the various polymers, is highly toxic. Acrylamide is absorbed through many routes, including transdermally and trans-bronchially. The transdermal route is believed to be more important than inhalation in the development of neuropathy (47).

Acrylamide toxicity causes a length-dependent sensory and motor neuropathy with distal weakness involving the hands and feet and sensory loss to all modalities. Ataxia and generalized hyporeflexia are more prominent that in other axonal neuropathies. Data from animal models suggest that this is due to a direct toxic effect on muscle spindles (48,49). An important diagnostic clue is the frequent development of an exfoliative dermatitis involving the hands prior to the onset of neuropathy (50). Patients may develop bother-some hyperhidrosis of the hands and feet, a finding unusual in other causes of peripheral neuropathy (51).

The pathology of acrylamide neuropathy has been established primarily in animal models. There is a loss of large fibers without evidence of demyelination. The character-istic finding is axonal swellings, particularly at the nerve terminals and the prenodal spaces. This is the result of accumulation of neurofilaments due to impaired axonal trans-port (52). This may give the appearance of paranodal demyelination. Limited data from human pathology is consistent with the animal data (53). There is more recent data suggesting there is also prominent injury to small unmeylinated cutaneous nerve fibers and sudomotor fibers (54,55).

In humans, the electrophysiological studies are in keeping with an axonal neuro-pathy. The sensory nerve action potential and compound muscle action potential ampli-tudes are reduced with preservation of the conduction velocities and distal latencies. The findings are in general symmetrical. CSF examination is usually normal (51).

Treatment is limited to removing the offending exposure. Recovery generally depends on the severity of the deficits. Those with mild deficits may recover without sequelae. Those with more advanced deficits are typically left with some residual distal motor and sensory deficits.

2.3.2. Carbon Disulfide

Carbon disulfide is used primarily in the production of synthetic polymers and cellophane. Toxicity results from inhalation. In acute high-dose exposures, psychosis and delirium are the principal manifestations. With chronic low dose exposure, a peripheral neuropathy is common. This may or may not occur in the setting of an extrapyramidal disorder (56).

The neuropathy associated with chronic low-dose exposure is a length-dependent axonal neuropathy. There is distal loss of sensation to all modalities and weakness in a symmetrical fashion. The electrophysiological features are consistent with axonal loss. Peripheral nerve pathology is similar to acrylamide neuropathy including axonal swelling secondary to neurofilament accumulation. There also appears to be some central effects with loss of fibers in the spinal cord tracts (57). There is no treatment other than removal from the exposure. As with acrylamide neuropathy, recovery depends on the severity of the deficits. Residual deficits are common in more severely affected patients.

2.3.3. Ethylene Oxide

Ethylene oxide is an epoxide used to sterilize materials that are otherwise heat sensitive and cannot be sterilized in other manners. Toxic exposure in humans is believed to occur via inhalation. An outbreak has been reported among operating room staff exposed to residual ethylene oxide from sterilization of operating room gowns (58). A sensory and motor neuropathy may be the only manifestation of this agent's toxicity, but encephalopathy also occurs (58,59). Residual ethylene oxide within dialyzers following sterilization may contribute to the peripheral neuropathy in chronic renal failure patients undergoing dialysis, and there are some data from cell culture models supporting this hypothesis (60,61). Electrodiagnostic studies are consistent with an axonal neuropathy. Pathology from animal models demonstrates a distal axonopathy (62,63).

2.3.4. Triorthocresylphosphate

Triorthocresylphosphate (TOCP) is an organophosphate ester. Because of its industrial use and similarities to the other industrial neurotoxins, it is discussed here rather than with the organophosphates above. TOCP is used primarily as a softener and a lubricant in industrial plastics production. Toxic exposure may occur transdermally, via inhalation or through the gastrointestinal tract. Currently, the most common source of intoxication is by ingestion of contaminated cooking oil (64). TOCP is of significant historical interest in the USA. In the early 1930s, there was a large outbreak of paralysis due to ingestion of a ginger extract (Jamaica Ginger of "Jake") containing TOCP that was intended to circumvent alcohol prohibition, and many thousands were left with permanent paralysis before the association with the "Jake" was confirmed (65). Acute exposure may cause gastrointestinal distress due to cholinergic overactivity, although neuromuscular blockade does not occur. One to two weeks after exposure, a motor greater than sensory axonal peripheral neuropathy develops. Spasticity and gait ataxia develop following the neuropathy due to a superimposed myelopathy. Although some recovery is possible, most patients are left with distal weakness and spasticity. As with other organophosphates, TOCPs neurotoxicity likely due to inhibition of neurotoxic esterase.

3. RECREATIONAL SUBSTANCE ABUSE

Substance abuse commonly causes central nervous system toxicity. However, the frequency and importance of peripheral neuropathy is underappreciated. Several agents including alcohol, n-hexane, and nitrous oxide have been associated with peripheral nerve disease. As with most toxic neuropathies, a high index of suspicion and a careful history will disclose a possible association. The medical history may be particularly challenging in a suspected substance abuser and establishing a trusting relationship with the patient is particularly important.

3.1. Alcohol

The association between heavy alcohol use and peripheral neuropathy has been recognized for over 200 years. It has been estimated that peripheral neuropathy occurs in ~10% of chronic alcoholics (66). The most common form of alcoholic neuropathy is an indolently progressive sensory predominant axonal neuropathy. Severe dysesthetic pain is common and sural nerve biopsy confirms prominent small fiber injury (67). As the neuropathy progresses, motor weakness and atrophy may develop in a length-dependent fashion.

More recently it has been recognized alcoholics may develop an acute neuropathy resembling the Guillain–Barré syndrome (67,68). Acute neuropathy is typically painful and is often associated with other systemic features of malnutrition and hepatic dysfunction. Differentiation from Guillain–Barré syndrome is made by the spinal fluid findings (normal protein and cell count with alcohol) and by electrophysiology (axonal loss rather than demyelination with alcohol) (68). Sural nerve biopsies typically show loss of large and small myelinated and unmyelinated fibers without evidence of demyelination or inflammation. In one series, five subjects were treated with oral vitamin supplementation and abstinence of alcohol and all improved (68).

The etiology of alcoholic neuropathy continues to be debated. Chronic alcohol use is associated with a number of possible confounding co-morbidities including alcoholic liver disease and malnutrition. The extent to which neuropathy is directly due to the toxic effects of alcohol as opposed to chronic illness and malnutrition is unclear. Animal models have resulted in conflicting evidence. In one rat model, alcohol induces minor axonal injury when nutritional status is controlled (69). In another rat model, no peripheral nerve abnormalities could be induced with chronic alcohol ingestion (70). Primate models have also failed to demonstrate any evidence of neurotoxicity with chronic ethanol ingestion (71). There is substantial evidence to suggest that in humans malnutrition is a major contributor to the peripheral neuropathy in alcoholics, on the basis of similarities of the clinical findings between alcoholic neuropathy and beri–beri (66,72,73). The link was further supported when beri–beri was found to be due to thiamine deficiency and the well known risk of thiamine deficiency in chronic alcoholics.

More recent clinical and pathological data indicate that patients with alcoholic neuropathy are clinically and pathologically distinct from non-alcoholic patients with thiamine deficiency. The former have prominent pain and small fiber loss on biopsy, whereas the latter have a more acute, motor predominant neuropathy with large fiber loss on nerve biopsy. Alcoholic patients with thiamine deficiency have variable pathological and clinical features (67). These data suggests both direct toxicity and nutritional deficiency are important clinical factors.

Treatment of alcohol-associated neuropathy is directed at improving nutritional intake and abstinence from alcohol. In the acute setting, intravenous or intramuscular vitamin therapy should be given.

3.2. Hexacarbons

N-Hexane is a commonly used organic solvent that has industrial application as a solvent and degreaser, and household application in glues, rubber cement, and spray paint. Chronic exposure in an industrial setting leads to a progressive sensory neuropathy followed by progressive distal weakness. Pain is common. The electrophysiological features are those of axonal loss. A wide variety of industries use n-hexane and outbreaks have been reported in the automotive maintenance, printing, ball manufacturing, roofing, and shoe industries among others (74–78).

The most common route of exposure of n-hexane is via recreational inhalation of glue, rubber cement, or spray paint. Abuse of these substances is gaining in popularity because they are legal and inexpensive. Patients typically present with a subacute progressive neuropathy with prominent weakness and amyotrophy (3). Workers who are exposed to large quantities may have neuropathy similar to that seen in huffers. In extreme cases, there may be confusion with Guillain–Barré syndrome. A characteristic feature of n-hexane neuropathy is continued progression for weeks after removal from exposure (coasting) (3).

In the subacute setting, multifocal conduction block is commonly observed on electrodiagnostic studies, presumably due to thinning of the myelin over areas of axonal enlargements (79,80). A failure to recognize this pattern may lead to a misdiagnosis of acute or chronic inflammatory demyelinating polyradiculoneuropathy. As the neuropathy progresses, conduction block resolves and there is a progressive decline in motor amplitudes are observed because of axonal injury.

The diagnosis should be suspected in any individual with a subacute neuropathy or in those with a progressive neuropathy and a plausible source of exposure. In the subacute setting, nerve conduction studies may be very useful. 2–5 Hexanedione, the toxic metabolite of *n*-hexane, may be measured in acid hydrolyzed urine samples (81). This test is only useful in patients with ongoing exposure. Unlike most other toxic neuropathies, nerve biopsy is of significant diagnostic utility. In addition to a loss of large myelinated axons, prominent axonal swellings are observed (Fig. 20.3). These "giant axons" are morphologically similar to those seen in acrylamide and inherited giant axonal neuropathy (53). They are due to cross linking of intermediate neurofilaments by 2–5 hexanedione. The crosslinking of neurofilaments leads to neuropathy by disrupting axonal transport.

Treatment of *n*-hexane neuropathy is directed at removal of the offending inhalant. As with other forms of substance abuse, this can prove challenging. Recovery from mild neuropathy is excellent (82). Patients with more severe neuropathy may have incomplete recovery.

3.3. Nitrous Oxide

Abuse of nitrous oxide, a commonly used inhalational anesthetic, may cause a length-dependent peripheral neuropathy and myelopathy clinically indistinguishable from the

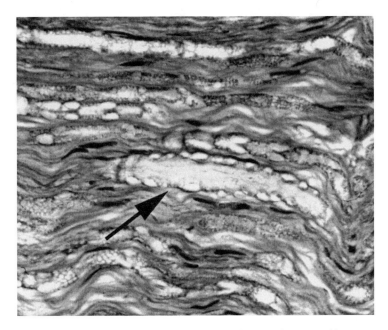

Figure 20.3 Axonal swellings are observed in several neuropathies, most prominently *n*-hexane toxicity and giant axonal neuropathy. Sural nerve biopsy from a patient with *n*-hexane toxicity demonstrates axonal enlargements due to accumulation of neurofilaments (arrow).

severe combined degeneration of vitamin B_{12} deficiency, despite normal serum B_{12} levels (83). Patients presents with progressive sensory loss, myelopathic findings, and other describe a Lhermitte's sign (83). It has been proposed that nitrous oxide interferes with the metabolism or effect of vitamin B_{12}; an animal model supports this hypothesis (84). Given ease of access, dentists represent the majority of subjects with nitrous oxide induced neuropathy due to abuse. However, recreation inhalation of nitrous oxide canisters used in whipped cream dispensers represents an increasingly common source of exposure (85,86). Patients with unrecognized B_{12} deficiency may be at high risk of developing a malignant form of severe combined degeneration following nitrous oxide anesthesia. A complete evaluation for subclinical B_{12} deficiency should be undertaken prior to nitric oxide exposure in any individual with symptoms of neuropathy or laboratory findings suggesting B_{12} deficiency (mild macrocytosis) (87–90).

Treatment of nitrous oxide myeloneuropathy includes replacement of vitamin B_{12} in those patients who are deficient. There is one report that methionine therapy may be beneficial (91).

4. IATROGENIC TOXIC NEUROPATHIES

Peripheral neuropathy is a reported side effect for a large number of medications, and iatrogenic neuropathies have become increasingly prevalent as the number of pharmacological agents increases (Table 20.3). The following section focuses on agents for which the peripheral neuropathy is a prominent complication and, in many instances, the dose-limiting side effect.

Table 20.3 Commonly Used Drugs Known to Induce Peripheral Neuropathy

Allopurinol	Indomethacin
Amiodarone	Isoniazid
Amitriptyline	Levamisole
Carbamide	Levodopa
Carboplatin	Lithium
Chlorambucil	Metronidazole
Chloramphenicol	Nitrofurantoin
Chloroquine	Oxaliplatin
Cisplatin	Pentazocine
Colchicine	Perhexiline
Cyclobenzaprine	Phenelzine
Dapsone	Phenytoin
Disopyramide	Procainamide
Disulfiram	Propafenone
Ethanol	Propranolol
Fluorouracil	Pyridoxine
Gentamycin	Sulfasalazine
Glutethimide	Suramin
Gold	Thalidomide
Hydralazine	Vancomycin
Hydroxyurea	Vincristine
Imipramine	

4.1. Antineoplastic Agents

Many cancer chemotherapeutic agents cause a peripheral neuropathy. The neuropathy is frequently dose-dependent and in many cases dose limiting. The neuropathy often improves following discontinuation of treatment; however, the degree of recovery depends on the magnitude of the maximal deficit, and in more severe cases recovery is incomplete.

4.1.1. Platinum Agents

The prototypical agent is cisplatin. Cisplatin exerts its antitumor effects by binding to DNA and preventing replication. It is commonly used to treat ovarian and other germ line tumors. Neuropathy is dose-dependent, and the incidence of neuropathy approaches 100% with high doses (92). The clinical features are distinctive. Sensory loss occurs in a length-dependent fashion, and in severe cases, a gait ataxia results that may leave the patient wheelchair bound. Weakness does not occur. Neuropathy often worsens for months after therapy has been discontinued (93). Although most patients improve, residual signs and symptoms are common. The electrophysiological findings are consistent with an exclusively sensory axonal neuropathy (reduced amplitude or absent sensory nerve action potentials).

There are cell culture, animal, and pathologic data suggesting cisplatin is directly toxic to dorsal root ganglia (94–96). The mechanism of neurotoxicity is unknown but likely involves binding of platinum to sensory neuron DNA causing apoptotic cell death (96,97). There is also experiment evidence of abnormal axonal transport and protein synthesis (96,98,99).

There is interest in preventing cisplatin neuropathy to allow higher doses to be given. Preclinical data suggest a fragment of adrenal corticotrophic hormone (ACTH 4–9) is effective (100), but clinical trials have provided mixed results (101,102). More recent data suggest delivery of nerve growth factor (NGF) or neurotrophic factor 3 (NT3) to dorsal root ganglia neurons by infection with a herpes simplex virus vector may prevent neuropathy in a rat model (103). No controlled human studies of NT3 or NGF have been performed to date.

Carboplatin is another platinum based anti-tumor agent that also causes peripheral neuropathy similar to that due to cisplatin, however, it is much less common and less severe when it occurs. Furthermore, unlike with cisplatin neuropathy, motor involvement occasionally occurs with carboplatin toxicity (104).

4.1.2. Vinca Alkaloids

Vincristine is the most neurotoxic of the vinca alkaloids. Vincristine is derived from the periwinkle plant and is used predominately against myelogenous neoplasms. Vincristine disrupts microtubule assembly and degradation, thus interfering with axonal transport. The neuropathy associated with vincristine can be severe and may limit its use. The neuropathy is typically length dependent affecting both motor and sensory modalities. A prominent feature is the early loss of reflexes due to direct muscle spindle toxicity. Despite this, the H-reflex is preserved on electrodiagnostic testing, a finding distinct from other neuropathies (105). Although cranial neuropathies are uncommon, they may occur (106). The neuropathy typically improves after treatment has been discontinued. The degree of improvement is dependent on the magnitude of the maximum deficit. Nerve conduction studies are consistent with an axonal neuropathy. Very early in the neuropathy, there is the unique finding of a preserved H-reflex with an absent Achilles tendon reflex due to isolated muscle spindle injury.

Patients with Charcot–Marie–Tooth disease type 1 may be at risk to develop a very severe neuropathy when exposed to vincristine (7,107–109). Patients with a family history of CMT 1 should have genetic testing.

4.1.3. Taxanes

Paclitaxel and its synthetic analog, decetaxel, are taxanes that have tumorcidal properties against a variety of solid and myelogenous neoplasms. With development of bone marrow stimulating proteins, peripheral neuropathy has become a dose limiting side effect. Like vincristine, these agents interfere with microtubule processing. Unlike vincristine, the neuropathy is sensory-predominant (110). As with cisplatin the neuropathy may progress after therapy has been discontinued; however, progression typically does not occur beyond ~1 month (111). The electrophysiology is consistent with an axonal sensory greater than motor peripheral neuropathy.

4.1.4. Suramin

Suramin was initially used as an anti-parasitic agent, but recently it has been used to treat a variety of cancers. The mechanism of its anti-tumor effects is uncertain but is believed to be based on its interaction with trophic pathways (112). Its mechanism of neurotoxicity is unknown. Suramin causes two types of peripheral neuropathy: a more common chronic axonal length-dependent sensory and motor neuropathy, and an uncommon subacute demyelinating polyradiculoneuropathy. It is not clear whether the chronic form is a toxic effect of a high peak level or a cumulative effect of an ongoing exposure, but it is typically mild and resolves slowly after the suramin is discontinued (113).

The subacute demyelinating polyradiculoneuropathy is more severe and occurs in ~10% of patients treated with suramin (113). The clinical syndrome and pathology are indistinguishable from acute inflammatory demyelinating polyradiculoneuropathy (Guillain–Barré syndrome). The response to immunotherapy has been indeterminate (113–115).

4.1.5. Cytosine Arabinoside

Cytosine Arabinoside, or Ara-C, is an anti-neoplastic agent used to treat myelogenous neo-plasms. Although neuropathy is a rare complication, it can be severe and disabling. The peripheral neuropathy typically occurs in one of two forms: a pure sensory neuropathy or an acute demyelinating polyradiculoneuropathy. The acute demyelinating polyradicu-loneuropathy may be severe and, as with suramin, is indistinguishable from acute inflam-matory demyelinating polyradiculoneuropathy (Guillain–Barré syndrome). Sural nerve biopsy demonstrates segmental demyelination mixed with axonal degeneration with Wallerian degeneration (116). The mechanism of neurotoxicity is not known.

4.1.6. Thalidomide

Thalidomide was approved in the early 1960s as a sedative. Reports of neurotoxicity at that time were overshadowed by its teratogenic effects, leading to its withdrawal from the market in 1962 (117). It is now prescribed for treatment of hematological malignancies and dermatitis herpetaformis. Peripheral neuropathy is common and is frequently the dose-limiting side effect (118). In one series, 53% of subjects receiving thalidomide had to stop treatment because of peripheral neuropathy (119). The risk for neuropathy appears to be dose dependent (119,120).

The neuropathy is primarily sensory with distal painful paresthesias. Motor involvement may occur, but is less prominent (121). There is evidence suggesting involvement of the dorsal root ganglia (122). Recovery following removal of the thalidomide is variable; in one series of long-term follow-up (4–6 years) approximately one-forth recovered completely, one-fourth improved with residual deficits and one-half failed to improve (123). Nerve conduction studies have been proposed as a means to screen for the early development of peripheral neuropathy. Baseline nerve conduction studies should be obtained within 3 months of starting and every 3–6 months thereafter. If sensory nerve action potential amplitudes drop by $\geq 50\%$ then the thalidomide should be discontinued (124). However, in one series clinical features preceded electrophysiological findings in 41% of their subjects, indicating careful clinical examinations are necessary so that treatment can be discontinued prior to the development of a more clinically significant neuropathy (119).

4.2. Amphiphilic Cationic Drugs

Amphiphilic cationic drugs are a group of lipophilic agents that are resistant to lysosomal degradation; drugs in this class include amiodarone, perhexiline, and chloroquine. These agents may cause a peripheral neuropathy, and while the clinical features vary, each agent causes the accumulation of osmiophilic lamellar lysosomal inclusions in fibroblasts and Schwann cells (125). Amiodarone and perhexline are distinctive in that they cause demyelinating neuropathy, likely because of direct Schwann cell injury due to lysosomal dysfunction (126). Chloroquine primarily causes a prominent myopathy and will not be discussed further.

4.2.1. Amiodarone

Amiodarone is a potent anti-arrhythmic used in cardiac disease. It is unique in that it has an extremely long half-life, exceeding 30 days in most individuals. The neuropathy typically begins months after treatment has begun and because of the long half-life continues to worsen for months after the drug is discontinued. Numbness and tingling of the feet are the first symptoms. Progressive weakness may follow and in extreme cases can become quite severe. Reflexes are reduced or absent. Other manifestations include a tremor and ataxia (127–130). Unlike most toxic neuropathies, electrophysiologic testing reveals a demyelinating neuropathy. CSF examination may show mildly elevated protein. Because of these findings, severe cases of amiodarone induced neuropathy may be confused with CIDP (131). Serum creatinine phosphokinase levels may be increased due to a concomitant myopathy. Patients may experience significant improvement, although recovery is slow because of the prolonged half-life.

4.2.2. Perhexiline

Perhexiline is used to treat coronary artery disease. The neuropathy involves both sensory and motor fibers, and like amiodarone neuropathy it can become very severe, resulting in both proximal and distal weakness. Facial weakness of papilledema may occur. Electrodiagnostic testing reveals a demyelinating neuropathy (132–134). Pathologic examination reveals segmental demyelination in addition to axonal loss. Lysosomal lamellar inclusions are observed in Schwann cells (135). The neuropathy improves with discontinuation of the perhexiline.

4.3. Other Drugs

4.3.1. Anti-human Immunodeficiency Virus Drugs

There are several classes of anti-HIV drugs including nucleoside analog reverse transcriptase inhibitors, non-nucleoside analog reverse transcriptase inhibitors, and protease inhibitors. All members of the first class cause peripheral neuropathy, except for zidovudine, which causes a myopathy (Table 20.4) (136). The neuropathy is clinically similar to the painful sensory neuropathy of HIV. Weight loss, low CD4 count, diabetes, pre-existing neuropathy and substance use may be predisposing factors (137,138). Symptoms may have a rapid onset, a useful feature in distinguishing toxic from HIV neuropathy (4). Symptoms improve after discontinuation of the suspected agent, although a several week period of coasting is expected. Electrodiagnostic testing reveals sensory predominant axonal loss and nerve biopsy has revealed preferential injury to small nerve fibers. The mechanism of nerve injury is thought to be related to toxicity to mitochondrial DNA (136,139). Zidovudine, which does not cause a peripheral neuropathy, causes a myopathy with features of mitochondrial dysfunction.

Non-nucleoside analogs and protease inhibitors do not cause neuropathy. The combination of two reverse transcriptase inhibitors and a protease inhibitors (highly active antiretroviral therapy—HAART) has resulted in a dramatic reduction in HIV related disease. HAART therapy may cause a lipodystrophy that consists of central adiposdity and peripheral fat wasting. Peripheral neuropathy may be observed. A prospective study of 112 patients suggested the combination of dadanosine (ddI) and stavudine (d4T) may be particularly prone to cause neuropathy.

4.3.2. Colchicine

Colchicine is a potent inhibitor of microtubule assembly and as a result has anti-mitotic properties. Its use in high doses commonly causes a unique neuromuscular syndrome consisting of a mild length-dependent sensory and motor peripheral neuropathy in combination with a severe proximal myopathy (140–142). Electrodiagnostic testing reveals an axonal neuropathy with fibrillations in proximal muscles where there is increased recruitment of myopathic appearing motor units (143). Because of the neuropathy and proximal weakness, the unwary examiner may mistakenly conclude the patient suffers from a polyradiculopathy. Serum CPK is elevated an muscle biopsy confirms the presence of the myopathy with vacuolar inclusions distributed centrally within the fibers or in the subsarcolemma zone. The neuropathy is not a significant cause of disability. Both the neuropathy and myopathy improve following discontinuation of colchicine.

4.3.3. Pyridoxine

Pyridoxine, vitamin B_6, is an over-the-counter nutritional supplement. Pyridoxine has been prescribed as a treatment for a variety of ailments including carpal tunnel syndrome

Table 20.4 Nucleoside Analog Reverse Transcriptase Inhibitors Known to Cause Peripheral Neuropathy

Stavudine
Fialuridine
Didanosine
Emtricitabine
Lamivudine
Zalcitabine

and pre-menstrual syndrome. High doses of pyridoxine (grams per day) may cause a severe sensory ganglionopathy with little recovery after discontinuation of the agent (144,145). Patients present with rapidly progressive loss of large fiber sensory modalities including joint position sense resulting in sensory ataxia and pseudoathetosis. The pathology demonstrates profound neuronal loss in the dorsal root ganglion the presumed site of action for the pyridoxine induced toxicity. Chronic lower dose exposure (several hundred milligram per day) may cause a less severe length-dependent sensory neuropathy. As with other toxic neuropathy, continued progression of symptoms following discontinuation has been described (5,146). The mechanism of sensory neuron injury is unknown. Data from a rat model suggest gene therapy with transfer of NT3 to dorsal root ganglia using herpes simplex virus is protective (147).

4.3.4. Nitrofurantoin

Nitrofurantoin is a commonly used antibiotic in the treatment of urinary tract infections. Neuropathy is a rare complication (148). Its importance is out of proportion to its frequency because the neuropathy causes rapidly progressive large fiber sensory loss and weakness (149,150). Elderly patients with renal failure are at highest risk (151). The only therapy is withdrawal of the agent. Early recognition of the neuropathy is very important given recovery is typically incomplete. The mechanism is not known.

5. SUMMARY

Toxins are an important cause of peripheral neuropathy. Exposure can occur in the workplace, from medical therapy or from substance abuse. Most toxins cause an axonal sensory predominant neuropathy. In these cases, diagnosis rests on the recognition of associated systemic features and the history of exposure. Some toxic neuropathies (e.g., high dose pyridoxine) cause a characteristic clinical syndrome that should suggest the correct diagnosis. Typically, once the appropriate exposure is recognized, the diagnosis is easy to confirm. While specific therapy is available for some toxins, treatment for most consists of removing the patient from the offending exposure. Prevention is the most important approach to toxic neuropathy. Industry and the Federal Government have made considerable progress in the last 50 years if efforts to protect workers from occupational exposure to known neurotoxins. Education of medical professionals regarding the neurotoxic side effects of commonly used medications is an important preventative strategy. Future treatment options may include growth factor therapy such as NT3 or NGF.

REFERENCES

1. Hill A. The environmental and disease: association or causation. Proc Royal Soc Med 1965; 58:295–300.
2. Greenberg RS, Daniels SR, Flanders WD, Eley JW, Boring JR. Interpretation of Epidemiological Literature. McGraw-Hill Companies, 2002.
3. Smith AG, Albers JW. *n*-Hexane neuropathy due to rubber cement sniffing. Muscle Nerve 1997; 20(11):1445–1450.
4. Berger AR, Arezzo JC, Schaumburg HH et al. 2′,3′-dideoxycytidine (ddC) toxic neuropathy: a study of 52 patients. Neurology 1993; 43(2):358–362.
5. Berger AR, Schaumburg HH, Schroeder C, Apfel S, Reynolds R. Dose response, coasting, and differential fiber vulnerability in human toxic neuropathy: a prospective study of pyridoxine neurotoxicity. Neurology 1992; 42(7):1367–1370.

6. Chaudhry V, Chaudhry M, Crawford TO, Simmons-O'Brien E, Griffin JW. Toxic neuropathy in patients with pre-existing neuropathy. Neurology 2003; 60(2):337–340.

7. Hogan-Dann CM, Fellmeth WG, McGuire SA, Kiley VA. Polyneuropathy following vincristine therapy in two patients with Charcot–Marie–Tooth syndrome. J Am Med Assoc 1984; 252(20):2862–2863.

8. Agency for Toxic Substances and Disease Registry (ATSDR). Case Studies in Environmental Medicine, Lead Toxicity. Atlanta: Public Health Service US, 1992.

9. Richards RT. Lead poisoning. Rocky Mt Med J 1967; 64(4):59–65.

10. Wu PB, Kingery WS, Date ES. An EMG case report of lead neuropathy 19 years after a shotgun injury. Muscle Nerve 1995; 18(3):326–329.

11. Goyer RA, Rhyne BC. Pathological effects of lead. Int Rev Exp Pathol 1973; 12:1–77.

12. Seto DS, Freeman JM. Lead neuropathy in childhood. Am J Dis Child 1964; 107:337–342.

13. Rubens O, Logina I, Kravale I, Eglite M, Donaghy M. Peripheral neuropathy in chronic occupational inorganic lead exposure: a clinical and electrophysiological study. J Neurol Neurosurg Psychiatry 2001; 71(2):200–204.

14. Ohnishi A, Schilling K, Brimijoin WS, Lambert EH, Fairbanks VF, Dyck PJ. Lead neuropathy. (1) Morphometry, nerve conduction, and choline acetyltransferase transport: new finding of endoneurial edema associated with segmental demyelination. J Neuropathol Exp Neurol 1977; 36(3):499–518.

15. Hyslop GH, Draus WM. The pathology of motor paralysis by lead. Arch Neurol Psychiatry 1923; 10:444.

16. Reiders F. Current concepts in the therapy of lead poisoning. In: Metal Binding in Medicine. Philadelphia: JB Lippincott, 1960:143.

17. Force UPST. Guide to Clinical Preventive Services. Baltimore, MD: Lippincott, Williams and Wilkins, 1996.

18. Sassa S, Kappas A. Prenatal diagnosis of acute intermittent porphyria. N Engl J Med 1976; 295(24):1381.

19. Devalin TM. Biochemistry with Clinical Correlations. Wiley Medical Publications, 1986.

20. Blom S, Lagerkvist B, Linderholm H. Arsenic exposure to smelter workers. Clinical and neurophysiological studies. Scand J Work Environ Health 1985; 11(4):265–269.

21. Feldman RG, Niles CA, Kelly-Hayes M et al. Peripheral neuropathy in arsenic smelter workers. Neurology 1979; 29(7):939–944.

22. Gerr F, Letz R, Ryan PB, Green RC. Neurological effects of environmental exposure to arsenic in dust and soil among humans. Neurotoxicology 2000; 21(4):475–487.

23. Mukherjee SC, Rahman MM, Chowdhury UK et al. Neuropathy in arsenic toxicity from groundwater arsenic contamination in West Bengal, India. J Environ Sci Health Part A Tox Hazard Subst Environ Eng 2003; 38(1):165–183.

24. Mathieu D, Mathieu-Nolf M, Germain-Alonso M, Neviere R, Furon D, Wattel F. Massive arsenic poisoning—effect of hemodialysis and dimercaprol on arsenic kinetics. Intensive Care Med 1992; 18(1):47–50.

25. Kyle RA, Pease GL. Hematologic aspects of arsenic intoxication. N Engl J Med 1965; 273:18–23.

26. Le Quesne PN, McLeod JG. Peripheral neuropathy following a single exposure to arsenic. Clinical course in four patients with elecetrophysiological and histological studies. J Neurol Sci 1977; 32(3):437–451.

27. Uede K, Furukawa F. Skin manifestations in acute arsenic poisoning from the Wakayama curry-poisoning incident. Br J Dermatol 2003; 149(4):757–762.

28. Mees RA. Een verschijnsel Bij polyneuritis arsenicosa. Nederl T Geneesk 1919; 1:391.

29. Guha Mazumder DN. Chronic arsenic toxicity: clinical features, epidemiology and treatment: experience in West Bengal. J Environ Sci Health Part A Tox Hazard Subst Environ Eng 2003; 38(1):141–163.

30. Albers JW, Wald JJ. Industrial and environmental toxic neuropathies. In: Brown WF, Bolton CF, Aminoff MJ, eds. Neuromuscular Function and Disease: Basic, Clinical and Electrodiagnostic Aspects. Philadelphia: WB Saunders Publishing, 2002:1143–1168.

31. Abernathy CO, Liu YP, Longfellow D et al. Arsenic: health effects, mechanisms of actions, and research issues. Environ Health Perspect 1999; 107(7):593–597.

32. Muckter H, Liebl B, Reichl FX, Hunder G, Walther U, Fichtl B. Are we ready to replace dimercaprol (BAL) as an arsenic antidote? Hum Exp Toxicol 1997; 16(8):460–465.

33. Atsmon J, Taliansky E, Landau M, Neufeld MY. Thallium poisoning in Israel. Am J Med Sci 2000; 320(5):327–330.

34. Tromme I, Van Neste D, Dobbelaere F et al. Skin signs in the diagnosis of thallium poisoning. Br J Dermatol 1998; 138(2):321–325.

35. Hoffman RS. Thallium toxicity and the role of Prussain blue in therapy. Toxicol Rev 2003; 22(1):29–40.

36. Satoh H. Occupational and environmental toxicology of mercury and its compounds. Ind Health 2000; 38(2):153–164.

37. Ohnishi A, Murai Y, Ikeda ML, Koroiwa Y. Experimental methylmercury intoxication. Morphometric analysis of the nerve fiber of the sural nerve, lumbar spinal roots, and Goll's tract. Neurol Med 1978; 9:564.

38. Korogi Y, Takahashi M, Okajima T, Eto K. MR findings of Minamata disease—organic mercury poisoning. J Magn Reson Imaging 1998; 8(2):308–316.

39. Longcope WT, Luetschar JA Jr. The uses of BAL (British Anit-Lewisite) in the treatment of the injurious effects of arsenic, mercury, and other metallic poisons. Ann Intern Med 1949; 31:545–554.

40. Aposhian HV, Aposhian MM. N-Acetyl-DL-penicillamine, a new oral protective agent against the lethal effects of mercuric chloride. J Pharmacol Exp Ther 1959; 126(2):131–135.

41. Hu H. Heavy metal poisoning. In: Braunwald, Fauci, Isselbacher et al., eds. Harrison's Principles of Internal Medicine. New York: McGraw-Hill, 2001.

42. Marrs TC. Organophosphate poisoning. Pharmacol Ther 1993; 58(1):51–66.

43. Kwong TC. Organophosphate pesticides: biochemistry and clinical toxicology. Ther Drug Monit 2002; 24(1):144–149.

44. Cavanagh JB. The toxic effects of tri-ortho-cresyl phosphate on the nervous system. J Neurol Neurosurg Psychiatry 1954; 17:163.

45. Van de Neucker K, Vanderstraeten G, De Muynck M, De Wilde V. The neurophysiologic examination in organophosphate ester poisoning. Case report and review of the literature. Electromyogr Clin Neurophys 1991; 31(8):507–511.

46. Eddleston M, Szinicz L, Eyer P, Buckley N. Oximes in acute organophosphorus pesticide poisoning: a systematic review of clinical trials. Q J Med 2002; 95(5):275–283.

47. Schaumberg HH, Spencer PS. Human toxic neuropathy due to industrial agents. In: Dyck PJ, Thomas PK, Griffin JW, Low PA, Poduslo JF, eds. Peripheral Neuropathy. Philadelphia: WB Saunders Publishing, 1993.

48. Lowndes HE, Baker T, Michelson LP, Vincent-Ablazey M. Attenuated dynamic responses of primary endings of muscle spindle: a basis for depressed tendon responses in acrylamide neuropathy. Ann Neurol 1978; 3(5):433–437.

49. Summer AJ, Asbury AK. Physiological studies of the dying–back phenomenon. Muscle stretch afferents in acrylamide neuropathy. Brain 1975; 98(1):91–100.

50. He FS, Zhang SL, Wang HL et al. Neurological and electroneuromyographic assessment of the adverse effects of acrylamide on occupationally exposed workers. Scand J Work Environ Health 1989; 15(2):125–129.

51. Kulig B. Acrylamide. In: de Wolff F, ed. Handbook of Clinical Neurology. Amsterdam: Elsevier, 1994:63–80.

52. Prineas J. The pathogenesis of dying–back polyneuropathies. II. An ultrastructural study of experimental acrylamide intoxication in the cat. J Neuropathol Exp Neurol 1969; 28(4):598–621.

53. Davenport JG, Farrell DF, Sumi M. "Giant axonal neuropathy" caused by industrial chemicals: neurofilamentous axonal masses in man. Neurology 1979; 26(10):919–923.

54. Navarro X, Verdu E, Guerrero J, Buti M, Gonalons E. Abnormalities of sympathetic sudomotor function in experimental acrylamide neuropathy. J Neurol Sci 1993; 114(1):56–61.

55. Ko MH, Chen WP, Hsieh ST. Neuropathology of skin denervation in acrylamide-induced neuropathy. Neurobiol Dis 2002; 11(1):155–165.

56. Vigliani EC. Carbon disulphide poisoning in viscose rayon factories. Br J Ind Med 1954; 11(4):235–244.

57. Spencer PS, Schaumberg HH. Central-peripheral distal axonopathy—the pathology of dying–back polyneuropathies. In: Zimmerman H, ed. Progress in Neuropathology. New York: Grune and Stratton, 1976:253.

58. Brashear A, Unverzagt FW, Farber MO, Bonnin JM, Garcia JG, Grober E. Ethylene oxide neurotoxicity: a cluster of 12 nurses with peripheral and central nervous system toxicity. Neurology 1996; 46(4):992–998.

59. Gross JA, Haas ML, Swift TR. Ethylene oxide neurotoxicity: report of four cases and review of the literature. Neurology 1979; 29(7):978–983.

60. Garnaas KR, Windebank AJ, Blexrud MD, Kurtz SB. Ultrastructural changes produced in dorsal root ganglia *in vitro* by exposure to ethylene oxide from hemodialyzers. J Neuropathol Exp Neurol 1991; 50(3):256–262.

61. Windebank AJ, Blexrud MD. Residual ethylene oxide in hollow fiber hemodialysis units is neurotoxic *in vitro*. Ann Neurol 1989; 26(1):63–68.

62. Ohnishi A, Inoue N, Yamamoto T et al. Ethylene oxide neuropathy in rats. Exposure to 250 ppm. J Neurol Sci 1986; 74(2–3):215–221.

63. Ohnishi A, Inoue N, Yamamoto T et al. Ethylene oxide induces central-peripheral distal axonal degeneration of the lumbar primary neurons in rats. Br J Ind Med 1985; 42(6):373–379.

64. Senanayake N. Tri-cresyl phosphate neuropathy in Sri Lanka: a clinical and neurophysiological study with a three year follow up. J Neurol Neurosurg Psychiatry 1981; 44(9):775–780.

65. Morgan JP, Penovich P. Jamaica ginger paralysis. Forty-seven-year follow-up. Arch Neurol 1978; 35(8):530–532.

66. Victor M, Adams RD. The effect of alcohol on the nervous system. Res Publ Assoc Res Nerv Ment Dis 1953; 32:526–573.

67. Koike H, Iijima M, Sugiura M et al. Alcoholic neuropathy is clinicopathologically distinct from thiamine-deficiency neuropathy. Ann Neurol 2003; 54(1):19–29.

68. Wohrle JC, Spengos K, Steinke W, Goebel HH, Hennerici M. Alcohol-related acute axonal polyneuropathy: a differential diagnosis of Guillain–Barré syndrome. Arch Neurol 1998; 55(10):1329–1334.

69. Bosch EP, Pelham RW, Rasool CG et al. Animal models of alcoholic neuropathy: morphologic, electrophysiologic, and biochemical findings. Muscle Nerve 1979; 2(2):133–144.

70. Lieber CS, DeCarli LM. The feeding of alcohol in liquid diets: two decades of applications and 1982 update. Alcohol Clin Exp Res 1982; 6(4):523–531.

71. Hallett M, Fox JG, Rogers AE et al. Controlled studies on the effects of alcohol ingestion on peripheral nerves of macaque monkeys. J Neurol Sci 1987; 80(1):65–71.

72. Victor M, Adams RD. On the etiology of the alcoholic neurologic disease with special reference to the role of nutrition. Am J Clin Nutr 1961; 9:379–397.

73. Wright H. On the Classification and Pathology of Beri-Beri. London: John Bale Sonsand Danielleson, 1903.

74. Chang CM, Yu CW, Fong KY et al. *N*-Hexane neuropathy in offset printers. J Neurol Neurosurg Psychiatry 1993; 56(5):538–542.

75. Chang AP, England JD, Garcia CA, Summer AJ. *n*-Hexane-related peripheral neuropathy among automotive technicians—California, 1999–2000. Focal conduction block in *n*-hexane polyneuropathy. MMWR Morb Mortal Wkly Rep 2001; 50(45):1011–1013.

76. Cianchetti C, Abbritti G, Perticoni G, Siracusa A, Curradi F. Toxic polyneuropathy of shoe-industry workers. A study of 122 cases. J Neurol Neurosurg Psychiatry 1976; 39(12):1151–1161.

77. Herbert R, Gerr F, Luo J, Harris-Abbott D, Landrigan PJ. Peripheral neurologic abnormalities among roofing workers: sentinel case and clinical screening. Arch Environ Health 1995; 50(5):349–354.

78. Huang CC, Shih TS, Cheng SY, Chen SS, Tchen PH. *n*-Hexane polyneuropathy in a ball-manufacturing factory. J Occup Med 1991; 33(2):139–142.

79. Pastore C, Izura V, Marhuenda D, Prieto MJ, Roel J, Cardona A. Partial conduction blocks in *N*-hexane neuropathy. Muscle Nerve 2002; 26(1):132–135.

80. Chang AP, England JD, Garcia CA, Summer AJ. Focal conduction block in *n*-hexane polyneuropathy. Muscle Nerve 1998; 21(7):964–969.

81. Cardona A, Marhuenda D, Marti J, Brugnone F, Roel J, Perbellini L. Biological monitoring of occupational exposure to *n*-hexane by measurement of urinary 2,5-hexanedione. Int Arch Occup Environ Health 1993; 65(1):71–74.

82. Chang YC. Patients with *n*-hexane induced polyneuropathy: a clinical follow up. Br J Ind Med 1990; 47(7):485–489.

83. Layzer RB, Fishman RA, Schafer JA. Neuropathy following abuse of nitrous oxide. Neurology 1978; 28(5):504–506.

84. Dinn JJ, McCann S, Wilson P, Reed B, Weir D, Scott J. Animal model for subacute combined degeneration. Lancet 1978; 2(8100):1154.

85. Sahenk Z, Mendell JR, Couri D, Nachtman J. Polyneuropathy from inhalation of N$_2$O cartridges through a whipped-cream dispenser. Neurology 1978; 28(5):485–487.

86. Diamond AL, Diamond R, Freedman SM, Thomas FP. "Whippets"-induced cobalamin deficiency manifesting as cervical myelopathy. J Neuroimaging 2004; 14(3):277–280.

87. Sesso RM, Iunes Y, Melo AC. Myeloneuropathy following nitrous oxide anesthaesia in a patient with macrocytic anaemia. Neuroradiology 1999; 41(8):588–590.

88. Marie RM, Le Biez E, Busson P et al. Nitrous oxide anesthesia-associated myelopathy. Arch Neurol 2000; 57(3):380–382.

89. Nestor PJ, Stark RJ. Vitamin B12 myeloneuropathy precipitated by nitrous oxide anaesthesia. Med J Aust 1996; 165(3):174.

90. Holloway KL, Alberico AM. Postoperative myeloneuropathy: a preventable complication in patients with B12 deficiency. J Neurosurg 1990; 72(5):732–736.

91. Stacy CB, Di Rocco A, Gould RJ. Methionine in the treatment of nitrous-oxide-induced neuropathy and myeloneuropathy. J Neurol 1992; 239(7):401–403.

92. Gregg RW, Molepo JM, Monpetit VJ et al. Cisplatin neurotoxicity: the relationship between dosage, time, and platinum concentration in neurologic tissues, and morphologic evidence of toxicity. J Clin Oncol 1992; 10(5):795–803.

93. LoMonaco M, Milone M, Batocchi AP, Padua L, Restuccia D, Tonali P. Cisplatin neuropathy: clinical course and neurophysiological findings. J Neurol 1992; 239(4):199–204.

94. Muller LJ, Gerritsen van der Hoop R, Moorer-van Delft CM, Gispen WH, Roubos EW. Morphological and electrophysiological study of the effects of cisplatin and ORG.2766 on rat spinal ganglion neurons. Cancer Res 1990; 50(8):2437–2442.

95. Walsh TJ, Clark AW, Parhad IM, Green WR. Neurotoxic effects of cisplatin therapy. Arch Neurol 1982; 39(11):719–720.

96. Gill JS, Windebank AJ. Cisplatin-induced apoptosis in rat dorsal root ganglion neurons is associated with attempted entry into the cell cycle. J Clin Invest 1998; 101(12):2842–2850.

97. Meijer C, de Vries EG, Marmiroli P, Tredici G, Frattola L, Cavaletti G. Cisplatin-induced DNA-platination in experimental dorsal root ganglia neuronopathy. Neurotoxiciology 1999; 20(6):883–887.

98. Cece R, Petruccioli MG, Cavaletti G, Barajon I, Tredici G. An ultrastructural study of neuronal changes in dorsal root ganglia (DRG) of rats after chronic cisplatin administrations. Histol Histopathol 1995; 10(4):837–845.

99. Russell JW, Windebank AJ, McNiven MA, Brat DJ, Brimijoin WS. Effect of cisplatin and ACTH4-9 on neural transport in cisplatin induced neurotoxicity. Brain Res 1995; 676(2):258–267.

100. Windebank AJ, Smith AG, Russell JW. The effect of nerve growth factor, ciliary neurotrophic factor, and ACTH analogs on cisplatin neurotoxicity *in vitro*. Neurology 1994; 44(3 Pt 1): 488–494.

101. van der Hoop RG, Vecht CJ, van der Burg ME et al. Prevention of cisplatin neurotoxicity with an ACTH(4-9) analogue in patients with ovarian cancer. N Engl J Med 1990; 322(2):89–94.

102. Roberts JA, Jenison EL, Kim K, Clarke-Pearson D, Langleben A. A randomized, multicenter, double-blind, placebo-controlled, dose-finding study of ORG 2766 in the prevention or delay

of cisplatin-induced neuropathies in women with ovarian cancer. Gynecol Oncol 1997; 67(2):172–177.

103. Chattopadhyay M, Goss J, Wolfe D et al. Protective effect of herpes simplex virus-mediated neurotrophin gene transfer in cisplatin neuropathy. Brain 2004; 127(Pt 4):929–939.

104. Canetta R, Rozencweig M, Carter SK. Carboplatin: the clinical spectrum to date. Cancer Treat Rev 1985; 12(suppl A):125–136.

105. Pal PK. Clinical and eletrophysiological studies in vincristine induced neuropathy. Electromyogr Clin Neurophys 1999; 39(6):323–330.

106. Legha SS. Vincristine neurotoxicity. Pathophysiology and management. Med Toxicol 1986; 1(6):421–427.

107. Mercuri E, Poulton J, Buck J et al. Vincristine treatment revealing asymptomatic hereditary motor sensory neuropathy type 1A. Arch Dis Child 1999; 81(5):442–443.

108. Moudgil SS, Riggs JE. Fulminant peripheral neuropathy with severe quadriparesis associated with vincristine therapy. Ann Pharmacother 2000; 34(10):1136–1138.

109. Graf W, Chance P, Lensch M, Eng L, Lipe H, Bird T. Severe vincristine neuropathy in Charcot–Marie–Tooth disease type 1A. Cancer 1996; 77:1356–1362.

110. Forsyth PA, Balmaceda C, Peterson K, Seidman AD, Brasher P, DeAngelis LM. Prospective study of paclitaxel-induced peripheral neuropathy with quantitative sensory testing. J Neurooncol 1997; 35(1):47–53.

111. van den Bent MJ, van Raaij-van den Aarssen VJ, Verweij J, Doorn PA, Sillevis Smitt PA. Progression of paclitaxel-induced neuropathy following discontinuation of treatment. Muscle Nerve 1997; 20(6):750–752.

112. Sullivan KA, Kim B, Buzdon M, Feldman EL. Suramin disrupts insulin-like growth factor-II (IGF-II) mediated autocrine growth in human SH-SY5Y neuroblastoma cells. Brain Res 1997; 744(2):199–206.

113. Chaudhry V, Eisenberger MA, Sinibaldi VJ, Sheikh K, Griffin JW, Cornblath DR. A prospective study of suramin-induced peripheral neuropathy. Brain 1996; 119(Pt 6):2039–2052.

114. La Rocca RV, Meer J, Gilliatt RW et al. Suramin-induced polyneuropathy. Neurology 1990; 40(6):954–960.

115. Soliven B, Dhand UK, Kobayashi K et al. Evaluation of neuropathy in patients on suramin treatment. Muscle Nerve 1997; 20(1):83–91.

116. Paul M, Joshua D, Rahme N et al. Fatal peripheral neuropathy associated with axonal degeneration after high-dose cytosine arabinoside in acute leukaemia. Br J Haematol 1991; 79(3):521–523.

117. Cohen S. Thalidomide polyneuropathy. Nord Hyg Tidskr 1962; 266:1268.

118. Wulff CH, Hoyer H, Asboe-Hansen G, Brodthagen H. Development of polyneuropathy during thalidomide therapy. Br J Dermatol 1985; 112(4):475–480.

119. Bastuji-Garin S, Ochonisky S, Bauche P et al. Incidence and risk factors for thalidomide neuropathy: a prospective study of 135 dermatologic patients. J Invest Dermatol 2002; 119(5):1020–1026.

120. Offidani M, Corvatta L, Marconi M et al. Common and rare side-effects of low-dose thalidomide in multiple myeloma: focus on the dose-minimizing peripheral neuropathy. Eur J Haematol 2004; 72(6):403–409.

121. Tseng S, Pak G, Washenik K, Pomeranz MK, Shupack JL. Rediscovering thalidomide: a review of its mechanism of action, side effects, and potential used. J Am Acad Dermatol 1996; 35(6):969–979.

122. Giannini F. Volpi N, Rossi S, Passero S, Fimiani M, Cerase A. Thalidomide-induced neuropathy: a ganglionopathy? Neurology 2003; 60(5):877–878.

123. Fullerton PM, O'Sullivan DJ. Thalidomide neuropathy: a clinical electrophysiological, and histological follow-up study. J Neurol Neurosurg Psychiatry 1968; 31(6):543–551.

124. Gardner-Medwin JM, Smith NJ, Powell RJ. Clinical experience with thalidomide in the management of severe oral and genital ulceration in conditions such as Behçet's disease: use of neurophysiological studies to detect thalidomide neuropathy. Ann Rheum Dis 1994; 53(12):828–832.

125. Jacobs JM, Costa-Jussa FR. The pathology of amiodarone neurotoxicity. II. Peripheral neuropathy in man. Brain 1985; 108(Pt 3):753–769.

126. Fardeau M, Tome FM, Simon P. Muscle and nerve changes induced by perhexiline maleate in man and mice. Muscle Nerve 1979; 2(1):24–36.

127. Palakurthy PR, Iyer V, Meckler RJ. Unusual neurotoxicity associated with amiodarone therapy. Arch Intern Med 1987; 147(5):881–884.

128. Silva Oropeza E, Peralta Rosado HR, Valero Elizondo C, Sadowinski E, Magana Serrano JA. A case of amiodarone and neuromyopathy. Rev Invest Clin 1997; 49(2):135–139.

129. Charness ME, Morady F, Scheinman MM. Frequent neurologic toxicity associated with amiodarone therapy. Neurology 1984; 34(5):669–671.

130. Abarbanel JM, Osiman A, Frisher S, Herishanu Y. Peripheral neuropathy and cerebellar syndrome associated with amiodarone therapy. Isr J Med Sci 1987; 23(8):893–895.

131. Zea BL, Leonard JA, Donofrio PD. Amiodarone producing an acquired demyelinating and axonal polyneuropathy. Muscle Nerve 1985; 8:612.

132. Goble AJ, Horowitz JD. Perhexilene neuropathy: a report of two cases. Aust NZ J Med 1984; 14(3):279.

133. Mandelcorn M, Murphy J, Colman J. Papilledema without peripheral neuropathy in a patient taking perhexiline maleate. Can J Ophthalmol 1982; 17(4):173–175.

134. Lorentz IT, Shortall M. Perhexilene neuropathy: a report of two cases. Aust NZ J Med 1983; 13(5):517–518.

135. Said G. Perhexiline neuropathy: a clinicopathological study. Ann Neurol 1978; 3(3):259–266.

136. Dalakas MC. Peripheral neuropathy and antiretroviral drugs. J Peripher Nerv Syst 2001; 6(1):14–20.

137. Blum AS, Dal Pan GJ, Feinberg J et al. Low-dose zalcitabine-related toxic neuropahy: frequency, natural history, and risk factors. Neurology 1996; 46(4):999–1003.

138. Lopez OL, Becker JT, Dew MA, Caldararo R. Risk modifiers for peripheral sensory neuropathy in HIV infection/AIDS. Eur J Neurol 2004; 11(2):97–102.

139. Dalakas MC, Semino-Mora C, Leon-Monzon M. Mitochondrial alterations with mitochondrial DNA depletion in the nerves of AIDS patients with peripheral neuropathy induced by 2′,3′-dideoxycytidine (ddC). Lab Invest 2001; 81(11):1537–1544.

140. Altiparmak MR, Pamuk ON, Pamuk GE, Hamuryudan V, Ataman R, Serdengecti K. Colchicine neuromyopathy: a report of six cases. Clin Exp Rheumatol 2002; 20(4 suppl 26):S13–S16.

141. Kuncl RW, Duncan G, Watson D, Alderson K, Rogawski MA, Peper M. Colchicine myopathy and neuropathy. N Engl J Med 1987; 316(25):1562–1568.

142. Younger DS, Mayer SA, Weimer LH, Alderson LM, Seplowitz AH, Lovelace RE. Colchicine-induced myopathy and neuropathy. Neurology 1991; 41(6):943.

143. Kuncl RW, Cornblath DR, Avila O, Duncan G. Electrodiagnosis of human colchicine myoneuropathy. Muscle Nerve 1989; 12(5):360–364.

144. Albin RL, Albers JW, Greenberg HS et al. Acute sensory neuropathy–neuronopathy from pyridoxine overdose. Neurology 1987; 37(11):1729–1732.

145. Schaumburg H, Kaplan J, Windebank A et al. Sensory neuropathy from pyridoxine abuse. A new megavitamin syndrome. N Engl J Med 1983; 309(8):445–448.

146. Parry GJ, Bredesen DE. Sensory neuropathy with low-dose pyridoxine. Neurology 1985; 35(10):1466–1468.

147. Chattopadhyay M, Wolfe D, Huang S et al. In vivo gene therapy for pyridoxine-induced neuropathy by herpes simplex virus-mediated gene transfer of neurotrophin-3. Ann Neurol 2002; 51(1):19–27.

148. Holmberg L, Boman G, Bottiger LE, Eriksson B, Spross R, Wessling A. Adverse reactions to nitrofurantoin. Analysis of 921 reports. Am J Med 1980; 69(5):733–738.

149. White WT, Harrison L, Dumas J II. Nitrofurantoin unmasking peripheral neuropathy in a type 2 diabetic patient. Arch Intern Med 1984; 144(4):821.

150. Toole JF, Parrish ML. Nitrofurantoin polyneuropathy. Neurology 1973; 23(5):554–559.

151. Yiannikas C, Pollard JD, McLeod JG. Nitrofurantoin neuropathy. Aust NZ J Med 1981; 11(4):400–405.

Hereditary Neuropathies

21

Inherited Peripheral Neuropathies: Charcot–Marie–Tooth Disease

Michael E. Shy, Richard A. Lewis, and Jun Li
Wayne State University School of Medicine, Detroit, Michigan, USA

ABSTRACT

Charcot–Marie–Tooth disease (CMT) refers to a spectrum of inherited peripheral neuropathies. They affect approximately one in 2500 people, and are one of the most common inherited neurological disorders. The genetic mutations follow autosomal dominant, recessive, and X-linked inheritance patterns, and spontaneous mutations also occur. CMT has been divided into two broad forms based on electrophysiological and morphologic criteria, with demyelinating forms associated with slow conduction velocities and axonal forms with normal or mildly slowed conduction velocities. However, this likely represents an oversimplification as genotyping reveals overlap in conduction velocities in some families. The clinical features of CMT follow a length-dependent pattern with distal weakness and sensory loss and reduced or absent reflexes. Some patients may be minimally affected, obscuring a familial pattern without a high index of suspicion. The discovery of new mutations has focused on physiologic mechanisms, but a clear understanding of pathologic mechanisms has remained elusive. At this time there is no effective treatment for CMT.

1. INTRODUCTION

Charcot–Marie–Tooth disease (CMT) refers to inherited peripheral neuropathies named for three investigators who described them in the late 1800s (1,2). CMT neuropathies affect approximately one in 2500 people, and are among the most common inherited neurological disorders. The majority of CMT patients have autosomal dominant inheritance, although X-linked dominant and autosomal recessive forms also exist. Apparent sporadic cases occur, since dominantly inherited disorders may begin as a new mutation in a given patient. The majority of CMT neuropathies are demyelinating, although up to one-third appear to be primary axonal disorders. Most patients have a "typical" CMT phenotype characterized by onset in childhood or early adulthood, distal weakness, sensory loss, foot deformities (pes cavus and hammer toes), and absent reflexes. However, some patients develop severe disability in infancy (Dejerine–Sottas Disease or congenital hypomyelination), while others develop few if any symptoms of disease. Thus far at least 30 genes are known to cause inherited neuropathies, and more than 50 distinct loci have been identified. A summary of the genes associated with CMT neuropathies can be found online at http://molgen-www.uia.ac.be/CMTMutations/. Genetic testing for several forms of CMT is now available, which, in addition to providing accurate diagnosis, also provides for genotypic–phenotypic correlations. Progress has been made toward understanding how particular mutations cause disease, but full details are open.

2. CLASSIFICATION

In landmark studies, Dyck and Lambert subdivided hereditary motor and sensory neuropathies (HMSNs) into dominantly inherited demyelinating HMSN I (CMT1) and dominantly inherited axonal HMSN II (CMT2) forms, based on electrophysiological and neuropathological criteria (3). Other types were then classified as HMSN III–VII, depending on inheritance pattern and accompanying features. When specific genetic causes for different forms of CMT began to be identified, the classification had to be expanded and modified (Table 21.1). In this chapter, we classify CMT into CMT1 if the patient has an autosomal dominantly inherited demyelinating neuropathy; CMT2 if

Table 21.1 Inherited Motor and Sensory Neuropathies

CMT1			
CMT1A	AD	17p11.2	PMP22 duplication and mutation
CMT1B	AD	1q21–23	MPZ
CMT1C	AD	16p13.1–12.3	LITAF/SIMPLE
CMT1D	AD	10q21–22	EGR2
HNPP	AD	17p11.2	PMP22 deletion
CMT2			
CMT2A	AD	1p35–36	KIF1Bβ
CMT2B	AD	3q13–22	RAB 7
CMT2C	AD	12q23–24	?
CMT2D	AD	7p15	GARS
CMT2E	AD	8p21	NF-light
CMTX1	AD	Xq13–22	GJB1 (Connexin 32)
DSD	AD	1q22–23	MPZ mutation
	AD	17p11.2	PMP22 mutation
	AD	10q21–22	EGR2 mutation
	AR		
CMT4			
CMT4A (demyelinating form)	AR	8q13	GDAP1
	AR	8q24	N-my-downstream regulated gene 1 mutation
			?
CMT4B1	AR	11q23	MTMR2
CMT4B2	AR	11p15	SBF2
CMT4C	AR	5123–33	KIAA1985
CMT4D	AR	8q24	NDRG1
CMT4F	AR	19q13.13–13.2	Periaxin
HMSNR	AR	10q23.2	?
Distal hereditary motor neuropathies			
dHMN1	AD	Unknown	?
dHMN2	AD	12q24.3	dHSP22
dHMN3	AR	1q21–23	?
dHMNV	AD	7p15	GARS
dHMNVI	AR	Unknown	?
dHMNVII	AD	Unknown	?
dHMN (also "CMT2F")	AD	7q11–q21	dHSP27
dHMN Jerash	AD	9p21.1	?
ALS4	AD	9q34	SETX
HMN Dynactin	AD	2p13′	Dynactin

the neuropathy is dominantly inherited and axonal; CMTX if the patient has an X-linked neuropathy; and CMT4 if the neuropathy is recessive. In addition, cases of CMT1, CMT2, and CMT4 are further subdivided based on differences in genetic abnormalities or linkage studies.

Dyck and Lambert classified Dejerine Sottas Disease (DSD) as a severe and disabling neuropathy beginning in infancy with an autosomal recessive inheritance pattern. Subsequently, it has been shown that many presumed DSD patients have autosomal dominant mutations in genes for peripheral myelin 22 (PMP22), myelin protein zero (MPZ), and early growth response 2 (EGR2) (see what follows). Although nerve conduction velocities in DSD patients are usually extremely slow (<15 m/s) some severely disabled children do not have slow velocities. Moreover, sural nerve biopsies in many DSD children reveal severe demyelination, while others reveal predominantly axonal loss. To minimize confusion, we use the term DSD to define patients who have onset by 2 years of age; delayed motor milestones; and severe motor sensory and skeletal deficits with frequent extension to proximal muscles; sensory ataxia; and scoliosis.

3. GENETIC, CLINICAL, AND PATHOLOGIC FEATURES

3.1. CMT1

Beginning in 1991, specific genetic mutations were identified that cause distinct forms of CMT1. As predicted, mutations have been found in genes expressed in myelinating Schwann cells.

3.1.1. CMT1A

This form is caused by a duplication on chromosome 17, containing the gene encoding PMP22 (4,5). It is the most common form of CMT, and $\sim$60% of CMT1 patients have this duplication. The function of PMP22 in Schwann cells remains unknown. Evidence that the duplication of PMP22 causes CMT1A includes:

1. Missense mutations in PMP22 causing the Trembler (*Tr*) and TremblerJ (*Tr^J*) naturally occurring mouse models of CMT1.
2. Transgenic mice and rats bearing extra copies of PMP22 developing a CMT1A-like neuropathy.
3. Some patients with missense mutations in PMP22 also developing a similar phenotype.

CMT1A represents a "typical" CMT phenotype. Patients are slow runners in childhood, develop foot problems in their teenage years due to high arches and hammer toes, and often require orthotics for ankle support as adults. Variable degrees of hand weakness occur, typically lagging $\sim$10 years behind the development of foot weakness. Sensory loss is variable and affects both large (vibration and proprioception) and small (pain and temperature) fiber modalities. Almost all patients with CMT1A have absent deep tendon reflexes. Enlarged nerve trunks may be palpated in the arm. While the combination of weak ankles and decreased proprioception often leads to problems with balance, the vast majority of patients remain ambulatory throughout their life, which is not shortened by their disease (6,7). Additional features, including postural tremor (referred as Roussy–Levy syndrome) and muscle cramps, may also occur. Occasional patients develop a severe phenotype in infancy, while others develop minimal disability throughout life. Since phenotypic variability occurs within the same generation within the same family, it is not possible to predict who will have more disabling forms of the disease.

There is overlap in the pathology among different forms of CMT1, and their pathology will be considered together. Segmental demyelination, remyelination, and axonal loss are characteristic features. Demyelination is severe in DSD. Onion bulbs of concentric Schwann cell lamellae are less frequent in children than in adults, and may be the predominate pathology. Axonal loss varies with individual patients. There is a loss of both small and large diameter myelinated fibers. Some fibers have relatively thickened myelin sheaths, resulting in lowered mean *g* ratios (axon diameter/fiber diameter). Focal, sausage-like thickenings of the myelin sheath (tomaculi) may be present in various types of CMT1, though their numbers have been said to be higher in patients with

CMT1B. However, neither disorder has tomaculi present to the extent seen in hereditary predisposition to pressure palsies (HNPP).

Immuno-electronmicroscopic analysis of sural nerve biopsies from CMT1A patients demonstrates increased PMP22 labeling when compared with controls. The effect of the duplication on other myelin proteins is unclear. P0 and myelin basic protein (MBP) levels were found to be similar to controls in three CMT1A patients, but P0 levels were reduced by 50% in a fourth patient. In a patient with a PMP22 missense mutation, causing the formation of a truncated protein, P0 and PMP22 levels were reduced. Immuno-electronmicroscopic studies on two CMT1B patients demonstrated normal levels of PMP22 and MBP but reduced levels of P0 (8). The clinical, physiologic, and pathologic findings suggest that different mutations of the same gene leads to different clinical phenotypes, and that alterations in expression patterns of other myelin genes may depend on the particular mutation in question.

3.1.2. CMT1B

CMT1B is due to assorted mutations in the gene encoding MPZ on chromosome 1 (9). MPZ is the major myelin protein in the peripheral nervous system, and is a member of the immunoglobulin superfamily. It has a single transmembrane domain, and is necessary for the adhesion of concentric myelin wraps in the internode.

Patients with CMT1B were initially thought to have the typical CMT phenotype described for CMT1A patients, but perhaps with more pronounced calf wasting. It is now evident that patients with MPZ mutations have a wide range of phenotypes, including very severe forms with congenital hypomyelination, presenting *in utero*, and DSD presenting in infancy, to milder CMT2-like cases, presenting in adulthood (10). The type and location of the mutation on the MPZ coding region appear to determine the severity of the neuropathy although genotype–phenotype correlations remain to be performed. In our experience, many neuropathies caused by MPZ mutations tend to cluster with very early onset, presenting prior to 1 year of age, or late onset neuropathies, presenting well into adulthood (11).

3.1.3. CMT1C

CMT1C has been shown to be due to mutations in a putative protein degradation gene LITAF/SIMPLE (12). There is limited clinical information on these patients, but they develop distal muscle weakness and atrophy, sensory loss, and slow nerve conduction velocities in the range of 20–25 m/s (12).

3.1.4. CMT1D

CMT1D is due to mutations in the early growth response 2 (EGR2, also called krox20), on chromosome 10 (13). EGR2 is a transcription factor involved in the regulations of as yet unspecified genes in the myelinating Schwann cell. It is associated with variable phenotypes, probably depending on the site and nature of the specific mutation. Most mutations cause severe disease, classified as Dejerine–Sottas or congenital hypomyelination, but recent examples have been described with milder phenotypes which do not present until adulthood (14,15).

3.2. CMTX1

CMTX1 is the second most common form of CMT, accounting for 10 and 16% of cases. It is caused by missense mutations in the connexin 32 kd (*Cx32*) gene, also known as gap junction beta one (*GJβ1*), located on the X chromosome (16). Cx32 is localized in uncompacted myelin of the paranodal loops and Schmidt–Lanterman incisures, and presumably functions as a gap junction protein permitting the passage of small molecules and ions between adjacent loops of the paranode or incisures. Currently, over 250 different mutations of Cx32 have been identified. Because they have a single X-chromosome, men tend to develop CMTX more severely than their female counterparts. Women are usually affected to a milder degree, probably because of X-inactivation of the abnormal chromosome (discussed subsequently).

Patients with CMTX usually develop symptoms in late teenage years or young adulthood. Several patients we have evaluated have been varsity athletes in high school, though they were never fast runners. Abnormalities are usually slowly progressive, limited to the distal legs and hands. Wasting of calf muscles is often more pronounced in CMTX than in CMT1A patients. Among the many mutations, few if any appear to have severe DSD or congenital hypomyelination phenotypes. Occasional female patients have presented in adulthood with a chronic inflammatory demyelinating polyradiculoneuropathy (CIDP)-like neuropathy (17).

Pathological features are an age-related loss of myelinated nerve axons. The demyelinating nature of the neuropathies is demonstrated by abnormally thin myelin ensheathing large caliber axons. Onion bulb formations are infrequent (18). Teased fiber analysis reveals frequent widening at the nodal gap, paranodal retractions, and, less frequently, segmental demyelination.

3.3. HNPP

HNPP is interesting in that a duplication of the PMP22 gene causes CMT1A, a deletion of the same 1.4 Mb region causes HNPP, an entirely different disorder (19). Patients with HNPP typically present with transient episodes of focal weakness or sensory loss that lasts from hours to days. Some patients have also been reported to develop symptoms of length dependent neuropathy, although in our experience this is unusual and is encountered in older patients. When patients are examined between episodes their neurological examination is often normal or only minimally abnormal. Occasionally, a brachial plexopathy may be the presenting symptom, but HNPP is distinct from hereditary brachial plexus neuropathy, which is discussed subsequently.

Segmental demyelination, remyelination, and some loss of large diameter axons have been described in nerve biopsies. Tomaculi are the hallmark of HNPP, and have been identified in at least one patient prior to the development of clinical symptoms (20). Immuno-electronmicroscopic studies of sural nerve biopsies have demonstrated the predicted under-expression of PMP22 (8).

3.4. CMT2

CMT2 represents axonal forms that are dominantly inherited, and include approximately one-third of autosomal dominant CMT. CMT2 is heterogeneous, and at least five subtypes (CMT 2A, B, C, D, E) have been identified by linkage analysis (21). The phenotype is similar to CMT1, with distal weakness, atrophy, sensory loss, and foot deformities. CMT2 patients have a wider age range of symptom onset and degree of disability than those with CMT1, and CMT2 patients are more likely to maintain their deep tendon reflexes. However, it is not possible to accurately distinguish CMT1 from CMT2 clinically, and electrodiagnostic testing is necessary. Reduced CMAP and SNAP amplitudes with normal or mildly slow conduction velocities are distinguishing features of

CMT2. Needle EMG shows evidence of active denervation and partial re-innervation. The electrophysiological features are consistent with pathological findings from sural nerve biopsies of axonal loss without evidence of demyelination.

3.4.1. CMT2A

CMT2A patients have typical CMT clinical presentations with sensorimotor peripheral neuropathies. The locus of CMT2A is at chromosome 1p36. Zuchner et al. (22) have reported that mutations in the nuclear encoded mitochondrial GTPase mitofusin (MFN) 2 cause most cases of CMT2A.

3.4.2. CMT2B

CMT2B is a predominantly sensory disorder and there is debate as to whether cases should be considered under pure sensory neuropathies. Recently, the gene causing CMT2B has been shown to be the small GTP-ase late endosomal protein *RAB7*, on chromosome 3q21 (23).

3.4.3. CMT2C

CMT2C is a rare disorder in which patients have diaphragmatic paresis of vocal cords in addition to other characteristics of CMT2. Although vocal cord and diaphragmatic paresis are not unique to CMT2C (e.g., CMT4A), recently linkage has been established to chromosome 12 in families with CMT2C, suggesting that it is at least a genetically distinct disorder (24).

3.4.4. CMT2D

CMT2D is a somewhat confusing disorder because some patients appear to have sensori-motor neuropathies while others have pure motor syndromes characterized as hereditary motor neuropathy type V (HMNV). At least one family has been described with some individuals having the pure motor syndrome and others also having sensory loss, suggesting that the two disorders are likely to be different phenotypes of the same disease (25). The CMT2D locus is on chromosome 7p14, and the genetic cause of CMT4D (HMNV) has been identified as mutations in the glycyl tRNA synthetase (GARS) gene, the GARS protein is involved in ligating glycine to its cognate tRNAs (26).

3.4.5. CMT2E

CMT2E has been established with linkage to chromosome 8p21, and subsequent studies have identified mutations in the neurofilament light (NF-L) gene (27). Since the NF-L protein is an important constituent of the neurofilaments used in axonal transport systems, and neurofilament phosphorylation is known to be abnormal in demyelinating forms of CMT, CMT2E may provide important clues into mechanisms of axonal damage not only in CMT2 but also in CMT1 (28).

3.5. CMT4

CMT4 represent recessively inherited forms, and are rare. They have heterogeneous phenotypes, and usually more severe than the autosomal dominantly inherited disorders. They may have systemic symptoms, such as cataracts and deafness. CMT4 is separable into demyelinating (4A and 4B) and axonal (4C) forms.

3.5.1. CMT4A

CMT4A is linked to 8q13–q21.1, and is caused by mutations in ganglioside-induced differentiation associated protein 1 (*GDAP1*), a novel protein of unknown function (29,30). The disorder was first described in four highly inbred families in Tunisia. Clinical onset began in the first two years of life, with delayed developmental milestones of sitting or walking, and weakness spreads to proximal muscles by the end of the first decade of life and many patients became wheelchair dependent. Sensory loss is mild, and deep tendon reflexes absent. Nerve conduction velocities (NCVs) are slow (average of 30 m/s). Sural nerve biopsies reveal loss of large diameter myelinated fibers and hypomyelination, but no abnormalities of myelin folding. Basal lamina onion bulbs, characterized by concentric layers of basal lamina without intervening regions of Schwann cell cytoplasm, have also been described (31). The gene was originally identified in a neuronal cell line (32), but MRNA studies suggest that the *GDAP1* gene is expressed in Schwann cells (29,30). The mutations appear to cause either demyelinating (29) or axonal (30) neuropathies, and may disrupt signaling between Schwann cells and axons.

3.5.2. CMT4B

CMT4B1 is a recessively inherited disorder characterized clinically by an unique pathological feature; the presence of focally folded myelin sheathes in nerve biopsy. The genetic locus is on chromosome 11q23, and encodes a gene called myotubularin-related protein-2 (*MTMR2*) (33). Affected patients become symptomatic early, with an average age of onset of 34 months, unlike most forms of CMT, proximal as well as distal weakness is prominent. Motor conduction velocities are severely reduced with temporal dispersion, CMAPs are reduced, and SNAPs are frequently absent. Segmental demyelination is also found in nerve biopsies.

Four children in a Turkish inbred family were identified with neuropathies characterized by focally folded myelin, a characteristic of CMT4B as described previously. However homozygosity mapping demonstrated linkage to a distinct locus on chromosome 11p15, leading to the designation of the locus as CMT4B2. Recently, mutations have been identified in a large, novel gene, named SET binding factor 2 (*SBF2*), that lies within the interval on 11p15 and segregates with the neuropathy in affected families, suggesting that the mutations are responsible for the disease (35). SBF2 is a member of the pseudo-phosphatase branch of myotubularins with striking homology to *MTMR2*.

3.5.3. CMT4C

CMT4C is a childhood-onset demyelinating form of hereditary motor and sensory neuropathy associated with an early-onset scoliosis and a distinct Schwann cell pathology. CMT4C is inherited as an autosomal recessive trait and is caused by homozygous or compound heterozygous mutations in the previously uncharacterized *KIAA1985* gene (35). Scoliosis is prominent early on and may precede weakness or sensory loss. Mean median motor NCV was 22.6 m/s, and nerve biopsy, when obtained, showed demyelination, onion bulb formation, and, most typically, large cytoplasmic extensions of Schwann cells. The translated protein defines a new protein family of unknown function with putative orthologues in vertebrates. Comparative sequence alignments indicate that members of this protein family contain multiple SH3 and TPR domains that are likely involved in the formation of protein complexes.

3.5.4. CMT4D

Kalaydjieva et al. (36) have reported a separate disorder with linkage to chromosome 8q24 in a gypsy population with an autosomal recessive inheritance pattern that is now recognized as CMT4D. The neuropathy has presented with distal muscle wasting and weakness, sensory loss, both foot and hand deformities, and the loss of deep tendon reflexes. Deafness is invariant and usually develops by the third decade. Brainstem auditory evoked responses (BAERs) are markedly abnormal with prolonged interpeak latencies. NCVs are severely reduced in younger patients and unobtainable after 15 years of age. A subsequent study has identified mutations in what is termed the "N-myc downstream-regulated gene" (*NDRG1*) in these patients (36). How the gene abnormality leads to the disorder is unknown.

3.5.5. CMT4F

CMT4F is a severe form of recessive CMT that has been defined in a large Lebanese family with mutations in the periaxin (*PRX*) gene on chromosome 19. PRX is expressed in Schwann cells and encodes two proteins which contain "PDZ" domains that usually interact with other PDZ domain-bearing proteins in intracellular signal transduction pathways. Binding partners for PRX in Schwann cells have not yet been identified, nor have the signal transduction pathways involving PRX been delineated. Nerve conduction studies are markedly slowed and onion bulbs are observed on sural nerve biopsies (37).

3.6. HMSNR

Hereditary motor and sensory neuropathy-Russe (HMSNR) has been localized to 10q23.2, a small interval telomeric to the *EGR2* gene (38). Patients develop primarily severe sensory loss, although motor conduction velocities are moderately reduced (average: 32 m/s).

4. DISTAL HEREDITARY MOTOR NEURONOPATHIES

Distal HMNs comprise ~10% of all HMNs and have been tentatively classified into seven subtypes based on clinical manifestations, age at onset, and mode of inheritance. Genetic loci for several subtypes of distal HMN have been identified. Distal HMN II has been linked in a large Belgian family to chromosome 12q24.3. Patients typically develop weakness in foot dorsiflexion by their late teens and some, but not all, become wheelchair bound in later years. Occasional patients have been described with decreased vibratory sensation. NCVs are normal while needle EMG demonstrates evidence of chronic denervation. It has been recently demonstrated that mutations in the α-crystallin domain of the small heat shock protein dHSP22 cause dHMN type II (39). Moreover, mutations in the α-crystallin and C-terminal tail of another sHSP, dHSP27, cause either an additional form of dHMN or a novel form of CMT2 (40). sHSPs constitute a protein superfamily in which members share an approximately 85 amino acid residue C-terminal region known as the α-crystallin domain. Family members typically form oligomers with other members of the superfamily. sHSP function is not well understood, but is thought to involve signal transduction pathways, protection from apoptosis, and the stabilization of cytoskeletal systems. Mutations in family members have previously been shown to cause myopathies and congenital cataracts. sHSP22 and sHSP27 have previously been found to interact with each other; therefore both disorders probably involve common mechanisms. What these mechanisms are, however, remains to be elucidated. As both sHSP22 and sHSP27 have chaperone-like properties, they may participate in processing proteins for intracellular trafficking, such as discussed earlier. However, they have also been shown to inhibit apoptosis and to stabilize cytoskeletal systems. In this regard, it is noteworthy that mutations in sHSP27 disrupt neurofilament assembly. Mutations in the neurofilament light chain gene

(*NEFL*) cause CMT2E. Taken together, these results suggest that the sHSPs may play critical roles in regulating or maintaining the axonal cytoskeleton and axonal transport. Upregulation of sHSP27 is also necessary for the survival of injured motor or sensory neurons, and sHSP27 is overexpressed in motor neurons of the SOD1 mouse model of familial amyotrophic lateral sclerosis (ALS). Therefore, sHSP-mediated pathways may also ultimately prove to play important roles in many neurodegenerative disorders.

Distal HMN V has been localized to chromosome 7p. It is the same disorder as CMT2D, and is caused by mutations in the glycyl tRNA synthetase gene on chromosome 7p15. In a Bulgarian family with 30 affected members, hand weakness and wasting usually occur in the late teenage years. While foot weakness ultimately develop in 40% of cases, this was usually mild and patients were still walking by age 60. One branch of the family had mild pyramidal features including Babinski signs. NCVs were normal except for reduced CMAP amplitudes in wasted muscles.

A recessive distal HMN has been termed the Jerash type based on a large Jordanian family with a locus mapped to chromosome 9p21.1–p12. Patients develop gait instability and foot drop prior to the age of 10 and a few years later develop wasting and weakness of hand muscles. Occasionally, milder phenotypes have been identified in patients over the age of 50. Initially, patients have presented with upper motor neuron signs including hyperreflexia, spasticity and up going toes. Subsequently, ankle reflexes are lost and plantar responses were described as down going. The ultimate course of this disorder is relatively benign, with the oldest affected patient ambulatory at age 80.

An additional distal motor syndrome has been mapped to 9q34 and has been classified as an autosomal dominant form of ALS (ALS4) because most patients have both upper and lower motor neuron signs including brisk reflexes and upgoing toes. However, the clinical course of these patients is much milder than typical ALS. The disease is characterized by a clinical onset in childhood, a slow rate of progression and a normal lifespan. Patients develop distal muscle weakness and atrophy and pyramidal signs but have normal sensation. The disorder is caused by missense mutations in the senataxin gene (*SETX*) (41). The function of *SETX* is unknown but the gene contains a DNA/RNA helicase domain with strong homology to human *RENT1* and *IGHMBP2*, two genes encoding proteins involved in RNA processing. It is hypothesized that mutations in *SETX* may cause neuronal degeneration through dysfunction of the helicase activity or other steps in RNA processing in motor neurons.

Puls and colleagues showed linkage of a lower motor neuron disorder to a region of 4 Mb at chromosome 2p13 (26). Mutation analysis of a gene in this interval that encodes the largest subunit of the axonal transport protein, dynactin, showed a single base-pair change resulting in an amino-acid substitution that is predicted to distort the folding of dynactin's microtubule-binding domain. Binding assays show decreased binding of the mutant protein to microtubules, suggesting that dysfunction of dynactin-mediated transport caused the motor neuron degeneration.

5. HEREDITARY BRACHIAL PLEXUS NEUROPATHY

Hereditary brachial plexus neuropathy (HBPN) has been mapped to chromosome 17q24–25. This unusual autosomal dominant disorder presents with episodes of acute onset pain, weakness and sensory loss in the upper extremities. Recovery usually occurs, beginning several weeks to months after the onset of symptoms. Subsequent attacks may occur in the same or opposite arm. Minor dysmorphic features, including short stature, hypotelorisms, epicanthal folds, and cleft palate, are frequent associated findings. Nerve conduction studies indicate normal values, entrapment syndromes, or asymmetrically reduced CMAP and SNAP amplitudes. Nerve biopsies have demonstrated tomaculi leading to the other name for this disorder, "tomaculous neuropathy." This disorder is genetically distinct from HNPP (42,43).

6. DIAGNOSIS

There are several steps in diagnosing an inherited neuropathy. The first is establishing whether the patient has symptoms and examination findings of length-dependent weakness and sensory loss in a symmetrical pattern. The neurological examination typically reveals weakness of foot dorsiflexion and eversion that is out of proportion to plantar flexion and inversion weakness. Patients often have abnormalities in dorsiflexion their fingers and performing fine movements of their hands. Muscle wasting in feet and hands is frequent. Tendon reflexes are often, but not always decreased. Foot abnormalities, such as pes cavus, and scoliosis are frequent. Autonomic symptoms or signs are usually not found in most forms of inherited neuropathies, excluding that disorder in which autonomic abnormalities are part of the disease criteria, such as the Hans.

Nerve conduction studies have an important role in characterizing CMT disorders since their initial use in separating CMT1 from CMT2 by conduction velocity. In the early 1980s, Lewis and Sumner (44) demonstrated that most cases of inherited neuropathies had uniformly slow conduction velocities, whereas acquired demyelinating neuropathies had asymmetric slowing with abnormal temporal dispersion. The pattern of slowing could thus be used, along with a patient's pedigree, to distinguish between inherited and acquired neuropathies. Over the past decade, this approach has had to be qualified. Most CMT1 patients, particularly those with CMT1A, have uniformly slow conduction velocities of about 20 m/s (although 38 m/s is used as a "cut off" value) (5). Conduction velocities in CMT1B tend to cluster at < 10 m/s in early onset cases or > 30 m/s in late onset cases (with only occasional examples in the range of 20 m/s) (11). Asymmetric slowing is characteristic of HNPP, and also may be found in patients with missense mutations in PMP22, MPZ, EGR-2 and Cx32 (45). Since all of these disorders may present without a clear family history of neuropathy, one must be cautious in using conduction velocity to distinguish acquired from inherited demyelinating neuropathies. Forms of inherited neuropathies associated with uniform and non-uniformly slowed conduction velocity are illustrated in Table 21.2 (45).

HNPP is also unique in that distal motor latencies are prolonged, markedly so for the median and peroneal nerves, and less so for the ulnar and tibial nerves, Conduction velocities across common sites of nerve entrapment are slow, but velocities over other segments are normal or near normal (46).

The distinction between demyelinating and axonal features is particularly confusing in CMTX. Nerve conduction velocities in CMTX patients are faster than in most patients with CMT1, often with prominent reductions in compound muscle action potential (CMAP) and sensory nerve action potential (SNAP) amplitudes. Thus, CMTX has been described as an axonal neuropathy, but analysis of conduction data reveals primary demyelinating features, and the disease is caused by mutations in Cx32, which is expressed in the myelinating Schwann cell. Conduction velocities in men are usually between 30 and 40 m/s, values that would be considered intermediate between CMT1 and CMT2. Distal motor latencies and F-wave latencies are usually prolonged (47,48). Female carriers usually have normal conduction velocities, but some have slowed velocities, probably do to inactivation of their mutant X chromosome.

Table 21.2 Electrophysiologic Findings of Inherited Demyelinating
Neuropathies

Inherited disorders with uniform conduction slowing
  Charcot–Marie–Tooth 1A
  Charcot–Marie–Tooth 1B
  Dejerine–Sottas
  Metachromatic leukodystrophy
  Cocaine's disease
  Krabbe's
Inherited disorders with multifocal conduction slowing
  Hereditary neuropathy with liability to pressure palsies
  Charcot–Marie–Tooth X
  Charcot–Marie–Tooth 1B
  Adrenomyeloneuropathy
  Pelizeus–Merzbacher disease with proteolysis protein null mutation
  Refsum's
Inherited disorders with electrophysiology that has not been characterized
  PMP 22 point mutations
  Adult onset leukodystrophies
  Me rosin deficiency
  Early growth response 2 (EGR2) gene mutations
  Myotubularin related protein 2 mutations
  Neurofilament light mutations
  LITAF/SIMPLE mutations
  Ganglioside induced differentiation associated protein 1

It is important to appreciate that although hereditary neuropathies are classified as demyelinating and axonal, all forms, including CMT1A, have axonal loss. Patient disability correlates better with axonal loss than with conduction velocity (6,28). Thus reductions in CMAP and SNAP amplitudes are found in most CMT1 patients, and in our series of 43 CMT1A patients, 34 had unobtainable peroneal CMAPs and 41 unobtainable sural SNAPs (6).

Nerve conduction velocities are essential to determine whether patients are likely to have demyelinating forms of neuropathy. We emphasize the importance of evaluating nerve conduction studies carefully for subtle signs of demyelination, such as prolonged distal motor latencies or F-wave latencies in determining whether the underlying cause is likely to be axonal or demyelinating. In our opinion, sural nerve biopsies are rarely helpful in diagnosing inherited neuropathies although they may prove invaluable for future research studies investigating pathogenic mechanisms of disease.

Typically, inherited neuropathies are chronic diseases with symptoms extending back into childhood although some atypical forms can have their onset in adulthood. Obtaining a careful pedigree is critical in the diagnosis of inherited neuropathies, not only to determine that there is an inherited neuropathy but also to determine who is at risk for developing the neuropathy. Careful pedigrees require going back carefully at least three generations. Identifying male-to-male transmission is the only way to exclude X-linked inheritance. While positive pedigrees may prove invaluable, caution must be taken in interpreting negative pedigrees; even dominantly inherited diseases can start in a particular patient. Similarly, family histories will usually be negative in recessive disorders. In some circumstances, genetic testing is necessary to determine the genetic cause of the neuropathy and to predict at risk family members.

Genetic testing has therefore become an important tool in the diagnosis of CMT. A full characterization of the neuropathy is critical for determining whether a genetic test will be informative. At present, we feel that a reasonable approach is to order testing when nerve conduction velocities are slow. However, mutations in myelin genes may have relatively normal conduction velocities. When one family member with CMT1 has been genotyped, it is usually not necessary to test other family members, and they can be screened by clinical examination and nerve conduction studies.

7. MANAGEMENT

There are no specific cures for inherited neuropathies. Most patients will benefit from of physical or occupational therapy. Foot care and orthotics, including ankle bracing, is most important, and if done well, can help patients ambulate independently throughout their lives. Difficulties with fine movements of the fingers are frequent, and occupational therapy can help with techniques to aid in buttoning, zippering and other hand movements requiring dexterity.

Genetic counseling is critical in the management of patients. Many patients are uninformed about genetic patterns in CMT, particularly concerning who is at risk in the family and what reproductive options are available. Genetic counselors can be invaluable in the time consuming task of obtaining careful pedigrees from patients.

A final point concerns medications and their affects on CMT patients. In general medications that have clear neurotoxic affects such as vincristine or cis platinum should be avoided, if medically possible, in CMT patients because they are likely to exacerbate the already existing neuropathy. There have been reports of severe, Guillain–Barré type weakness in patients with CMT who were given vincristine (49,50). For other medications the situation is less clear. The Charcot–Marie–Tooth Association (CMTA) publishes a list of medications that may exacerbate CMT. The degree of risk varies with the individual medication and in some cases; the risk may be small compared to the medical need. Good judgment by the physician on the risk/benefit ratio of a given medication can probably surmise as a useful guide for the use of these medicines.

ACKNOWLEDGMENTS

This material was supported in part by grants from the NIH, MDA, and Charcot–Marie–Tooth Association.

REFERENCES

1. Charcot J, Marie P. Sue une forme particulaire d'atrophie musculaire progressive souvent familial debutant par les pieds et les jamber et atteingnant plus tard les mains. Re Med 1886; 6:97–138.
2. Tooth H. The peroneal type of progressive muscular atrophy. London: Lewis, 1886.
3. Dyck PJ, Lambert EH. Lower motor and primary sensory neuron diseases with peroneal muscular atrophy. II. Neurologic, genetic, and electrophysiologic findings in various neuronal degenerations. Arch Neurol 1968; 18(6):619–625.
4. Lupski JR, de Oca-Luna RM, Slaugenhaupt S et al. DNA duplication associated with Charcot–Marie–Tooth disease type 1A. Cell 1991; 66(2):219–232.

5. Raeymaekers P, Timmerman V, Nelis E et al. Duplication in chromosome 17p11.2 in Charcot–Marie–Tooth neuropathy type 1a (CMT 1a). The HMSN Collaborative Research Group. Neuromuscul Disord 1991; 1(2):93–97.

6. Krajewski KM, Lewis RA, Fuerst DR et al. Neurological dysfunction and axonal degeneration in Charcot–Marie–Tooth disease type 1A. Brain 2000; 123(Pt 7):1516–1527.

7. Thomas PK, Marques W Jr, Davis MB et al. The phenotypic manifestations of chromosome 17p11.2 duplication. Brain 1997; 120(Pt 3):465–478.

8. Anani T, Sindou P, Richard L, Diot M, Vallat JM. Ultrastructural immunocytochemical abnormalities of peripheral myelin proteins in hereditary sensory-motor neuropathies: 12 cases. Ann N Y Acad Sci 1999; 883:186–195.

9. Hayasaka K, Ohnishi A, Takada G, Fukushima Y, Murai Y. Mutation of the myelin P0 gene in Charcot–Marie–Tooth neuropathy type 1. Biochem Biophys Res Commun 1993; 194(3):1317–1322.

10. Warner LE, Hilz MJ, Appel SH et al. Clinical phenotypes of different MPZ (P0) mutations may include Charcot–Marie–Tooth type 1B, Dejerine–Sottas, and congenital hypomyelination. Neuron 1996; 17(3):451–460.

11. Shy ME, Jani A, Krajewski K et al. Phenotypic clustering in MPZ mutations. Brain 2004; 127(Pt 2):371–384.

12. Street VA, Bennett CL, Goldy JD et al. Mutation of a putative protein degradation gene LITAF/SIMPLE in Charcot–Marie–Tooth disease 1C. Neurology 2003; 60(1):22–26.

13. Warner LE, Mancias P, Butler IJ et al. Mutations in the early growth response 2 (EGR2) gene are associated with hereditary myelinopathies. Nat Genet 1998; 18(4):382–384.

14. De Jonghe P, Timmerman V, Nelis E et al. A novel type of hereditary motor and sensory neuropathy characterized by a mild phenotype. Arch Neurol 1999; 56(10):1283–1288.

15. Yoshihara T, Kanda F, Yamamoto M et al. A novel missense mutation in the early growth response 2 gene associated with late-onset Charcot–Marie–Tooth disease type 1. J Neurol Sci 2001; 184(2):149–153.

16. Bergoffen J, Scherer SS, Wang S et al. Connexin mutations in X-linked Charcot–Marie–Tooth disease. Science 1993; 262(5142):2039–2042.

17. Tabaraud F, Lagrange E, Sindou P, Vandenberghe A, Levy N, Vallat JM. Demyelinating X-linked Charcot–Marie–Tooth disease: unusual electrophysiological findings. Muscle Nerve 1999; 22(10):1442–1447.

18. Hahn AF, Ainsworth PJ, Naus CC, Mao J, Bolton CF. Clinical and pathological observations in men lacking the gap junction protein connexin 32. Muscle Nerve 2000; 9(suppl):S39–S48.

19. Chance PF, Alderson MK, Leppig KA et al. DNA deletion associated with hereditary neuropathy with liability to pressure palsies. Cell 1993; 72(1):143–151.

20. Gabreels-Festen A, Wetering RV. Human nerve pathology caused by different mutational mechanisms of the PMP22 gene. Ann N Y Acad Sci 1999; 883:336–343.

21. Vance JM. The many faces of Charcot–Marie–Tooth disease. Arch Neurol 2000; 57(5):638–640.

22. Zuchner S, Mersiyanova IV, Muglia M et al. Mutations in the mitochondrial GTPase mitofusin 2 cause Charcot–Marie–Tooth neuropathy type 2A. Nat Genet 2004; 36(5):449–451.

23. Verhoeven K, De Jonghe P, Coen K et al. Mutations in the small GTP-ase late endosomal protein RAB7 cause Charcot–Marie–Tooth type 2B neuropathy. Am J Hum Genet 2003; 72(3):722–727.

24. Klein CJ, Cunningham JM, Atkinson EJ et al. The gene for HMSN2C maps to 12q23-24: a region of neuromuscular disorders. Neurology 2003; 60(7):1151–1156.

25. Sambuughin N, Sivakumar K, Selenge B et al. Autosomal dominant distal spinal muscular atrophy type V (dSMA-V) and Charcot–Marie–Tooth disease type 2D (CMT2D) segregate within a single large kindred and map to a refined region on chromosome 7p15. J Neurol Sci 1998; 161(1):23–28.

26. Antonellis A, Ellsworth RE, Sambuughin N et al. Glycyl tRNA synthetase mutations in Charcot–Marie–Tooth disease type 2D and distal spinal muscular atrophy type V. Am J Hum Genet 2003; 72(5):1293–1299.

27. Mersiyanova IV, Perepelov AV, Polyakov AV et al. A new variant of Charcot–Marie–Tooth disease type 2 is probably the result of a mutation in the neurofilament-light gene. Am J Hum Genet 2000; 67(1):37–46.

28. Kamholz J, Menichella D, Jani A et al. Charcot–Marie–Tooth disease type 1: molecular pathogenesis to gene therapy. Brain 2000; 123(Pt 2):222–233.

29. Baxter RV, Ben Othmane K, Rochelle JM et al. Ganglioside-induced differentiation-associated protein-1 is mutant in Charcot–Marie–Tooth disease type 4A/8q21. Nat Genet 2002; 30(1):21–22.

30. Cuesta A, Pedrola L, Sevilla T et al. The gene encoding ganglioside-induced differentiation-associated protein 1 is mutated in axonal Charcot–Marie–Tooth type 4A disease. Nat Genet 2002; 30(1):22–25.

31. Ben Othmane K, Hentati F, Lennon F et al. Linkage of a locus (CMT4A) for autosomal recessive Charcot–Marie–Tooth disease to chromosome 8q. Hum Mol Genet 1993; 2(10):1625–1628.

32. Liu H, Nakagawa T, Kanematsu T, Uchida T, Tsuji S. Isolation of 10 differentially expressed cDNAs in differentiated Neuro2a cells induced through controlled expression of the GD3 synthase gene. J Neurochem 1999; 72(5):1781–1790.

33. Bolino A, Muglia M, Conforti FL et al. Charcot–Marie–Tooth type 4B is caused by mutations in the gene encoding myotubularin-related protein-2. Nat Genet 2000; 25(1):17–19.

34. Senderek J, Bergmann C, Weber S et al. Mutation of the SBF2 gene, encoding a novel member of the myotubularin family, in Charcot–Marie–Tooth neuropathy type 4B2/11p15. Hum Mol Genet 2003; 12(3):349–356.

35. Senderek J, Bergmann C, Stendel C et al. Mutations in a gene encoding a novel SH3/TPR domain protein cause autosomal recessive Charcot–Marie–Tooth type 4C neuropathy. Am J Hum Genet 2003; 73(5):1106–1119.

36. Kalaydjieva L, Gresham D, Gooding R et al. N-myc downstream-regulated gene 1 is mutated in hereditary motor and sensory neuropathy-Lom. Am J Hum Genet 2000; 67(1):47–58.

37. Boerkoel CF, Takashima H, Stankiewicz P et al. Periaxin mutations cause recessive Dejerine–Sottas neuropathy. Am J Hum Genet 2001; 68(2):325–333.

38. Rogers T, Chandler D, Angelicheva D et al. A novel locus for autosomal recessive peripheral neuropathy in the EGR2 region on 10q23. Am J Hum Genet 2000; 67(3):664–671.

39. Irobi J, Van Impe K, Seeman P et al. Hot-spot residue in small heat-shock protein 22 causes distal motor neuropathy. Nat Genet 2004; 36(6):597–601.

40. Evgrafov OV, Mersiyanova I, Irobi J et al. Mutant small heat-shock protein 27 causes axonal Charcot–Marie–Tooth disease and distal hereditary motor neuropathy. Nat Genet 2004; 36(6):602–606.

41. Chen YZ, Bennett CL, Huynh HM et al. DNA/RNA Helicase Gene Mutations in a Form of Juvenile Amyotrophic Lateral Sclrosis (ALS4). Am J Hum Genet 2004; 74(6):1128–1135 Epub 2004 Apr 21.

42. Chance PF. Survey of inherited peripheral nerve diseases. Electroencephalogr Clin Neurophysiol 1999; 50(suppl):121–128.

43. Kuhlenbaumer G, Stogbauer F, Timmerman V, De Jonghe P. Diagnostic guidelines for hereditary neuralgic amyotrophy or heredofamilial neuritis with brachial plexus predilection. On behalf of the European CMT Consortium. Neuromuscul Disord 2000; 10(7):515–517.

44. Lewis RA, Sumner AJ. The electrodiagnostic distinctions between chronic familial and acquired demyelinative neuropathies. Neurology 1982; 32(6):592–596.

45. Lewis RA, Sumner AJ, Shy ME. Electrophysiological features of inherited demyelinating neuropathies: a reappraisal in the era of molecular diagnosis. Muscle Nerve 2000; 23(10):1472–1487.

46. Li J, Krajewski K, Shy ME, Lewis RA. Hereditary neuropathy with liability to pressure palsy: the electrophysiology fits the name. Neurology 2002; 58(12):1769–1773.

47. Lewis RA, Shy ME. Electrodiagnostic findings in CMTX: a disorder of the Schwann cell and peripheral nerve myelin. Ann N Y Acad Sci 1999; 883:504–507.
48. Nicholson G, Nash J. Intermediate nerve conduction velocities define X-linked Charcot–Marie–Tooth neuropathy families. Neurology 1993; 43(12):2558–2564.
49. Hildebrandt G, Holler E, Woenkhaus M et al. Acute deterioration of Charcot–Marie–Tooth disease IA (CMT IA) following 2 mg of vincristine chemotherapy. Ann Oncol 2000; 11(6):743–747.
50. Uno S, Katayama K, Dobashi N et al. Acute vincristine neurotoxicity in a non-Hodgkin's lymphoma patient with Charcot–Marie–Tooth disease. Rinsho Ketsueki 1999; 40(5):414–419.

22

Hereditary Sensory Autonomic Neuropathies

Victoria H. Lawson

University of Utah, Salt Lake City, Utah, USA

ABSTRACT

Hereditary sensory autonomic neuropathies constitute a rare and heterogeneous group of disorders. Hereditary patterns are most commonly autosomal dominant, but recessive and X-linked inheritance is also observed. Clues to the diagnosis come from the history and examination findings of recurrent distal limb injuries, insensitivity to noxious stimuli, episodes of acral infections, and autonomic symptoms such as abnormal sweating, skin blotching, postural hypotension, gastrointestinal disturbances, and loss of normal tearing. Supportive laboratory testing includes abnormal autonomic and sweat tests and gastrointestinal cinesoradiography and manometry. Treatment is supportive to prevent infections from acral ulcers and manage autonomic dysfunction. Prognosis is worse for those with prominent autonomic features, but is strongly modified by the quality of supportive care. Genetic analysis is evolving and is beginning to elucidate pathogenetic mechanisms.

1. INTRODUCTION

Hereditary sensory and autonomic neuropathies (HSAN) are a group of disorders with primary involvement of neurons subserving sensation and autonomic functions. A classification system includes five main types based on clinical, electrophysiologic, and pathologic features and on modes of inheritance (1). Linkage analysis has been established for some and associated genes identified for type 1, type 3, and type 4. A sixth type that is X-linked has been described in a single case (2). Clinical features of the five main types are similar, with profound loss of sensory modalities with little or no loss of strength, but specific features of autonomic dysfunction vary according to type.

2. CLINICAL FEATURES

2.1. HSAN1

HSAN type 1 (also referred to as hereditary sensory radicular neuropathy) is the most common form (3) and is distinguished from other types by its older age of onset. Patients typically become symptomatic in the second to fourth decades (4), although extremes of age at onset have been reported (5). Classic symptoms are dissociated sensory loss (predominantly pain and temperature loss with relative preservation of touch) in a distal distribution. In the most severe and neglected cases, the tissue complications from painless plantar ulcers have led to neurotrophic arthropathy and mutilating acropathy (1,6,7). Although acral pain sensation is impaired, pain can still occur as a result of secondary osteomyelitis or cellulitis (1,6) or as a late manifestation of the neuropathy in the form of lancinating pain (1,4,8). Both anhidrosis and hyperhidrosis occur, with areas of abnormal sweating corresponding roughly to the regions of sensory loss ("sweaty feet") (5). Other autonomic features of orthostasis, sphincter dysfunction, and sexual dysfunction do not occur in HSAN1. Hearing loss severe enough to cause complete deafness has been described and is thought to be due to cell loss in the organ of corti and spiral ganglia (4,8–10). Less consistent findings include spastic gait (11,12) and tonic pupils (13).

On examination, foot deformities, such as thinning of the ankles, peroneal muscle atrophy (7,14), high arched feet (7,14), steppage gait, frequent ankle injuries (15), and the presence of calluses or corns (4) with or without pain, may be observed. In severe cases, mutilation may shorten the feet to the point that the patient can no longer ambulate (7,14). However, patients who have meticulously cared for their feet may have only mild pes cavus and hammer toes without plantar ulcers. Joint enlargement, effusion, ligament laxity, excessive mobility, and crepitus suggest neurogenic arthropathy (6). Loss of pain and temperature sensation is profound in a symmetric distribution, predominantly affecting the distal portions of the lower extremities and occasionally the upper extremities. There is relative preservation of light touch and pressure perception (1). Distal weakness is minimal. Ankle jerks are reduced or absent, but reflexes are normal elsewhere.

HSAN1 is the only type with an autosomal dominant pattern of inheritance. The gene has been mapped to chromosome 9 (9q22) and codes for serine palmitoyltransferase, long-chain base subunit 1 (SPTLC1). SPTLC1 is an enzyme important for the generation of the sphingolipids ceramide, and sphingomyelin (16,17) and mutation may disrupt a modulatory function of sphingolipids or, given that ceramide is a signaling factor in programed cell death, disrupt apoptosis of differentiating neurons (17,18). There is genetic heterogeneity within the HSAN1 phenotype as two families with the phenotype have not been linked to the 9q locus, suggesting at least one additional locus for HSAN1 (2,16,19,20).

2.2. HSAN2

HSAN2 is inherited in an autosomal recessive manner (1,21–23) and presents during infancy or early childhood. It tends to affect the limbs more proximally as well as the trunk and involves the upper extremities to a greater extent than the lower extremities (22–24). Lower extremity manifestations are recurrent foot fractures, pressure point ulcers, and limb deformations (1,22,24). Autonomic dysfunction becomes prominent with neurogenic bladder or impotence (22). Tonic pupils have been observed (13). The autosomal recessive inheritance, early onset, and truncal sensory loss distinguish this type from HSAN1.

Examination findings include paronychia, painless whitlows, and ulcers of the fingers and plantar surfaces of the feet. Acral mutilation may be observed in the hands as well as the feet due to secondary osteomyelitis and may lead to shortened or clubbed fingers. Sensory loss involves all modalities but touch-pressure and position senses are affected earlier and more significantly than pain or temperature and occurs in a more proximal distribution than that in HSAN1. Deep tendon reflexes are absent but muscle strength is preserved. Hearing loss has been reported (22,25).

HSAN2 remains unlinked to a chromosomal locus. Genes for one of the neurotrophins, brain derived neurotrophic factor (BDNF), and genes for three of the neurotrophin receptors [tyrosine kinase A (TRKA), TRKB, and p75] have been screened and excluded as candidate genes for HSAN2 (26).

2.3. HSAN3

HSAN3 [also referred to as familial dysautonomia or the Riley–Day syndrome] (27) is an autosomal recessive disorder, which presents in infancy and predominantly in Ashkenazi Jews (28). This is a severe disorder with marked autonomic symptoms. Infants suffer from decreased lacrimation (alacrima or "tearless cry"), hyperhidrosis (which may vary from erratic to excessive sweating), labile blood pressure, skin blotching, and difficulties with body temperature control (29–31). A set of five criteria have been proposed, which include (i) lack of axon flare following intradermal histamine administration, (ii) pupillary miosis following instillation of 2.5% methacholine chloride, (iii) alacrima, (iv) absence of fungiform papillae on the tongue, and (v) diminished deep tendon reflexes (32).

There are other clinical issues. Infants have difficulties in sucking and swallowing, failure to thrive, recurrent pulmonary infections, episodic fever, and episodic vomiting. The oral problems may improve with age, but give way to continued delays in development and growth. Alacrima can lead to corneal abrasions (33). Recurrent pulmonary infections are related to autonomic gastrointestinal dysfunction with aspiration. Even when the gastric symptoms are well managed to minimize aspiration, respiratory control difficulties occur with abnormal responses to hypercapnia and hypoxia (34). These difficulties may manifest as drowning or near-drowning during underwater swimming, syncope and convulsions with high altitude or air travel, and cyanosis or decerebrate posturing with breath-holding (34).

Examination findings in older children may include kyphoscoliosis from compression fractures of the vertebra, neurogenic arthropathy relating to recurrent fractures of the feet and long bones, and absence of fungiform papillae on the tongue (35,36). Cranial nerve examination may reveal a diminished gag reflex and corneal insensitivity and abrasions (28,37) as well as defective taste perception and hypersalivation. Pain and temperature perception is reduced. Strength is normal but deep tendon reflexes are absent. Autonomic dysfunction is indicated by skin color changes such as generalized erythema or blotching (the latter related to emotional upset), redness and cold of the hands (from peripheral vasoconstriction), and rubor of the feet. If the patient is anxious or agitated, excessive sweating may be noted as well as hypertension and orthostatic hypotension (38). Sphincter and sexual function are usually normal (1).

HSAN3 is linked to chromosome 9q31. Mutations in the gene IKBKAP (inhibitor of kappa light polypeptide gene enhancer in B cells, kinase complex-associated protein), which codes for a protein thought to be involved in transcriptional elongation, have been identified (39,40).

2.4. HSAN4

HSAN4 (also referred to as congenital insensitivity to pain with anhidrosis) is autosomal recessive with onset at birth or during early childhood. It is characterized by episodic fever, anhidrosis, absence of response to painful stimuli, oral/acral mutilation (with associated neurogenic arthropathy), and mental retardation (1,41). The episodic fever is due to loss of thermoregulation from anhidrosis, and recurrent febrile episodes are related to exposure to heated environments. The more diffuse nature of the anhidrosis may help to distinguish HSAN4 from HSAN1 and 2 in which anhidrosis is coincident with areas of sensory loss. Typical patient reports include "biting off the tip of the tongue," "burning the tips of fingers with an automobile lighter," and "burning hands and fingers on a hot oven" due to the inability to perceive pain (41). Normal lacrimation separates HSAN4 from HSAN3. Although the features described earlier are typical for HSAN4, it may present at any time from birth to the seventh decade with symptoms so mild as to remain unrecognized by the affected individual (42). Whether this phenotypic heterogeneity corresponds to genetic heterogeneity has yet to be determined.

Clinical examination may reveal mutilation or loss of fingers, toes, tongue, or ears, and there may be joint deformities. Responses to superficial pain (pinprick and burning heat) and deep pain (testicular/tendon compression, ischemia, esophageal balloon dilatation, cold water immersion of a limb) are absent, but touch, vibration, and position sensation are relatively intact. Cranial nerves, strength, and deep tendon reflexes are normal. There is a risk of spinal cord compression related to compression fractures of spinal vertebral bodies (43).

HSAN4 is due to mutations of the NTRK1 or *TRKA* gene on chromosome 1q22. NTRK1 encodes a receptor (tyrosine kinase) for nerve growth factor and may be important for the development of small, primary neurons. Nerve growth factor released from target cells such as skin, muscle, and glandular tissues recognize this receptor in neural crest cells and stimulate their survival. Mutations in the receptor disrupt this interaction and result in the developmental defect responsible for the phenotype (44–46).

2.5. HSAN5

HSAN5 is the least common and well defined of the HSAN types. It is thought to be autosomal recessive, but may include dominant inheritance. Clinical features are similar to HSAN4 with no response to painful stimuli, but is differentiated from other types by an absence of autonomic dysfunction (particularly anhidrosis) and mental retardation (47). Symptom onset is at birth or infancy with the typical features of ulceromutilating changes of the limbs and joints.

Examination reveals acral ulcerations, painless fractures, and neuropathic joint degeneration. There is absent pain and temperature sensation over the limbs with preservation of other sensory modalities. Muscle strength, tone, and deep tendon reflexes are normal.

The phenotypes of HSAN5 and HSAN4 are similar with the exception of anhidrosis and mental retardation, but mutations in the *TRKA* gene have not been demonstrated (48), and chromosomal linkage remains to be established.

3. LABORATORY EVALUATION

3.1. Electrodiagnostic Studies

Routine nerve conduction studies should include sensory and motor nerve testing. Needle EMG is less informative.

3.2. Nerve Biopsy Studies

A nerve biopsy may be indicated. Histologic evaluation should include both a distal lower extremity nerve (sural nerve) and muscle (such as gastrocnemius). Cryostat sections of muscle may be taken for standard histochemical reactions and visualization with light and electron microscopies. Semi-thin sections of nerve should be evaluated by light microscopy for the density of myelinated fibers. Electron microscopy is necessary to assess unmyelinated fibers, axonal contents, myelin sheath structure, and the endoneurial space (49). Histologic changes parallel electrophysiologic changes with marked reduction of unmyelinated fibers (C-fibers) and milder degrees of loss of small myelinated fibers (A δ-fibers). Large myelinated fibers (A α-fibers) are least affected (50). Fiber loss is greater distally than proximally in the lower limb (1).

3.3. Autonomic Studies

The history should include inquiries about sweating abnormalities, skin blotching, temperature instability, trouble swallowing, episodic vomiting, bowel/bladder incontinence, and impotence. Physical examination should include assessment of the skin for blotching, excessive sweatiness, or dryness as well as assessment for postural hypotension and absent compensatory tachycardia.

A battery of autonomic tests, which may only be available in special laboratories, will be reviewed. Figure 22.1 presents an algorithm of the main features of autonomic testing.

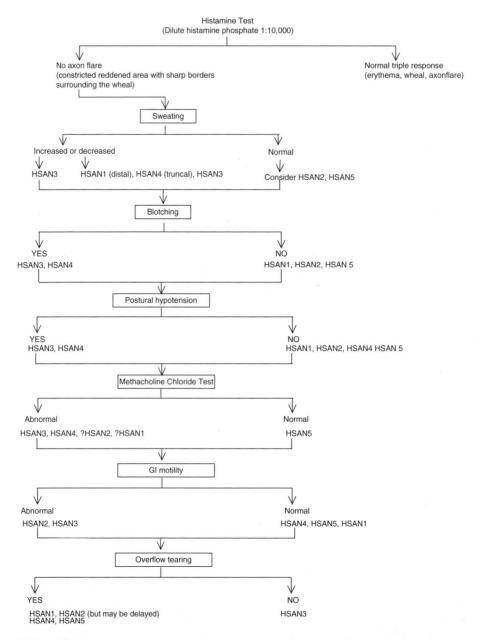

Figure 22.1   Algorithm of the main features of autonomic testing in the setting of a suspected HSAN.

3.3.1.   Histamine test

Intradermal histamine injection is used to demonstrate the dermal autonomic response. The resulting axonal flare may be absent in any disorder with a sensory dysfunction and therefore lacks specificity, but is useful to establish that sensory dysfunction exists (51). The test should be performed with dilute (1:10,000) histamine phosphate to avoid false-normal results with more concentrated solutions (52). Equivocal results may occur in children <6 weeks old and in children on antihistamines (51,53).

3.3.2. Sudomotor Function

The pattern of sweating under conditions of stress or agitation can be assessed by four auto-nomic reflex tests: (i) quantitative sudomotor axon reflex test (QSART) (54,55); (ii) sympath-etic skin response (SSR) (56); (iii) silastic imprints of sweat glands (57,58); and (iv) the thermoregulatory sweat test (59). QSART relies on the orthodromic propagation of an action potential from the unmyelinated post-ganglionic axon of an eccrine sweat gland in response to iontophoresis of acetylcholine. The sweat response is quantified using a capsule adherent to the skin that is connected to a sudorometer. The response is obtained at specific distal and proximal sites on the lower extremity and compared to normative values. Sudo-motor axon damage is indicated by a reduced or excessive response.

The SSR refers to a change in skin surface voltage as a result of sudomotor activity in response to deep inspiration or noxious stimuli (60). It can be easily performed during routine nerve conduction studies using disc electrodes on the dorsal and ventral surfaces of the hand or foot. Only the absence of a response is considered to be abnormal.

The sweat gland is stimulated directly by inotophoresis of 1% pilocarpine or acetyl-choline in the silastic imprint test. Silastic is then spread onto the skin and allowed to harden to obtain a cast of the sweat droplets emerging from the ducts. Because it assesses the response of the sweat gland itself without relying on the axon reflex, the silastic imprint test less directly reflects nerve fiber status when compared with QSART.

The thermoregulatory test assesses sweating of the whole body using a covering of ali-zarin red, cornstarch, and sodium carbonate, while the subject is heated in a hot chamber. The body pattern of anhidrosis indicates the anatomic distribution of affected efferent sympathetic nerves (59). Sweating is decreased distally in HSAN1, decreased diffusely in HSAN4, increased or decreased diffusely in HSAN3, and normal in HSAN2 and HSAN5.

3.3.3. Postural Hypotension

Postural hypotension is defined as a difference of at least 20 mmHg in systolic blood pressure or 10 mmHg in diastolic blood pressure between reclining and standing. Although this may be performed in the office, it may be difficult for patients with arthroses or other orthopedic problems and does not assess sympathetic modulation alone (61). In the setting of physical disability, cardiac disturbances, or other non-neurologic causes of postural hypotension (Table 22.1), referral to an autonomic testing laboratory is

Table 22.1 Non-neurologic Causes of Postural Hypotension

Cardiac	Venous pooling
Cardiac output block	Pregnancy
Mitral valve prolapse	Varicose veins
Aortic stenosis	Drugs
Hypertrophic cardiomyopathy	Endocrine/metabolic disorders
Cardiac myxoma or thrombus	Diabetes
Cardiac dysrhythmias	Addison's disease
Congestive heart failure	Hypopituitarism
Non-cardiac	Myxedema
Effective blood volume	Thyrotoxicosis
depletion	Pheochromocytoma
Dehydration	Hypokalemia
Hyponatremia	Carcinoid syndrome
Addison's disease	Increased age

indicated. The presence of postural hypotension supports the diagnosis of HSAN3 and 4; its absence suggests HSAN1, 2 or 5, but does not rule out HSAN4.

3.3.4. Pupil Abnormalities

HSAN3, HSAN4, and sometimes HSAN1 result in parasympathetic pupillary denervation. Application of low dose parasympathetic agents (2.5% methacholine chloride or 0.0625% pilocarpine) results in pupillary constriction due to denervation supersensitivity. However, corneal lesions and reduced drug dilution because of lack of tearing may cause false-abnormal responses (51,62). Pupillary function can also be assessed with infrared pupillometry.

3.3.5. Gastrointestinal Motility

An early and frequent sign of gastric autonomic dysfunction is oropharyngeal incoordination. Gastric and esophageal dysmotility as well as oropharyngeal incoordination may be assessed using cinesophagrams and manometric studies (34).

3.3.6. Lacrimation

Lacrimation can be assessed using Schirmer's test for eye moisture. In this test, sterile filter paper is placed over the border of the lower eyelid and the degree of moisture is measured after 5 min; <8 mm wetting is abnormal (63). Parenteral methacholine can also be used to distinguish whether alacrima is due to neurogenic pathology, because methacholine will produce tears in a neurogenic lesion but not in a glandular lesion.

4. LABORATORY FINDINGS

4.1. HSAN1

Nerve conduction studies reveal reduced or absent sensory nerve action potentials with relatively preserved motor nerve action potentials. Mild slowing of conduction velocities or prolongation of distal latencies may be seen (3,10,13,64,65). Needle EMG may include abnormal spontaneous activity and large polyphasic motor units suggestive of chronic partial denervation (13,64). *In vitro* study of excised sural nerve segments shows striking reduction of C-fibers (unmyelinated) and lesser reductions of A α-fibers (large myelinated) and A δ-fibers (small myelinated) (50). Histologic changes parallel electrophysiologic changes with marked reduction of unmyelinated C-fibers and milder degrees of loss of small myelinated fibers (A δ-fibers). Numbers of large myelinated fibers (A α-fibers) are least reduced (50). Fiber loss is greater distally than proximally in the lower limb (1). Anhidrosis is observed in the distribution of sensory loss.

4.2. HSAN2

Nerve conduction findings include absent sensory nerve action potentials with mildly decreased amplitude and increased latency motor potentials (24,66,67). Mild needle EMG abnormalities have been reported, including minimal fibrillation potentials and polyphasic, large motor units, suggesting some chronic motor axon loss. *In vivo* sural and superficial peroneal nerve studies reveal undetectable A δ- (small myelinated), A α- (large myelinated), and C (unmyelinated)-fiber potentials (24). Pathologic findings are marked loss of myelinated fibers with ballooned fibroblasts in the endoneurium

(1,21,24,65,67). This loss is more pronounced distally with evidence of ongoing segmental demyelination and remyelination in a small proportion of fibers. Unmyelinated fibers are also lost but to a variable degree and, in some instances, displaying histological evidence of abortive regeneration. These findings suggested an active, slowly progressive process rather than a static, congenital defect (1,24). Sweating is usually absent.

4.3. HSAN3

Nerve conduction studies reveal reduced sensory nerve action potential amplitudes in the lower extremities with mildly slowed motor nerve conduction velocities (68). Sural nerve biopsy reveals decreased numbers of nerve fibers of all sizes. Larger unmyelinated nerve fibers are most severely reduced, whereas the larger myelinated fibers ($>12~\mu m$) are relatively less affected. There is no evidence for fiber degeneration or segmental demyelination (68,69). Loss of autonomic, small sensory, and γ-motoneurons have been demonstrated (69–74). Despite near-normal numbers of α-motoneurons, inspection reveals distal axonal atrophy (73,74). Autopsy studies reported volume loss in the brainstem and cranial nerves of severely affected children (75,76). Volume loss in neuronal populations without pathologic hallmarks of active degeneration is a consistent finding and has been interpreted as a disturbance in early neuronal differentiation. Sweating may be increased or decreased.

4.4. HSAN4

Electrodiagnostic evaluation reveals intact sensory and motor responses, although entrapment neuropathies may occur secondary to neurogenic arthropathy and recurrent fractures. Nerve biopsy shows an absence of unmyelinated afferent sensory neurons (C-fibers) and an absence of sympathetic fibers to sweat glands, supporting the idea that HSAN4 is due a defect during neural crest differentiation, rather than a neurodegenerative process (41,77–80). SSR is absent (81).

4.5. HSAN5

Sensory and motor nerve action potentials are normal (47,82). Sural nerve biopsy reveals a selective severe decrease in the numbers of small myelinated fibers and a less severe decrease in the numbers of unmyelinated fibers (47,82,83). Sweating studies are normal.

5. MANAGEMENT

5.1. Tissue Complications

Plantar ulcerations, fractures, cellulitis, osteomyelitis, osteolysis, and neurogenic arthropathy can be avoided with proper attention to foot care (1). Patients should be advised to regularly and meticulously examine their feet, seek proper fitting shoes, minimize activities that will put them at risk for foot injury (excessive standing or walking; heavy lifting), and seek medical attention early in the event of an ulcer. Patients with HSAN4 may require specific devices to prevent injury to their mouth and tongue, such as soft polyvinyl mouth guards (84).

5.2. Pain Control

Lancinating and burning pain should be treated with pharmacologic agents that are appropriate for neuropathic pain, whereas pain associated with cellulitis and osteomyelitis is more appropriately treated with analgesics.

5.3. Autonomic Dysfunction

Anhidrosis can lead to life-threatening hyperthermia and febrile episodes, and individuals should be advised to avoid heated environments, sun exposure, and intense physical activity. Oropharyngeal incoordination should be treated with a gastrotomy tube to prevent aspiration and dehydration. Dysmotility and reflux should be treated conservatively with H2-blockers, thickened feeds, and appropriate positioning. If these interventions fail, fundoplication should be considered (85). Vomiting crises may be treated with avoidance of physical or emotional stress as well as pharmacologically with diazepam (0.2 mg/kg q3h up to maximum dose of 10 mg) and chloral hydrate suppositories (30 mg/kg q6h up to a maximum dose of 2 g) (34). Postural hypotension may be alleviated by elastic stockings, hydration, exercise of the lower extremities, and pharmacologically with fludrocortisone or midodrine (86). Increased blood pressure can be treated with avoidance of precipitants (pain and anxiety) but may also be treated with clonidine or diazepam (34). Profound hypotension and cardiac arrest may occur during general anesthesia and this should be performed only with a knowledgeable anesthetist and with pretreatment with adequate hydration (34,87). Corneal ulcerations from defective lacrimation and corneal insensitivity can be prevented with good general hydration, artificial tears, and soft contact lenses (which also promote healing). In refractory cases, procedures that block tear drainage (tear duct puncta cautery) or tarsorrhaphy may be required (34).

6. PROGNOSIS

Data on prognosis are anecdotal, with the exception of HSAN3 for which there are two detailed survival studies. HSAN1 is slowly progressive, and survival has been linked to appropriate and meticulous care of foot ulcers with prevention of secondary severe and life-threatening infections (1). HSAN2 does not show a clinical progression, but pathologic data point to a slow progression (1). HSAN3 is progressive but survival has been shown to be longer when patients participate in a specialized clinic (88,89). Sudden death is common, particularly during sleep, and sudden deaths that occur during the day are thought to be due to cardiac or vasovagal causes. HSAN4 is a static condition related to a defect during embryogenesis (3), but episodes of hyperpyrexia may be life-threatening, especially in the first 3 years of life (90). Data on survival and progression of disease in HSAN5 is lacking given its rare occurrence.

7. DIFFERENTIAL DIAGNOSIS

The clinical features of HSAN are distinctive, but other diagnoses should be considered in the setting of mild symptoms (Tables 22.2–22.4). The presence of marked distal weakness and wasting with ulceromutilation also suggests hereditary motor and sensory neuropathy (HMSN or CMT) type 2B (91). Marked atrophy and weakness without ulceromutilating changes suggest CMT. Porphyric neuropathy is a familial disorder and involves both

Table 22.2 Differential Diagnosis of HSAN

	Inherited	Non-inherited
HSAN1	Autosomal dominant amyloidosis CMT2B HSAN3 Porphyria	Syringomyelia Diabetes AIDP Distal small fiber neuropathy
HSAN2	Congenital sesnsory neuropathy with skeletal dysplasia Congenital autonomic dysfunction with universal pain loss	
HSAN3	Biemond congenital and familial analgesia HSAN4	
HSAN4	Amyloid neuropathy Diabetic small fiber neuropathy Acute pandysautonomia HSAN5 HSAN3	Fabry disease Tangier disease Anhidrotic ectodermal dysplasia
HSAN5	Amyloid neuropathy Diabetic small fiber neuropathy Acute pandysautonomia HSAN4	Fabry disease Tangier disease Anhidrotic ectodermal dysplasia

small myelinated and unmyelinated nerve fibers, but is characterized by episodic attacks of psychosis, abdominal pain, weakness, and constipation. Fabry disease is an X-linked disorder due to the deficiency of α-galactosidase A and presents with burning pain and dysesthesias along with angiokeratoses of the skin and corneal opacities. Skin biopsy

Table 22.3 Clinical Differentiation of the HSAN Patient

	HSAN1	HSAN2	HSAN3	HSAN4	HSAN5
Inheritance	AD	AR	AR	AR	AR
Fungiform papillae of the tongue	No	No	Yes	May be present	No
Corneal reflexes	Yes	No	No	Yes	Yes
DTRs	Reduced/ absent	Reduced/ absent	Reduced/ absent (normal in 5%)	Normal	Normal
Visceral pain appreciation	Normal	Abnormal	Normal	Abnormal	Abnormal
Paronychia	No	Yes	No	Yes	Yes
Sensory loss	Pain/ temperature	All	Pain/ temperature	Pain/ temperature	Pain/ temperature
Self-mutilation	Intermediate	Intermediate	Rare	Prominent	Prominent
Mental retardation	No	Rare	No	Mild	No
Sphincter/sexual dysfunction	No	No	May be present	No	No

Table 22.4 Clinical Autonomic Evaluation of the HSAN Patient

	Sweating	Blotching	Postural hypotension	Methacholine chloride test	Gastric motility	Overflow tearing
HSAN1	Decreased distally	No	No	Variable response	Normal	Yes
HSAN2	Normal	No	No	Variable response	Abnormal	Yes
HSAN3	Increased or decreased diffusely	Yes	Yes	Abnormal response	Abnormal	No
HSAN4	Decreased diffusely	Yes	Yes	Abnormal response	Normal	Yes
HSAN5	Normal	No	No	Normal response	Normal	Yes

shows lipid inclusions in vascular epithelial cells, but the diagnosis is made from measurements of enzyme activity in serum (92). Tangier disease is an autosomal recessive disorder characterized by progressive sensorimotor neuropathy during childhood in association with enlarged orange tonsils. Serum lipid analysis shows reduced cholesterol, reduced high-density lipoproteins, and normal or increased triglycerides. Nerve biopsy may reveal lipid-laden histiocytes (93).

In the absence of a family history, acquired disorders, such as syringomyelia, can affect the decussating spinothalamic tract fibers conveying pain and temperature, but leads to a "cape-like" distribution of anesthesia rather than the typical lower extremity, distal predominant pattern of HSAN. Orthostatic hypotension, impotence, bladder or bowel incontinence, and heart rate variability may be seen in diabetes (94,95).

REFERENCES

1. Dyck P. Neuronal atrophy and degeneration predominantly affecting peripheral sensort and autonomic neurons. In: Dyck PJ, Griffin JW, Low PA, Poduslo JF, eds. Peripheral Neuropathy. Vol. 2. Philadelphia: WB Saunders, 1993:1557–1598.
2. Jestico JV, Urry PA, Efphimiou J. An hereditary sensory and autonomic neuropathy transmitted as an X-linked recessive trait. J Neurol Neurosurg Psychiatry 1985; 48:1259–1264.
3. Mendell JR. Hereditary sensory and autonomic neuropathies. In: Jerry R Mendell, John T Kissel, David R Cornblath, eds. Diagnosis and Management of Peripheral Nerve Disorders. New York: Oxford University Press, 2001:376–460.
4. Hicks EP. Hereditary perforating ulcer of the foot. Lancet 1922; 1:319.
5. Burg D, Pongratz D, Burg G. Hereditary and autonomic neuropathies—classification and clinical characteristics. In: Asbury AKB, H, Sluga E, eds. Sensory Neuropathies. Wien, New York: Springer Verlag, 1995:57–73.
6. Dyck PJ, Stevens JC, O'Brien PC et al. Neurogenic arthropathy and recurring fractures with subclinical inherited neuropathy. Neurology 1983; 33:357–367.
7. Dyck PJK, Magal AJ IV, Kraybill EN. A virginia kinship with herditary sensory neuropathy: peroneal muscular atrophy and pes cavus. Mayo Clin Proc 1965; 40:685.
8. Reimann HA, McKechnie WG, Stanisavljevic S. Hereditary sensory radicular neuropathy and other defects in a large family. Am J Med 1958; 573:259.
9. Denny-Brown D. Hereditary sensory radicular neuropathy. J Neurol Neurosurg 1951; 14:237–252.

10. Horoupian DS. Hereditary sensory neuropathy with deafness: a familial multisystem atrophy. Neurology 1989; 39:244–248.

11. Van Epps C, Kerr HD. Familial lumbosacral syringomyelia. Radiology 1940; 35:160–173.

12. Spillane JD, Wells CEC. Acrodystrophic Neuropathy: A Critical Review of the Syndrome of Trophic Ulcers, Sensory Neuropathy, and Bony Erosion, Together with an Account of 16 Cases in South Wales. London: Oxford University Press, 1969.

13. Miller RG, Nielsen SL, Sumner AJ. Hereditary sensory neuropathy and tonic pupils. Neurology 1976; 26:931–935.

14. England AC, Denny-Brown D. Severe sensory changes, and trophic disorder, in peroneal muscular atrophy (Charcot–Marie–Tooth type). Arch Neurol Psychiatry 1952; 67:1.

15. Riley HA. Syringomyelia or myelodysplasia. J Nerv Ment Dis 1930; 72:1.

16. Dawkins JL, Hulme DJ, Brahmbhatt SB, Auer-Grumbach M, Nicholson GA. Mutations in SPTLC1, encoding serine palmitoyltransferase, long chain base subunit-1, cause hereditary sensory neuropathy type I. Nat Genet 2001; 27:309–312.

17. Bejaoui K, Wu C, Scheffler MD et al. SPTLC1 is mutated in hereditary sensory neuropathy, type 1. Nat Genet 2001; 27:261–262.

18. Kolesnick RK, M. Annu Rev Physiol 1998; 60:643–655.

19. Kwon JM, Elliott JL, Yee WC et al. Assignment of a second Charcot–Marie–Tooth type II locus to chromosome 3q. Am J Hum Genet 1995; 57:853–858.

20. Auer-Grumbach M, Wagner K, Timmerman V, de Jonghe P, Hartung HP. Ulcero-mutilating neuropathy in an Austrian kinship without linkage to hereditary motor and sensory neuropathy IIB and hereditary sensory neuropathy I loci. Neurology 2000; 54:45–52.

21. Ogryzlo M. A familial peripheral neuropathy of unknown etiology resembling Morvan's disease. Can Med Assoc J 1946; 54:547–553.

22. Nukada H, Pollock M, Haas LF. The clinical spectrum and morphology of type II hereditary sensory neuropathy. Brain 1982; 105(Pt 4):647–665.

23. Heller IH, Robb P. Hereditary sensory neuropathy. Neurology 1955; 5:15–29.

24. Ota M, Ellefson RD, Lambert EH, Dyck PJ. Hereditary sensory neuropathy, type II. Clinical, electrophysiologic, histologic, and biochemical studies of a Quebec kinship. Arch Neurol 1973; 29:23–37.

25. Munro M. Sensory radicular neuropathy in a deaf child. Br Med J 1956; 1:541–544.

26. Davar G, Shalish C, Blumenfeld A, Breakfield XO. Exclusion of p75NGFR and other candidate genes in a family with hereditary sensory neuropathy type II. Pain 1996; 67:135–139.

27. Riley CM, Day RL, Greeley DM, Langford WS. Central autonomic dysfunction with defective lacrimation. I. Report of five cases. Pediatrics 1949; 3:468.

28. Brunt PW, McKusick VA. Familial dysautonomia. A report of genetic and clinical studies, with a review of the literature. Medicine (Baltimore) 1970; 49:343–374.

29. Riley CMR. Familial dysautonomia differentiated from related disorders: case reports and discussion of current concepts. Pediatrics 1966; 37:435–446.

30. Riley C. Familial dysautonomia. Advances Pediat 1957; 9:157–190.

31. Moses SW, Rotem Y, Jagoda N, Talmor N, Eichbom F, Levin S. A clinical, genetic and biochemical study of familial dysautonomia in Israel. Israel J Med Sci 1967; 3:358–371.

32. Axelrod FB, Nachtigal R, Dancis J. Familial dysautonomia: diagnosis, pathogenesis and management. Adv Pediatr 1974; 21:75–96.

33. Mahloudji M, Brunt PW, McKusick VA. Clinical neurologic aspects of familial dysautonomia. J Neurol Sci 1970; 11:383.

34. Axelrod FB. Familial dysautonomia. In: Low PA, ed. Clinical Autonomic Disorders. New York: Lippincot–Raven Publishers, 1997:525–535.

35. Henkin RKI. Abnormalities of taste and smell thresholds in familial dysautonomia: improvement with methacholine. Life Sci 1964; 3:1319–1325.

36. Dancis JSAA. Familial dysautonomia. J Pediatr 1970; 77:174.

37. Fogelson MH, Rorke LB, Kaye R. Spinal cord changes in familial dysautonomia. Arch Neurol 1967; 17:103.

38. Fellner MJ. Manifestations of familial autonomic dysautonomia: report of a case, with an analysis of 125 cases in the literature. Arch Dermatol 1964; 89:190.

39. Anderson SL, Coli R, Daly IW et al. Familial dysautonomia is caused by mutations of the *IKAP* gene. Am J Hum Genet 2001; 68:753–758.

40. Slaugenhaupt SA, Blumenfeld A, Gill SP et al. Tissue-specific expression of a splicing mutation in the *IKBKAP* gene causes familial dysautonomia. Am J Hum Genet 2001; 68:598–605.

41. Swanson AG. Congenital insensitivity to pain with anhidrosis. Arch Neurol 1963; 8:299–306.

42. Thrush DC. Congenital insensitivity to pain. Brain 1973; 96:369–386.

43. Piazza MR, Bassett GS, Bunnell WP. Neuropathic spinal arthropathy in congenital insensitivity to pain. Clin Orthop 1988; 175–179.

44. Greco A, Villa R, Fusetti L, Orlandi R, Pierotti MA. The Gly571Arg mutation, associated with the autonomic and sensory disorder congenital insensitivity to pain with anhidrosis, causes the inactivation of the NTRK1/nerve growth factor receptor. J Cell Physiol 2000; 182:127–133.

45. Smeyne RJ, Klein R, Schnapp A et al. Severe sensory and sympathetic neuropathies in mice carrying a disrupted Trk/NGF receptor gene. Nature 1994; 368:246–249.

46. Indo Y, Tsuruta M, Hayashida Y et al. Mutations in the TRKA/NGF receptor gene in patients with congenital insensitivity to pain with anhidrosis. Nat Genet 1996; 13:485–488.

47. Low PA, Burke WJ, McLeod JG. Congenital sensory neuropathy with selective loss of small myelinated fibers. Ann Neurol 1978; 3:179–182.

48. Toscano E, Simonati A, Indo Y, Andria G. No mutation in the TRKA (NTRK1) gene encoding a receptor tyrosine kinase for nerve growth factor in a patient with hereditary sensory and autonomic neuropathy type V. Ann Neurol 2002; 52:224–227.

49. Gherardi RK. Neuromusuclar pathology. In: Poirier J, Gray F, Escourolle R, eds. Manual of Basic Pathology. Philadelphia: WB Saunders, 1990.

50. Dyck PJ, Lambert EH, Nichols PC. Quantitative measurement of sensation related to compound action potential and number and sizes of myelinated and unmyelinated fibers of sural nerve in health, Friedreich's ataxia, hereditary sensory neuropathy, and tabes dorsalis. In: Cobb WA, ed. Handbook of Electroencephalography and Clinical Neurophysiology. Vol. 9. Amsterdam: Elsevier Publishing Co., 1971.

51. Axelrod FB, Pearson J. Congenital sensory neuropathies. Diagnostic distinction from familial dysautonomia. Am J Dis Child 1984; 138:947–954.

52. Smith AAD, J. Response to intradermal histamine in familial dysautonomia: a diagnostic sign. J Pediatr 1963; 64:889–894.

53. Perlman M, Benady S, Saggi E. Neonatal diagnosis of familial dysautonomia. Pediatrics 1979; 63:238–241.

54. Low PA, Opfer-Gehrking TL, Proper CJ, Zimmerman I. The effect of aging on cardiac autonomic and postganglionic sudomotor function. Muscle Nerve 1990; 13:152–157.

55. Low PA, Caskey PE, Tuck RR, Fealey RD, Dyck PJ. Quantitative sudomotor axon reflex test in normal and neuropathic subjects. Ann Neurol 1983; 14:573–580.

56. Shahani BT, Halperin JJ, Boulu P, Cohen J. Sympathetic skin response—a method of assessing unmyelinated axon dysfunction in peripheral neuropathies. J Neurol Neurosurg Psychiatry 1984; 47:536–542.

57. Kennedy WR, Sakuta M, Sutherland D, Goetz FC. Quantitation of the sweating deficiency in diabetes mellitus. Ann Neurol 1984; 15:482–488.

58. Kennedy WR, Navarro X. Sympathetic sudomotor function in diabetic neuropathy. Arch Neurol 1989; 46:1182–1186.

59. Fealey R. The thermoregulatory sweat test. In: Low P, ed. Clinical Autonomic Disorders: Evaluation and Management. Boston: Little, Brown, 1993:217–229.

60. Novak V, Mendell JR. Evaluation of the peripheral neuropathy patient using autonomic reflex tests. In: Jerry R Mendell, John T Kissel, David R Cornblath, eds. Diagnosis and Managment of Peripheral Nerve Disorders. New York: Oxford University Press, 2001:43–66.

61. Hilz MJ, Axelrod FB, Braeske K, Stemper B. Cold pressor test demonstrates residual sympathetic cardiovascular activation in familial dysautonomia. J Neurol Sci 2002; 196:81–89.

62. Korczyn AD, Rubenstein AE, Yahr MD, Axelrod FB. The pupil in familial dysautonomia. Neurology 1981; 31:628–629.

63. Holland NR, Crawford TO, Hauer P, Cornblath DR, Griffin JW, McArthur JC. Small-fiber sensory neuropathies: clinical course and neuropathology of idiopathic cases. Ann Neurol 1998; 44:47–59.

64. Danon MJ, Carpenter S. Hereditary sensory neuropathy: biopsy study of an autosomal dominant variety. Neurology 1985; 35:1226–1229.

65. Schoene WC, Asbury AK, Astrom KE, Masters R. Hereditary sensory neuropathy. A clinical and ultrastructural study. J Neurol Sci 1970; 11:463–487.

66. Johnson RH, Spalding JM. Progressive sensory neuropathy in children. J Neurol Neurosurg Psychiatry 1964; 27:125.

67. Winkelman RK, Lambert EH, Hayles AB. Congenital absence of pain: report of a case and experimental studies. Arch Dermatol 1962; 85:325.

68. Aguayo AJ, Nair CP, Bray GM. Peripheral nerve abnormalities in the Riley–Day syndrome. Findings in a sural nerve biopsy. Arch Neurol 1971; 24:106–116.

69. Pearson J, Dancis J, Axelrod F, Grover N. The sural nerve in familial dysautonomia. J Neuropathol Exp Neurol 1975; 34:413–424.

70. Pearson J, Pytel BA. Quantitative studies of sympathetic ganglia and spinal cord intermediolateral gray columns in familial dysautonomia. J Neurol Sci 1978; 39:47–59.

71. Pearson J, Pytel B. Quantitative studies of ciliary and sphenopalatine ganglia in familial dysautonomia. J Neurol Sci 1978; 39:123–130.

72. Pearson J, Pytel BA, Grover-Johnson N, Axelrod F, Dancis J. Quantitative studies of dorsal root ganglia and neuropathologic observations on spinal cords in familial dysautonomia. J Neurol Sci 1978; 35:77–92.

73. Low PA. Clinical autonomic disorders. Philadelphia: Lippincot–Raven Publishers, 1997.

74. Dyck PJ, Kawamura Y, Low PA, Shimono M, Solovy JS. The number and sizes of reconstructed peripheral autonomic, sensory and motor neurons in a case or dysautonomia. J Neuropathol Exp Neurol 1978; 37:741–755.

75. Cohen PS, Solomon NH. Familial dysautonomia: case report with autopsy. J Pediatr 1955; 46:663.

76. Brown WJ, Beauchemin JA, Linde LM. A neuropathological study of familial dysautonomia (Riley–Day syndrome) in siblings. J Neurol Neurosurg Psychiatry 1964; 27:131.

77. Goebel HH, Veit S, Dyck PJ. Confirmation of virtual unmyelinated fiber absence in hereditary sensory neuropathy type IV. J Neuropathol Exp Neurol 1980; 39:670–675.

78. Sztriha L, Lestringant GG, Hertecant J, Frossard PM, Masouye I. Congenital insensitivity to pain with anhidrosis. Pediatr Neurol 2001; 25:63–66.

79. Rafel E, Alberca R, Bautista J, Navarrete M, Lazo J. Congenital insensitivity to pain with anhidrosis. Muscle Nerve 1980; 3:216–220.

80. Langer J, Goebel HH, Veit S. Eccrine sweat glands are not innervated in hereditary sensory neuropathy type IV. An electron-microscopic study. Acta Neuropathol (Berl) 1981; 54:199–202.

81. Shorer Z, Moses SW, Hershkovitz E, Pinsk V, Levy J. Neurophysiologic studies in congenital insensitivity to pain with anhidrosis. Pediatr Neurol 2001; 25:397–400.

82. Dyck PJ, Mellinger JF, Reagan TJ et al. Not "indifference to pain" but varieties of hereditary sensory and autonomic neuropathy. Brain 1983; 106(Pt 2):373–390.

83. Donaghy M, Hakin RN, Bamford JM et al. Hereditary sensory neuropathy with neurotrophic keratitis. Description of an autosomal recessive disorder with a selective reduction of small myelinated nerve fibres and a discussion of the classification of the hereditary sensory neuropathies. Brain 1987; 110(Pt 3):563–583.

84. Littlewood SJ, Mitchell L. The dental problems and management of a patient suffering from congenital insensitivity to pain. Int J Paediatr Dent 1998; 8:47–50.

85. Axelrod FB, Gouge TH, Ginsburg HB, Bangaru BS, Hazzi C. Fundoplication and gastrostomy in familial dysautonomia. J Pediatr 1991; 118:388–394.

86. Axelrod FB, Krey L, Glickstein JS, Allison JW, Friedman D. Preliminary observations on the use of midodrine in treating orthostatic hypotension in familial dysautonomia. J Auton Nerv Syst 1995; 55:29–35.
87. Axelrod FB, Donenfeld RF, Danziger F, Turndorf H. Anesthesia in familial dysautonomia. Anesthesiology 1988; 68:631–635.
88. Axelrod FB, Abularrage JJ. Familial dysautonomia: a prospective study of survival. J Pediatr 1982; 101:234–236.
89. Axelrod FB, Goldberg JD, Ye XY, Maayan C. Survival in familial dysautonomia: impact of early intervention. J Pediatr 2002; 141:518–523.
90. Rosenberg S, Marie SKN, Kleimann S. Congenital insensitivity to pain with anhidrosis (hereditary sensory and autonomic neuropathy type IV). Pediatr Neurol 1994; 11:50–56.
91. Auer-Grumbach M, De Jonghe P, Wagner K, Verhoeven K, Hartung HP, Timmerman V. Phenotype–genotype correlations in a CMT2B family with refined 3q13–q22 locus. Neurology 2000; 55:1552–1557.
92. Onishi A, Dyck PJ. Loss of small peripheral sensory neurons in Fabry disease. Histologic and morphometric evaluation of cutaneous nerves, spinal ganglia, and posterior columns. Arch Neurol 1974; 31:120–127.
93. Yao JK, Herbert PN, Fredrickson DS et al. Biochemical studies in a patient with a Tangier syndrome. J Neuropathol Exp Neurol 1978; 37:138–154.
94. Brown MJ, Martin JR, Asbury AK. Painful diabetic neuropathy. A morphometric study. Arch Neurol 1976; 33:164–171.
95. Low PA, Walsh JC, Huang CY, McLeod JG. The sympathetic nervous system in diabetic neuropathy. A clinical and pathological study. Brain 1975; 98:341–356.

23

Other Hereditary Neuropathies

Jun Li
Wayne State University, Detroit, Michigan, USA

A. Gordon Smith
University of Utah, Salt Lake City, Utah, USA

ABSTRACT

There are a number of rare inherited diseases with prominent peripheral nerve involvement. They include porphyria, leukodystrophies, Krabbe's disease, Fabry disease, hereditary amyloidosis, giant axonal neuropathy, and Tangier disease. Although uncommon, each disorder has distinctive features, and familiarity with them aids in their recognition. Porphyria typically presents in an acute fashion, leukodystrophies include upper motor neuron findings (spasticity, exaggerated deep tendon reflexes) and some are associated with a demyelinating polyneuropathy with slowed nerve conduction velocity, whereas Fabry disease and hereditary amyloidosis preferentially affect small caliber unmyelinated sensory and autonomic nerves resulting in prominent pain and autonomic dysfunction. Systemic symptoms or signs of involvement of other organ systems often provide diagnostic clues. Abdominal pain and psychosis are common in porphyria, characteristic skin lesions occur in Fabry disease, and heart and renal failure suggests amyloidosis. Diagnostic conformation is aided by nerve biopsy, biochemical enzymatic assay, or genetic testing.

1. INTRODUCTION

Most hereditary neuropathies involve only peripheral nerve, but there are rare hereditary neuropathies that also involve the central nervous system and other organs. These include porphyria, leukodystrophies, Krabbe's disease (KD), Fabry disease, hereditary amyloidosis, giant axonal neuropathy, and Tangier disease. Although they are rare, familiarity with their clinical features is important. They have distinctive clinical presentation, differential diagnosis, and diagnostic approaches.

2. PORPHYRIC NEUROPATHY

The term porphyria is derived from the Greek word *porphuros*, meaning purple, and refers to the reddish-purple color of urine owing to excessive excretion of pigmented porphyrins. Although rare, this disease has captured public interest because King George III and van Gogh may have had porphyria (1,2). The first description of an acute porphyric attack, occurring secondary to exposure to a sedative drug (sulfonal) dates to 1889 (3). Two decades later, this disorder was recognized as an inborn error of metabolism (4). However, a full appreciation of the clinical and biochemical features did not occur until the mid 20th century with analysis of high prevalence populations (5–7). The genes coding for enzymes of the porphyrin synthetic pathway have been identified and sequenced, and genotype–phenotype correlations are clarifying the pathogenesis (8).

2.1. Clinical Features

Porphyrias are autosomal dominant or autosomal recessive and owing to mutations affecting genes encoding enzymes in the biosynthetic pathway of heme. There are seven types of porphyria, and the nervous system may be affected in four of them (Table 23.1). Neuroporphyrias may be further divided into two groups: 1) neurovisceral porphyrias, including acute intermittent porphyria (AIP) and δ-aminolevulinate dehydratase (ALAD) deficiency and 2) neurocutaneous porphyrias, including hereditary coproporphyria (HCP) and variegate porphyria (VP) which often cause skin lesions (1), which are absent in the neurovisceral porphyries (Fig. 23.1). AIP is the most common type of porphyria in North America (prevalence of 1–2 per 100,000), whereas ALAD is extremely rare (nine reported cases). VP is rare in most regions of the world, but has high prevalence in others, particularly South Africa (prevalence of 3 per 1000) (9–11).

Regardless of the specific form of porphyria, neuropathy usually presents with single or intermittent acute attacks. Abdominal pain, vomiting, and constipation are almost

Table 23.1   The Classification of Neuro-Porphyria

Disorder	Defective enzyme	Gene location	Mutations	Porphyrin profile
AIP	Porphobilinogen deaminase	AD 11q24	>90	↑↑↑ PBG, ALA in urine; normal in feces.
HCP	Coproporphyrinogen oxidase	3q12	16	↑↑ PBG, ALA, COPRO in urine; ↑↑↑ COPRO in feces.
VP	Protoporphyrinogen oxidase	1q23	5	↑↑ PBG, ALA, COPRO in urine; ↑↑ PROTO > COPRO
ALAD deficiency	ALAD	9q34	9	↑↑↑ ALA, ↑or normal PBG in urine; normal in feces.

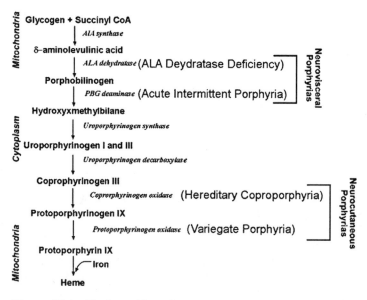

Figure 23.1 The heme biosynthetic pathway. The enzyme defects responsible for the various forms of porphyria are noted. The neurovisceral porphyrias result in accumulation of water soluble, upstream, metabolites that may be measured in urine. The neurocutaneous porphyrias result in accumulation of fat soluble metabolites best measured in stool.

universal features during the attacks, often leading to extensive inconclusive gastroenterological evaluations (12,13). Autonomic instability, including tachycardia and hypertension, is common, but often overlooked.

Acute attacks may progress to include acute motor neuropathy, similar to the acute motor sensory axonal neuropathy variant of the Guillain–Barré Syndrome (GBS). However, weakness may start in proximal upper extremity muscles, a pattern atypical for GBS. After several recurrent attacks, distal weakness may occur. Mild neuropathic sensory symptoms, such as numbness and tingling, may occur, but usually do not represent a major complaint. Sensory disturbances often have a "bathing trunk" distribution, with reduced touch and pin-prick over the trunk and thighs, a pattern atypical for GBS (10). Deep tendon reflexes may be normal in some patients.

Factors which increase heme synthesis may provoke porphyric attacks. Cytochrome P450 contains heme, and any substance that stimulates synthesis of this enzyme may provoke an attack. Drugs are the most common provocative factors, (Table 23.2) (9,10,14). Estrogen and progesterone compounds induce cytochrome P450, and oral contraceptives or pregnancy may also provoke attacks. Reduced caloric intake and stress are also risk factors (15).

Recognition of dermatological abnormalities may facilitate the diagnosis. Photosensitivity is a hallmark of neurocutaneous porphyrias, with fragile skin and development of bullous lesions after exposure to sunlight (Fig. 23.2). Facial hypertrichosis and hyperpigmentation may also be observed (9,10).

Psychiatric symptoms are common in porphyria, but are frequently ignored. Because these symptoms are unusual in other acute neuropathies, their recognition may expedite the diagnosis. Anxiety, restlessness, insomnia, and psychosis are common and may occur years prior to the acute attack. During the attack, confusion, delusion, hallucinations, and agitation are common (16). Other central nervous system manifestations including seizures and inappropriate secretion of anti-diuretic hormone (SIADH) (17,18). Care must be

Table 23.2 Drugs that may Precipitate the Acute Porphyria

Unsafe	Safe
Barbiturates	Narcotic analgesics
Sulfonamide antibiotics	Aspirin
Meprobamate	Acetaminophen
Glutethimide	Phenothiazines
Chlorpropamide	Penicillin and derivatives
Diphenylhydantoin	Streptomycin
Mephenytoin	Glucocorticoids
Succinimide	Propranolol
Carbamazepine	Digoxin
Valproic acid	Bromides
Pyrazolones	Insulin
Griseofulvin	Atropine
Ergots	Diazepam
Synthetic estrogens	Diphenhydramine
and progestins	Ether
Danazol	Nitrous oxide
Alcohol	Neostigmine

Source: Modified from Barohn et al. (14).

taken when treating seizures because many anticonvulsants can exacerbate porphyria (Table 23.2).

2.2. Laboratory Evaluation

Electrodiagnostic evaluation is consistent with an axonal motor polyneuropathy (19–21). Compound muscle action potential (CMAP) amplitudes are reduced, whereas conduction velocities are normal or mildly slowed. Sensory nerve action potential amplitudes are normal or minimally reduced. Needle electromyography (EMG) reveals fibrillations and positive waves and decreased motor unit recruitment. Denervation changes may be widespread, including proximal muscles. Differentiation from acute inflammatory demyelinating polyradiculoneuropathy (AIDP) is straightforward because the electrodiagnostic features are indicative of a primary acquired demyelinating lesion. However, distinction from axonal variants of GBS may be difficult on the basis of electrodiagnostic testing alone.

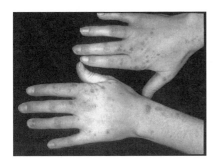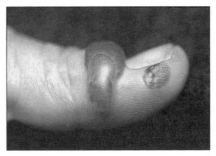

Figure 23.2 Porphyric skin lesions. Neurocutaneous porphyrias case photosensitive skin lesions that may be bullous (right panel). (Image courtesy of Dr John Zone, University of Utah Department of Dermatology.)

Nerve biopsy is not required, and axonal degeneration and regeneration are the primary pathologic features (21,22).

Laboratory evaluation may reveal leukocytosis during acute attacks. Hyponatremia may be secondary to SIADH (9,13). Cerebrospinal fluid (CSF) is usually acellular with normal or elevated protein (9,10). A definitive diagnosis relies on the identification of excessive porphyrins in urine or feces. The Watson–Schwartz test is a qualitative test for urinary porphyrins but has low sensitivity, and a negative result does not exclude the diagnosis. Quantitative porphyrins in a 24 h urine or feces collection should be performed when the diagnosis is suspected. The pattern of porphyrins in urine and feces may allow differentiation among porphyria types (Table 23.1). Porphyrins in the first half of the synthetic pathway are water-soluble, and thus appear in the urine, but the interpretation of urine results may be problematic and measurement of stool levels may be necessary to make a conclusive diagnosis. Porphyrins from the later half of the pathway are fat-soluble and may only be measured in stool. Patients with suspected cutaneous porphyrias should have stool sampled first. Lead may interfere with heme biosynthesis, resulting in elevated porphyrins with lead poisoning, and a lead level may need to be checked when lead poisoning is also being considered (9).

2.3.   Genetics

The genes responsible for each relevant enzyme have been identified, cloned, and sequenced, and leading to mouse models (23,24). Urinary or fecal porphyrins may be increased in genetically involved, but clinically nonpenetrant, family members (9), and genetic testing may be the most accurate means of determining if other family members are affected (8). DNA testing is not available for routine clinical use and is only available in research laboratories.

2.4.   Management and Prognosis

Patients with porphyria may be asymptomatic until a precipitating factor is encountered. When the disease is known, avoidance of provocative factors is most important. During an acute attack, hydration is important, but with attention to possible hyponatremia from SIADH. Fasting increases δ-aminolevulinic acid (ALA) synthase activity and carbohydrate intake reduces it, therefore glucose infusion represents a therapy during the acute attack. Pain is managed with analgesics or opiates. Seizures may be controlled with safe medications (Table 23.2). Cardiovascular function should be monitored because of possible dysautonomia. Specific treatment with hematin, a hydroxide of heme, suppresses the accumulation of porphyrins by down-regulating ALA synthase. Although a randomized trial did not show significant clinical benefit (25), most clinicians still use hematin to treat acute porphyric attacks. Hematin is administered intravenously at a dose of 1–4 mg/kg daily for several days to two weeks depending on response.

Prediction of subsequent attacks is not possible. VP with homozygosity tends to have an earlier onset and more severe phenotype. In general, recurrent attacks are more common in AIP than in other types of porphyrias. Porphyrias may be associated with an increased incidence of hepatocellular carcinoma (9,10).

2.5.   Pathogenesis

Porphyrins are intermediate products in the biosynthesis of heme, which is a critical component of multiple proteins essential to human life, including cytochrome P-450 oxidase, hemoglobin, and myoglobin (Fig. 23.1) (8). Heme biosynthesis starts in the mitochondria. Glycine and succinyl CoA are converted to ALA, a step catalyzed by the rate-limiting enzyme ALA synthase. ALA moves to the cytoplasm where additional steps occur. When coproporphyrinogen III is synthesized, it re-enters the mitochondria, where protoporphyrin IX is produced. Heme forms with the insertion of an iron into the center of the protoporphyrin IX ring. Once produced, heme exerts a negative feedback on ALA synthase activity. For this reason, a defect in any of the synthetic enzymes results in reduced heme formation and reduced negative feedback, resulting in an increased activity of ALA synthase. There is overproduction of the porphyrins upstream from the deficiency and underproduction down-stream.

The pathophysiologic mechanisms in the development of porphyric neuropathy are unclear, but it is assumed that excessive accumulation of intermediate porphyrins is toxic to peripheral nerve. Acute porphyric attacks are always accompanied by increased activity of ALA synthase and excessive urinary excretion of ALA. These biochemical features also occur in the lead toxicity, which may cause a motor neuropathy with prominent upper extremity involvement. The toxic porphyrins may be taken up by nerve terminals and transported to the cell body via retrograde axonal transport. This hypothesis would explain why proximal upper extremity muscles are preferentially involved because they are supplied by the shortest motor nerves (26).

The toxic hypothesis does not explain the observation of excessive ALA concentrations in asymptomatic patients, and other mechanisms may contribute. Reduced levels of heme may result in reduced activity of heme containing enzymes relevant for peripheral nerve function.

3. LEUKODYSTROPHIES

Clinically significant peripheral neuropathy may occur in several leukodystrophies, including adrenomyeloneuropathy (AMN), metachromatic leukodystrophy (MLD), and KD. Because peripheral nerves are normal or minimally abnormal in early-onset forms of adrenoleukodystrophy, only AMN is discussed in this chapter. The leukodystrophies share several common features (Table 23.3) (27). Motor symptoms or signs, including slowly progressive spasticity, weakness, ataxia, and pyramidal tract signs, usually dominate the clinical presentation. Patients may manifest cortical abnormalities such as seizures and cognitive and behavioral disturbances. Urinary symptoms are common. Despite these similarities, the differences among the leukodystrophies are considerable, and the distinctive features of each disorder will be reviewed.

The genes responsible for the three leukodystrophies have been characterized, but genetic testing for these disorders is presently performed only in research laboratories (28).

3.1. Adrenomyeloneuropathy

3.1.1. Clinical Features

AMN is one of the two most common phenotypes of X-linked adrenoleukodystrophy. Neurological manifestations mainly involve the spinal cord and peripheral nerve. Men typically present in the third decade with slowly progressive spasticity. Proximal leg weakness contributes to the gait disturbance. Bowel and bladder dysfunction are common. Peripheral nerve manifestations are subtle, and symptoms of tingling and pain are uncommon. Sensation is reduced to all modalities, and proprioceptive loss can be

Table 23.3 Clinical and Laboratory Features of Leukodystrophies

Leukodystrophies	AMN	MLD	KD
Age of onset	3rd–4th decade	Infantile or juvenile or adult	Infantile (90%) or juvenile + adult (10%)
Inheritance and gene location	X-linked, Xq28 >406 mutations	AR, ch 22q13 >70 mutations	AR, ch 14q31 >60 mutations
Unique clinical features	Adrenal insufficiency, skin hyperpigmentation, gynecomastia	Prominent behavior disturbance and dementia	Seizures and vision loss with optic disc pallor
MRI	Symmetric increased signals of T2-weighted image in parietal-occipital region, which may not occur in AMN	Diffuse and symmetric high signals in the deep white matter of bilateral hemispheres with U-fiber sparing	Similar to MLD
Electrophysiology	Axonal in most cases	Demyelinating with uniform slowing	Demyelinating with uniform slowing
CSF	Normal or mildly elevated	Elevated	Highly elevated in many cases
Biochemical analysis	Serum VLCFA elevated	Low arylsulfatase-A activity and excessive sulfatides in urine	Low galactocerebrosidase activity in leukocytes or skin fibroblasts
Nerve biopsy	Axonal degeneration as the dominant feature, may have some demyelinating changes	Segmental demyelination and remyelination. "Tuffstone" bodies and lamellated inclusions with periodicity under EM	Segmental demyelination and remyelination. Nonorientated straight or curved prismatic inclusions in Schwann cells under EM

severe (27,28). A milder set of symptoms can be seen in 20% of female carriers, with onset in the fourth or later decades (28).

Central nervous system dysfunction eventually occurs in half of patients in the form of cognitive impairment (28–30). Occasional patients may present with a progressive cerebellar disorder imitating spinocerebellar ataxia (SCA) (28).

Microscopic evidence of adrenal involvement is observed in all patients, but in a substantial number adrenal insufficiency remains asymptomatic. Symptoms of adrenal insufficiency include weakness, fatigue, weight loss, and dermatological changes, including increasing pigmentation of the oral mucosa and skin around the nipples and over the elbows, knees, and scrotum (28,31). Women carriers do not develop adrenal insufficiency or hyperpigmentation (28).

3.1.2. Laboratory Evaluation

The diagnosis is suggested by neuroradiologic findings of demyelination affecting posterior white matter on brain MRI in half of patients with AMN (Table 23.3) (28).

Spinal cord imaging usually reveals atrophy of the thoracic cord (32). CSF examination is normal, differentiating it from multiple sclerosis (33).

Nerve conduction studies reveal evidence for an axonal neuropathy, but some patients demonstrate features of demyelinating polyneuropathy (34). Somatosensory evoked potentials are usually abnormal in asymptomatic female carriers. Brainstem auditory evoked potentials are abnormal in most men and 50% of women. Visual evoked potentials are abnormal in one-fifth of patients (35–37).

Nerve biopsy findings are consistent with axonal loss with some associated demyelination (38).

The diagnosis is made by documenting elevated very long chain fatty acids (VLCFA) in serum (28). Approximately 10% of female carriers have normal VLCFA levels (28).

3.1.3. Differential Diagnosis

Other disorders with chronic spastic paraparesis and peripheral neuropathy include HIV-induced myelopathy/neuropathy, syphilis myelopathy, HTLV1, vitamin B12 or vitamin E deficiency, transverse myelitis, and hereditary spastic paraparesis.

3.1.4. Management and Prognosis

Patients without clinical or neuroimaging evidence of CNS involvement may live a normal lifespan, although wheelchair dependency is common. Patients with cognitive deficits and an abnormal brain MRI scan may have a more aggressive course, reminiscent of childhood adrenoleukodystrophy. Female carriers have a benign course (28).

There is no effective treatment for AMN. Bone marrow transplantation (BMT) results in normalization of VLCFA levels, with encouraging results in patients with adrenoleukodystrophy without cerebral involvement, but the risks of BMT are significant. Patients with more severe manifestations may not be appropriate candidates because they may not tolerate the risk of BMT (39,40).

Dietary modification with restricted VLCFA intake and glyceroltrioleate supplementation ("Lorenzo's oil") has been evaluated in both childhood adrenoleukodystrophy and AMN. Although the treatment results in significant reduction of VLCFA levels, there is no effect on clinical manifestations or progression (41). Treatment of adrenal insufficiency with steroids is essential (28).

3.1.5. Pathogenesis

The ALD protein is a peroxisomal membrane protein belonging to the ATP-binding cassette (ABC) protein family. ALD protein may be involved in the transportation of VLCFA into peroxisomes, where VLCFA are oxidized. Mutation of the *ALD* gene may impair the degradation of VLCFA and lead to the accumulation of VLCFA (42). Although VLCFA levels correlate with adrenal dysfunction, there is a poor correlation with neurologic manifestations (43,44). A variety of immunologic derangements have been described, but treatment with immune modulating therapy has been unsuccessful, suggesting these findings may be a secondary process (45,46).

3.2. Metachromatic Leukodystrophy

3.2.1. Clinical Features

MLD has three broad phenotypes, infantile, the juvenile, and the adult forms. The infantile form presents with progressive mental regression and ataxia, and features of a myelopathy that are similar to those in adrenoleukodystrophy. Peripheral neuropathy occurs in almost every case, resulting in decreased or absent deep tendon reflexes (27,31). Clinical manifestations in the juvenile and adult forms are similar to the infantile form, except for severity and age of onset. MLD may present with isolated peripheral neuropathy, resulting in slowly progressive distal weakness, sensory loss, and pes cavus (47).

3.2.2. Laboratory Evaluation

Brain MRI is useful in diagnosing MLD, showing diffuse, symmetric demyelination with sparing of U fibers. Nerve conduction studies reveal uniformly slow conduction velocities which differs from the multifocal pattern observed with acquired demyelinating neuropathies, such as CIDP (48). Characteristic abnormalities are segmental demyelination and remyelination and metachromic aggregates in Schwann cells apparent with toluidine blue staining, and "tuffstone" bodies and lamellated inclusions with periodicity observed with electron microscopy (Fig. 23.3) (38).

Patients with MLD have excessive sulfatides in urine, and arylsulfatase-A activity is absent or reduced in leukocytes. However, the activity of arylsulfatase-A may be reduced in patients with arylsulfatase-A pseudodeficiency, a condition caused by mutations affecting the polyadenylation of the arylsulfatase-A mRNA. Patients with pseudodeficiency are usually normal clinically. A definitive diagnosis of MLD may be more easily established by nerve biopsy.

3.2.3. Differential Diagnosis

Peripheral neuropathy is not usually a dominant feature in patients with early onset MLD, and the differential diagnosis for these patients includes many hereditary neurodegenerative

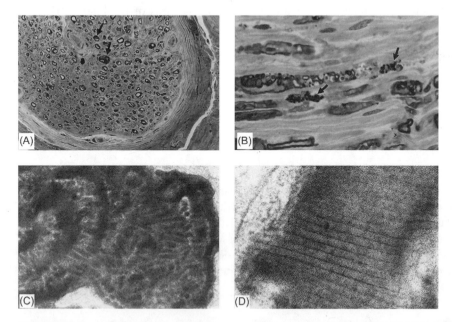

Figure 23.3 Metachromatic leukodystrophy pathology. Semithin transverse ($\times 400$) and longitudinal ($\times 1000$) sections stained with toluidine blue show a mild reduction in myelinated fibers, many thinly myelinated fibers, and Schwann cell inclusions (arrows). (C) Electron microscopy demonstrates prismatic inclusions within a Schwann cell ($\times 39,000$ before reduction). (D) At higher magnification, these inclusions show a periodicity of 5.6–5.8 nm ($\times 73,000$ before reduction). [From Felice et al. (110) with permission.]

and metabolic disorders. The diagnosis of MLD should be considered in an adult patient with dementia, psychiatric disturbances, spasticity, and peripheral neuropathy. The differential diagnosis is similar to that for AMN. Occasionally, MLD causes an isolated peripheral neuropathy, and consideration should be given to demyelinating forms of Charcot–Marie–Tooth (CMT1) disease (47).

3.2.4. Management and Prognosis

There is no specific treatment available for MLD. Management is mainly symptomatic with physical therapy and orthotics. Psychiatric treatment is often required. BMT is under investigation (49).

3.2.5. Pathogenesis

Mutations of arylsulfatase-A are causative for MLD. Impairment of arylsulfatase-A results in the accumulation of excessive sulfatides, which lead to neuronal degeneration and demyelination by unknown mechanisms (50).

3.3. Krabbe's Disease

3.3.1. Clinical Features

KD has four phenotypes: infantile, late-infantile, juvenile, and adult-onset forms. The infantile form represents 90%, and affected children are irritable and rigid with tonic spasms, and gradually develop spasticity, dysarthria, weakness, visual loss, seizures, and mental regression. Peripheral neuropathy is common, resulting in reduced or absent deep tendon reflexes, but is clinically over-shadowed by manifestations of central nervous system involvement. Late-onset forms have a similar presentation, but long track signs may be more prominent (27,31). Several cases of KD have been described with slowly progressive isolated peripheral neuropathy with pes cavus deformities (51).

3.3.2. Laboratory Evaluation

Nerve conduction studies reveal uniform slowing of motor conduction velocity, differentiating it from acquired demyelinating neuropathies (38,48). CSF protein is very high (52). Nerve biopsy is helpful with the finding of nonorientated straight or curved prismatic inclusions in Schwann cells visualized with electron microscopy (Fig. 23.4) (38).

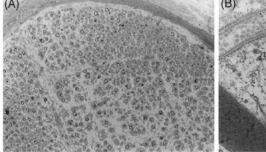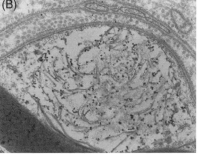

Figure 23.4   KD. (A) A transverse section of the sural nerve reveals moderate reduction in myelinated fibers and with uniformly thin myelin sheaths. The interstitial space in the endoneurium is enlarged. (B) An electron micrograph of Schwann cell cytoplasm reveals curvilinear lamellar inclusions, with low density granular material. [From Matsumoto (111) with permission.]

Biochemical diagnosis is by demonstrating deficient β-galactocerebrosidase (GALC) activity (27,31).

3.3.3. Differential Diagnosis

The differential diagnosis includes other types of leukodystrophies, inherited neurodegenerative, and metabolic diseases. For patients with isolated peripheral neuropathy, the phenotype is similar to, but distinguished from CMT1 by genetic testing (51,53).

3.3.4. Management and Prognosis

There is no specific treatment available for KD, but BMT is investigational.

3.3.5. Pathogenesis

KD is caused by the mutations of *GALC* gene. Dysfunction of GALC leads the accumulation of excessive galactosylceramides, which may cause neuronal degeneration and demyelination (31).

4. FABRY DISEASE AND HEREDITARY AMYLOIDOSIS

Fabry disease and hereditary amyloidosis are distinct in that they are small fiber neuropathies. In both, pain is a cardinal feature, and autonomic dysfunction is common.

4.1. Fabry Disease (FD)

4.1.1. Clinical Features

FD is an X-linked disorder that usually presents in childhood with attacks of severe burning pain with elevation of temperature and associated with anhidrosis or hypohidrosis. The distribution of symptoms does not follow a length-dependent nerve pattern, and pain may occur in any location, including the trunk or face. Heat intolerance is common. Motor nerve function is spared. Neurologic examination is surprisingly normal aside from subtle sensory findings, reduced ankle reflexes and diminished sweating (54,55).

Systemic manifestations are common and of diagnostic importance. Cutaneous angiokeratomas are small reddish lesions that may be slightly raised, and do not blanch with pressure. Lesions are most frequent in a "bathing trunk" distribution, including the periumbilical, gluteal, and perineal regions (Fig. 23.5). Their density increases with age. A variety of characteristic eye findings may also herald the diagnosis. Corneal glyosphingolipid deposits forming whorls are seen in most patients and carriers. Characteristic lens deposits forming "spokes" or "propellers" may be observed, but do not cause symptomatic visual loss (56,57).

Symptomatic involvement of other organ systems develops with disease progression, and may occasionally represent the presenting complaint. Cerebral small vessel disease develops at a young age and may result in strokes similar to those associated with diabetes and hypertension (55,58,59). Renal failure develops with age. Late in the disease, glycosphingolipids accumulate within neurons, resulting in cognitive decline (60).

Occasional patients with residual α-galactosidase-A activity present later in life with a milder phenotype, sometimes with isolated cardiac involvement (61,62). Occasional female carriers develop sensory complaints or cardiomyopathy (63).

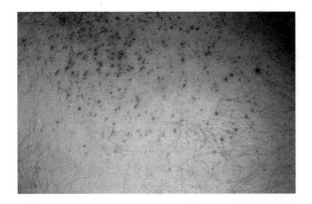

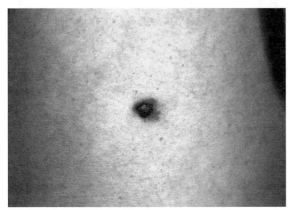

Figure 23.5 Angiokeratomas: Angiokeratomas are small red lesions, typically located in a "bathing trunk" distribution (umbilicus, gluteal cleft, scrotum). Although many may be observed in one location (upper panel), isolated lesions occur, and a detailed skin examination should be performed on every patient with a painful sensory neuropathy, particularly those of young age.

4.1.2. Laboratory Evaluation

Nerve conduction studies are usually normal or conduction velocity may be mildly reduced (64). Sympathetic skin response may be diminished or absent. Other autonomic testing may reveal evidence of orthostatic tachycardia and abnormal sweating (65), suggesting a small fiber axonal sensory polyneuropathy that can be confirmed by skin biopsy showing reduced epidermal nerve fiber density (64,66).

Nerve biopsy reveals axonal loss. Electron microscopy demonstrates lamellar inclusions in pericytes and endothelial, smooth muscle and perineurial cells (Fig. 23.6). Similar inclusions may also be demonstrated in other tissues including muscle and kidney (38,54,58).

A definitive diagnosis is usually made by measuring α-galactosidase-A activity in serum, plasma, leukocytes, or skin fibroblasts. The diagnosis is strengthened with the demonstration of accumulation of globotriaosylceramides, the most redundant metabolites in FD (54,58). The enzymatic activity is usually absent in hemizygotes (affected males), but may have some activity in heterozygotes (female carriers). Occasional male patients may have a mutation allowing expression of some α-galactosidase-A. Genetic testing may be necessary to confirm the diagnosis in manifesting carriers or males with atypical mutations, but DNA testing is limited to research laboratories (66).

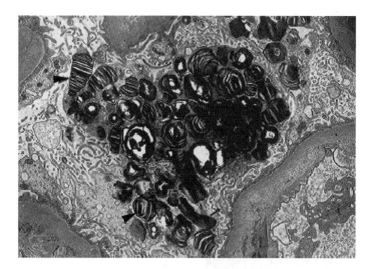

Figure 23.6 Fabry disease pathology. An electron micrograph reveals lamellar osmiophilic inclusions in glomerular visceral epithelial cell (arrowheads). Similar inclusions may be seen in a sural nerve biopsy (original magnification ×20,000). [From Branton et al., Medicine 2002, with permission.] Lower: Depiction of the bluish-purple, macular rash in the "bathing trunk" distribution typical of Fabry disease. [From Menkes (112) with permission.]

4.1.3. Differential Diagnosis

Neuropathies that affect small fibers include hereditary sensory autonomic neuropathy (HSAN), diabetic neuropathy, and idiopathic painful sensory neuropathy. The age of onset, clinical and electrodiagnostic features usually allow easy differentiation from diabetic neuropathy. Every patient with a painful sensory neuropathy should undergo a thorough dermatologic examination for angiokeratomas. Ophthalmologic evaluation may also be illustrative. Biochemical testing should be pursued in selected patients. Nerve biopsy and genetic testing may be helpful in rare individuals.

4.1.4. Management and Prognosis

Neuropathic pain may be debilitating and should be aggressively treated. Because of systemic involvement, cardiac and renal consultation is important, and many patients may require dialysis or renal transplantation (58,59).

There has been progress in the enzymatic treatment of FD. Replacement with recombinant α-galactosidase-A has been evaluated in a double-blind trial with successful removal of microvascular endothelial deposits of globotriaosylceramide from the kidneys, heart, and skin (67).

4.1.5. Pathogenesis

Mutations are distributed in all exons and are usually unique to a specific family. A hemizygous male manifests typical FD, whereas a heterozygous carrier may or may not be symptomatic depending on the lyonization (random inactivation) of the X chromosome (66). When the enzyme is deficient, glycosphingolipids accumulates in different tissues. The primary deposit is globotriaosylceramide, whereas galabiosylceramide is less common. These deposits may injury organs and cause abnormalities, such as neuropathy, renal insufficiency, or vascular endothelial cell damage (54,59,67).

5. HEREDITARY AMYLOIDOSIS

Amyloidosis as a diagnostic entity may cause confusion, partly because the term "amyloidosis" is used to refer to a variety of acquired and genetic disorders. Further, the nomenclature of genetic amyloidosis is confusing because of recent advances in the understanding of the genetic basis of the different forms. Although this chapter will focus on hereditary amyloidosis, a brief review of amyloidosis in general will provide a useful foundation.

All forms of amyloidosis involve deposition of fibrillary protein aggregates in the extracellular space of multiple tissues. Amyloid deposits may be comprised of a number of proteins, and 18 amyloidogenic proteins have been identified so far (68). All forms of amyloid share a similar beta pleated sheet conformation, and it is this conformation that explains the affinity of amyloid for Congo red dye as well as its birefringence under polarized light (Fig. 23.7). There are different forms of amyloidosis. Acquired

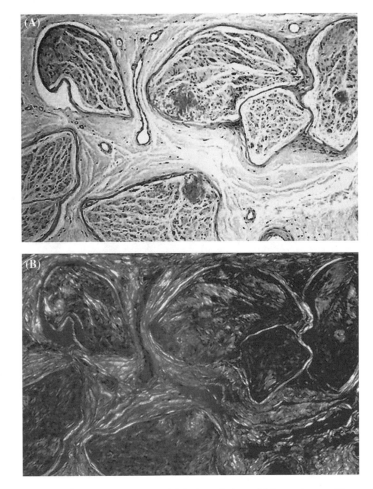

Figure 23.7 Hereditary amyloidosis pathology: This sural nerve biopsy demonstrates endoneurial deposits of amyloid using both H&E staining (A) and Congo red staining with polarized views (B). [From Yazaki et al. (82) with permission.]

amyloidosis is due to light chain disease (AL), and has been termed primary amyloidosis. Reactive systemic amyloidosis (AA) refers to amyloid deposition secondary to a systemic inflammatory condition, and does not result in peripheral nerve injury.

Hereditary amyloidosis refers to a group of autosomal dominant genetic disorders involving alterations to proteins resulting in the formation and deposition of amyloid in various organs. Like amyloidosis in general, the nomenclature of hereditary amyloidosis is confusing. Traditionally, different forms were named for the geographic area where the particular forms were endemic. A different classification system based on clinical syndromes has also been used, and divides forms involving peripheral nerve into familial amyloid polyneuropathy (FAP) types I–IV. Although this classification has advantages over the geographic designations, it also has drawbacks. For example, not every patient with a mutation known to cause a particular type of FAP has polyneuropathy. There is also significant phenotypic overlap. Now that the genetic and protein products underlying each form are better understood, the preferred classification system is based on the protein name itself with reference to the specific mutation. Although recognition of the different clinical patterns is important, this system is most reflective of the underlying pathophysiology. Table 23.4 summarizes the different classification systems and the salient clinical features of each clinical subtype. The overwhelming majority of patients with hereditary amyloidosis have mutations in the transthyretin (TTR) gene. This section will focus on TTR, but other forms will be briefly reviewed.

The prevalence of hereditary amyloidosis varies geographically. In northern Portugal, gene frequency is estimated at 1/538, whereas in the USA it is between 1/100,000 and 1/1,000,000 (69). However, hereditary amyloidosis may be frequently misdiagnosed as AL amyloidosis, and in one series of patients who carried the diagnosis of AL, 10% were found to have hereditary amyloidosis.

Table 23.4   Hereditary Amyloidosis

Protein	Gene	Protein function	Syndrome	Geography	Clinical features
Transthyretin	18q11.2	Transports thyroxine and retinol	FAP I	Portuguese Swedish Japanese	Painful neuropathy, autonomic dysfunction CTS, cardiac, vitreous opacity
			FAP II	Indiana Maryland Swiss German	Painful neuropathy, CTS, early vitreous opacity, cardiac
Apolipoprotein A1	11q23	Major apoprotein of HDL Transports cholesterol from tissue to the liver	FAP III	Iowa	Renal failure, gastric ulcer, neuropathy
Gelsolin	9q34	Calcium binding protein that helps clear actin from plasma	FAP IV	Finnish	Cranial neuropathies, corneal lattice dystrophy, neuropathy

5.1. Transthyretin Amyloidosis (TTR)

5.1.1.   Clinical Features

TTR amyloidosis usually presents in early adulthood (third to fourth decade) with a painful sensory neuropathy. The syndrome is relentlessly progressive, leading to death in 10–15 years without treatment. In the Portuguese population, the mean age of onset is 33 years of age, although 10% present during their 40s or 50s or later (70). Late onset is more frequently observed in sporadic cases and in other endemic regions, including Sweden, France, and the UK (69). Unlike FD, sensory symptoms are length-dependent. Symptomatic carpal tunnel syndrome is common. The neuropathy progresses over years, eventually involving motor nerves as well. Autonomic dysfunction is very common, consistent with prominent early small fiber injury. Autonomic gastrointestinal symptoms include alternating diarrhea and constipation, severe constipation, and gastroparesis. Orthostatic hypotension may be severe. Impotence occurs early and other bladder complaints may follow later in the disease (69,71,72).

Nonneurologic manifestations are common. Cardiac dysfunction includes arrhythmias and direct cardiac involvement with congestive heart failure. Patients may present with an isolated cardiomyopathy (73–75). Mild renal impairment is rare in TTR. Vitreous opacities may also be observed early in the disease course.

In rare instances, amyloid deposition may occur in the meninges and brain, and dementia, strokes, ataxia and seizures have been described (76–78).

There is great phenotypic variability among patients from distinct endemic regions, with specific mutations tending to have similar syndromes. Patients from Portugal, Sweden, and Japan (FAP I) present as described earlier, whereas cardiac disease and vitreous opacities are more frequently observed in kindreds from Indiana and Maryland (FAP II). However, even within one kindred, phenotypic manifestations may overlap substantially.

5.1.2.   Other Forms of Hereditary Amyloidosis

Hereditary amyloidosis can be due to abnormalities of proteins unrelated to TTR. Mutations in the gene for apolipoprotein A1 (FAP III) results in a progressive peripheral neuropathy similar to that seen with TTR mutations, but with prominent gastric ulcers and renal involvement (79). Mutations in the gene encoding gelsolin, a calcium binding protein important in the clearing of actin filaments, results in a characteristic syndrome of cranial polyneuropathy, starting with weakness of the upper part of the face. Corneal lattice dystrophy occurs due to amyloid deposition in corneal nerves (69,80). Other forms that do not involve the peripheral nervous system resulting from mutations in a variety of unrelated genes (Fibrinogen Aα, lysozyme, amyloid precursor protein, and cystatin C).

5.1.3.   Laboratory Evaluation

Nerve conduction studies reveal reduced sensory and motor amplitudes with normal or mildly slowed conduction velocities (81,82). Needle EMG reveals signs of denervation and reinnervation that may involve distal and proximal limb muscles, supporting a polyradiculopathy likely due to meningeal amyloid deposition. Cardiovagal and sudomotor testing may also be abnormal, supporting small fiber involvement (81).

Definitive testing requires demonstration of amyloid deposition or identification of a causative mutation. Although nerve biopsy is the logical choice in a patient with peripheral neuropathy, diagnostic sensitivity may not be as high as other tissues (83). Full thickness rectal biopsy may be the most sensitive procedure and should be performed if nerve biopsy fails to reveal amyloid deposition (69). Aspiration of abdominal fat pad tissue provides a noninvasive diagnostic test. Tissue amyloid deposition is demonstrated by Congo red staining with an "apple green" birefringence when viewed under polarized light (Fig. 23.4). Scintigraphy with specific ligand to amyloids can be used to confirm cardiac or hepatic accumulation of amyloids (72).

Histologic tests do not distinguish between different forms of amyloidosis (82,84). Genetic testing is commercially available. For the *TTR* gene, a substitution of methionine for valine at position 30 is the most prevalent mutation, although other mutations have been identified. Mutations for Apolipoprotein A-I or Gelsolin-related amyloidosis are relatively few (69,85,86). In certain situations, genetic testing may be used as the first line diagnostic test. Patients who are from an endemic area, have a suggestive clinical scenario or positive family history should undergo genetic testing.

5.1.4. Differential Diagnosis

Amyloid neuropathy must be differentiated from other causes of predominantly small fiber neuropathy, including HSAN, diabetic neuropathy, and idiopathic painful sensory neuropathy. Prominent autonomic dysfunction is usually seen only in diabetes and amyloidosis.

5.1.5. Management and Prognosis

Liver transplantation is the only therapy currently available that directly influences disease progression, and has been used primarily in patients with TTR amyloidosis (69,87). TTR is synthesized in the liver, and transplantation results in normalization of serum TTR levels within days (87). The survival rates in the several years following transplantation are between 60% and 80%, with most deaths resulting from cardiac or septic complications (69,87). Transplantation results in stabilization of peripheral neuropathy and improved overall outcome, but cardiac disease and autonomic dysfunction do not respond (87–89). Neuropathic pain and orthostatic hypotension should be aggressively treated. Cardiovascular and renal function should be monitored and treated (72,90). Vitrectomy in patients with vitreous opacities may restore vision.

5.1.6. Pathogenesis

The mechanisms of protein aggregation and amyloid deposition, and how amyloid deposits result in tissue injury are unknown (69,72,91). Vascular deposition may result in nerve ischemia (71). A variety of biochemical and immunologic derangements may contribute to axonal loss, and TTR amyloid deposits result in oxidative stress and stimulation of the receptor for advanced glycation end products (92,93). There is also evidence of complement deposition on amyloid deposits in peripheral nerve (94).

6. GIANT AXONAL NEUROPATHY

6.1. Clinical Features

Giant axonal neuropathy (GAN) is an autosomal recessive disorder that usually presents prior to age seven with clumsy gait, poor motor skills and imbalance. Distal weakness and impaired sensation develop along with reduced or absent tendon reflexes. Cranial nerves may be affected with facial weakness, ptosis or vocal cord paralysis. Central nervous system involvement occurs later with dysarthria, tremor, nystagmus, seizures and cognitive decline. Pale and tightly curled hair ("kinky hair") is distinctive, but is not always present.

6.2. Laboratory Evaluation

Nerve conduction studies show significantly reduced sensory and motor amplitudes with preserved conduction velocities, consistent with an axonal sensory motor neuropathy (95–98). Brain MRI scan may show scattered areas of dysmyelination. Most cases have mild to moderated cerebral atrophy (97–99).

Nerve biopsy shows "giant" swollen axons. The axonal enlargements tend to occur at paranoidal regions, and overlying myelin is absent or thin. Large axons are filled with packed neurofilaments displacing other axonal organelles to the peripheral areas of axoplasm (Fig. 23.8) (95,97–99).

6.3. Management and Prognosis

There is no specific treatment. Pain should be treated aggressively. The disease is relentlessly progressive and most patients die by the third decade (95–99).

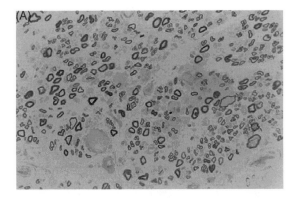

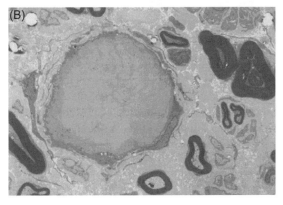

Figure 23.8   Giant axonal neuropathy pathology: (A) Semithin sections reveal numerous giant axons (original magnification ×100). (B) An electron micrograph reveals a giant axon filled with neurofilaments: no myelin sheath is visible (bar = 5 mm). [From Zemmouri et al. (97) with permission.]

6.4. Pathogenesis

GAN is due to mutations in the gene coding for gigaxonin, on chromosome 16q24 (96,100). Gigaxonin belongs to the kelch-repeat superfamily and is thought to have roles in the sidearm orientation of intermediate filaments (100–102).

7. TANGIER DISEASE

7.1. Clinical Features

Tangier disease (TD) is an autosomal recessive disorder with onset from first to seventh decades, and peripheral neuropathies occurs in about two-thirds of cases. Multiple patterns of neuropathy have been reported, including mononeuropathy (oculomotor, long thoracic, limb nerves), mononeuropathy multiplex, (brachial plexus), and a unique syringomyelia-like syndrome. A mild symmetric sensorimotor polyneuropathy may concur, but is usually over-shadowed by the symptoms in arms and trunk (103,104).

Non-neurological manifestations are unusual, and include enlarged tonsils with a yellowish lobulated appearance (but many patients have had a prior tonsillectomy), splenomegaly and atherosclerosis leading to cardiovascular diseases at young age (103–105).

7.2. Laboratory Evaluation

Electrodiagnostic studies show evidence for sensorimotor axonal loss, with controversy over demyelination (103). Complete blood counts may reveal thrombocytopenia and CSF protein may be elevated. Nerve biopsy confirms axonal loss and lipid accumulation in nonmembrane-bound vacuoles (104,106,107). Definitive diagnosis relies on serum lipid assay with absent or reduced HDL, reduced cholesterol, elevated triglycerides and reduced apolipoprotein A-I (103,105).

7.3. Management and Prognosis

The role of lipid lowering agents in the disease is unclear.

7.4. Pathogenesis

The gene for TD is an ATP binding cassette transporter 1 (*ABC*) gene located on chromosome 9q31 (108,109). ABC1 protein forms a channel-like structure across the cellular membrane, and is required for the transportation of cholesterol from cells to HDL. Mutations of the *ABC1* gene impair cholesterol clearance. Excessive cholesterol accumulates in tissues or cells resulting in premature atherosclerotic disease (105). The mechanism underlying the neuropathy is unknown, but biopsy findings of lipid deposits in Schwann cells suggests that impaired lipid clearance from Schwann cells and neurons may result in toxicity and axonal loss (107).

REFERENCES

  1. Mc Alpine I, Hunter R. The "insanity" of George III: a classic case of porphyria. Br Med J 1966; 65–71.

2. Loftus L, Arnold W. Vincent van Gogh's illness: acute intermittent porphyria? Br Med J 1991; 303:1589–1591.

3. Stokvis B. Over twee zeldsame Kleuerstoffen in Urine van Zieken. Ned Tijdschr Geneeskd 1889; 13:409–411.

4. Garrod A. Inborn errors of metabolism. 2nd ed. Hodder and Sloughton, 1923.

5. Waldenstrom J. The porhyria as inborn errors of metabolism. Am J Med 1957; 22:758–772.

6. Dean G. The porphyries—a story of inheritence and environment. 2nd ed. New York: Lippincott, 1971.

7. Eales L. Porphyrias as seen in Cape Town—a survey of 250 cases and some recent studies. S Afr J Lab Med 1963; 9:145–151.

8. Shreiber W. A molecular view of the neurologic porphyries. Clin Lab Med 1997; 17:73–83.

9. Tefferi A, Colgan J, Solberg LJ. Acute porphyrias: diagnosis and management. Mayo Clin Proc 1994; 69:991–995.

10. Elder G, Hift R, Meissner P. The acute porphyrias. Lancet 1997; 349:1613–1617.

11. Maruno M, Furuyama K, Akagi R et al. Highly heterogeneous nature of delta-aminolevulinate dehydratase (ALAD) deficiencies in ALAD porphyria. Blood 2001; 97:2972–2978.

12. McEneaney D, Hawkins S, Trimble E, Smye M. Porphyric neuropathy—a rare and often neglected differential diagnosis of Guillain–Barré Syndrome. J Neurol Sci 1993; 114:231–232.

13. Suarez J, Cohen M, Larkin J et al. Acute intermittent porphyria: clinicopathologic correlation. Report of a case and review of the literature. Neurology 1997; 48:1678–1683.

14. Barohn R, Sanchez J, Anderson K. Acute peripheral neuropathy due to hereditary coproporphyria. Muscle Nerve 1994; 17:793–799.

15. Felsher B, Redeker A. Acute intermittent porphyria: effect of diet and griseofulvin. Medicine (Baltimore), 1967; 46:217–223.

16. Crimlisk H. The little imitator—porphyria: a neuropsychiatric disorder. J of Neurol Neurosurg Psychiatry 1997; 62:319–328.

17. Scane A, Wright J, Godwin-Austen R. Acute intermittent porphyria presenting as epilepsy. Br Med J 1986; 292:946–947.

18. Muraoka A, Suehiro I, Fuji M, Murakami K. Aminoelvulinic acid dehydratase deficiency porphyria (ADP) with syndrome of inappropriate secretion of antidiuretic hormone (SIADH) in a 69-year-old woman. Kobe J Med Sci 1995; 41:23–31.

19. Albers J, Robertson WJ, Daube J. Electrodiagnostic findings in acute porphyric neuropathy. Muscle Nerve 1978; 1:292–296.

20. Flugel K, Druschky K. Electromyogram and nerve conduction in patients with acute intermittent porphyria. J Neurol 1977; 214(4):267–279.

21. Defanti C, Sghirlanzoni A, Bottachhi E, Peluchetti D. Porphyric neuropathy: a clinical, neurophysiological and morphological study. Ital J Neurol Sci 1985; 6:521–526.

22. Thorner P, Bilbao J, Sima A, Briggs S. Porphyric neuropathy: an ultrastructural and quantitative case study. Can J Neurol Sci 1981; 8(4):281–287.

23. Lindberg R, Porcher C, Grandchamp B et al. Porphobilinogen deaminase deficiency in mice causes a neuropathy resembling that of human hepatic porphyria. Nat Genet 1996; 12(2):195–199.

24. Lindberg R, Martini R, Baumgartner M et al. Motor neuropathy in porphobilinogen deaminase-deficient mice imitates the peripheral neuropathy of human acute porphyria. J Clin Invest 1999; 103(8):1127–1134.

25. Herrick A, McColl K, Moore M, Cook A, Goldberg A. Controlled trial of haem arginate in acute hepatic porphyria. Lancet 1989; 1:1295–1297.

26. Case Reports of the Massachusetts General Hospital (case 39-1984). N Engl J Med 1984; 311:839–847.

27. Aicardi J. The inherited leukodystrophies: a clinical overview. J Inherit Metab Dis 1993; 16(4):733–743.

28. Moser H. Adrenoleukodystrophy: phenotype, genetics, pathogenesis and therapy. Brain 1997; 120:1485–1508.

29. Edwin D, Speedie L, Kohler W et al. Cognitive and brain magnetic resonance imaging findings in adrenomyeloneuropathy. Ann Neurol 1996; 40:675–678.
30. Edwin D, Speedie L, Naidu S, Moser H. Cognitive impairment in adult-onset adrenoleukodystrophy. Mol Chem Neuropathol 1990; 12:167–176.
31. Kaye E. Update on genetic disorders affecting white matter. Pediatr Neurol 2001; 24:11–24.
32. Kumar A, Kohler W, Kruse B et al. MR findings in adult-onset adrenoleukodystrophy. Am J Neuroradiol 1995; 16:1227–1237.
33. Griffin J, Li C, Ho T et al. Pathology of the motor-sensory anobal Guillain–Barré syndrome. Ann Neurol 1996; 39:17–28.
34. vanGeel B, Koelman J, Barth P, Ongerboer de Visser B. Peripheral nerve abnormalities in adrenomyeloneuropathy: a clinical and electrodiagnostic study. Neurology 1996; 46:112–118.
35. Tobimatsu S, Fukui R, Kato M et al. Multimodality evoked potential in patients and carries with adrenoleukodystrophy and adrenomyeloneuropathy. Electroenceph Clin Neurophsiol 1985; 62:18–24.
36. Kaplan P, Tusa R, Rignani J, Moser H. Somatosensory evoked potentials in adrenomyeloneuropathy. Neurology 1997; 48:1662–1667.
37. Kaplan P, Kruse B, Tusa R et al. Visual system abnormalities in adrenomyeloneuropathy. Ann Neurol 1995; 37:550–552.
38. Graham D, Lantos P. Greenfield's neuropathology. Vol. 2. 6th ed. New York: Arnold, 1997.
39. Moser H. Clinical and therapeutic aspects of adrenoleukodystrophy and adrenomyeloneuropathy. J Neuropathol Exp Neurol 1995; 54(5):740–745.
40. Aubourg P, Blanche S, Jambaque I et al. Reversal of early neurologic and neuroradiologic manifestations of X-linked adrenoleukodystrophy by bone marrow transplantation. N Engl J Med 1990; 322:1860–1866.
41. Aubourg P, Adamsbaum C, Lavallard-Rousseau M et al. A two-year trial of oleic acid and erucic acids ("Lorenzo's oil") as treatment for adrenomyeloneuropathy. N Engl J Med 1993; 329:745–752.
42. Tanaka A, Tanabe K, Morita M. ATP binding/hydrolysis by and phosphorylation of peroxisomal ATP-binding cassette proteins PMP70 (ABCD3) and adrenoleukodystrophy protein (ABCD1). J Biol Chem 2002; 277:40142–40147.
43. Powers J, Schaumburg H, Johnson A, Raine C. A correlative study of the adrenal cortex in adrenoleukodystrophy: evidence for a fatal intoxication with very long chain fatty acids. Invest Cell Pathol 1980; 3:353–376.
44. Chaudhry V, Moser H, Cornblath D. Nerve conduction in adrenomyeloneuropathy. J Neurol Neurosurg Psychiatry 1996; 61:181–185.
45. Moser H, Moser A, Smith K et al. Adrenoleukodystrophy: phenotypic variability and implications for therapy. J Inherit Metab Dis 1992; 15:645–664.
46. Naidu S, Bresnan M, Griffin D et al. Intensive immunosuppression fails to alter neurological progression in childhood adrenoleukodystrophy. Arch Neurol 1988; 45:846–848.
47. Comabella M, Waye J, Raguer N et al. Late-onset metachromatic leukodystrophy clinically presenting as isolated peripheral neuropathy: compound heterozygosity for the IVS2 + 1G → A Mutation and a newly identified missense mutation (Thr408IIe) in a Spanish Family. Ann Neurol 2001; 50:108–112.
48. Lewis R, Sumner A, Shy M et al. Electrophysiological features of inherited demyelinating neuropathies: A reappraisal in the era of molecular diagnosis. Muscle Nerve 2000; 23:1472–1487.
49. Koc O, Day J, Nieder M et al. Allogeneic mesenchymal stem cell infusion for treatment of metachromatic leukodystrophy (MLD) and Hurler syndrome (MPS-IH). Bone Marrow Transplant 2002; 30:215–222.
50. Hageman A, Gabreels F, de Jong J et al. Clinical symptoms of adult metachromatic leukodystrophy and arylsulfatase A pseudodeficiency. Arch Neurol 1995; 52:408–413.
51. Marks H, Scavina M, Kolodny E, Palmieri M, Childs J. Krabbe's disease presenting as a peripheral neuropathy. Muscle Nerve 1997; 20:1024–1028.

52. Lyon G, Hagberg B, Evrard P et al. Symptomatology of late onset Krabbe's leukodystrophy: the European experience. Dev Neurosci 1991; 13:240–244.

53. Krajewski K, Lewis R, Fuerst D et al. Neurological dysfunction and axonal degeneration in Charcot–Marie–Tooth disease type 1A. Brain 2000; 123:1516–1527.

54. Brady R, Schiffmann R. Clinical features of and recent advances in therapy for Fabry disease. JAMA 2000; 284:2771–2775.

55. Menkes D. The cutaneous stigmata of Fabry disease. Arch Neurol 1999; 56:487.

56. Spaeth G, Frost P. Fabry's disease. Its ocular manifestations. Arch Ophthalmol 1965; 74(6):760–769.

57. Sher N, Letson R, Desnick R. The ocular manifestations of Fabry's disease. Arch Ophthalmol 1979; 97(4):641–646.

58. Branton M, Schiffmann R, Sabnis S et al. Natural history of Fabry renal disease: influence of alpha-galactosidase A activity and genetic mutations on clinical course. Medicine (Baltimore) 2002; 81:122–128.

59. Dashe J. Case records of the Massachusetts General Hospital. N Engl J Med 1998; 339:1914–1923.

60. deVeber G, Schrwarting G, Kolodny E, Kowall N. Fabry disease: immunocytochemical characterization of neuronal involvement. Ann Neurol 1992; 31(4):409–415.

61. Clarke J, Knaack J, Crawhall J, Wolfe L. Ceramide trihexosidosis (Fabry's disease) without skin lesions. N Engl J Med 1971; 284(5):233–235.

62. Ogawa K, Sugamata K, Funamoto N et al. Restricted accumulation of globotiaosylceramide in the hearts of atypical cases of Fabry disease. Hum Pathol 1990; 21:1067–1073.

63. Broadbent J, Edwards W, Gordon H et al. Fabry cardiomyopathy in the female confirmed by endomyocardial biopsy. Mayo Clin Proc 1981; 56:623–628.

64. Sheth K, Swick H. Peripheral Nerve conduction in Fabry disease. Ann Neurol 1980; 7:319–323.

65. Luciano CA, Russell JW, Banerjee TK et al. Physiological characterization of neuropathy in Fabry's disease. Muscle Nerve 2002; 26(5):622–629.

66. Ashton-Prolla P, Tong B, Shabbeer J et al. Fabry disease: twenty-two novel mutations in the alpha-galactosidase A gene and genotype/phenotype correlations in severely and mildly affected hemizygotes and heterozygotes. J Investig Med 2000; 48:227–235.

67. Eng C, Guffon N, Wilcox W et al. Safety and efficacy of recombinant human alpha-galactosidase A—replacement therapy in Fabry's disease. N Engl J Med 2001; 345:9–16.

68. Buxbaum J, Tagoe C. The genetics of the amyloidoses. Annu Rev Med 2000; 51:543–569.

69. Hund E, Linke R, Willig F, Grau A. Transthyretin-associated neuropathic amyloidosis. Pathogenesis and treatment. Neurology 2001; 56(4):431–435.

70. Sousa A, Coelho T, Barros J. Genetic epidemiology of familial amyloidotic polyneuropathy (FAP_-type I in Povoa do Varzim and Vila do Conde (north of Portugal). Am J Med Genet 1995; 60:512–521.

71. Adams D. Hereditary and acquired amyloid neuropathies. J Neurol 2001; 248:647–657.

72. Falk R, Comenzo R, Skinner M. The systemic amyloidosis. N Engl J Med 1997; 898–909.

73. De Freitas F. The heart in Portuguese amyloidosis. Postgrad Med J 1986; 62:601–605.

74. Jacobson D, Pan T, Kyle R. Transthyretin Ile20, a new variant associated with late-onset cardiac amyloidosis. Human Mutat 1997; 9:83–85.

75. Jacobson D, Pastore R, Yaghoubian R. Variantsequence transthyretin (insoleucine 122) in late-onset cardiac amyloidosis in black Americans. N Engl J Med 1997; 336:466–473.

76. Benson M. Leptomeningeal amyloid and variant transthyretins [comment]. Am J Pathol 1996; 148:351–354.

77. Garzuly F, Vidal R, Wisniewski T. Familial meningocerebrovascular amyloidosis, Hungarian type, with mutan transthyretin (TTR Asp18Gly). Neurology 1996; 47:1562–1567.

78. Petersen R, Goren H, Cohen M. Transthyretin amyloidosis: a new mutation associated with dementia. Ann Neurol 1997; 41:307–313.

79. Van Allen M, Frohlick J, Davis J. Inherited predisposition to generalized amyloidosis. Neurology 1969; 19:10–25.

80. Yin H, Kwiatkowski D, Mole J et al. Structure and biosynthesis of cytoplasmic and secreted variants of gelsolin. J Biol Chem 1984; 259:5271–5276.

81. Montagna P, Marchello L, Plasmati R et al. Electromyographic findings in transthyretin (TTR)-related familial amyloid polyneuropathy (FAP). Electroenceph Clin Neurophysiol 1996; 101(5):423–430.

82. Yazaki M, Yamashita T, Kincaid J et al. Rapidly progressive amyloid polyneuropathy associated with a novel variant transthyretin serine 25. Muscle Nerve 2002; 25:244–250.

83. Simmons Z, Blaivas M, AJ A. Low diagnostic yield of sural nerve biopsy in patients with peripheral neuropathy and primary amyloidosis. J Neurol Sci 1993; 120:60–63.

84. Gorson K. Case Records of the Nassachusetts General Hospital. N Engl J Med 2001; 344:917–923.

85. Booth D, Tan S, Booth S et al. Hereditary hepatic and systemic amyloidosis caused by a new deletion/insertion mutation in the apolipoprotein Al gene. J Clin Invest 1996; 97:2714–2721.

86. Maury C, Liljestrom M, Boysen G et al. Danish type gelsolin related amyloidosis: 654G-T mutation is associated with a disease pathogenetically and clinically similar to that caused by the 654G-A mutation (familial amyloidosis of the Finnish type). J Clin Pathol, 2000; 53:95–99.

87. Adams D, Samuel D, Goulon-Goeau C et al. The course and prognostic factors of familial amyloid polyneuropathy after liver transplantation. Brain 2000; 123(Pt 7):1495–1504.

88. Dubrey S, Davidoff R, Skinner M et al. Progression of ventricular wall thickening after liver transplantation for familial amyloidosis. Transplantation 1997; 64:74–80.

89. Pomfret E, Lewis W, Jankins R et al. Effect of orthotic liver transplantation on the progression of familial amyloidotic polyneuropathy. Transplantation, 1998; 65:918–925.

90. Low P. Autonomic neuropathies. Curr Opin Neurol 2002; 15:605–609.

91. Sousa M, Cardoso I, Fernandes R, Guimaraes A, Saraiva M. Deposition of transthyretin in early stages of familial amyloidotic polyneuropathy: evidence for toxicity of nonfibrillar aggregates. Am J Pathol 2001; 159(6):1993–2000.

92. Sousa M, Du Yan S, Fernandes R et al. Familial amyloid polyneuropathy: receptor for advanced glycation end products-dependent triggering of neuronal inflammatory and apoptotic pathways. J Neurosci 2001; 21(19):7576–7586.

93. Nyhlin N, Anan I, El S, Ando Y, Suhr O. Reduction of free radical activity in amyloid deposits following liver transplantation for familial amyloidotic polyneuropathy. J Internal Med 2002; 251(2):136–141.

94. Hafer-Macko C, Dyck PJ, Koski C. Complement activation in acquired and hereditary amyloid neuropathy. J Peripher Nerv Syst 2000; 5(3):131–139.

95. Ben Hamida M, Hentati F, Ben Hamida C. Giant axonal neuropathy with inherited multisystem degernation in a Tunisian kindred. Neurology 1990; 40:245–250.

96. Flanigan K, Crawford T, Griffin J et al. Localization of the giant axonal neuropathy gene to chromosome 16q24. Ann Neurol 1998; 43:143–148.

97. Zemmouri R, Azzedine H, Assami S et al. Charcot–Marie–Tooth 2-like presentation of an Algerian family with giant axonal neuropathy. Neuromuscul Disord 2000; 10:592–598.

98. Kuhlenbaumer G, Young P, Oberwittler C et al. Giant axonal neuropathy (GAN): case report and two novel mutations in the gigaxonin gene. Neurology 2002; 58:1273–1276.

99. Malandrini A, Dotti M, Battisti C et al. Giant axonal neuropathy with subclinical involvement of the central nervous system: case report. J Neurol Sci 1998; 158:232–235.

100. Bomont P, Cavalier L, Blondeau F et al. The gene encoding gigaxonin, a new member of the cytoskeletal BTB/kelch repeat family, is mutated in giant axonal neuropathy. Nat Genet 2000; 26(3):370–374.

101. Timmerman V, De Jonghe P, Van Broeckhoven C. Of giant axons and curly hair. Nat Genet 2000; 26(3):254–255.

102. Herrmann D, Griffin J. Intermediate filaments: a common thread in neuromuscular disorders. Neurology 2002; 58:1141–1143.

103. Siao P, Cros D. Case records of the Massachusetts General Hospital. Weekly clinicopathological exercises. Case 16-1996. A 36-year-old woman with bilateral facial and hand weakness and impaired truncal sensation. N Engl J Med 1996; 334(21):1389–1394.

104. Pietrini V, Rizzuto N, Vergani C, Zen F, Ferro Milone F. Neuropathy in Tangier disease: A clinicopathologic study and a review of the literature. Acta Neurol Scand 1985; 72(5):495–505.

105. Oram JF. Molecular basis of cholesterol homeostasis: lessons from Tangier disease and ABCA1. Trends Mol Med 2002; 8(4):168–173.

106. Gibbels E, Schaefer HE, Runne U et al. Severe polyneuropathy in Tangier disease mimicking syringomyelia or leprosy. Clinical, biochemical, electrophysiological, and morphological evaluation, including electron microscopy of nerve, muscle, and skin biopsies. J Neurol 1985; 232(5):283–294.

107. Dyck PJ, Ellefson RD, Yao JK, Herbert PN. Adult-onset of Tangier disease: 1. Morphometric and pathologic studies suggesting delayed degradation of neutral lipids after fiber degeneration. J Neuropathol Exp Neurol 1978; 37(2):119–137.

108. Remaley AT, Rust S, Rosier M et al. Human ATP-binding cassette transporter 1 (ABC1): genomic organization and identification of the genetic defect in the original Tangier disease kindred. Proc Natl Acad Sci USA 1999; 96(22):12685–12690.

109. Brousseau ME, Schaefer EJ, Dupuis J et al. Novel mutations in the gene encoding ATP-binding cassette 1 in four tangier disease kindreds. J Lipid Res 2000; 41(3):433–441.

110. Felice KJ, Gomez Lira M, Natowicz M et al. Adult-onset MLD: a gene mutation with isolated polyneuropathy. Neurology 2000; 55(7):1036–1039.

111. Matsumoto R, Oka N, Nagahama Y, Akiguchi I, Kimura J. Peripheral neuropathy in late-onset Krabbe's disease: histochemical and ultrastructural findings. Acta Neuropathol (Berl) 1996; 92(6):635–639.

112. Menkes DL. Images in neurology. The cutaneous stigmata of Fabry disease: an X-linked phakomatosis associated with central and peripheral nervous system dysfunction. Arch Neurol 1999; 56(4):487.

Focal Peripheral Neuropathy

24
Radiculopathy

Firas G. Saleh and Rahman Pourmand
Stony Brook University Hospital, Stony Brook, New York, USA

ABSTRACT

Pain in the neck, low back, and limbs are common clinical complaints. Presentations may be acute or chronic with weakness and sensory loss. It is important to distinguish among those diverse symptoms that are related to radiculopathies and those that are not, and those that are emergencies. Distinctions can be reliably made through a thoughtful history and examination with help from carefully selected diagnostic tests. An orderly and efficient approach is presented to evaluate spine and limb pain.

1. INTRODUCTION

Radiculopathy is defined as disease of spinal nerve roots, which typically results in back or neck pain that radiates down the extremities, and is associated with neurological signs and symptoms that follow a dermatomal or myotomal pattern. Dermatome in Greek means a skin slice and refers to a specific area of skin supplied by a single nerve root, while a

439

myotome is the motor equivalent to a dermatome and is used to refer to a group of muscles innervated by one root.

Back and neck pain is the most common cause of disability in individuals <45 years of age and is the second leading cause of physician visits and the third leading cause of work absenteeism (1–3). Lumbosacral (LS) radiculopathy is the most common type and accounts for almost two-third of cases, while cervical (C) radiculopathy is less common and accounts for about one-third of cases, and thoracic (T) nerve roots are rarely involved (<1%). The thoracic spine is more stable because of its mechanical connection to the chest wall. L5 and S1 roots together represent >90% of cases in the LS spine, while C7 followed by C6 roots represent >85% of cases in the cervical spine, and T11 and T12 roots have the highest incidence of lesions in the thoracic spine.

The most common etiology of radiculopathy in young patients is herniation of a single soft intervertebral disc. In adults >50 years of age, the most common etiology is degenerative changes from spondylosis and osteophyte formation. These changes eventually result in spinal canal stenosis and narrowing of the intervertebral foramina.

Despite the frequency of symptomatic disk and degenerative disease other less common but more serious etiologies must also be considered in individual patients. These include infectious, inflammatory, traumatic, vasculitic, metabolic, and neoplastic pathologies. Diabetes mellitus and herpes are two disorders that cause focal thoracic radiculopathies. Table 24.1 includes a full differential diagnosis of radiculopathy.

2. ANATOMY AND PHYSIOLOGY

The spinal cord is incased in the vertebral column, which is a rigid bony canal made of 33 vertebrae. It forms 31 pairs of nerve root segments: eight cervical, 12 thoracic, five lumbar, five sacral, and one coccygeal. Cervical and lumbar roots are the largest. Every segment is made of ventral and dorsal nerve roots. Ventral roots are made of motor fibers from the anterior horn of the spinal cord gray matter. In the thoracic and upper lumbar segments, ventral roots also include preganglionic sympathetic fibers from the intermediolateral horn, while lateral cells in the sacral area supply preganglionic parasympathetic fibers. Dorsal roots are made of sensory fibers from dorsal root ganglia (DRG) cells that lie outside of the spinal cord in the dorsal root ganglia. The ganglia are located in the intervertebral foramina that are bordered superiorly and inferiorly by pedicles of vertebral bodies, and anteriorly by intervertebral discs and vertebral bodies. Posteriorly, they are bordered by the facet joints, and laterally by the denticulate ligament which is part of the pia mater located midline between the ventral and dorsal roots.

Ventral and dorsal nerve roots of the same level join to form a short spinal nerve that emerges through the intervertebral foramen giving rise to recurrent meningeal branches before dividing into two rami. The larger ventral ramus forms the plexuses and ultimately innervates the extremities and trunk including the intercostal and abdominal wall muscles. The lesser dorsal ramus innervates paraspinal muscles, the skin of neck, trunk, and gluteal area, and the soft tissue structures surrounding the nerve roots including the periosteum, the joint capsule, and the ligaments.

The spinal nerve roots receive their blood supply from a network of capillaries formed from radicular arteries that enter the spinal canal through the intervertebral foramina and then divide, passing along the ventral and dorsal nerve roots, within a common sheath that is continuous with the covering meningeal layers. The major portion of the venous drainage is carried out through the intervertebral foramina corresponding in part to the arterial supply.

Table 24.1 Differential Diagnosis of Radiculopathy

Mechanical[a]
    Disc herniation (soft or hard)
    Spinal canal stenosis (ideopathic or acquired)
    Spondylosis or spondylolesthesis
    Ligamental hypertrophy
    Trauma
Infections[b]
    Viral: herpes simplex, herpes zoster, cytomegalovirus, Epstein–Barr virus
    Lyme disease
    Neurosyphilis
    Tuberculosis (Potts disease)
    Mycoplasma
Tumors
    Intradural[a]: astrocytoma, ependymoma, schwannoma, meningioma, neurofibroma
    Extradural[b]: metastasis, lymphoma, multiple myeloma, sarcoma
Inflammatory
    Guillain–Barré syndrome[c]
    Sarcoidosis[b]
    Vasculitis[b]
    Ankylosing Spondylitis[a]
    Arachnoiditis[a]
    Pachymeningitis[a]
    Radiculitis[a]
Metabolic
    Diabetes Mellitus[b]
    Adrenal insufficiency[c]
    Vitamin B_{12} defficiency[b]
    Porphyria[c]
Arteriovenous malformations[a]
Spinal radiation[a]

[a]Could be associated with myelopathy.
[b]Could be associated with both myelopathy and neuropathy.
[c]Could be associated with neuropathy.

    The vertebrae are separated by fibrocartilagenous plates called discs, that are present at all levels, except between C1 and C2 and below S1. The discs are made of an internal gelatinous core called nucleus pulposus that absorbs compressive forces, distributing them equally to an external fibrous surrounding structure called the annulus fibrosus, which provides tensile strength.

    Early in life, the nucleus pulposus is well hydrated, but with time, the water content is lost. Degenerative changes in combination with underlying genetic factors alter the way compressive forces are transmitted. The transmission of forces may become asymmetric, resulting in weakening, tearing, and fissuring of the annulus through which the nucleus pulposus can protrude. In addition, by early adulthood, most of the disc loses its blood and nerve supply, sparing only a thin outer layer of the annulus fibrosus. Thus, if herniation takes place, it may not produce pain from within the nucleus because of the loss of nerve supply. The pain produced may result from either mechanical compression on the spared outer layer of the disc or compression of nearby nerve roots. Chemical irritation of roots may also occur, because the constituents of the nucleus pulposus can serve as inflammatory mediators, or can stimulate such mediators to act.

Ordinarily, when disk protrusion occurs, it tends to do so through the weakest point of the surrounding tissues, which is the posterolateral portion of the annulus fibrosus and posterior longitudinal ligament. Less frequently, protrusion or herniation is central or medial, which usually has more serious consequences involving the spinal cord with resultant myelopathy due to compression of the ascending and descending tracts.

The spinal cord extends from the foramen magnum as a continuation of the medulla oblongata, and ends in most adults between the L1 and L2 vertebrae. Accordingly, LS spinal nerve roots below L2 descend down almost vertically in the spinal canal to exit through their corresponding intervertebral foramina. The descending bundle of nerve roots is called the cauda equina.

It is important to remember that cervical nerve roots exit through intervertebral foramina above their matching vertebrae, for example, C6 nerve root exits between C5 and C6, but the C8 nerve root exits between C7 and T1 vertebrae because there are only seven cervical vertebrae. Below this level, roots emerge below the level of their corresponding vertebrae, for example, L4 nerve root exits between L4 and L5.

Another relevant point is that protrusion of an intervertebral disc tends to compress the nerve root originating one level below, especially if the protrusion is medial, for example, a disc that protrudes between L4 and L5 vertebrae may affect L5 nerve root rather than the L4 root that exits at the L4–L5 level.

3. APPROACH AND EVALUATION

Five questions should be addressed in a suspected radiculopathy. The most important is whether the patient's symptoms could be related to a serious and critical cause that requires urgent or emergent management. The second is whether the patient's symptoms represent disease of the spine or are they related to peripheral structures, like joints, peripheral nerves, or muscles. If the symptoms originate from the spine, the third question is whether they generated by a neurogenic or a nonneurogenic event. The fourth, relates to the level of the pathology. A final question that always needs to be considered is whether a patient's symptoms could be related to a functional rather than an organic cause.

These questions can be readily answered in most cases from a complete and thorough clinical history and comprehensive but focused physical examination. Laboratory workup, imaging studies, and neurophysiologic tests should be chosen based on information from history and examination, and their results interpreted to correlate with the clinical presentation.

3.1. Clinical History

The classic chief complaint with a radiculopathy is radicular pain emanating from the neck or back. This pain is usually intermittent with properties described as lancinating, stabbing, aching, or shooting in nature that radiate down the extremities in a partial or complete dermatomal pattern depending on the nerve root involved. For example, in L5 or S1 radiculopathies, pain usually radiates down the posterior and lateral aspects of the thigh extending below the knee. Some patients describe neurogenic intermittent claudication or pseudoclaudication especially if an underlying spinal stenosis is present. In L1–L3 radiculopathies, pain radiates over the anterior and proximal medial parts of the thigh, usually terminating above the knee. Pain can be more marked in the leg than in the back. When pain is bilateral and symmetrically affects the trunk, it is called girdle pain.

Pain frequently worsens with spinal extension, walking, sitting, and conditions that can increase the intraspinal pressure such as coughing, sneezing, laughing, crying, or strained lifting. Pain tends to lessen with flexion of the spine, standing upright, and leaning forward. In particular, a patient may report that the pain is markedly relieved when leaning over a shopping cart. Pain frequently is less with lateral bending or rotation to the opposite direction from the involved nerve root ascribed to increasing the intervertebral foraminal space available for the root to pass through, and thus decreasing the degree of compression and irritation.

Spinal pain is often associated with other positive sensory symptoms such as tingling, pins and needles, and burning, or negative symptoms as numbness. These symptoms are in a dermatomal distribution, especially distally in the hands or feet where pain is usually minimal.

Less frequently, patients complain of weakness in certain muscles of the same myotome. Overall, sensory and motor symptoms are usually mild with lesions involving a single root, due to the fact that dermatomes and myotomes are usually innervated by multiple nerve roots.

Autonomic sympathetic fibers may be involved. If the lesion is at the C8–T1 level, a Horner's syndrome may occur (ptosis, meiosis, enophthalmus, and anhydrosis). In the thoracolumbar area, there may be a loss of sweating with increased skin temperature. If L1–L3 roots are affected, ejaculation may be impaired; lesions at the S3–S4 level may result in parasympathetic dysfunction with loss of erection and dysfunctional bladder.

Symptoms suggestive of a central disc herniation causing a myelopathy or cauda equina syndrome are important to recognize. They include recent urinary frequency, urgency, or incontinence, constipation, impotence, saddle area (rectal and genital) pain or tingling, gait disturbance, and progressively worsening motor or sensory changes.

Constitutional symptoms such as fever, chills, night sweats, unexplained weight loss, fatigue, persistent severe pain at night, skin rash, and involvement of other joints or other body organs raise the possibility of underlying systemic diseases like infections, malignancies with possible metastasis, or connective tissue diseases. Other historical features of possible importance are trauma with the possibility of a fracture, alcohol or intravenous drug abuse, recurrent infections suggesting an immune compromised state, previous malignancies, medicines that might accelerate osteoporosis. These features have been published as "red flags" by the Agency for Health Care Policy and Research on December 1994. Table 24.2 includes a complete list.

It should kept in mind that neck or back pain can be referred from extraspinal sources. Referred pain to the neck includes posterior lower lobe pneumonia, pericarditis, or coronary artery disease. Referred pain from the abdomen to the thoracic spine includes kidney and gall bladder infections or stones, ruptured aortic aneurysms, retroperitoneal bleeding, or malignancies. Pelvic sources referred to the LS spine are prostatitis or endometriosis. Pain from joint pathology and arthralgias can be referred to the spine and misinterpreted as originating from the spine.

An inquiry into a patient's social and work situations and any psychiatric history may reveal emotional issues that might influence the patient's views of their pain and outcome. Finally, a history of doctor "shopping" for pain medications is an indication of a functional component.

3.2. Physical Examination

The goal of the physical examination is to focus on the diagnostic process by confirming findings predicted from the history and determining the level of spinal nerve root

Table 24.2   Red Flags for Potentially Serious Conditions Causing Neck or Back Pain

From medical history
Possible fracture
   Major trauma, such as vehicle accident or fall from height
   Minor trauma or even strenuous lifting (in older or potentially osteoporotic patient)
Possible tumor or infection
   Age >50 or <20
   History of cancer
   Constitutional symptoms, such as recent fever or chills or unexplained weight loss
   Risk factors for spinal infection: recent bacterial infection (e.g., urinary tract infection); IV drug
      abuse; or immune suppression (from steroids, transplant, or HIV)
   Pain that worsens when supine; severe nighttime pain
Possible cauda equina syndrome
   Saddle anesthesia
   Recent onset of bladder dysfunction, such as urinary retention, increased frequency, or overflow
      incontinence
   Severe or progressive neurologic deficit in the lower extremity
From physical examination
Possible cauda equina syndrome
   Unexpected laxity of the anal sphincter
   Perianal/perineal sensory loss
   Major motor weakness: quadriceps (knee extension weakness); ankle plantar flexors, evertors, and
      dorsiflexors (foot drop)

Source: Bigos et al. (13).

pathology. Determination of the level of the lesion is facilitated by knowledge of root anatomy and associated symptoms and signs (Table 24.3).

The physical exam should include the general appearance, vital signs, and general neurologic examination to exclude a serious underlying condition with referred symptoms to the spine or secondary involvement of the spine.

Focusing on true root lesions, initial examination of station and gait provides information. Alteration in stance or posture may include leaning away or flexing the spine from the affected root. Similarly, when sitting, flexion of the knees or resting weight on the opposite buttock may open disk spaces. Neri's sign is flexion at the knees while bending forward to alleviate the pain induced by stretching of nerves. Minor's sign is bending the affected leg while supporting the body on the unaffected side upon rising from seated position (12). Trendelenburg gait is secondary to weakness of the gluteus medius muscle on one side, which results in failure to raise the pelvis on the contralateral side during standing. Sometimes there may be no significant weakness, but walking will be with caution to avoid or alleviate the pain with short slow steps with semiflexed knees, or walking on toes to avoid dorsiflexion of the foot (antalgic or analgesic gait).

General inspection should include the neck and back for alignment, signs of trauma, surgery, infections, inflammations, or developmental disorders like midline sinuses or café au lait spots. Loss of normal cervical or lumbar lordosis due to involuntary spasm of paraspinal muscles is not specific. Similarly, palpation or percussion for tender points is not specific but point tenderness may be encountered with infectious, metastatic, or traumatic lesions. Other signs that can be caused by root lesions are muscle atrophy and fasciculations in muscles supplied by that root.

Motor examination should focus on finding a myotomal pattern of involvement, and this can be achieved by examining different muscles innervated by the same spinal nerve

Table 24.3   Common Clinical Features Associated with Specific Root Lesions

C5

 Sensory disturbance: shoulder, lateral arm

 Motor deficit: subclavius, rhomboids, rotator cuff muscles except subscapularis, (biceps, deltoid)[a]

 Stretch reflex: (scapulohumeral, deltoid)[b], biceps, brachioradialis

 Superficial reflex: interscapular

C6

 Sensory disturbance: lateral forearm, thumb and index

 Motor deficit: biceps, brachioradialis, serratus anterior, subscapularis, coracobrachialis, teres major, latissimus dorsi, pectoralis, (deltoid, pronator teres, triceps)[a]

 Stretch reflex: biceps, brachioradialis, (deltoid, pectoralis)[b]

 Superficial reflex: palmar

C7

 Sensory disturbance: volar and dorsal forearm, middle finger

 Motor deficit: triceps, pronator teres, forearm extensors, serratus anterior, latissimus dorsi, pectoralis, anconeus

 Stretch reflex: triceps, (pectoralis, pronator)[b]

 Superficial reflex: palmar

C8 & T1

 Sensory disturbance: medial 2 fingers and hypothenar area (C8), and medial forearm (T1)

 Motor deficit: forearm flexors, hand muscles, pectoralis

 Stretch reflex: triceps, (wrist extension/flexion, thumb flexion, pectoralis)[b]

 Superficial reflex: palmar

L1–L2

 Sensory disturbance: inguinal region, inner proximal thigh

 Motor deficit: iliopsoas, pectineus, graciles, iliacus

 Stretch reflex: patellar (minimal)

 Superficial reflex: cremasteric, hypogastric (Bechterew's)

L3–4

 Sensory disturbance: anterior thigh (L3), lateral thigh and medial leg (L4)

 Motor deficit: quadriceps femoris, adductors, obturator externus, (iliopsoas, tibialis anterior)[a]

 Stretch reflex: patellar, thigh adductor[b]

 Superficial reflex: gluteal, plantar

L5

 Sensory disturbance: lateral leg, medial dorsum of foot including big toe

 Motor deficit: gluteus medius/minimus, tibialis anterior, obturator internus, semitendinosus, semimembranosus, peroneus longus/brevis, tibialis posterior, toes extensors

 Stretch reflex: (tibialis posterior, medial hamstring)[b]

 Superficial reflex: gluteal, plantar

S1

 Sensory disturbance: lateral dorsum and sole of foot, little toe, distal dorsal leg

 Motor deficit: hamstrings, gastrocnemius, soleus, obturator internus, gemelli, toes extensors, peronei

 Stretch reflex: achilles

 Superficial reflex: gluteal, plantar

S2

 Sensory disturbance: middle dorsal leg and thigh

 Motor deficit: toes flexors, gastrocnemius, soleus

 Stretch reflex: achilles

 Superficial reflex: bulbocavernous, clitorocavernous, anal sphincter

Note: Clinical features vary in existence and severity secondary to the overlap among dermatomes and myotomes.

[a]These muscles may be affected but to a lesser extent.

[b]These reflexes may be absent in normal individuals.

root but by different peripheral nerves. However, weakness is not common in root lesions due to the overlap of myotomes with multiple roots innervating the same muscle. When weakness is found, both distal and proximal muscles that belong to the same myotome should be studied to confirm that the lesion is proximal to the origin of a peripheral nerve and cannot be explained by an injury to that nerve.

Common motor deficits noted in specific root lesions include the following weakness C5 and C6: weakness of arm abduction and external rotation plus scapular instability; C4: weakness of the diaphragm that can be life threatening if ventilation is compromised; and C7: weakness of arm adduction, and extension of arm, wrist, and fingers. Beevor's sign is upward movement of the umbilicus with attempted sit up due to weakness of inferior abdominal wall muscles. It is typically observed with thoracic myelopathies. Thoracic segments: weakness of abdominal muscles detected by bulging of the affected portion of the abdominal wall. Beevor's sign is movement of the umbilicus with tightening of the abdominal muscles. L1–L4: weakness of hip flexion and adduction and leg extension; L5 and S1: weakness of hip extension, knee flexion, and foot dorsi/plantarflexion (mild L5 weakness can be detected by difficulty heel walking and mild S1 weakness by difficulty with toe walking); S2: weakness of small muscles of the foot; and S3 and S4: weakness of bladder and bowel sphincters and erectile dysfunction.

The sensory examination can confirm a dermatomal pattern but is limited by root overlap and by the subjective nature of sensory perception. Sensory loss can involve some modalities and spare others. Common sensory deficits include the following. C6: sensory abnormalities along the lateral forearm and thumb; C7: sensory loss of middle finger; C8 sensory loss along medial forearm and little finger; T3–T5: sensory loss at the level of the nipples; T9–T11: sensory loss in periumbilical area; L4: sensory loss along medial thigh. L5: sensory loss over medial dorsum of foot and big toe; S1: loss over little toe and sole of the foot.

Muscle stretch reflexes examination is valuable for demonstrating asymmetry variation because radiculopathies are commonly unilateral. Informative reflexes include the following. C4–C5: scapulohumeral (rhomboids); C5–T1: pectoralis; C6: biceps and brachioradialis; C7: triceps. L2–L3: thigh adductors; L4: patellar; L5: medial hamstring; and S1: ankle.

Superficial skin reflexes may be abnormal in ipsilateral root lesions, especially if the spinal cord is also involved. C4–C5: interscapular reflex (scratching the skin over the interscapular area results in contraction of scapular muscles); C6–T1: palmar reflex (stroking the palm of hand results in flexion of fingers); T5–T11: superficial abdominal reflexes may be divided into epigastric (T5–T7), supraumbilical (T7–T9), umbilical (T9–T11), and infraumbilical (T11–L1). Bechterew's hypogastric reflex (T11 through L2) is elicited by stroking the inner surface of thigh leading to contraction of lower abdominal muscles on the same side. L1–L2: cremasteric reflex; L4–S2: gluteal reflex (contraction of gluteal muscles by scratching the skin of the buttocks) and plantar reflex; S2–S3: anal sphincter reflex and bulbocavernous reflex.

Special maneuvers can be performed to induce pain related to nerve root irritation or compression. Tests for cervical nerve roots include the following. Spurling maneuver is extending, tilting, and rotating the head toward the suspected nerve root to reproduce or aggravate pain. A test to relieve pain is abduction of the shoulder ipsilateral to the diseased nerve root. Lhermitte's sign is defined as an electrical shock down the body elicited by neck flexion secondary to either intrinsic (e.g. multiple sclerosis) or extrinsic (spondylosis) cervical spinal cord compression. Tests for LS roots include the following. Laseque sign is defined as radicular leg pain elicited by elevation of the leg while in the supine position. A more specific but less sensitive test than straight leg raising is the crossed straight leg raising test that is considered positive when pain is induced in the leg by lifting the opposite asymptomatic leg. Pain can be aggravated by dorsiflexion of ankle or big toe and also by adduction and internally rotating thigh and leg. Buckling sign represents the involuntary knee flexion while carrying out the straight leg raising test to decrease the tension and stretching of nerve roots.

It is important during the examination to be alert to signs indicating a myelopathy requiring more urgent and aggressive management. Signs include progressively worsening motor or sensory deficits, hyperreflexia, Babinski or Hoffmann signs, spastic gait, clumsiness and loss of coordination, rectal sphincter dysfunction, and urinary retention with overflow incontinence (assessed by measuring the post void bladder residual volume).

When the history and examination do not support a radiculopathy or other cause a functional etiology should be considered. Waddell signs are common indicators of a factitious or a malingering patient (13) and include tenderness to superficial palpation, reaction to simulation tests as if they are real, loss of positive tests with distraction, overreaction, and examination findings that do not follow neuroanatomical distributions. Additional signs include camptospasm (static forward flexion of trunk) and coccygodynia (pain in the coccyx region) (11).

3.3. Workup

A differential diagnosis should be clear after completing the history and physical examination, and the workup will depend upon specific questions that need to be answered.

3.3.1. Laboratory Tests

Tests that focus on causes of radiculopathy are few. Fasting and 2-h glucose tolerance tests screen for undiagnosed diabetes that can present as a thoracic radiculopathy. A spinal tap for CSF analysis is helpful if Lyme disease or neurosyphilis is suspected.

3.3.2. Imaging Studies

Plain spine X-ray is helpful in diagnosing bony deformities or congenital defects, sublaxation, fractures, malignment lesions, or infectious processes. Degenerative changes with narrowing of the intervertebral foramina have high false positive rates since almost half the patients who show these findings are asymptomatic.

MRI is the most informative imaging study for showing spinal soft tissue details including disc herniation, degenerative changes, annular tears, and changes associated with infectious, malignant, or demyelination processes. In addition, MRI is helpful in differentiating postsurgical scarring from recurrent disc disease, particularly if gadolinium is used.

CT-scan is better than MRI for detecting boney details and abnormalities. When combined with myelography, it provides more anatomical details than MRI for nerve roots at the level of the intervertebral foramina. Drawbacks that limit its use include the invasive lumbar puncture with possible side effects of headache and hematoma, and risk of reaction to contrast material. However, it is an alternative when implanted metal hardware and claustrophobia are contraindications to MRI.

Both MRI and CT with myelography have comparable false positive findings in up to one-third of patients >60 years of age (12–14). Further, the size of the herniated disc does not always correlate with the severity of signs and symptoms.

Other imaging modalities are used infrequently. Bone scan may be helpful for assessing malignant, ischemic, infectious, or traumatic changes. Single-photon emission computed tomography (SPECT) scanning is similar to bone scan but provides three-dimensional images.

3.3.3.   Electrophysiological Studies

An electrophysiologic workup includes nerve conduction studies (NCS), electromyography (EMG), and infrequently somatosensory evoked potentials (SSEP). These studies do not have the ability to define the underlying pathology, but can confirm the presence of a lesion, determine the level and severity of axonal damage, and differentiate radiculopathy from peripheral neuropathy or plexopathy. They can be used for postoperative follow up evaluation, and in determining the age and severity of a radiculopathy, which can be important in medico-legal cases.

NCS assess the distal portion of sensory nerves and both the distal and proximal portions of motor fibers. In a radiculopathy, NCS are usually normal for several reasons. The lesion site in a radiculopathy is proximal to the dorsal root ganglion, and the distal segment of sensory nerves will be unaffected. The distal portion of motor nerve conduction lesion will be normal because the severity of denervation in one root is insufficient to reduce the motor potential. The proximal portion of motor nerves is assessed by F-wave and H-wave testing, but the region of nerve damage from a radiculopathy is usually too small to demonstrably prolong either response and can be abnormal in any lesion along the way.

The needle EMG is the most important electrophysiological test because it is sensitive to motor nerve damage and can be applied to any muscle to delimit radicular involvement. The principles are to demonstrate denervation in several muscles innervated by the suspected root and not by a single nerve. There are temporal factors to consider with needle EMG. The first EMG finding in an acute radiculopathy is decreased motor unit recruitment. Within 1–2 weeks, denervation changes consisting of fibrillation potentials and positive sharp waves occur in paraspinal muscles, with gradual spread over the next 2–3 weeks to distal muscles. Within 1–2 months, reinnervation begins, marked by complex (polyphasic) motor unit potentials. These changes occur in the same order, from proximal to distal. In chronic radiculopathies, fibrillation potentials and positive sharp waves will be reduced or absent and motor units will be of high amplitude. Although sensitive for denervation, the degree of damage may be mild and not detectable. In some situations, comparison with the unaffected side may reveal subtle changes.

SSEP's are used to evaluate large sensory nerve fiber pathways from the level of the peripheral nerve through the nerve root, spinal cord, and brain. In general, they are not useful in the evaluation of radiculopathy because the nerves stimulated carry nerve fibers originating at several spinal root levels. Furthermore, the length of nerve compression represents only a very short segment of the much longer sensory pathway, resulting in only minimal slowing of the response.

4.   MANAGEMENT AND PROGNOSIS

Management of a radiculopathy must consider a large number of variables. No precise management protocol covers all variables, and the main issue is indications for surgery (Table 24.4). Fortunately, 80–90% of patients recover completely and spontaneously with conservative management, within 6 weeks (1,2). However, relapse may occur in a certain percentage of patients, and a low but significant percentage of patients continue

Table 24.4 Common Indications for Surgery in Radiculopathy

Progressive neurological deficit(s)[a]
Cauda equina syndrome[a]
Persistent neurologic deficits and/or pain that significantly interfere with patients daily function, and fail to improve despite all possible non-surgical measures
Positive imaging studies that correlate with the patient's clinical presentation

[a]Usually requires emergent surgical intervention.

to have symptoms despite all measures, and they may eventually develop chronic pain syndrome.

After excluding serious etiologies that might need a more aggressive approach or special treatment modalities, pain and conservative rehabilitation are appropriate. Initial bed rest or limiting mobility to decrease mechanical root irritation is appropriate. Complete bed rest for more than few days, however, should be discouraged and the patient should be advised to resume activities as soon as possible, if tolerated (25). Spine immobilization via neck collars or back corsets or braces can be used, but for not much more than few weeks to prevent deconditioning and dependence on such devices.

Nonsteroidal anti-inflammatory drugs are appropriate for their analgesic as well as their anti-inflammatory effects. Others that target neuropathic pain, such as gabapentin or tricyclic antidepressants, are used. Opiate use should be restricted secondary to the risk of tolerance and dependence. Muscle relaxants, including botulinum toxin, may help relieve paraspinal muscle spasm that is believed to be a significant source of pain. A short course of oral steroids to help decrease nerve root edema may be effective. A more aggressive approach includes epidural injections of steroids or local anesthetics to speed up the resolution of inflammation and reduce pain.

Physical therapy modalities including hot pads, ultrasound, electrical stimulation, and massaging can be helpful, in conjunction with exercises aimed at strengthening spinal muscles may be helpful with pain relief and aid mobility. Chiropractic maneuvers should be discouraged in the acute phase because they could result in worsening of disc herniation and further compression of nerve roots with possible serious consequences, especially in the cervical region.

Emergent surgical assessment and intervention is indicated when neurologic deficits are progressively and rapidly deteriorating or there are signs of cauda equina syndrome. Elective surgery is governed by the degree of disc herniation and bone formation in the canal and foramena in conjunction with muscle weakness, sensory loss, and needle EMG changes. Surgery for persistent and severe pain is most uncertain. Spinal surgery is not without risk, which include arachnoiditis and fibrosis of nerve roots which may lead to recurrence of symptoms and failure of surgery. Other common possible causes of surgery failure are listed in Table 24.5.

Table 24.5 Possible Causes of Spinal Surgery Failure

Recurrent disc herniation at operation level, or at a close level with similar symptoms
Surgical complications including arachnoiditis, bleeding, infection, scarring, or direct root injury
Wrong diagnosis
Technical errors and instruments failure
Spinal instability or failure to fuse
Underlying functional, non-organic etiology
Inappropriate postoperative rehabilitation and physical therapy process

REFERENCES

1. Anderson GBJ. The epidemiology of spinal disorders. In: Frymoyer JW, ed. The Adult Spine: Principles and Practice. Philadelphia: Lippincot-Raven, 1997:93–141.
2. Anderson GBJ. Epidemiologic features of chronic low back pain. Lancet 1999; 354:581–585.
3. Hart LG, Deyo RA, Cherkin DC. Physician office visits for low back pain: frequency, clinical evaluation, and treatment patterns from a U.S. national survey. Spine 1995; 20:11–19.
4. Keith LM. Clinically Oriented Anatomy. 3rd ed. Baltimore: Williams & Wilkins, 1992.
5. Peter LW, Roger W. Functional Neuroanatomy of Man. Philadelphia: WB Saunders Company, 1975.
6. Randall LB. Evaluation and management of neck and back pain. In: Rahman P, ed. Neuromuscular Disease: Expert Clinicians' Views. Woburn: Butterworth–Heinemann, 2001:529–561.
7. David AC. Disorders of nerve roots and plexuses. In: Walter GB, Robert BD, Gerald MF, Marsden CD, eds. Neurology in Clinical Practice. Vol. 2. 3rd ed. Woburn: Butterworth–Heinemann, 2000:2019–2032.
8. Deyo RA, Weinstein JN. Low Back Pain. N Engl J Med 2001; 344:363–370.
9. Della-Giustina DA. Emergency Department Evaluation and Treatment of Back Pain. Emerg Med Clin North Am 1999; 17(4):877–893.
10. Vroomen PC, de Krom MC, Knottnerus JA. Diagnostic value of history and physical examination in patients suspected of sciatica due to disc herniation: a systematic review. J Neurol 1999; 246:899–906.
11. Vroomen PC, de Krom MC, Wilmink JT, Kester AD, Knottnerus JA. Diagnostic value of history and physical examination in patients suspected of lumbosacral nerve root compression. J Neurol Neurosurg Psychiatry 2002; 72:630–634.
12. DeJong RN. The Neurologic Examination: Incorporating the Fundamentals of Neuroanatomy and Neurophysiology. 4th ed. Hagerstown: Harper & Row, 1979.
13. Bigos S, Bowyer O, Braen G, Brown K, Deyo R, Haldeman S, Hart J, Johnson E, Keller R, Kido D, Liang M, Nelson R, Nordin M, Owen B, Pope M, Schwartz R, Stewart D Jr, Susman J, Triano J, Tripp L, Turk D, Watts C, Weinstein J. Acute Low Back Problems in Adults: Assessment and Treatment. Clinical Practice Guideline No. 14. AHCPR Publication No. 95-0643, Rockville, MD: Agency for Health Care Policy and Research, Public Health Service, U.S. Department of Health and Human Service. December 1994.
14. Waddell G, McCulloch JA, Kummel E, Venner RM. Nonorganic physical signs in low back pain. Spine 1980; 5:117–125.
15. Humphreys SC, Eck JC. Radiologic decision-making: neuroimaging in low back pain. Am Fam Physician 2002; 65(11):2299–2306.
16. Boden SD, Davis DO, Dina TS, Patronas NJ, Wiesel SW. Abnormal magnetic-resonance scans of the lumbar spine in asymptomatic subjects: a prospective investigation. J Bone Joint Surg Am 1990; 72:403–408.
17. Weishaupt D, Zanetti M, Hodler J, Boos N. MR imaging of the lumbar spine: prevalence of intervertebral disk extrusion and sequestration, nerve root compression, end plate abnormalities, and osteoarthritis of the facet joints in asymptomatic volunteers. Radiology 1998; 209:661–666.
18. Lomen-Hoerth C, Aminoff MJ. Clinical neurophysiologic studies: which test is useful and when? Neurol Clin 1999; 17(1):65–74.
19. Robinson LR. Electromyography, magnetic resonance imaging, and radiculopathy: it's time to focus on specificity. Muscle Nerve 1999; 22:149–150.
20. Levin KH. Electrodiagnostic approach to the patient with suspected radiculopathy. Neurol Clin 2002; 20(2):397.
21. Kenneth CG. Approach to Radiculopathies. 53rd Annual Meeting for the American Academy of Neurology, Philadelphia, May 5–11, 2001.

22. David CP, Barbara ES. Radiculopathy. In: Electromyography and Neuromuscular Disorders: Clinical-Electrophysiologic Correlations. 1st ed. Butterworth–Heinemann Medical, 1998:413–433.

23. Humphreys SC, Eck JC. Clinical evaluation and treatment options for herniated lumbar disc. Am Fam Physician 1999; 59(3):575–582, 587.

24. Patel AT, Ogle AA. Diagnosis and management of acute low back pain. Am Fam Physician 2000; 61(6):1779–1786, 1789–1790.

25. Hall S, Bartleson JD, Onofrio BM, Baker HL Jr, Okazaki H, O'Duffy JD. Lumbar spinal stenosis: clinical features, diagnostic procedures, and results of surgical treatment in 68 patients. Ann Intern Med 1985; 103:271–275.

26. Malmivaara A, Häkkinen U, Aro T, Heinrichs ML, Koskenniemi L, Kuosma E, Lappi S, Paloheimo R, Servo C, Vaaranen V, Hernberg S. The treatment of acute low back pain— bed rest, exercises, or ordinary activity? N Engl J Med 1995; 332:351–355.

27. van Tulder MW, Koes BW, Bouter LM. Conservative treatment of acute and chronic non-specific low back pain: a systematic review of randomized controlled trials of the most common interventions. Spine 1997; 22:2128–2156.

28. Atlas SJ, Keller RB, Robson D, Deyo RA, Singer DE. Surgical and nonsurgical management of lumbar spinal stenosis: four-year outcomes from the Maine Lumbar Spine Study. Spine 2000; 25:556–562.

25
Plexopathies

John C. Kincaid

Indiana University School of Medicine, Indianapolis, Indiana, USA

ABSTRACT

Plexopathies are lesions that affect the major interchanging segments between the nerve roots and the peripheral nerves. Plexopathy should be considered when the pattern of nerve dysfunction cannot be explained by a lesion of a single nerve root or peripheral nerve. Plexopathies usually occur as recognizable syndromes. In most instances the diagnosis is made clinically, with support from electrodiagnostic and imaging studies. Treatment and prognosis depend on the underlying condition.

1. INTRODUCTION

The diagnosis of a plexopathy can be challenging because of the complexity of the underlying axonal interchanges. A firm grasp of anatomy is essential. However, the basic diagnostic principle is to distinguish radicular and peripheral nerve trunk lesions. There are clinical patterns of neuropathy that can be recognized as likely reflecting a plexopathy, and will be outlined subsequently.

Electrodiagnostic studies have an important role in making these distinctions. The lesion site in plexopathies is distal to the sensory ganglion cell, and both motor (compound muscle action potential: CMAP) and sensory (sensory nerve action potential: SNAP) responses will be reduced or absent. Lesions proximal to the level of the sensory ganglion cells, such as radiculopathies or nerve root avulsions, affect the CMAP but not the SNAP. Needle EMG examination in a plexopathy will usually be abnormal in anterior myotomes (limb muscles), but normal in posterior myotomes (paraspinal muscles). Plexopathies can also include damage to nerve roots, in the settings of trauma, and diabetes. Needle EMG is essential in determining the territory of involvement, and can help estimate severity, chronology, prognosis. In acute plexopathies, it may take up to 4 weeks for the full extent of denervation to become evident. Low amplitude polyphasic, unstable motor unit potentials indicate re-innervation. Long duration, high amplitude, stable configuration motor unit potentials indicate complete re-innervation. Mixed populations of complex and simple potentials suggest ongoing denervation and re-innervation. Myokymic discharges, in the appropriate clinical context, support radiation-induced plexopathy.

Magnetic resonance imaging (MRI) may identify lesion sites within the plexus either by hyperintense signals in the nerve or by demonstrating compressive structures such as hematomas or neoplasm (1). Spinal MRI or myelography followed by a postmyelogram CT is helpful to determine whether radiculopathy is present.

2. BRACHIAL PLEXUS

2.1. Anatomy and Function

The brachial plexus is formed from axons arising from the ventral rami of C5–T1 spinal levels (Fig. 25.1). The innervation of dermatomes follows an orderly pattern through the trunks and cords of the plexus. The C5 root innervates the radial side of the forearm and C6 root the thumb and index finger. The axons pass through the upper trunk and lateral or posterior cords of the plexus. The C7 root innervates in the middle and ring fingers, and axons pass through the middle trunk and lateral cord. The C8 root supplies the fifth finger and ulnar side of the hand and T1 the ulnar side of the forearm. The axons pass through the lower trunk and medial cord.

The innervation of myotomes is less logical, but conforms to an understandable pattern. The long thoracic nerve originates directly from C5–C7 roots (proximal to the plexus) and innervates the serratus anterior muscle, which stabilizes the shoulder blade. The dorsal scapular, suprascapular, axillary, and musculocutaneous nerves originate from C5–C6 roots and innervate muscles that control shoulder motion and elbow flexion. These nerves are derivatives of the upper trunk. The median and radial nerves originate from C6–C7 roots and innervate muscles that extend and flex the wrist. Axons pass through the upper and middle trunks and the lateral and posterior cords. The C7 root is the major innervation of elbow extension. Axons pass through the middle trunk and posterior cord into the radial nerve. The median and radial nerves innervate the muscles that flex and extend the fingers, respectively, and are innervated

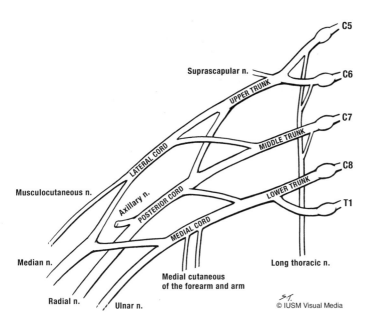

Figure 25.1   Anatomy of the brachial plexus.

by C7–C8 roots, the axons pass through the middle and lower trunks and posterior and medial cords. The median and ulnar nerves innervate intrinsic hand muscles. They are supplied by C8–T1 roots and derived from lower trunk and medial cord.

2.2.   Brachial Plexopathies

Etiologies of brachial plexus lesions include trauma, inflammation, genetic, neoplastic infiltration, prior therapeutic radiation, and thoracic outlet syndrome (2,3).

2.2.1.   Traumatic Causes

Obstetric brachial plexus palsy is the most common traumatic cause, with an incidence of 0.5–2.0 per thousand births. Weakness is detected at or shortly after birth when an arm is noted not to move properly (4,5). Patterns of plexus injury may involve the upper, middle or lower trunks. Upper trunk lesions, Erb's palsy, produce deficits in abduction of the shoulder, external rotation of the arm, and flexion of the elbow. Deficits of both upper and middle trunk function are common in this setting. Lower plexus lesions, Klumpke's palsy, produce impairment of finger function. Isolated deficits of this type are rare, and impairment of finger function are more often encountered with pan-plexus lesions.

Traumatic plexopathies can be caused by motor vehicle accidents, falls associated with shoulder dislocations, and penetrating knife or gun shot wounds (2,3). Any portion of the plexus is susceptible in such circumstances. Surgical procedures which require the arm to be positioned in an externally rotated and abducted posture while the head is rotated to the opposite side may damage the plexus. Lower trunk deficits can occur after median sternotomy. These can be confused initially with postoperative ulnar neuropathy, but abnormalities of median and ulnar-innervated hand muscles confirm a lower trunk pattern. Plexopathies can develop during the postoperative period, when positioning or the operative site are not factors. The clinical course is similar to that of an idiopathic inflammatory type plexopathy.

"Stingers or burners" are another type of traumatic plexopathy, occurring most often during contact sports, like football (6). The player performing a block or tackle experiences sudden downward force on the shoulder and reports an immediate stinging or burning sensation in the arm. Sensory and motor symptoms tend to clear over a few minutes. Motor deficits in shoulder abduction and elbow flexion may occur, but long-lasting sensory and motor deficits are unusual.

Heavy, improperly fitting back packs worn for several consecutive days can cause plexopathy by combined downward and retracting forces on the shoulders and plexus.

With acute skeletal and penetrating injuries, neurological deficits may not be fully assessable in the immediate medical setting. Plain X-ray films can identify fractures and dislocations of the vertebrae, upper ribs, and shoulders that may impinge on the plexus. The scope of neurological deficit should be defined as soon as conditions permit. Pain should be managed with appropriate levels of analgesics.

Pathologic features vary with the nature of the injury. Traction forces act on myelin sheaths, axons, perineurium and epineurium, and vasculature structures of the plexus. In some circumstances, forces act maximally at the nerve root level, rather than in the plexus, and avulsion of nerve rootlets from the spinal cord may occur in extreme circumstances. Severe lesions may produce a combination of plexus and nerve root injury.

The course of recovery varies based on the etiology. Myelin sheath damage tends to clear over days to weeks, and recovery will likely be good. Axonal injury requires months to years to improve, and may not be complete. Deficits due to nerve root avulsion do not improve. Penetrating injures due to a sharp object may be considered for early surgical exploration and repair. Blunt force and traction type injuries are usually observed for several months before surgical intervention is considered. Obstetric palsies which have not shown improvement by 3 months should be considered for surgical intervention. If motor and sensory deficits are still present 2–3 weeks after onset, electrodiagnostic studies can help to determine the extent and nature of the lesions. Needle EMG can also be helpful for following the course by detecting signs of re-innervation.

Occupational and physical therapy for maintaining range of joint motion is important for enhancing recovery. Splinting may be required to prevent contracture and to maximize the function of other portions of the involved limb. Active exercise should be started as soon as recovery of strength permits.

2.2.2. Inflammatory Causes

Brachial plexopathy arising secondary to systemic inflammatory responses has been given the eponym Parsonage–Turner syndrome or neuralgic amyotrophy (7,8). These plexopathies begin most often with spontaneous pain in the upper and posterior regions of the shoulder and proximal arm. The pain, which may be excruciating, increases over a few days to weeks, may worsen with arm and shoulder motion, but not with coughing, sneezing, or straining. The pain is bilateral in one-third of cases.

Weakness and sensory symptoms become apparent between a few days or weeks after onset. Weakness is most often found in shoulder abduction, external rotation, and elbow flexion. Scapular winging is common. Localization is usually to several nerves of the upper portion of the plexus, but occasionally one nerve is affected in apparent isolation. Sensory loss is most often along the radial side of the forearm or hand and in the distribution of the axillary nerve.

Pain severity lessens over weeks to several months, but some degree of pain may linger for months, and may be at least partly related to shoulder motion abnormalities that have developed secondary to weakness. Motor and sensory deficits tend to improve over several months to several years. A small percent of patients have permanent deficits. Recurrence is rare and raises the question of an inherited form of brachial plexopathy.

Cervical radiculopathy and lesions of the shoulder joint are the main considerations. The onset of weakness and sensory symptoms concurrent with pain somewhat favors acute radiculopathy over plexopathy. Significant worsening of pain with active or passive motions of the shoulder favors an intrinsic shoulder lesion over plexopathy. A confident diagnosis of an idiopathic plexopathy may require several weeks for the typical syndrome of pain and then weakness plus sensory loss to evolve.

Sensory nerve conduction studies may reveal postganglion involvement, but the nerve affected may be challenging to study. Needle EMG provides information on the distribution and severity of denervation. Muscles showing the greatest abnormality in the symptomatic limb should be sampled contralaterally, as bilateral involvement may be present at a subclinical level. Follow-up studies in several months can help define prognosis by demonstrating signs of re-innervation. MRI or myelogram can exclude a radicular lesion that could produce the same clinical deficits. MRI may directly support the diagnosis of plexopathy by showing local enlargement and increased T2 signals in the involved portions of the plexus (1).

There are no controlled trials for the use of immune modulating therapy such as corticosteroids. One challenge in assessing treatment is that a secure diagnosis often cannot be made until several weeks after onset, thus missing a therapeutic time window. If steroid therapy is used, a high dose intravenous regimen similar to that used for an acute attack of multiple sclerosis, followed by an oral taper should likely be chosen. Management focuses on treating the pain and maintaining range of motion. Narcotic analgesics are frequently needed, but may be only partly effective. Pain may severely limit the patient's willingness to move the involved limb. Active strengthening therapy should be started when signs of recovery appear.

The pathogenesis is presumed to be an autoimmune inflammatory attack on the plexus. There are no abnormalities in serum characteristic of an inflammatory process. Support for an inflammatory etiology is the acute onset and that in a number of patients, the onset is within days to weeks after a systemic infection or vaccination. Plexopathies with these same clinical characteristics may also occur after an episode of overly vigorous exertion, or after a surgical procedure in which limb positioning cannot be easily linked to the lesion. The primary target of the inflammatory response is presumed to be the vascular supply of the plexus or intramuscular nerves. It has been suggested that it is a localized form of mononeuritis multiplex which affects individual nerves arising from the plexus.

2.2.3. Inherited Brachial Plexopathy

A familial form of brachial plexopathy occurs as a dominantly inherited disorder (9). There are associated mild dysmorphic features including hypotelorism and epicanthal folds. The clinical characteristics of acute episodes are similar to those described earlier for inflammatory plexopathies. Systemic infections or overly vigorous exertion, and women giving birth, can precipitate an attack. Recurrences are unique to this form of plexopathy. This entity is distinguished clinically from hereditary liability to pressure palsy, where weakness involves individual nerves, and is usually in association with maintenance of a position that compresses the nerve. There is much less pain than in the plexopathy.

Biopsies of upper extremity nerves during an attack show inflammatory changes in vascular structures and axonal degeneration. The genetic basis of this type of plexopathy has not yet been fully established. Linkage with a locus on chromosome 17 has been demonstrated in some but not in all families (10).

When the diagnosis of hereditary plexopathy is established, immune modulating treatment can be started much earlier than in the sporadic form. Treatment with high dose intravenous methylprednisolone has shown some benefit in terms of lessening the pain (11). It is not clear, though, whether this treatment alters the course of the motor and sensory deficits. A case report describes benefit from intravenous gamma globulin treatment in this condition (12).

2.2.4. Neoplastic Causes

Primary nerve tumors of the brachial plexus are exceedingly rare, but metastatic spread occurs primarily from breast and lung cancers (13). A neoplastic plexopathy may develop at any time as part of the original symptom complex, or months to years later as a tumor recurrence. The inferior portion of the plexus tends to be most often involved, and pain is an early symptom, usually located in the axilla, medial arm, or shoulder. The pain tends to be less severe compared with idiopathic plexopathies. Weakness occurs in both ulnar and median innervated intrinsic hand muscles and forearm muscles. Sensory symptoms of parasthesia and numbness occur in the fourth and fifth fingers and the medial forearm. A Horner's syndrome may be present.

The diagnosis may be suspected in the setting of a known cancer. Plain X-ray films of the spine can detect signs of bone erosion, as the vertebral body is a common site of metastasis. CT and MRI can demonstrate a mass lesion in the plexus, and contrast enhancement may identify the lesion site. Electrodiagnostic studies can help differentiate between lesions of the nerve root, lower plexus, and ulnar nerve. Lower plexus lesions may result in reduced or absent SNAP responses in the ulnar and medial antebrachial cutaneous nerves. Ulnar and median motor conduction studies tend to show mild diffuse slowing of velocity and more marked reduction in CMAP amplitude. Needle EMG should show denervation in limb muscles supplied by the involved portion of the plexus but spare paraspinal muscles.

If a mass lesion is demonstrated in the plexus by imaging and a primary neoplasm has not been found, or if the primary is thought to be in remission, biopsy of the plexus lesion may be required to clarify the diagnosis.

The differential diagnosis includes cervical radiculopathy at the C8 or T1 level, combined ulnar and median neuropathy, and lesions of the shoulder joint. The latter does not produce neurological signs, but can cause shoulder, axillary, and arm pain. When a plexopathy develops years after previous treatment of the neoplasm, both tumor recurrence and plexopathy secondary to previous radiation treatment should be considered.

Management is dictated by the biology of the primary neoplasm. Additional chemotherapy and local radiation therapy may be options. Evaluation and treatment by the rehabilitation services will help improve the patient's ability to deal with the deficits.

The pathogenesis of neoplastic plexopathy is most often direct invasion of the plexus from adjacent structures such as the apex of the lung or a vertebral body, or by metastatic spread through the lymphatics.

2.2.5. Postradiation Causes

Therapeutic radiation treatment can cause a brachial plexopathy, with a latency of 5–10 years (14,15). The condition is characterized by insidious progressive weakness, muscle atrophy, fasciculations, and sensory loss. Pain is usually not severe. The upper trunk is most often involved, with weakness most prominent in shoulder and elbow flexor muscles. Sensory loss is most often located in the musculocutaneous, superficial radial, and median sensory areas. These features can inexorably worsen over years to complete limb dysfunction.

Laboratory evaluation is directed to determine whether there is recurrent tumor or a radiculopathy. The absence of anatomic findings on MRI of the plexus and neck is against these and for post-radiation plexopathy. Needle EMG is supportive of a postradiation cause if myokymic discharges can be demonstrated. Myokymic discharges are spontaneous, time-locked groups of motor unit potential discharges that recur in a rhythmic pattern.

The pathogenesis is thought to be a small caliber vasculopathy affecting the vasa nervorum of the nerves located in the radiation portals. Susceptibility of the upper trunk is not understood, and can occur when treatment is within accepted radiation dosage ranges. A similar process can involve the lumbo-sacral plexus. There is no direct treatment for this condition at this time.

2.2.6. *Thoracic Outlet Syndrome*

This is a loosely defined entity, often invoked to account for otherwise unexplainable activity-related pain, weakness, fatigability, and sensory disturbance in the arm. Within this symptom complex is a clearly definable entity termed true neurogenic thoracic outlet syndrome (1,2,16). This is a very rare condition, but has a consistent, clinical, and electrodiagnostic pattern. It typically occurs in women, and includes a long history of unilateral axillary and medial arm pain. Weakness and atrophy of intrinsic hand and medial forearm muscles is obvious, with greater weakness of median-innervated thenar muscles than ulnar-innervated muscles. Many patients have had carpal tunnel surgery, without benefit. Sensory loss occurs in the ulnar aspect of the hand and the medial forearm.

Electrodiagnostic evaluation is remarkable for reduced or absent SNAP responses in ulnar and medial antebrachial nerves, but normal median nerve SNAP responses. Median CMAP responses are lower than ulnar responses. Needle EMG shows chronic neurogenic abnormalities in median, ulnar, and radial muscles innervated by the lower trunk of the plexus.

Plain X-rays of the neck demonstrate either a cervical rib or an elongated transverse process of the seventh cervical vertebra. These anatomic variations are usually present bilaterally but may be somewhat asymmetric. The cervical rib, or a fibrous band which extends from the elongated transverse process to the first rib, impinges abnormally on the lower portion of the plexus.

Surgical removal of the cervical rib, or the fibrous band which extends from the vertebral body's lateral process down to the first rib, may improve pain, but usually does not improve motor or sensory deficits. One reason for the relatively poor response to surgery may be that the deficits have accumulated over a many year time span and have produced significant axonal pathology.

3. LUMBO-SACRAL PLEXUS

3.1. Anatomy and Function

The lumbar and sacral plexes arise on different sides of the pelvic brim and have some what distinct functions, see Fig. 25.2. Motor functions of the lumbar plexus are hip

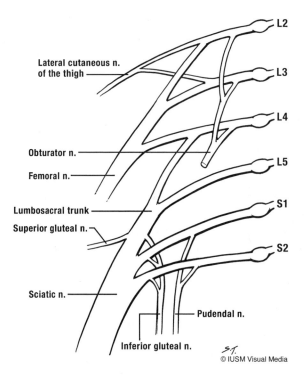

Lateral cutaneous n.
of the thigh

Obturator n.

Femoral n.

Lumbosacral trunk

Superior gluteal n.

Sciatic n.

Inferior gluteal n.

L2

L3

L4

L5

S1

S2

Pudendal n.

© IUSM Visual Media

Figure 25.2 Anatomy of the lumbosacral plexus. The lumbar portion arises for L2–L4, whereas the sacral portion arises for L4–S2. The lumbosacral trunk carries lumbar axons into the sacral plexus.

flexion, leg adduction, and knee extension. The psoas and iliacus muscles are the major flexors of hip flexion, and rectus femoris a lessor flexor. The psoas is innervated by branches arising at the most proximal aspect of the plexus, whereas the iliacus is supplied by branches from the proximal portion of the femoral nerve in the pelvis. The rectus femoris is supplied by the femoral nerve distal to the inguinal ligament. Leg adduction is controlled by the adductor muscle group via the obturator nerve. All of these muscles are innervated by roots from L2, L3, and L4. Knee extension is controlled by the quadriceps muscle group which is innervated by the femoral nerve L3 and L4 nerve roots.

Dermatomes of the lumbar plexus begin in the groin with the illio-inguinal and genito-femoral nerves, which are from L1 and L2 roots. The lateral surface of the thigh is innervated by the lateral cutaneous nerve, which is from L2 and L3 roots. This nerve passes under the inguinal ligament. The anterior and anterior-medial aspects of the thigh are supplied by the femoral nerve. A portion of the medial aspect of the thigh is also innervated by the obturator nerve. The saphenous branch of the femoral nerve innervates the medial aspect of the lower leg down to about the level of the medial malleolous. The sensory portion of the femoral nerve is predominantly L3 and L4 in origin.

The L5, and to some degree L4 nerve root, make major contributions to the nerves which arise from the sacral portion of the plexus. The lumbo-sacral trunk conveys the lumbar nerve root component into the sacral plexus. The motor functions of the sacral plexus are hip abduction and extension, knee flexion, ankle extension and flexion, foot eversion and inversion, and toe flexion and extension. Hip abduction and external rotation are done by the gluteus medius, minimus, and tensor fasciae lata muscles all of which are innervated by the superior gluteal nerve. This nerve arises directly from the plexus and is predominatly L5. Hip extension is done by the gluteus maximus which is supplied by the inferior gluteal nerve. This nerve also arises directly from the plexus and is mainly of S1 origin.

The sacral plexus then gives rise to the sciatic nerve which contains components from the L4 through S2 nerve roots. The sciatic nerve contains axons which will become the peroneal and posterior tibial nerves. In the upper leg the sciatic nerve innervates the hamstring muscles. The peroneal division of the sciatic nerve supplies the short head of the biceps femoris muscle, whereas the other hamstring muscles are innervated by the posterior tibial division. L5 is the predominant nerve root supplying these muscles except for the short head of biceps femoris, which some consider to be predominantly S1 innervated. Proximal to the knee the peroneal and posterior tibial divisions separate into individual nerves. The peroneal nerve controls ankle and toe extension, and ankle eversion. L5 and S1 are the major nerve roots. The posterior tibial nerve controls ankle flexion and inversion, and toe flexion. L5–S2 are the contributing nerve roots.

The sensory pattern of the sacral plexus derived nerves include the posterior aspect of the thigh, the lateral and posterior areas of the lower leg, and both the dorsal and plantar aspects of the foot.

3.2. Lumbo-Sacral Plexopathies

Etiologies include trauma, gun shot wounds, pelvic fractures, compression by hematomas, inflammation with or without concomitant diabetes, invasion by neoplasms, and damage from prior therapeutic radiation (17,18).

3.2.1. Traumatic Causes

Major trauma to the abdomen or pelvis can also injure the lumbo-sacral plexus (19–21). Neurological deficits may not be apparent initially in the setting of severe injury. Gun shot wounds tend to involve the lumbar portion of the plexus and produce deficits of femoral and obturator nerve function. A shielding effect of the bony pelvis may explain why the sacral portion of the plexus is less likely to be involved. Crush injuries of the pelvis can produce deficits in both the lumbar and sacral plexus, with the latter being more commonly involved. Pelvic fractures in the region of the sacro-illiac joint can involve axons of the sacral plexus with weakness in the distribution of L4–S1 roots.

Plain X-rays can assess fractures, but CT or MRI is necessary to assess soft tissue lesions. Electrodiagnostic evaluation can help define the distribution and severity of plexus involvement, but will not be informative until about 2–4 weeks after the injury. Follow-up studies at several month intervals can also be helpful for defining the longer term prognosis and course of recovery.

3.2.2. Hematoma

Hematoma in the retroperitoneal space can produce lumbar plexopathy (22,23). Anticoagulated patients with therapeutic levels are the most susceptible, and hemophiliacs are also at risk. Bleeding may be spontaneous, associated with minor trauma, or follow diagnostic procedures which require vascular access through the femoral vessels. Unilateral pain in the back, lower abdomen, or groin is the initial symptom. Pain may intensify over hours to a day or so. Movement of the hip, active or passive, often worsens the pain. Unilateral weakness of hip flexion, knee extension, and often hip adduction appears in the same time-frame. The patellar reflex is reduced or is absent. Sensory loss and parasthesia occur in the anterior thigh and medial lower leg. Signs of hypovolemia and anemia due to blood loss from the hemorrhage may be present.

Diagnosis is confirmed by CT or MRI studies of the pelvis. Anti-coagulation therapy should be stopped. Transfusion may be required. It is not clear if surgical evacuation of the hematoma improves the neurological outcome. The level of pain can be significant and should be treated with appropriate analgesics. Electrodiagnostic studies performed 3–4 weeks after onset can define prognosis. Evaluation by rehabilitative services is appropriate as soon as stability of the clinical status permits. The neurological deficits tend to improve but may be long lasting in some.

The pathogenesis is compression of the lumbar plexus or femoral nerve secondary to the hematoma formation. A combination of demyelination and axonopathy likely occurs. The hematoma forms in the retroperitoneal space either within the psoas muscle, or beneath the illiacus fascia in the groove between the psoas and illiacus muscles in the pelvis. The proximal lesion tends to produce deficits in both femoral and obturator nerve territories, whereas the more distal one involves only the femoral territory.

3.2.3. Inflammatory Causes

Lumbo-sacral plexopathies can arise secondary to a presumed inflammatory attack on the plexus, as in the brachial plexus (24–26). The clinical features are similar to those described subsequently for diabetes-associated plexopathy. The upper, lower, or both portions of the plexus can be involved.

Patients may have an elevated sedimentation rate, and some will have evidence of a systemic process like Wegener's granulomatosis or polyarteritis nodosa. Biopsy of the sural, superficial peroneal, or lateral femoral cutaneous nerves may aid the diagnosis by showing inflammatory cells in epineural vessels. The electrodiagnostic findings are similar to those of diabetes-associated plexitis described in the following section.

Weakness improves spontaneously over months. There is some support for treatment with immune-modulating drugs. As with inflammatory brachial plexitis there may be a several week delay between onset and the confirmation of the diagnosis, making it difficult to judge the efficacy of therapy. The choice of agents is dictated by whether a systemic condition is present, and corticosteroids plus cyclophosphamide may be required. If the inflammatory process appears to be limited to the plexus alone, single agent treatment with a corticosteroid or intravenous gamma globulin may be adequate.

3.2.4. Diabetes-Associated Plexopathy

Diabetic plexopathy is the most common lumbosacral plexopathy. Symptoms usually begin with spontaneous pain in the back, hip, or proximal leg (27–29). The pain is perceived "deep in the muscles or bone," and tends to be unilateral initially. It intensifies over days to weeks, and often reaches a very high level that is incompletely responsive to major oral analgesics. The intensity decreases after 2–6 weeks, and can linger at a lower level for several months.

Within a few weeks after onset of the pain, weakness and sensory loss develop in the affected limb. Weakness is most commonly in the territory of the lumbar plexus, and produces deficits of hip flexion, adduction, and knee extension. Weakness can also occur more caudally and produce a sciatic distribution deficit. Occasionally, both lumbar and sacral territories are involved concurrently. Weakness evolves for several months, often to a severe degree, and significant muscle atrophy occurs. Patients may become wheelchair bound due to the severe proximal weakness. Muscle stretch reflexes are reduced or lost in the involved territories. Sensory deficits occur most often in the anterior thigh and medial lower leg. Loss of sensation tends to be more prominent than paresthesia.

Some patients develop a similar syndrome on the opposite side several months later. Thoracic radiculopathies, characterized by band-like truncal pain and sensory loss, may also develop in the same time frame as the leg symptoms. Symptoms and signs of polyneuropathy are often absent or present to only a minimal degree.

Patients may experience significant anorexia and weight loss during the period of maximum pain. It is not clear whether this is an indirect effect of the severe pain or due to a concomitant enteropathy. It is possible that poor blood glucose control prior to onset of the plexopathy explains the associated weight loss. The onset of the plexopathy may occur shortly after the diagnosis of diabetes, or later when enhanced efforts at blood sugar control have been instituted. Overall, patients who experience this type of plexopathy do not have worse blood glucose control (29).

The type of plexopathy is common and readily recognized. Laboratory studies should be directed towards establishing the status of glucose control, and identifying systemic inflammatory conditions. When studied, spinal fluid protein level is usually mildly elevated. Electrodiagnostic studies demonstrate active denervation in clinically involved muscles. Contralateral muscles should also be evaluated, as subclinical involvement may be present. Interestingly, the lumbar paraspinals also often show active denervation at multiple levels, supporting a combined radicular and plexus process rather than a plexopathy alone. Nerve conduction studies usually show axonal type abnormalities in the involved nerves.

The condition tends to improve spontaneously over months to $\sim$2 years, but significant motor deficits may persist. Traditionally, management has been limited to pain control and rehabilitation. Treatment with immuno-modulators like corticosteroids or intravenous gamma globulin though may lessen the evolution of the deficits and shorten the course. Both oral and intravenous steroid treatment has been used.

The pathogenesis of this lesion is not completely established. Type II diabetics are much more commonly afflicted than Type I patients. Metabolic, ischemic, and inflammatory etiologies have been postulated. A multifocal vasculitis affecting small caliber vessels in the nerve roots and plexus is the current hypothesis, but the relationship of glucose and immune-mediated process is not currently understood.

3.2.5. Neoplastic Causes

The lumbo-sacral plexus can be infiltrated by neoplasms that arise locally from the colon, cervix, or bladder (30,31). Retroperitoneal lymphomas and sarcomas can also invade the plexus. Less common are metastatic lesions from breast cancers or melanomas. The cancer is usually known, and rarely the initial manifestation.

Pain is usually the initial symptom, and is located in the back, hip, or proximal leg. The intensity increases over days to a few weeks. Weakness and sensory loss usually develop several weeks later. The distribution of these signs corresponds with the portion of the plexus involved, lumbar, sacral, or diffuse. The lumbar portion is more often involved when the neoplasm directly infiltrates the plexus, whereas metastatic lesions tend to involve the sacral portion. Bilateral involvement occurs in $\sim$25% of cases. Leg edema may be present and is due to venous or lymphatic compromise.

The diagnosis is confirmed by CT or MRI imaging of the pelvis. MRI has a higher yield than CT. Biopsy may be required to determine the specific tissue type if the primary is not known. Electrodiagnostic testing will show a pattern of acute or subacute axonopathy in the involved territories.

Management is dictated by the biology of the neoplasm, and its responsiveness to chemotherapy and radiation. Input from rehabilitation services may help ease the physical burdens imposed by the lesions.

3.2.6. Postradiation Causes

Prior therapeutic radiation can cause lumbo-sacral plexopathy (30). The characteristics are similar to those described for postradiation brachial plexopathy. Weakness and sensory disturbance are the initial manifestations. Pain is also present but tends to be less prominent than with neoplastic infiltration of the plexus. Bilateral involvement is common. The mean time delay between radiation treatment and onset of the plexopathy is 5 years, but the range is 1–30 years. The most common tumors treated with radiation are lymphomas, gynecological, and testicular.

The differential diagnosis is recurrence of the original neoplasm, and an unrelated lesion such as a lumbar radiculopathy from disc disease, should be considered. Imaging and electrodiagnostic studies are helpful in making the diagnosis. Absence of a mass lesion in the plexus favors a post-radiation case. Myokymic discharges on EMG testing of clinically involved muscles strongly supports radiation plexopathy, but their absence is not exclusionary.

There is no direct treatment for the radiation related plexopathies. Management is only symptomatic.

REFERENCES

1. van Es HW. MRI of the brachial plexus. Eur Radiol 2001; 11:325–336.
2. Wilbourn AJ. Brachial plexus disorders. In: Dyck PJ, ed. Peripheral Neuropathy. Philadelphia: WB Saunders, 1993:911–950.
3. Wilbourn AJ. Brachial plexopthies. In: Brown WF, Bolton CF, Aminoff MJ, eds. Neuromuscular Function and Disease. Philadelphia: WB Saunders, 2002:831–851.
4. Bisinella GL, Birch R. Obstetric brachial plexus lesions. J Hand Surg (Br) 2003; 28(B):40–45.
5. Marcus JR, Clarke HM. Management of obstetrical brachial plexus palsy. Clin Plast Surg 2003; 30:289–306.
6. Weinberg J, Rokito S, Silber J. Etiology, treatment, and prevention of athletic "stingers." Clin Sports Med 2003; 21:493–500.
7. Parsonage J, Turner JWA. Neuralgia amyotrophy the shoulder-girdle syndrome. Lancet 1948; 1:973–978.
8. Tsairis P, Dyck PJ, Mulder D. Natural history of brachial plexus neuropathy. Arch Neurol 1972; 27:109–117.
9. Windebank AJ. Inherited recurrent focal neuropathies. In: Dyck PJ, ed. Peripheral Neuropathy. Philadelphia: WB Saunders, 1993:1137–1143.
10. Watts GDJ, O'Briant MS, Borreson TE, Windebank AJ, Chance PJ. Evidence for genetic herterogeneity in hereditary neuralgic amyotrophy. Neurology 2001; 56:675–678.
11. Klein CJ, Dyck PJB, Friedenberg SM, Burns TM, Windebank AJ, Dyck PJ. Inflammation and neuropathic attacks in hereditary brachial plexus neuropathy. J Neurol Neurosurg Psychiatry 2002; 73:45–50.
12. Ardolino G, Barbieri S, Prioir A. High dose intravenous immune globulin in the treatment of hereditary recurrent brachial plexus neuropathy. J Neurol Neurosurg Psychiatry 2003; 74:550–551.
13. Kori SH, Foley KM, Posner JB. Brachial plexus lesions in patients with cancer: 100 cases. Neurology 1981; 31:45–50.

14. Thomas JE, Colby MY. Radiation-induced or metastatic brachial plexopathy. J Am Med Assoc 1972; 11:1392–1395.

15. Harper CM, Thomas JE, Cascino TL, Litchy WJ. Distinction between neoplastic and radiation-induced brachial plexopathy, with emphasis on the role of EMG. Neurology 1989; 39:502–506.

16. Gilliatt RW, LeQuense PM, Logue V, Sumer AJ. Wasting of the hand associated with a cervical rib or band. J Neurol Neurosurg Psychiatry 1970; 33:615–624.

17. Donaghy M. Lumbosacral plexus disorders. In: Dyck PJ, ed. Peripheral Neuropathy. Philadelphia: WB Saunders, 1993:951–959.

18. Weber M. Lumbosacral plexopathies. In: Brown WF, Bolton CF, Aminoff MJ, eds. Neuromuscular Function and Disease. Philadelphia: WB Saunders, 2002:852–864.

19. Weis EB. Subtle neurological injuries in pelvic fractures. J Trauma 1984; 24:983–985.

20. Kutsy RL, Robinson LR, Routt ML. Lumbosacral plexopathy in pelvic trauma. Muscle Nerve 2000; 23:1757–1760.

21. Chou-Tan FY, Efenbaum M, Chan K-T, Song J. Lumbosacral plexopathy in gunshot wounds and motor vehicle accidents. Am J Phys Med Rehabil 2001; 80:280–285.

22. Chiu WS. The syndrome of retroperitoneal hemorrhage and lumbar plexus neuropathy during anticoagulant therapy. South Med J 1976; 69:595–599.

23. Emery S, Ochoa J. Lumbar plexus neuropathy resulting from retroperitoneal hemorrhage. Muscle Nerve 1978; 1:330–334.

24. Evans BA, Stevens JC, Dyck PJ. Lumbosacral plexus neuropathy. Neurology 1981; 31:1327–1330.

25. Bradley WG, Chad D, Verghese JP, Liu HC, Good P, Gabbai AA, Adelman LS. Painful lumbosacral plexopathy with elevated sedimentation rate: a treatable inflammatory syndrome. Ann Neurol 1984; 15:457–464.

26. Triggs WJ, Young MS, Eskin T, Valenstein E. Treatment of idiopathic lumbosacral neuropathy with intravenous immunoglobulin. Muscle Nerve 1997; 20:244–246.

27. Barohn RJ, Sahenk Z, Warmolts JR, Mendell JR. The Bruns–Garland syndrome (Diabetic Amytorophy) revisited 100 years later. Arch Neurol 1991; 48:1130–1135.

28. Krendel DA, Costigan DA, Hopkins LC. Successful treatment of neuropathies in patients with diabetes mellitus. Arch Neurol 1995; 2:1053–1061.

29. Dyck PJB, Windebank AJ. Diabetic and nondiabetic lumbosacral radiculoplexus neuropathies: new insights into pathophysiology and treatment. Muscle Nerve 2002; 25:477–491.

30. Thomas JE, Cascino TL, Earle JD. Differential diagnosis between radiation and tumor plexopathy of the pelvis. Neurology 1985; 35:1–7.

31. Jaeckle KA, Young DF, Foley KM. The natural history of lumbosacral plexopathy in cancer. Neurology 1985; 35:8–15.

26
Median Mononeuropathies

A. Gordon Smith
University of Utah, Salt Lake City, Utah, USA

ABSTRACT

The median nerve is the most frequently injured nerve. Median mononeuropathy at the wrist (carpal tunnel syndrome) is one of the most common referral questions for electro-diagnostic testing, and is a major cause of work-related disability. The median nerve may also be injured in the forearm, in the region of the pronator teres muscle, but the pronator syndrome is controversial. The anterior interosseous nerve may also be injured in the forearm. More proximal lesions of the median nerve in the arm and axilla are less common. This chapter reviews the anatomy of the median nerve and discusses the most common clinical syndromes. The role of electrodiagnostic testing and appropriate treatment are emphasized.

1. ANATOMY

The median nerve is formed by the C6-T1 nerve roots. The lateral and medial cords of the brachial plexus contribute to the median nerve in the lateral axilla. The nerve travels down the medial arm adjacent to the brachial artery and after crossing into the forearm dives between the heads of the pronator teres muscle. After innervating the pronator teres, flexor carpi radialis, and flexor digitorum superficialis muscles, the nerve passes through a fibrous arch in the flexor digitorum profundus (the "sublimus bridge"). The anterior interosseous nerve branches off in this region and innervates the flexor policus longus, flexor digitorum profudus (digits 2–3), and pronator quadratus muscles as well as providing sensory supply to the wrist joint. The anterior interosseous nerve may become entrapped as it passes under the sublimus bridge. The next branch, the palmar cutaneous branch, arises in the distal forearm and supplies sensation to the thenar region. This is the final branch before the median nerve traverses the carpal tunnel. The carpal bones form the floor of the carpal tunnel and the transverse carpal ligament forms the roof. The tendons of the flexor digitorum profundus, flexor digitorum superificialis, and the flexor pollicis longus muscles travel through the tunnel with the median nerve. Immediately after entering the palm, the nerve branches into the terminal motor branch that supplies the abductor pollicis brevis, opponens pollicis, and a portion of the flexor pollicis brevis. The remaining sensory fibers branch into two common palmar digital nerves, which then divide into the digital nerves supplying the first three and a half digits of the hand. Figure 26.1 summarizes median nerve anatomy schematically including common sites of injury and entrapment.

There are several normal anatomic variants of the median nerve. Appreciation of these anomalies is important in the interpretation of electrodiagnostic studies. The most common variants are the Martin–Gruber anastamoses, which involve the crossing-over

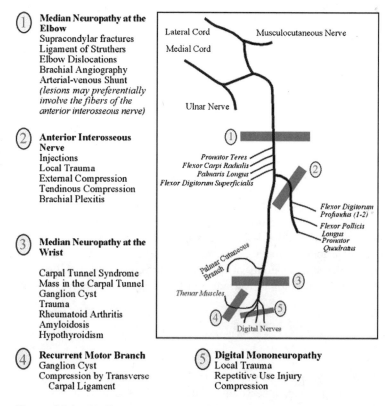

① **Median Neuropathy at the Elbow**
Supracondylar fractures
Ligament of Struthers
Elbow Dislocations
Brachial Angiography
Arterial-venous Shunt
(lesions may preferentially involve the fibers of the anterior interosseous nerve)

② **Anterior Interosseous Nerve**
Injections
Local Trauma
External Compression
Tendinous Compression
Brachial Plexitis

③ **Median Neuropathy at the Wrist**

Carpal Tunnel Syndrome
Mass in the Carpal Tunnel
Ganglion Cyst
Trauma
Rheumatoid Arthritis
Amyloidosis
Hypothyroidism

④ **Recurrent Motor Branch**
Ganglion Cyst
Compression by Transverse
  Carpal Ligament

⑤ **Digital Mononeuropathy**
Local Trauma
Repetitive Use Injury
Compression

Figure 26.1 Median nerve anatomy. This schematic representation of the median nerve demonstrates major nerve branches, the muscles they innervate, and common sites of injury. Important causes for median mononeuropathy are listed by anatomic site.

of fibers from the median to the ulnar nerve. Martin–Gruber anastamoses have an estimated prevalence of ~30% based on careful electrophysiologic evaluation (1), but are observed much less frequently during routine electrodiagonstic testing. There are several subtypes, all of which include a branch from the median nerve in the forearm in the region of the anterior interosseous nerve that joins the ulnar nerve in the forearm. The crossed fibers usually cross back to the median nerve after the wrist and supply thenar muscles. They may also supply hypothenar muscles. Patients with Martin–Gruber anastamoses supplying hyopthenar muscles may develop unexpected hand intrinsic weakness with lesions of the anterior interosseous nerve (2). Martin–Gruber anastamoses may create some confusion in the electrodiagnostic evaluation of carpal tunnel syndrome (CTS). When the crossed fibers innervate thenar muscles via the ulnar nerve, they are not slowed at the wrist. This results in inappropriately fast median motor conduction velocity in the forearm. Because the muscles innervated by the crossed fibers are usually not directly under the recording electrode, a small positive deflection may be seen when the median nerve is stimulated at the elbow. Observation of either pattern should prompt a careful evaluation for CTS. Crossovers in the palm innervating intrinsic hand muscles (Riche–Cannieu anastamoses) are less common.

2. CARPAL TUNNEL SYNDROME

Median nerve entrapment at the wrist, CTS, is the most common entrapment neuropathy and ~2–3% of the population suffers from CTS (3). Variability in prevalence data is likely due to variations in occupational and industrial work exposure. A majority of patients attribute their CTS to work exposure and CTS is a significant cause of work-related morbidity; 90% have a good treatment outcome and are able to return from work, but 10% are permanently disabled (4).

2.1. Clinical Features

CTS typically presents with paresthesias, numbness, and pain involving the wrist hand and fingers. Symptoms often awaken the patient and are worse in the morning. They are exacerbated by provocative activities involving repetitive flexion and/or extension of the wrist. Shaking of the hands often relieves the numbness and paresthesias (5). Driving, typing, writing, or using hand tools may worsen symptoms. Individuals working in industries that involve repetitive forceful wrist flexion and extension are at increased risk (6,7).

Most patients appreciate more significant symptoms in the first three digits. However, over half describe paresthesias involving the fifth digit and 40% have pain or paresthesias in the forearm or above, with a significant minority (7%) experiencing shoulder pain (Fig. 26.2) (8). Numbness may be limited to only one digit. Therefore, differentiation of CTS from other causes of limb pain can be problematic and careful physical and electrodiagnostic evaluation are of significant help.

Many patients also experience subjective hand weakness. This is typically described as a tendency to drop objects or a sense of incoordination with fine motor tasks. The weakness is often due to pain inhibition or sensory loss that impairs fine motor control.

The physical examination may be normal, particularly in mild CTS. Many patients have reduced sensation to pinprick in a median nerve sensory distribution. The finding of reduced pin on the lateral side of the fourth digit compared with the medial side is helpful, although not observed in all patients because the median nerve sometimes innervated both sides of the fourth finger. Typically, the skin over the thenar eminence has normal

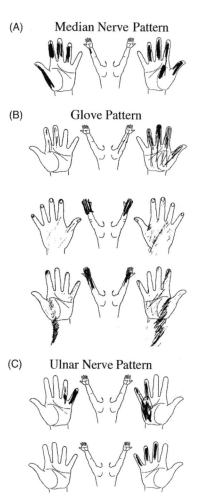

Figure 26.2   Distribution of sensory symptoms in CTS. This figure, modified from Stevens et al. (8), illustrates patterns of sensory complaints in patients with CTS. A patient completed each drawing. (A) Sensory symptoms may be limited to the median nerve distribution, or (B) may occur in a glove pattern or (C) ulnar nerve distribution. [Reproduced from Stevens et al. (8) with permission.]

sensation because the palmar cutaneous branch of the median nerve, which arises proximal to the carpal tunnel, provides sensory innervation to this region. Care must be taken not to over-interpret the sensory examination, as there is significant normal variation in sensory distributions. Furthermore, the sensory examination is inherently subjective, and patients may describe reduced sensation in unexpected areas (8). The finding of subjective sensory change in regions not supplied by the median nerve should not exclude the diagnosis or discourage further diagnostic evaluation in a patient with suggestive symptoms. Patients with more severe disease have weakness of thumb abduction and opposition and those with advanced disease have thenar atrophy. Elderly patients may present with thenar atrophy and weakness without significant sensory complaints or pain.

A variety of provocative physical examination maneuvers have been described. The most commonly sought is the Tinel's sign. Tinel first described paresthesias with nerve percussion in patients recovering from nerve injury (9). The "flick sign" refers to a history of shaking the hands after awakening with numbness or pain. Paresthesias provoked by arm extension and wrist flexion is termed the Phalen's sign. Other signs focus on reproduction of symptoms with compression over the carpal tunnel. The diagnostic accuracy of these various maneuvers is poor and their positive and negative predictive values are low (10). In one study of 142 patients referred for possible CTS, the negative predictive values were all <40% (11). Because many normal individuals have these signs, and many CTS patients do not, their clinical value is limited.

2.2. Diagnostic Evaluation

The diagnosis of CTS is complicated by neurologic co-morbidity. Patients with an underlying peripheral neuropathy are challenging because they often describe hand numbness that is worse at night, but they also have an increased risk of developing CTS. Patients with superimposed cervical spine disease or ulnar mononeuropathy also pose a clinical challenge because they have numbness, pain, and weakness that extends out of the median nerve distribution. Given the variability in clinical findings and complaints among patients with suspected CTS, supportive diagnostic studies play a very important role in the evaluation. Electrodiagnostic evaluation with nerve conduction studies (NCS) and electromyography (EMG) is the most commonly used study. A large variety of specific electrodiagnostic techniques have been described. This review focuses on the general principles and the most commonly employed techniques.

The earliest electrophysiological changes in CTS are due to demyelination of large sensory nerve fibers. Median sensory conduction velocity across the carpal tunnel is slowed, and thus the median sensory distal latency becomes prolonged. Diagnostic criteria are based on the difference between the median and ulnar sensory distal latency or conduction velocity (Fig. 26.3). The median sensory response may be recorded antidromically by stimulating proximal to the wrist and recording the sensory nerve action potential at the digit, or orthodromically by stimulating at the digit or in the palm, and recording above the wrist (Fig. 26.4). Use of a short segment orthodromic technique, stimulating at the palm and recording at the wrist, maximizes diagnostic sensitivity because the area of nerve conduction slowing across the carpal tunnel region represents a larger fraction of the total length of the nerve examined compared with studies investigating longer segments (12,13). Focal slowing can be detected by stimulating the nerve in 1 cm increments starting proximal to the wrist and extending into the palm ("inching"). Sensory nerve action potential amplitude may be reduced due to sensory conduction block at the wrist (which can be detected by inching). With more severe lesions, there is injury to the axons themselves. This is recognized as diminished sensory amplitudes, even when stimulating distally.

Motor NCS are usually normal in mild CTS. In more moderate disease, there is prolongation of the motor distal latency due to demyelination of motor nerve fibers. With severe CTS, there is a decline in the compound muscle action potential amplitude due to axonal injury. Because of the effects of reinnervation, the motor amplitude remains normal for some time despite ongoing axonal injury. For this reason, needle EMG is useful to demonstrate the presence of axonal loss.

A variety of specific NCS diagnostic criteria for CTS have been proposed. In general, NCS are reproducible and have a high sensitivity (>85%) and specificity (>95%) (14). A review of the literature demonstrated that the most sensitive and specific parameter was median sensory or mixed nerve conduction study from the palm to the wrist over a short distance (7–8 cm). The American Association of Neuromuscular Electrodiagnostic Medicine CTS Practice Parameter recommends starting the evaluation with a median sensory NCS across the wrist using a distance of 14 cm. If this is normal, the more sensitive palm to wrist study should be performed (14). It has been suggested that a combination of multiple median nerve studies maximizes diagnostic accuracy (15). However, if any individual parameter is significant abnormal (orthodromic palmar median versus ulnar

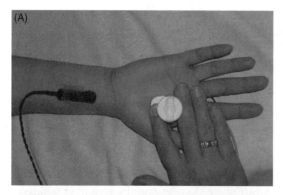

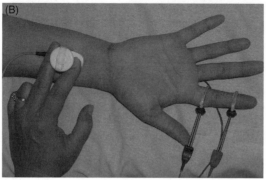

Figure 26.3 Median sensory nerve conduction technique. (A) An orthodromic sensory nerve con-duction study over a short segment (8 cm) is the most sensitive technique for detection of slowing across the wrist. The nerve is stimulated in the palm and the response recorded immediately proximal to the wrist. (B) A standard antidromic sensory study over a longer segment (14 cm) is often used as a screening study.

difference of >0.3 ms or antidromic ring difference of >0.4), further sensory studies are not necessary (16).

Electrodiagnostic studies serve several purposes in the diagnostic evaluation of sus-pected CTS. The first is to confirm the diagnosis of CTS. They are also used to exclude

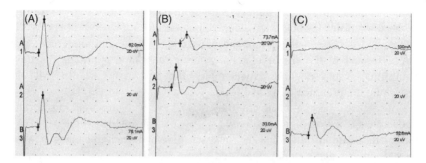

Figure 26.4 Sensory nerve conduction in CTS. Median (top) and ulnar (bottom) sensory nerve action potentials from (A) a normal subject, (B) a patient with moderate CTS with reduced median sensory amplitude (17 μV compared with 37 μV for the ulnar response) and prolonged distal latency (peak latency of 4.8 ms compared with 3.1 ms for the ulnar response), and (C) a patient with more severe CTS and an absent median sensory response.

other disorders (neuropathy, radiculopathy, other mononeuropathies). It is very important that the results of the electrodiagnostic study be interpreted in clinical context. The finding of slowed median nerve conduction across the wrist on NCS does not necessarily imply that CTS is the cause for the patient's symptoms. The electrodiagnostic consultant should try to place the findings in context and make a judgement concerning their clinical relevance. Electrodiagnostic studies can be used for prognostic purposes and to direct therapy. Mild CTS with pure sensory demyelination is likely to be more responsive to conservative therapy than more severe disease. Conversely, those with reduced motor amplitude and axonal loss on EMG have a poorer prognosis and should be treated aggressively. The electrodiagnostic evaluation for suspected CTS should therefore include motor conduction studies and needle examination of multiple limb muscles in order to exclude a superimposed radiculopathy or ulnar or radial mononeuropathy (14).

Although NCS are very useful, up to 25% of patients with clinically suspected CTS may have a normal study (17). Some authors, particularly in the surgical literature, have suggested NCS are not very useful because of this observation (18). A prospective study of sequential patients referred for CTS addressed this question. When the clinical history and examination were strongly suggestive of CTS, the NCS results were typically abnormal (92%). However, when the clinical data was less definitive, but CTS was still suspected (e.g., mild CTS), NCS results could not be predicted based on clinical data (positive predictive value of 67%). NCS were therefore often necessary to confirm the diagnosis of CTS (17). There is also evidence that patients with clinically suspected CTS but normal NCS are less likely to experience resolution of symptoms following surgical release (51%) when compared with those with abnormal NCS (65–77%). Patients with moderate CTS are most likely to respond and those with severe CTS are least likely to respond (19). This suggests many patients with suspected CTS but normal NCS probably do not have CTS. Although patients with normal NCS may still have true CTS, surgical intervention should only be considered in those who have failed conservative therapy and have a classic syndrome. A repeat NCS may be useful in patients whose initial NCS was normal.

Other procedures have been assessed for the diagnosis of suspected CTS. A variety of quantitative sensory testing devices have been studied and have been found to have a low diagnostic accuracy (20–22). Quantitative sensory testing is a psychophysiological test and results are significantly influenced by patient bias. For example, normal subjects without any training, can simulate neuropathic sensory loss (23).

Radiologic evaluation for CTS has shown greater promise. MRI of the carpal tunnel may be used to evaluate structural or anatomic abnormalities, although it is not necessary for the routine evaluation of idiopathic CTS (24). Patients with a mass in the wrist, trauma, or persistent symptoms following surgical evaluation may benefit from MRI. There are also data suggesting that ultrasound may be a useful diagnostic technique. Ultrasound typically demonstrates nerve swelling proximal to the site of compression with flattening distally (25). Careful measurement of nerve area may have a sensitivity of up to 67% with a specificity of 97% (26).

2.3. Prognosis and Management

Treatment of CTS should start by identification and modification of activities that provoke or exacerbate symptoms. Treatment of underlying diseases associated with CTS (rheumatoid arthritis, hypothyroidism) may result in improvement. Up to 10% or more of pregnant individuals develop CTS, presumably due to hand swelling or hypertension. Conservative therapy is generally warranted given most patients have complete resolution of symptoms within weeks of delivery (27,28). Most patients with idiopathic CTS of mild to moderate severity also respond to conservative therapy. However, patients with more severe symptoms, and particularly those with thenar atrophy, weakness, or denervation on electrodiagnostic testing should be referred for definitive surgical therapy.

The most commonly employed conservative therapy for CTS is wrist splinting. Up to 80% of patients with CTS have resolution of their symptoms within days to weeks of using splints at nighttime (29). A variety of off-the-shelf and custom wrist splints are available. Splinting in the neutral position reduces nocturnal intra-carpal tunnel pressures more than splinting in relative extension (30). Any wrist splint that is comfortable and in the neutral position is acceptable.

A course of nonsteroidal anti-inflammatory medication is often prescribed in combination with wrist splinting. However, this treatment has not been well studied. There has been only one randomized study comparing placebo, nonsteroidal anti-inflammatory medication, diuretic, and oral prednisolone. Only the prednisolone group, which took 20 mg daily for 2 weeks and 10 mg daily for 2 weeks noted a significant benefit. Patients were only followed for 4 weeks, so the long term outcome is unknown (31). Vitamin B6 (pyridoxine) has been suggested in the past but small studies suggest a lack of efficacy (32). Use of pyridoxine is discouraged, as high doses may result in a sensory neuropathy that can be very severe (33). Small studies of diuretics alone also failed to show evidence for efficacy (32).

For patients who fail neutral wrist splinting, local steroid injection into the carpal tunnel is a therapeutic option. It has been suggested that this approach is limited by a relatively low rate of long term success (34). However, several studies suggest a significant fraction of patients with mild to moderate disease have sustained benefit (35,36). One prospective study demonstrated that 10% of patients remained symptom free at 1 year (37). In another study patients, one-third had normal NCS at 1 year (38). There is a very small risk of injuring the median nerve during the injection. Local steroid injection is an appropriate therapy for patients with mild to moderate disease who wish to avoid carpal tunnel release. For those who have recurrent symptoms, up to 3 injections yearly may be safely performed (39). Because it is less invasive than surgery, steroid injection may also be more appropriate for patients with an uncertain diagnosis and can serve as a diagnostic procedure, for those who respond are more likely to respond to carpal tunnel release than those who do not respond (40). Iontophoresis of dexamethasone may be an effective and safe therapy. It involves applying a small electrical current to an electrode containing a medication, which propels it through the skin. In a prospective study of 19 patients who had failed splinting and anti-inflammatory medication, 58% had benefit at 6 months, a rate superior to that in most studies of local injection (41). Because repeat iontophoresis treatments are well tolerated and inexpensive, this therapy holds significant promise and deserves more careful study.

Patients who have failed conservative management, have severe disease with axonal injury, or wish immediate definitive therapy should be referred for carpal tunnel release. Surgical release is highly successful, with 90% of patients experiencing a successful outcome (42). A variety of techniques have been described, including endoscopic approaches and "mini" open release. Each technique works well. Proponents of endoscopic release argue that it results in an earlier return to work. However, there may also be a higher risk of injury to the median nerve (39). A recent meta-analysis of the literature suggests the various techniques may be essentially equivalent, both for long-term side effects and efficacy (43). The most prudent approach is to refer the patient to a surgeon with significant expertise in carpal tunnel release.

2.4. Pathophysiology

There are two general mechanisms underlying CTS: a reduced canal size and a predisposition to nerve compression. Any lesion within the carpal tunnel may compress the median nerve. Medical causes include rheumatoid arthritis and sarcoidosis. Structural causes include ganglion cysts, tumors, and vascular malformations. Wrist fractures or hematomas may result in acute CTS. A variety of medical conditions may predispose the median nerve to compression, including peripheral neuropathy, particularly that associated with diabetes (Table 26.1). As many as one in three patients with CTS have a predisposing condition (44).

It has been suggested that proximal nerve compression predisposes to a more distal injury along the nerve's course (the "double crush" hypothesis) (45). Although there has been significant debate about the double crush hypothesis, there is no convincing animal or clinical data to support it (46,47). An EMG examination to exclude a radiculopathy as a confounding clinical feature is suggested, but routine neuroimaging of the cervical spine is not recommended.

The etiology of idiopathic CTS is unknown. There has been significant debate as to whether patients with CTS have a congenitally smaller canal than those who do not. Although there are some data to support this concept (48), most evidence suggests congenital canal narrowing is not a predisposing factor (49,50). Occupational exposure is important, and repetitive forceful extension and flexion of the wrist places individuals at increased risk.

3. MEDIAN MONONEUROPATHIES IN THE REGION OF THE ELBOW

The second most common site for median nerve injury is in the proximal forearm and near the elbow. Supracondylar humeral fractures may injure the median nerve proximal to the elbow. Often, only the fascicles supplying the anterior interosseous nerve are involved (51). A significant minority of individuals have a bony spur above the medial humeral condyle (surpacondylar spur). There may be a ligament that runs from the spur to the humerus (ligament of Struthers) that can compress the median nerve (Fig. 26.5). In this instance, surgical removal of the ligament and spur may be necessary. Caution should be exercised when considering the diagnosis of median mononeuropathy due to

Table 26.1 Medical Conditions Associated with Carpal Tunnel Syndrome

Diabetes mellitus
Peripheral neuropathy
Hypothyroidism
Amyloidosis
Sarcoidosis
Gout
Rheumatoid arthritis
Pregnancy
Tumor
Fractures
Occupational exposures

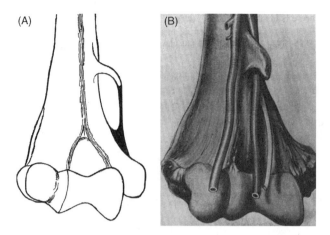

Figure 26.5   Supracondylar spur and ligament of Struthers. A reproduction of Struthers' original sketch demonstrates the bony and ligamentous anatomy (A). The brachial artery and median nerve may travel between the humerus and ligament (B). [With permission from Stewart (63).]

compression by a ligament of Struthers, for the rarity of the clinical syndrome is well exceeded by the frequency of the anatomic variant (2%).

Procedures in the antecubital fossa can injure the median nerve. Cardiac catheterization via the brachial artery may cause a severe median neuropathy (52). Poorly performed venipuncture may also injure the median nerve in this region. Often, only the fibers supplying the anterior interosseous nerve are involved. A variety of neuropathic complications of anterior-venous dialysis shunts have been described. Sometimes the median nerve may be affected in isolation, although other nerves are often involved. Injury may occur by direct compression or ischemia (53–55).

3.1.   Pronator Teres Syndrome

The "pronator teres syndrome" is a confusing clinical entity. Most reports of this entity emphasize aching pain in the flexor forearm that becomes worse with repeated pronation or following several specific provocative maneuvers (56). Proponents of the syndrome suggest that the pain is due to compression of the median nerve as it passes through the two heads of the pronator teres muscle. Reports of true neurogenic pronator teres syndrome are rare however. In one series, 39 patients underwent a thorough electrodiagnostic evaluation, and mild median nerve injury was found in only two individuals. Despite this, surgical decompression resulted in good improvement in 28, fair improvement in five, and no change in three patients (57). The explanation for the clinical improvement following decompression despite a lack of evidence for median nerve injury is uncertain. It has been suggested that pronator teres syndrome is really a forearm compartment syndrome rather than a nerve compression syndrome, and that release of the median nerve in the region is effective because the procedure includes a fasciotomy (58). Patients with suspected pronator teres syndrome should undergo a careful electrodiagnostic study. If there is evidence of median nerve injury, MRI neurography of the region may be useful and surgical decompression is a reasonable therapeutic option if there is significant axonal injury. In the absence of median nerve injury, conservative therapy should be pursued, and surgical intervention reserved for patients with severe symptoms refractory to this approach. Any surgical approach should include a fasciotomy.

3.2. Anterior Interosseous Neuropathy

Anterior interosseous mononeuropathies are the second most common median mono-neuropathy following CTS. As already noted, lesions in the elbow or distal arm may cause preferential injury to the fibers supplying the anterior interosseous nerve. Direct trauma to the nerve may also occur, as described earlier. External compression by a cast has also been described (59). The most common cause of anterior interosseous neuropathy is idiopathic. Patients may experience forearm pain due to involvement of sensory nerves supplying the wrist joint. However, the primary complaint is weakness of flexion of the first two fingers and the thumb affecting pinching. When patients attempt to make an O with their thumb and first finger, they are unable to do so. The distal thumb and first finger collapse against one another, forming a tear drop shape (the "pinch sign") (Fig. 26.6). Weakness of the third muscle supplied by the nerve, the pronator quadratus, does not cause clinical findings. In patients who have a Martin–Gruber anastamosis, intrinsic hand muscles may be weak because fibers innervating ulnar hand muscles travel with the crossed fibers in the anterior interosseous nerve (2). The cause for spontaneous anterior interosseous neuropathy is often difficult to define. The nerve may become compressed as it passes through the tendons of the pronator teres and flexor digitorum superficialis. Idiopathic brachial plexus neuropathy ("Parsonage–Turner Syndrome" or "brachial plexitis") may cause preferential injury to the anterior interosseous nerve (60). Clues to this diagnosis include patchy involvement of other muscles in the arm and the presence of shoulder pain. Most patients experience spontaneous improvement over several months. If there is no improvement, MRI of the region may be necessary to exclude an anatomic or structural abnormality. It is important to remember that more proximal lesions may cause isolated anterior interosseous injury, so exclusion of a ligament of Struthers and imaging of the entire median nerve course may be necessary.

4. OTHER CAUSES OF MEDIAN MONONEUROPATHY

The median nerve may be injured in the axilla. Generally, however, multiple nerves are involved and isolated median mononeuropathy is rare. Distal median nerve branches may also be injured. The recurrent motor branch of the median nerve arises just distal to the carpal tunnel and supplies thenar muscles. It may be compressed by the transverse

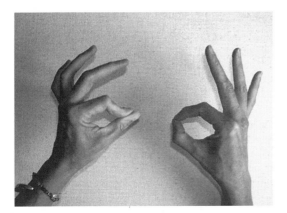

Figure 26.6 The pinch sign. Patients with anterior interosseous neuropathy are unable to form an O with the thumb and first finger due to weakness of deep finger and thumb flexors.

carpal ligament or by ganglion cysts (61). Electrodiagnostic studies demonstrate normal sensory nerve function in the presence of abnormal median motor nerve conduction and thenar EMG examination. Surgical exploration should be considered. The digital nerves in the palm may also be injured by local trauma, compression, or local anatomic abnormalities. For example, musicians may experience digital neuropathies due to overuse compression (62).

REFERENCES

1. Amoiridis G. Median–ulnar nerve communications and anomalous innervation of the intrinsic hand muscles: an electrophysiological study. Muscle Nerve 1992; 15(5):576–579.
2. Spinner M. The anterior interosseous-nerve syndrome, with special attention to its variations. J Bone Joint Surg Am 1970; 52(1):84–94.
3. Atroshi I, Gummesson C, Johnsson R, Ornstein E, Ranstam J, Rosen I. Prevalence of carpal tunnel syndrome in a general population. JAMA 1999; 282(2):153–158.
4. Bekkelund SI, Pierre-Jerome C, Torbergsen T, Ingebrigtsen T. Impact of occupational variables in carpal tunnel syndrome. Acta Neurol Scand 2001; 103(3):193–197.
5. Pryse-Phillips WE. Validation of a diagnostic sign in carpal tunnel syndrome. J Neurol Neurosurg Psychiatry 1984; 47(8):870–872.
6. Hales TR, Bernard BP. Epidemiology of work-related musculoskeletal disorders. Orthop Clin North Am 1996; 27(4):679–709.
7. Roquelaure Y, Mechali S, Dano C et al. Occupational and personal risk factors for carpal tunnel syndrome in industrial workers. Scand J Work Environ Health 1997; 23(5):364–369.
8. Stevens JC, Smith BE, Weaver AL, Bosch EP, Deen HG Jr, Wilkens JA. Symptoms of 100 patients with electromyographically verified carpal tunnel syndrome. Muscle Nerve 1999; 22(10):1448–1456.
9. Stewart JD, Eisen A. Tinel's sign and the carpal tunnel syndrome. Br Med J 1978; 2(6145):1125–1126.
10. Katz JN, Larson MG, Sabra A et al. The carpal tunnel syndrome: diagnostic utility of the history and physical examination findings. Ann Intern Med 1990; 112(5):321–327.
11. Hansen PA, Micklesen P, Robinson LR. Clinical utility of the flick maneuver in diagnosing carpal tunnel syndrome. Am J Phys Med Rehabil 2004; 83(5):363–367.
12. Kimura J. The carpal tunnel syndrome: localization of conduction abnormalities within the distal segment of the median nerve. Brain 1979; 102(3):619–635.
13. Ross MA, Kimura J. AAEM case report #2: the carpal tunnel syndrome. Muscle Nerve 1995; 18(6):567–573.
14. Practice parameter for electrodiagnostic studies in carpal tunnel syndrome: summary statement. Muscle Nerve 2002; 25(6):918–922.
15. Robinson LR, Micklesen PJ, Wang L. Strategies for analyzing nerve conduction data: superiority of a summary index over single tests. Muscle Nerve 1998; 21(9):1166–1171.
16. Kaul MP, Pagel KJ, Dryden JD. When to use the combined sensory index. Muscle Nerve 2001; 24(8):1078–1082.
17. Witt JC, Hentz JG, Stevens JC. Carpal tunnel syndrome with normal nerve conduction studies. Muscle Nerve 2004; 29(4):515–522.
18. Szabo RM, Slater RR Jr, Farver TB, Stanton DB, Sharman WK. The value of diagnostic testing in carpal tunnel syndrome. J Hand Surg [Am] 1999; 24(4):704–714.
19. Bland JD. Do nerve conduction studies predict the outcome of carpal tunnel decompression? Muscle Nerve 2001; 24(7):935–940.
20. Werner RA, Franzblau A, Johnston E. Comparison of multiple frequency vibrometry testing and sensory nerve conduction measures in screening for carpal tunnel syndrome in an industrial setting. Am J Phys Med Rehabil 1995; 74(2):101–106.

21. Werner RA, Franzblau A, Johnston E. Quantitative vibrometry and electrophysiological assessment in screening for carpal tunnel syndrome among industrial workers: a comparison. Arch Phys Med Rehabil 1994; 75(11):1228–1232.

22. Franzblau A, Werner RA, Johnston E, Torrey S. Evaluation of current perception threshold testing as a screening procedure for carpal tunnel syndrome among industrial workers. J Occup Med 1994; 36(9):1015–1021.

23. Freeman R, Chase K, Risk M. Quantitative sensory testing cannot differentiate simulated sensory loss from sensory neuropathy. Neurology 2003; 60:465–470.

24. Cosgrove J. Magnetic resonance imaging in the evaluation of carpal tunnel syndrome: a literature review. J Clin Neuromusc Dis 2000; 1:175–180.

25. Buchberger W, Schon G, Strasser K, Jungwirth W. High-resolution ultrasonography of the carpal tunnel. J Ultrasound Med 1991; 10(10):531–537.

26. Nakamichi K, Tachibana S. Ultrasonographic measurement of median nerve cross-sectional area in idiopathic carpal tunnel syndrome: Diagnostic accuracy. Muscle Nerve 2002; 26(6):798–803.

27. McLennan HG, Oats JN, Walstab JE. Survey of hand symptoms in pregnancy. Med J Aust 1987; 147(11–12):542–544.

28. Wand JS. Carpal tunnel syndrome in pregnancy and lactation. J Hand Surg [Br] 1990; 15(1):93–95.

29. Burke DT, Burke MM, Stewart GW, Cambre A. Splinting for carpal tunnel syndrome: in search of the optimal angle. Arch Phys Med Rehabil 1994; 75(11):1241–1244.

30. Gelberman RH, Hergenroeder PT, Hargens AR, Lundborg GN, Akeson WH. The carpal tunnel syndrome. A study of carpal canal pressures. J Bone Joint Surg Am 1981; 63(3):380–383.

31. Chang MH, Chiang HT, Lee SS, Ger LP, Lo YK. Oral drug of choice in carpal tunnel syndrome. Neurology 1998; 51(2):390–393.

32. O'Connor D, Marshall S, Massy-Westropp N. Non-surgical treatment (other than steroid injection) for carpal tunnel syndrome. Cochrane Database Syst Rev 2003(1):CD003219.

33. Schaumburg H, Kaplan J, Windebank A et al. Sensory neuropathy from pyridoxine abuse a new megavitamin syndrome. N Engl J Med 1983; 309:445–448.

34. Demirci S, Kutluhan S, Koyuncuoglu HR et al. Comparison of open carpal tunnel release and local steroid treatment outcomes in idiopathic carpal tunnel syndrome. Rheumatol Int 2002; 22(1):33–37.

35. Dammers JW, Veering MM, Vermeulen M. Injection with methylprednisolone proximal to the carpal tunnel: randomised double blind trial. BMJ 1999; 319(7214):884–886.

36. Ayhan-Ardic FF, Erdem HR. Long-term clinical and electrophysiological results of local steroid injection in patients with carpal tunnel syndrome. Funct Neurol 2000; 15(3):157–165.

37. Graham RG, Hudson DA, Solomons M, Singer M. A prospective study to assess the outcome of steroid injections and wrist splinting for the treatment of carpal tunnel syndrome. Plast Reconstr Surg 2004; 113(2):550–556.

38. Hagebeuk EE, de Weerd AW. Clinical and electrophysiological follow-up after local steroid injection in the carpal tunnel syndrome. Clin Neurophysiol 2004; 115(6):1464–1468.

39. Katz JN, Simmons BP. Clinical practice. Carpal tunnel syndrome. N Engl J Med 2002; 346(23):1807–1812.

40. Edgell SE, McCabe SJ, Breidenbach WC, LaJoie AS, Abell TD. Predicting the outcome of carpal tunnel release. J Hand Surg [Am] 2003; 28(2):255–261.

41. Banta CA, Bland JD, You H et al. A prospective, nonrandomized study of iontophoresis, wrist splinting, and antiinflammatory medication in the treatment of early-mild carpal tunnel syndrome. J Occup Med 1994; 36(2):166–168.

42. Scholten RJ, Gerritsen AA, Uitdehaag BM, van Geldere D, de Vet HC, Bouter LM. Surgical treatment options for carpal tunnel syndrome. Cochrane Database Syst Rev 2002(4):CD003905.

43. Thoma A, Veltri K, Haines T, Duku E. A systematic review of reviews comparing the effectiveness of endoscopic and open carpal tunnel decompression. Plast Reconstr Surg 2004; 113(4):1184–1191.

44. Atcheson SG, Ward JR, Lowe W. Concurrent medical disease in work-related carpal tunnel syndrome. Arch Intern Med 1998; 158(14):1506–1512.

45. Upton AR, McComas AJ. The double crush in nerve entrapment syndromes. Lancet 1973; 2(7825):359–362.

46. Morgan G, Wilbourn AJ. Cervical radiculopathy and coexisting distal entrapment neuropathies: double-crush syndromes? Neurology 1998; 50(1):78–83.

47. Wilbourn AJ, Gilliatt RW. Double-crush syndrome: a critical analysis. Neurology 1997; 49(1):21–29.

48. Horch RE, Allmann KH, Laubenberger J, Langer M, Stark GB. Median nerve compression can be detected by magnetic resonance imaging of the carpal tunnel. Neurosurgery 1997; 41(1):76–82.

49. Cobb TK, Bond JR, Cooney WP, Metcalf BJ. Assessment of the ratio of carpal contents to carpal tunnel volume in patients with carpal tunnel syndrome: a preliminary report. J Hand Surg [Am] 1997; 22(4):635–639.

50. Pierre-Jerome C, Bekkelund SI, Mellgren SI, Nordstrom R. Quantitative MRI and electrophysiology of preoperative carpal tunnel syndrome in a female population. Ergonomics 1997; 40(6):642–649.

51. Spinner M, Schreiber SN. Anterior interosseous-nerve paralysis as a complication of supracondylar fractures of the humerus in children. J Bone Joint Surg Am 1969; 51(8):1584–1590.

52. Kennedy AM, Grocott M, Schwartz MS, Modarres H, Scott M, Schon F. Median nerve injury: an underrecognised complication of brachial artery cardiac catheterisation? J Neurol Neurosurg Psychiatry 1997; 63(4):542–546.

53. Redfern AB, Zimmerman NB. Neurologic and ischemic complications of upper extremity vascular access for dialysis. J Hand Surg [Am] 1995; 20(2):199–204.

54. Ergungor MF, Kars HZ, Yalin R. Median neuralgia caused by brachial pseudoaneurysm. Neurosurgery 1989; 24(6):924–925.

55. Bolton CF, Driedger AA, Lindsay RM. Ischaemic neuropathy in uraemic patients caused by bovine arteriovenous shunt. J Neurol Neurosurg Psychiatry 1979; 42(9):810–814.

56. Tetro AM, Pichora DR. High median nerve entrapments. An obscure cause of upper-extremity pain. Hand Clin 1996; 12(4):691–703.

57. Hartz CR, Linscheid RL, Gramse RR, Daube JR. The pronator teres syndrome: compressive neuropathy of the median nerve. J Bone Joint Surg Am 1981; 63(6):885–890.

58. Stewart J, Jablecki C. Median nerve. In: Brown W, Bolton C, Aminoff MJ, eds. Neuromuscular Function and Disease Basic Clinical and Electrodiagnostic Aspects. 1st ed. Philadelphia: W.B. Saunders, 2002:873.

59. Gardner-Thorpe C. Anterior interosseous nerve palsy: spontaneous recovery in two patients. J Neurol Neurosurg Psychiatry 1974; 37(10):1146–1150.

60. Rennels GD, Ochoa J. Neuralgic amyotrophy manifesting as anterior interosseous nerve palsy. Muscle Nerve 1980; 3(2):160–164.

61. Bennett JB, Crouch CC. Compression syndrome of the recurrent motor branch of the median nerve. J Hand Surg [Am] 1982; 7(4):407–409.

62. Lederman RJ. Neuromuscular and musculoskeletal problems in instrumental musicians. Muscle Nerve 2003; 27(5):549–561.

63. Stewart JD. Focal Peripheral Neuropathies. 2nd ed. New York: Raven Press, 1993:164.

27
Radial Neuropathy

Michael Stanton
University of Rochester Medical Center, Rochester, New York, USA

ABSTRACT

Radial neuropathies are relatively infrequent, and may result from multiple causes. Depending on the site of lesion, they result in numbness in the arm, forearm, and hand in addition to weakness of extensor movements of the elbow, wrist, and digits. Knowledge of radial nerve anatomy aids in localizing lesion sites, and is aided by electrodiagnostic studies. Treatment depends upon underlying causes.

1. RADIAL NERVE ANATOMY

The radial nerve (1–3) is derived from C5 to C8 and occasionally T1 nerve roots. Fibers from these roots traverse the upper, middle, and lower trunks, and the posterior divisions of the brachial plexus (Fig. 27.1). In the infra-clavicular region, the fibers contribute to the posterior cord, which is named for its anatomic relationship to the axillary artery. The proper radial nerve arises from the posterior cord in the lower part of the axilla. The nerve descends into the arm along the junction of the latassimus dorsi and the long head of the triceps muscles. It then passes medially between the long and medial heads of the triceps muscle. The spiral groove is located at mid-humerus, and it is here that the radial nerve passes from the medial to lateral side of the arm. Below the spiral groove, the nerve pierces the lateral intermuscular septum, crossing the elbow joint anterior to the lateral epicondyle in its path, through the supinator muscle. The path from the lateral inter-muscular septum to the supinator muscle is known as the radial tunnel.

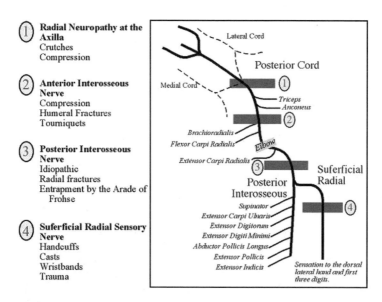

① **Radial Neuropathy at the Axilla**
Crutches
Compression

② **Anterior Interosseous Nerve**
Compression
Humeral Fractures
Tourniquets

③ **Posterior Interosseous Nerve**
Idiopathic
Radial fractures
Entrapment by the Arade of Frohse

④ **Suferficial Radial Sensory Nerve**
Handcuffs
Casts
Wristbands
Trauma

Figure 27.1 Diagram of radial nerve showing major points and branches to individual muscles. Major entrapment sites marked by gray bars, and associated numbers refer to table with differential diagnoses and causes.

The afferent fibers from the posterior cutaneous nerve of the arm join the radial nerve at the junction of the arm and axilla. Afferent fibers from the posterior cutaneous nerve of the forearm join the radial nerve just proximal to the spiral groove. The lower lateral cutaneous nerve of the arm joins the radial nerve at the spiral groove or in common with the posterior cutaneous nerve of the forearm. Afferent fibers from the posterior and lateral cutaneous nerves of the forearm join the radial nerve in the radial tunnel. In the distal portion of the radial tunnel (4,5), the afferent fibers of the superficial radial nerve join the efferent motor fibers of the posterior interosseous nerve. The superficial radial nerve remains anterior to the supinator. It receives cutaneous afferents from the dorsum of the lateral hand, posterolateral thumb, and proximal dorsal surface of digits (6–8).

The triceps is innervated by several branches of the nerve between the axilla and the upper arm, proximal to the spiral groove. Motor branches to the brachialis muscle, the brachioradialis muscle, and the extensor carpi longus muscle arise in the radial tunnel. The extensor carpi brevis has a variable innervation in the radial tunnel from either the radial nerve, posterior interosseous nerve or arising from the superficial radial nerve (9). The supinator muscle receives branches proximal to and within the supinator (9). The posterior interosseous nerve pierces the supinator muscle through a fibrous opening, the Arcade of Frohse (10,11). It then innervates the extensor digitorum communis, extensor carpi ulnaris, extensor digiti minimi, abductor pollicis longus, extensor pollicis longus and brevis, and the extensor indicis muscles.

2. CLINICAL FEATURES

Injury to the radial nerve in the axilla results in weakness in elbow extension, forearm supination, wrist extension, digit extension, and thumb abduction (Fig. 27.1). Sensation is lost in the dorsolateral hand and dorsal forearm, and dorsolateral arm. Injury to the nerve at the spiral groove results in weakness in wrist extension, elbow supination, digit extension, and thumb abduction. Sensation is lost as described earlier. Injury to the posterior interosseous nerve at the Arcade of Frohse results in mild wrist extensor weakness, with radial deviation, digit extension weakness, and thumb abduction weakness. There is no sensory loss. Injury to the superficial radial nerve in the forearm causes loss of sensation in the dorsolateral hand.

3. EVALUATION

Electrophysiologic evaluation is useful in the localization and has the ability to distinguish between weakness predominantly due to conduction block from that due to axonal injury. Evaluation includes sensory and motor nerve conduction studies and needle electromyography.

Motor nerve conduction studies can be carried out recording from the following muscles: extensor digitorum, extensor indicis proprius, middle of the abductor pollicis lungus, and extensor pollicis longus and stimulation can be carried out at the following sites (1,12–14): the elbow between the brachioradialis muscle and biceps tendon, below the spiral groove over the lateral humerus at approximately the distal one-third of the arm, above the spiral groove over the medial humerus at approximately the proximal one-third of the arm, and at Erb's point. Sensory responses are evaluated by distal stimulation of the radial sensory nerve along the lateral radius with recording from the snuff box (1). Assessment of the degree of axonal loss is made by side-to-side comparisons of distal sensory nerve action potential and compound muscle action potential amplitudes (15). Acute and subacute conduction block can be demonstrated by motor studies (12,15). Consensus criteria for partial conduction block requires either a 50% amplitude reduction or a 40% area reduction if there is mild temporal dispersion and >60% amplitude or 50% area if moderate temporal dispersion is present (16). Intra-operative nerve action potentials (NAPs) are useful in assessing axonal continuity for surgical intervention (17,18).

Ultrasound has been used to evaluate continuity of the nerve in the setting of humeral shaft fracture (19). MRI has been used to evaluate radial neuropathies at the elbow (20). Its advantage is that it can evaluate for intrinsic and extrinsic mass lesions. Focal and diffuse thickening and increased T2 signal are associated with nerve injury.

4. ETIOLOGIES

Etiologies of radial mononeuropathy and its branches include trauma, prolonged compression, entrapment, systemic illness, and neoplasia.

Trauma is the main cause of radial neuropathy proximal to the spiral groove. Traumatic injury to the radial nerve in the axilla can occur from stretch, contusion, or gunshot wound (17,18,21). Traumatic injury of the radial nerve at the arm or elbow can occur with mid-shaft and distal humerus fracture (22–25), blunt contusion, laceration, or gunshot wound. Risk of radial nerve transection is increased with oblique fracture of the distal one-third of the humerus (22). The radial nerve and posterior interosseous nerves can be injured from fracture near the head of the radius (3,17,21,25–27) and by a Monteggia lesion, a fracture of the proximal ulna with radial head dislocation (2,27,28). Entrapment in callus formation and at the lateral intermuscular septum can occur as a sequelae of humerus fracture (17,22,29). In the supinator syndrome, there is entrapment of the posterior interosseous nerve at the Arcade of Frohse either spontaneously (2,10,11,17,26,28), after trauma

(2,28), or in the setting of rheumatoid arthritis (30). Handcuff neuropathy most commonly involves the superficial radial nerve (31). Radial neuropathy in the arm is reported in athletes who use their arms in repetitive, strenuous activities (32–34).

Iatrogenic injury of the radial nerve has occurred from hematoma following transarterial axillary block (35), injection injury in the upper arm (21,28,36), and compression in the arm by automatic blood pressure cuffs (37). Venipuncture of the cephalic vein in the distal forearm can cause injury to the superficial radial nerve (38,39).

Acute retrohumeral radial neuropathy following prolonged compression is most commonly localized to the spiral groove (2,12,28). The key feature is marked conduction block and reduced conduction velocity across the injury (12).

Mononeuropathy has been described as an early component of immune or inflammatory mediated diseases of the peripheral nervous system such as vasculitis (40), neurosarcoidosis (41), multifocal motor neuropathy with conduction block (42), Lewis–Sumner neuropathy or multifocal acquired demyelinating sensory and motor neuropathy (43), and in early Guillain–Barre Syndrome (44). Historically, radial neuropathy was described in lead toxicity (45). Mononeuropathy can be secondary to intrinsic tumor, and compression by extrinsic tumors (10,17,26,28), and tumor-like masses in focal inflammatory myositis (6), and amyloidosis. Arteriovenous shunts can cause neuropathy (7,46). It is also described in individuals with hereditary neuropathy with pressure palsy (3,37).

5. TREATMENT

Good spontaneous recovery, within days to weeks, usually occurs in patients with radial palsy secondary to compression at the spiral groove; however, incomplete and prolonged recovery may take place when electrophysiologic studies are suggestive of significant axonal injury (12). With traumatic injury, repair of sharp transection has been recommended within 72 h, whereas for blunt transections delay of weeks to delineate the margin of injury is recommended (17). When the nerve is not transected, a high rate of spontaneous recovery does occur (17,18). When sufficient recovery does not occur, intra-operative NAPs can be used to determine whether neurolysis or resection is necessary for nerve repair (17,21). With arm level injuries, surgical treatment often results in good proximal function but digit and thumb extension may remain poor and require tendon transfer (17,18,47). Surgery for entrapment of the posterior interosseous nerve is reported to result in a high rate of good return of digit extension, although thumb extension may require tendon transfer (18,26). Painful neuralgia after injury to the superficial radial nerve can often be treated by resection with the proximal end left beneath the brachioradialis muscle (17,18). Radial tunnel syndrome (1,48–50) as a pain syndrome is controversial and recent studies have not shown benefit from surgical release (8,51). Immunotherapy is indicated for inflammatory causes (42,43).

REFERENCES

1. Carlson N, Logigian EL. Radial neuropathy. Neurol Clin 1999; 17(3):499–523, vi.
2. Dumitru D, Zwarts MJ. Focal peripheral neuropathy. In: Dumitru D, Amato AA, Zwarts MJ, eds. Electrodiagnostic Medicine. Philadelphia: Hanley & Belfus, Inc., 2002:1043–1126.
3. Shaw JL, Sakellarides H. Radial-nerve paralysis associated with fractures of the humerus. A review of forty-five cases. J Bone Joint Surg Am 1967; 49(5):899–902.

4. Ozkan M, Bacakoglu AK, Gul O, Ekin A, Magden O. Anatomic study of posterior interosseous nerve in the arcade of Frohse. J Shoulder Elbow Surg 1999; 8(6):617–620.

5. Thomas SJ, Yakin DE, Parry BR, Lubahn JD. The anatomical relationship between the posterior interosseous nerve and the supinator muscle. J Hand Surg [Am] 2000; 25(5):936–941.

6. Alzagatiti BI, Bertorini TE, Horner LH, Maccarino VS, O'Brien T. Focal myositis presenting with radial nerve palsy. Muscle Nerve 1999; 22(7):956–959.

7. Amato AA, Kissel JT, Mendel JR. Neuropathies associated with organ system failure. In: Mendel JR, Kissel JT, Cornblath DR, eds. Diagnosis and Management of Peripheral Nervous System Disorders. Oxford University Press, 2001:565–591.

8. Atroshi I, Johnsson R, Ornstein E. Radial tunnel release. Unpredictable outcome in 37 consecutive cases with a 1–5 year follow-up. Acta Orthop Scand 1995; 66(3):255–257.

9. Branovacki G, Hanson M, Cash R, Gonzalez M. The innervation pattern of the radial nerve at the elbow and in the forearm. J Hand Surg [Br] 1998; 23(2):167–169.

10. Eaton CJ, Lister GD. Radial nerve compression. Hand Clin 1992; 8(2):345–357.

11. Spinner M. The arcade of Frohse and its relationship to posterior interosseous nerve paralysis. J Bone Joint Surg Br 1968; 50(4):809–812.

12. Brown WF, Watson BV. AAEM case report #27: acute retrohumeral radial neuropathies. Muscle Nerve 1993; 16(7):706–711.

13. Dumitru D, Amato AA, Zwarts MJ. Nerve conduction studies. In: Dumitru D, Amato AA, Zwarts MJ, eds. Electrodiagnostic Medicine. Philadelphia: Hanley & Belfus, Inc., 2002:159–223.

14. Young AW, Redmond MD, Hemler DE, Belandres PV. Radial motor nerve conduction studies. Arch Phys Med Rehabil 1990; 71(6):399–402.

15. Watson BV, Brown WF. Quantitation of axon loss and conduction block in acute radial nerve palsies. Muscle Nerve 1992; 15(7):768–773.

16. Olney RK. Consensus criteria for the diagnosis of partial conduction block. Muscle Nerve 1999; 22(suppl 8):S225–S229.

17. Kim DH, Kam AC, Chandika P, Tiel RL, Kline DG. Surgical management and outcome in patients with radial nerve lesions. J Neurosurg 2001; 95(4):573–583.

18. Kline DG, Hudson HR. Acute injuries of peripheral nerves. In: Youmans JR, ed. Neurological Surgery: a Comprehensive Reference Guide to the Diagnosis and Management of Neurosurgical Problems. 4th ed. Philadelphia: WB Saunders Company, 1996:2103–2181.

19. Bodner G, Buchberger W, Schocke M et al. Radial nerve palsy associated with humeral shaft fracture: evaluation with US—initial experience. Radiology 2001; 219(3):811–816.

20. Rosenberg ZS, Bencardino J, Beltran J. MR features of nerve disorders at the elbow. Magn Reson Imaging Clin N Am 1997; 5(3):545–565.

21. Kline DG. Macroscopic and microscopic concomitants of nerve repair. Clin Neurosurg 1979; 26:582–606.

22. Bostman O, Bakalim G, Vainionpaa S, Wilppula E, Patiala H, Rokkanen P. Immediate radial nerve palsy complicating fracture of the shaft of the humerus: when is early exploration justified? Injury 1985; 16(7):499–502.

23. Mast JW, Spiegel PG, Harvey JP Jr, Harrison C. Fractures of the humeral shaft: a retrospective study of 240 adult fractures. Clin Orthop 1975; 112:254–262.

24. Pollock FH, Drake D, Bovill EG, Day L, Trafton PG. Treatment of radial neuropathy associated with fractures of the humerus. J Bone Joint Surg Am 1981; 63(2):239–243.

25. Sturzenegger M, Rutz M. Radial nerve paralysis—causes, site, and diagnosis. Analysis of 103 cases. Nervenarzt 1991; 62(12):722–729.

26. Cravens G, Kline DG. Posterior interosseous nerve palsies. Neurosurgery 1990; 27(3):397–402.

27. Galbraith KA, McCullough CJ. Acute nerve injury as a complication of closed fractures or dislocations of the elbow. Injury 1979; 11(2):159–164.

28. Stewart JD. Focal Peripheral Neuropathies. Philadelphia: Lippincott, Williams & Wilkins, 2000.

29. Chesser TJ, Leslie IJ. Radial nerve entrapment by the lateral intermuscular septum after trauma. J Orthop Trauma 2000; 14(1):65–66.

30. Fernandez AM, Tiku ML. Posterior interosseous nerve entrapment in rheumatoid arthritis. Semin Arthritis Rheum 1994; 24(1):57–60.
31. Grant AC, Cook AA. A prospective study of handcuff neuropathies. Muscle Nerve 2000; 23(6):933–938.
32. Prochaska V, Crosby LA, Murphy RP. High radial nerve palsy in a tennis player. Orthop Rev 1993; 22(1):90–92.
33. Sinson G, Zager EL, Kline DG. Windmill pitcher's radial neuropathy. Neurosurgery 1994; 34(6):1087–1089 (discussion 9–90).
34. Streib E. Upper arm radial nerve palsy after muscular effort: report of three cases. Neurology 1992; 42(8):1632–1634.
35. Ben-David B, Stahl S. Axillary block complicated by hematoma and radial nerve injury. Reg Anesth Pain Med 1999; 24(3):264–266.
36. Gaur SC, Swarup A. Radial nerve palsy caused by injections. J Hand Surg [Br] 1996; 21(3):338–340.
37. Lin CC, Jawan B, de Villa MV, Chen FC, Liu PP. Blood pressure cuff compression injury of the radial nerve. J Clin Anesth 2001; 13(4):306–308.
38. Sheu JJ, Yuan RY. Superficial radial neuropathy following venepuncture. Int J Clin Pract 2001; 55(6):422–423.
39. Vialle R, Pietin-Vialle C, Cronier P, Brillu C, Villapadierna F, Mercier P. Anatomic relations between the cephalic vein and the sensory branches of the radial nerve: how can nerve lesions during vein puncture be prevented? Anesth Analg 2001; 93(4):1058–1061.
40. Said G. Necrotizing peripheral nerve vasculitis. Neurol Clin 1997; 15(4):835–848.
41. Chapelon C, Ziza JM, Piette JC et al. Neurosarcoidosis: signs, course and treatment in 35 confirmed cases. Medicine (Baltimore) 1990; 69(5):261–276.
42. Parry GJ. AAEM case report 30: multifocal motor neuropathy. Muscle Nerve 1996; 19(3):269–276.
43. Saperstein DS, Amato AA, Wolfe GI et al. Multifocal acquired demyelinating sensory and motor neuropathy: the Lewis–Sumner syndrome. Muscle Nerve 1999; 22(5):560–566.
44. Baba M, Matsunaga M, Ozaki I. Posterior interosseous syndrome in acute Guillain–Barré syndrome. Electromyogr Clin Neurophysiol 1994; 34(6):367–371.
45. Erdem S, Kissel JT, Mendel JR. Toxic neuropathies: drugs, metals, and alcohol. In: Mendel JR, Kissel JT, Cornblath DR, eds. Diagnosis and Management of Peripheral Nervous System Disorders. Oxford University Press, 2001:297–343.
46. Arteriovenous shunts and nerve damage. Lancet 1981; 1(8213):211.
47. Shergill G, Bonney G, Munshi P, Birch R. The radial and posterior interosseous nerves. Results of 260 repairs. J Bone Joint Surg Br 2001; 83(5):646–649.
48. Lister GD, Belsole RB, Kleinert HE. The radial tunnel syndrome. J Hand Surg [Am] 1979; 4(1):52–59.
49. Roles NC, Maudsley RH. Radial tunnel syndrome: resistant tennis elbow as a nerve entrapment. J Bone Joint Surg Br 1972; 54(3):499–508.
50. Rosenbaum R. Disputed radial tunnel syndrome. Muscle Nerve 1999; 22(7):960–967.
51. Sotereanos DG, Varitimidis SE, Giannakopoulos PN, Westkaemper JG. Results of surgical treatment for radial tunnel syndrome. J Hand Surg [Am] 1999; 24(3):566–570.

28
Ulnar Mononeuropathies

John D. Steffens
University of Utah, Salt Lake City, Utah, USA

ABSTRACT

The ulnar nerve is the major nerve to the hand and is susceptible to injury at the elbow and wrist. Injury to the nerve may be associated with pain at the site of the lesion, although insidious atrophy and/or weakness of ulnar innervated muscles is common. Ulnar mononeuropathy should be considered when the fifth or fourth and fifth digits of the hand develop altered sensation; or when intrinsic hand muscles become weak and/or atrophic. Documentation of nerve injury and localization are aided by electrodiagnostic evaluation. The most common cause of injury is compression at the elbow, which generally responds well to conservative or simple decompressive interventions. Other disorders can be confused with ulnar neuropathies. Underlying metabolic, genetic, or acquired illnesses may be exacerbating factors.

1. INTRODUCTION

Ulnar mononeuropathies are common, and compression at the elbow is second in frequency to median nerve compression at the wrist. Compression of the ulnar nerve can also occur at other sites. There are a number of pathological processes that may injure the nerve. An understanding of normal ulnar nerve anatomy and common anatomic variants is important for correct interpretation of the clinical and electrodiagnostic examination, facilitates accurate lesion localization, and leads to a better understanding of underlying causes.

2. ANATOMY

The ulnar nerve is a mixed motor and sensory nerve. Motor fibers originate from cell bodies located in the cervical spinal cord, at the C8 and T1 levels. Sensory fibers originate from dorsal root ganglia at levels C7–8 and T1. Both motor and sensory fibers from C8 and T1 combine to form the lower trunk of the brachial plexus, whereas C7 fibers form the middle trunk (Fig. 28.1). Variations occur rarely (3–5%) and are associated with a prefixed or post-fixed brachial plexus. In these situations, the spinal root levels contributing to the brachial plexus and its branches may be one higher or one lower, respectively.

The anterior division of the lower trunk combines with C7 fibers from the middle trunk to form the medial cord, with the ulnar nerve proper as the largest branch. The nerve then travels through the axilla by crossing under the pectoralis minor and traverses along the medial arm to pass through the ulnar groove and then the cubital tunnel at the elbow. The latter structure is a fairly restrictive canal, bounded above by the aponeurosis between the olecranon and the medial epicondyle (the humeral–ulnar aponeurosis, composed of the tendinous arch of the two heads of the flexor carpi ulnaris) and below by the medial ligament of the elbow (Fig. 28.2). Movement at the elbow (especially flexion) narrows this canal and is an important mechanism for local nerve compression. The first two branches of the ulnar nerve arise at or below this point and provide innervation to the flexor carpi ulnaris and flexor digitorum profundus III and IV (proximal and distal branches, respectively). The nerve then continues through the forearm, crossing the wrist lateral to the tendon of the flexor carpi ulnaris, and enters the hand through Guyon's canal, which is a boney canal bounded medially by the pisiform, and laterally by the hook of the hamate. Sensory branches usually leave the nerve proximal to Guyon's canal, whereas the remaining motor nerve branches occur within or distal to the canal.

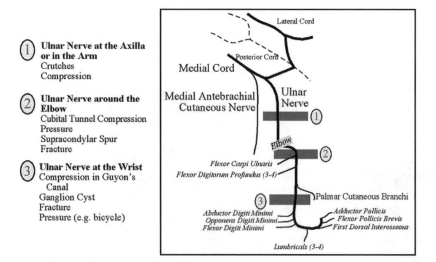

Figure 28.1 Diagram of ulnar nerve showing branches to individual muscles. Major entrapment sites marked by gray bars and associated numbers refer to table with differential diagnoses and causes.

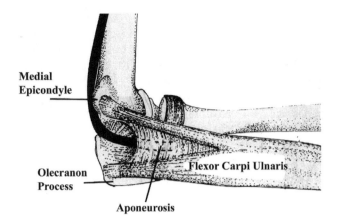

Medial
Epicondyle

Olecranon
Process

Flexor Carpi Ulnaris

Aponeurosis

Figure 28.2   Diagram of the ulnar nerve at the elbow showing the cubital tunnel.

The ulnar nerve innervates 10 muscles. Branches to the flexor carpi ulnaris and flexor digitorum profundus III and IV leave the nerve just below the elbow, distal to or within the cubital tunnel. All other muscular branches are given off distal to the wrist, in or near Guyon's canal. The hypothenar group consists of the abductor, opponens, and flexor digiti minimi. The thenar group consists of the adductor pollicis and deep head of the flexor pollicis brevis. The remaining muscles are the dorsal and volar interossei, lumbricals III, IV, and the palmaris brevis. All distal muscles are innervated by C8 and T1 roots, with the exception of the flexor carpi ulnaris and flexor digitorum profundus III and IV which have C7 and C8 fibers. The flexor carpi ulnaris also has variable T1 contributions.

Ulnar-to-median (1) and median-to-ulnar (Martin–Gruber anastamosis) communication in the forearm occur in ~17% of people (2). There are four variations of the Martin–Gruber anastamosis. Type I (60%) has median-to-ulnar motor crossover, with preservation of standard median and ulnar muscle innervation. Type II (35%) has median-to-ulnar motor crossover, with resultant median fibers innervating ulnar muscles. Type III (3%) and IV (1%) send motor fibers from the ulnar to the median nerve with ulnar innervation of median muscles (III) or ulnar innervation of ulnar muscles (IV) (3). There are occasional examples of ulnar-to-median communication of sensory fibers as variations to the pattern noted earlier (4).

Sensory branches of the ulnar nerve include (from proximal to distal) the palmar cutaneous, dorsal cutaneous [which arises an average of 5.5 cm proximal to the head of the ulna (5)], and superficial terminal branches. Similar to the distal motor branches, sensory nerves are largely of fibers of C8 origin. They mediate sensation to the skin overlying the hypothenar eminence, the dorsal ulnar portion of the hand, including half of the fourth and all the fifth digits, and palmar aspect of the fifth and half of the fourth digits.

3. CLINICAL FEATURES

Clinical symptoms and examination findings are dependent upon the location of the lesion (Fig. 28.1) (6). In the cubital syndrome, sensory symptoms predominate with paresthesias occurring in most patients but pain in less than half, whereas motor symptoms are noted in two-thirds. Physical examination findings parallel symptoms, with sensory deficits and motor weakness noted in 75–80% and atrophy noted in two-thirds (7). Early presentations may be restricted to motor symptoms with ill-defined loss of strength and dexterity.

Cold may exacerbate symptoms, and nonmotor symptoms may fluctuate or even disappear for periods of time. Severe injury to the ulnar nerve at or above the elbow may result in a "claw hand" deformity (*main en griffe*) with intrinsic muscle atrophy, hyperextension of the fourth and fifth digits (and sometimes the third digit) at the metacarpophalangeal joint and flexion at the interphalangeal joints, loss of ulnar flexion, and altered sensation over the ulnar aspect of the hand. Mild injury at the elbow can result in sparing of flexor carpi ulnaris function. Lesions in the forearm or hand may cause findings similar to those of more proximal lesions (i.e., be associated with intrinsic muscle wasting etc.), but will spare the flexor carpi ulnaris and flexor digitorum profundus III and IV, with variable sparing of ulnar sensation. Excluding post-operative or immediately post-traumatic situations, compressive etiologies are usually due to repetitive insults, such as in over-use syndromes, with manual labor activities. Tardy ulnar palsy refers to situations of remote trauma to the elbow that is thought to trigger arthritic changes, which in turn lead to compression at the elbow. With compression at Guyon's canal there may be similar symptoms and signs, but typically without sensory disturbance. Lesions to the ulnar nerve in the hand result in variable involvement of distal motor branches, thereby having a range of clinical presentations, which may include finger tremor (8). Some authors separate compressive lesions of the ulnar nerve in the hand into three (9) or four (10) groups based upon location of the compression relative to Guyon's canal. Group I refers to proximal lesions in Guyon's canal, with resultant muscle weakness in all innervated hand muscles and involvement of the superficial terminal branches of the ulnar nerve before they branch. Group II is divided into IIa and IIb by different authors (10). These groups are characterized by more distal lesions within Guyon's canal, resulting in weakness of ulnar innervated muscles but without sensory nerve involvement (group II or IIb) or weakness that spares hypothenar muscles (group IIa). The former involves lesions of the proximal portion of the deep motor branch of the nerve, and the latter involves more distal lesions after the branch to hypothenar muscles. Group III is very distal in Guyon's canal and involves only superficial terminal sensory nerves.

Historical factors are relevant in deciphering the etiology; repetitive movements associated with ulnar neuropathy include Nordic skiing (11), meat packing (12), wheel-chair athletes (13), some types of video game playing (14), and playing musical instruments [15–17], carrying mail (18), unusual sleep positions (19), telesales representatives (20), use of an axillary crutch (21), bicycling (22–24), and driving (25). Surgery is thought to be a risk factor, attributed to positioning during the procedure and tilting the patient (26), but a retrospective review of over 1 million patients undergoing diagnostic and noncardiac procedures at one institution (Mayo Clinic) revealed a rate of persistent (>3 months) ulnar neuropathy of 1 per 2729 patients. There was no relation to the type of anesthetic technique or patient positioning. Both very thin and obese body habitus were positive risk factors (27). Cardiac procedures were excluded from the study, as sternal splitting procedures are associated with a 5–37% rate of post-operative nerve damage, with 40% having an ulnar neuropathy, 40% a brachial plexopathy, and 20% both neuropathies (28,29). Fortunately, up to 92% (range 57–93%) of patients had full recovery by 3 months after surgery (30). Other iatrogenic causes of ulnar neuropathy include arteriovenous fistula for dialysis (31,32), injections (33), subdermal contraceptive implantation (34), liquid nitrogen cryotherapy (35), and one case of ulnar neuropathy of the hand after high pressure air injection (36).

4. LABORATORY EVALUATION

The electrodiagnostic evaluation is the first step in further evaluation. Nerve conduction practices have been reviewed and delineated by the American Association of

Neuromuscular Electrodiagnostic Medicine and the American Academy of Neurology (37). When performing studies, care should be taken to exclude measurement errors (38). The elbow should be in a position of moderate flexion (70–90° from horizontal), with stimulation and measurement performed in the same positions. Across-elbow distances should be ~10 cm, and stimulation of the ulnar nerve >3 cm distal to the medial epicondyle should be avoided as the nerve usually lies deep at this point. The diagnosis of a focal ulnar nerve lesion at the elbow is most convincing when several internally consistent abnormalities are noted, rather than an isolated abnormality (38). Abnormalities supportive of a lesion include: an absolute motor nerve conduction velocity (NCV) across the elbow of <50 m/s; NCV across the elbow segment that is at least 10 m/s slower than the NCV from below the elbow to the wrist segment; and a compound muscle action potential amplitude across the elbow segment that is at least 20% lower than that recorded at the wrist.

Needle EMG examination should include the first dorsal interosseous muscle, as this is the most frequent muscle to demonstrate abnormalities in ulnar nerve lesions. In addition, ulnar innervated forearm muscles, nonulnar C8 innervated muscles of the hand, and cervical paraspinous muscles may be tested in order to exclude a process involving the medial cord or lower trunk of the brachial plexus, cervical (C8) roots, or motor neurons. Note that changes limited to the first dorsal interosseous (i.e., sparing the forearm muscles) do not exclude an ulnar nerve lesion at or above the elbow.

Because of the long list of possible causes for compressive ulnar mononeuropathies (either at the elbow or at the wrist), imaging studies may be of use. Magnetic resonance imaging (MRI) may help to delineate a typical compression due to repetitive movements from other entities such as tophaceous gout or calcium pyrophosphate crystal deposition, intraneural or extraneural growths, accessory muscles, or other described entities. In ordinary compressive neuropathy, there is increased ulnar nerve signal within 3–4 cm of the compressed region in almost all cases and no signal change in normal controls (39).

5. DIFFERENTIAL DIAGNOSIS

The diagnosis of ulnar neuropathy may appear straightforward, but a wide range of entities can masquerade as or contribute to ulnar mononeuropathy. There is a wide range of etiologies. One large study of ulnar mononeuropathy at the elbow revealed that 33% had local or systemic factors contributing to or responsible for the lesion (7). Identified factors included diabetes, alcohol abuse, and polyneuropathy of uncertain cause. Compressive ulnar neuropathy is a common manifestation of hereditary neuropathy with a liability to pressure palsy, and other forms of hypertrophic neuropathies (40) including focal demyelinating neuropathy of the ulnar nerve presenting with a Guyon's canal compressive neuropathy (41). A painful ulnar neuropathy as paraneoplastic process has been described (42). Other systemic processes include systemic scleroderma (43), drug induced lupus syndrome with antiphospholipid antibodies (44), and cutaneous anthrax (45).

When symptoms are of sudden onset, especially when there is pain, vasculitic or ischemic process such as mononeuritis multiplex, diabetes, or acute trauma should be considered. These processes occur less commonly at sites of compression and are more likely in the forearm or above the elbow.

Local factors reported to be associated with the development of ulnar neuropathy are lipomas (46–48), ganglion cysts (49–51), accessory or anomalous muscles (52–54), schwannoma (55,56), lepromatous lesions (57), intraneural mucoid pseudocysts (58), medial triceps dislocation (59,60), intraneural cysts (61,62), tumoral calcium deposition processes (63,64), gouty tophi (65,66), intraneural metastases (67), intramuscular hemorrhage (68), ulnar artery aneurysm (69), and thrombosed ulnar vein (70), among others.

Remote causes mimicking ulnar neuropathy include, cervical syrinx (71), small infarcts of the hand knob of the precentral gyrus (72), injury to the teres minor through a conjectured referral pain pattern (73), and small localized tumors of the precentral gyrus (unpublished observation). Injuries to the C8 nerve root or lower trunk and/or medial cord of the brachial plexus have been addressed previously in this chapter, but must remain on the list of differential diagnostic possibilities.

6. MANAGEMENT AND PROGNOSIS

Addressing the cause of compression can result in a resolution or an arrest of progression. For some types of local factors, surgical decompression is effective. In one series, ulnar neurolysis was effective for pain relief, and 50% of patients had some sensory recovery, whereas 90% of patients had improvement or arrest of progression of loss of motor function (74). A management dilemma is what to do for uncomplicated ulnar neuropathy at the elbow, and there are few large prospective trials for guidance. Observational data suggest that symptomatic ulnar neuropathy at the elbow without physical examination findings or electrodiagnostic abnormalities can be effectively managed with conservative therapy; padding the elbow, reducing repetitive flexion and extension movements, use of anti-inflammatories, and reducing the amount of time spent with elbows flexed. Conservative management techniques will effectively prevent the need for surgery in up to 90% (75).

Those with motor findings or evidence for denervation on electrodiagnostic evaluations generally do not respond adequately to conservative therapy and will require surgical intervention. Despite surgery, the clinical outcome in one study was improvement in only 70% (76). Different types of surgical procedures do not clearly predict the outcome, although utilizing a stabilized subcutaneous ulnar nerve transposition with immediate range of motion allows patients to return to their occupation sooner than other methods; and 2 year follow-up data suggests that up to 70% have an excellent clinical outcome, with another 20% having a good outcome (77).

7. CONCLUSIONS

Ulnar neuropathy is common. Although there are many causes for compression, the most common are related to the anatomical constraints of the cubital tunnel and Guyon's canal, with repetitive flexion movements most typically the culprit for compression. In these conditions, electrodiagnostic evaluation is able to differentiate ulnar neuropathy from other conditions. MRI can help clarify the picture in unusual cases. Electrodiagnostic findings help guide decisions regarding conservative vs. surgical therapy. Patients with symptoms only, or nonlocalizing electrodiagnostic findings, can often be successfully managed with conservative measures. Early surgical decompression with anterior transposition is recommended for any patient with motor findings on physical examination or electrodiagnostic evaluation. Those who have surgery have a good to excellent outcome post-operatively.

REFERENCES

1. Streib EW. Ulnar-to-median anastamosis in the forearm: electromyographic studies. Neurology 1979; 29:1534–1537.
2. Leibovic SJ, Hastings H. Martin–Gruber revisited. J Hand Surg 1992; 17:47–53.

3. Gutmann L. AAEM minimonograph No. 2: important anomalous innervation of the extremities. Muscle Nerve 1993; 16:339–347.

4. Hopf HC. Forearm ulnar-to-median nerve anastamosis of sensory axons. Muscle Nerve 1990; 13:654–656.

5. Grossman JA, Yen L, Rapaport D. The dorsal cutaneous branch of the ulnar nerve. An anatomic clarification with six case reports. Chir Main 1998; 17(2):154–158.

6. Campbell WW, Pridgeon RM, Riaz G et al. Sparing of the flexor carpi ulnaris in ulnar neuropathy at the elbow. Muscle Nerve 1989; 12:965–967.

7. Artico M, Pastore FS, Nucci F, Giuffre R. 290 surgical procedures for ulnar nerve entrapment at the elbow: pathophysiology, clinical experience and results. Acta Neurochir (Wien) 2000; 142:303–308.

8. Streib EW. Distal ulnar neuropathy as a cause of finger tremor: a case report. Neurology 1990; 40(1):153–154.

9. Ebeling P, Gilliatt RW, Thomas PK. A clinical and electrical study of ulnar nerve lesions of the hand. J Neurol Neurosurg Psychiatry 1960; 23:1–9.

10. Cavallo M, Poppi M, Martinelli P, Gaist G. Distal ulnar neuropathy from carpal ganglion: a clinical and electrophysiologic study. Neurosurgery 1988; 22:902–905.

11. Fulkerson JP. Transient ulnar neuropathy from Nordic skiing. Clin Orthop 1980; 153:230–231.

12. Streib EW, Sun SF. Distal ulnar neuropathy in meat packers. An occupational disease? J Occup Med 1984; 26(11):842–843.

13. Burnham RS, Steadward RD. Upper extremity peripheral nerve entrapments among wheelchair athletes: prevalence, location, and risk factors. Arch Phys Med Rehabil 1994; 75(5):519–524.

14. Friedland RP, St John JN. Video-game palsy: distal ulnar neuropathy in a video game enthusiast. N Engl J Med 1984; 311(1):58–59.

15. Lederman RJ. Neuromuscular and musculoskeletal problems in instrumental musicians. Muscle Nerve 2003; 27(5):549–561.

16. Charness ME, Ross MH, Shefner JM. Ulnar neuropathy and dystonic flexion of the fourth and fifth digits: clinical correlation in musicians. Muscle Nerve 1996; 19(4):431–437.

17. Lederman RJ. AAEM minimonograph No. 43: neuromuscular problems in the performing arts. Muscle Nerve 1994; 17(6):569–577.

18. Massey EW. Dimple sign in mail carrier's ulnar neuropathy. Neurology 1989; 39(8):1132.

19. Finsterer J. Ulnar neuropathy at the elbow due to unusual sleep position. Eur J Neurol 2000; 7(1):115–117.

20. Lewis MB. Telesales neuropathy. Postgrad Med J 2000; 76(902):793–794.

21. Veerendrakumar M, Taly AB, Nagaraja D. Ulnar nerve palsy due to axillary crutch. Neurol India 2001; 49(1):67–70.

22. Eckman PB, Perstein G, Altrocchi PH. Ulnar neuropathy in bicycle riders. Arch Neurol 1975; 32(2):130–132.

23. Mellion MB. Common cycling injuries. Management and prevention. Sports Med 1991; 11(1):52–70.

24. Patterson JM, Jaggers MM, Boyer MI. Ulnar and median nerve palsy long-distance cyclists. A prospective study. Am J Sports Med 2003; 31(4):585–589.

25. Abdel-Salam A, Eyres KS, Cleary J. Drivers' elbow: a cause of ulnar neuropathy. J Hand Surg [Br] 1991; 16(4):436–437.

26. Lee CT, Espley AJ. Perioperative ulnar neuropathy in orthopaedics: association with tilting the patient. Clin Orthop 2002; 396:106–111.

27. Warner MA, Warner ME, Martin JT. Ulnar neuropathy. Incidence, outcome, and risk factors in sedated or anesthetized patients. Anesthesiology 1994; 81(6):1332–1340.

28. Morin JE, Long R, Elleker MG, Eisen AA, Wynands E, Ralphs-Thibodeau S. Upper extremity neuropathies following median sternotomy. Ann Thorac Surg 1982; 34(2):181–185.

29. Seyfer AE, Grammer NY, Bogumill GP, Provost JM, Chandry U. Upper extremity neuropathies after cardiac surgery. J Hand Surg [Am] 1985; 10(1):16–19.

30. Casscells CD, Lindsey RW, Ebersole J, Li B. Ulnar neuropathy after median sternotomy. Clin Orthop 1993; 291:259–265.

31. Klein C, Halevy A, Gandelman-Marton R, Halpern Z, Weissgarten J, Averbukh Z, Arlazoroff A. Nerve conduction abnormalities in the arms of patients with arteriovenous fistula. Ren Fail 1996 18(1):85–89

32. Knezevic W, Mastaglia FL. Neuropathy associated with Brescia–Cimino arteriovenous fistulas. Arch Neurol 1984; 41(11):1184–1186.

33. Geiringer SR, Leonard JA Jr. Injection related ulnar neuropathy. Arch Phys Med Rehabil 1989; 70(9):705–706.

34. Marin R, McMillian D. Ulnar neuropathy associated with subdermal contraceptive implant. South Med J 1998; 91(9):875–878.

35. Finelli PF. Ulnar neuropathy after liquid nitrogen cryotherapy. Arch Dermatol 1975; 111(10):1340–1342.

36. Markal N, Celebioglu S. Compression neuropathy of the hand after high-pressure air injection. Ann Plast Surg 2000 44(6):680–681.

37. Quality Assurance Committee of the AAEM and Quality Standards Subcommittee of the AAN. Practice parameter: Electrodiagnostic studies in ulnar neuropathy at the elbow. Neurology 1999; 52:688–690.

38. Landau ME, Diaz MI, Barner KC, Campbell WW. Changes in nerve conduction velocity across the elbow due to experimental error. Muscle Nerve 2002; 26:838–840.

39. Britz GW, Haynor DR, Kuntz C, Goodkin R, Gitter A, Maravilla K, Kliot M. Ulnar nerve entrapment at the elbow: correlation of magnetic resonance imaging, clinical, electrodiagnostic, and intraoperative findings. Neurosurgery 1996; 38:458–465.

40. Taras J, Melone CP. Hypertrophic neuropathy presenting with ulnar nerve compression: a case report. J Hand Surg [Am] 1995; 20(2):233–234.

41. Dhillon MS, Chu ML, Posner MA. Demyelinating focal motor neuropathy of the ulnar nerve masquerading as compression in Guyon's canal: a case report. J Hand Surg [Am] 2003; 28(1):48–51.

42. Sharief MK, Robinson SF, Ingram DA, Geddes JF, Swash M. Paraneoplastic painful ulnar neuropathy. Muscle Nerve 1999; 22(7):952–955.

43. Mouthon L, Halimi C, Muller GP, Cayre-Castel M, Begue T, Masquelet AC, Guillevin L. Systemic scleroderma associated with bilateral ulnar nerve entrapment at the elbow. Rheumatology (Oxford) 2000; 39(6):682–683.

44. Graham LE, Bell AL. Minocycline associated lupus-like syndrome with ulnar neuropathy and antiphospholipid antibody. Clin Rheumatol 2001; 20(1):67–69.

45. Terzioglu A, Aslan G. Ulnar nerve lesion due to cutaneous anthrax. Ann Plast Surg 1999; 43(6):644–645.

46. Zahrawi F. Acute compression ulnar neuropathy at Guyon's canal resulting from lipoma. J Hand Surg [Am] 1984; 9(2):238–239.

47. Galeano M, Colonna M, Risitano G. Ulnar tunnel syndrome secondary to lipoma of the hypothenar region. Ann Plast Surg 2001; 46(1):83–84.

48. Sakai K, Tsutsui T, Aoi M, Sonobe H, Murakami H. Ulnar neuropathy caused by a lipoma in Guyon's canal—case report. Neurol Med Chir (Tokyo) 2000; 40(6):335–338.

49. Shu N, Uchio Y, Ryoke K, Yamamoto S, Oae K, Ochi M. Atypical compression of the deep branch of the ulnar nerve in Guyon's canal by a ganglion. Case report. Scand J Plast Reconstr Surg Hand Surg 2000; 34(2):181–183.

50. Sharma RR, Pawar SJ, Delmendo A, Mahapatra AK. Symptomatic epineural ganglion cyst of the ulnar nerve in the cubital tunnel: case report and brief review of the literature. J Clin Neurosci 2000; 7(6):542–543.

51. Cavallo M, Poppi M, Martinelli P, Gaist G. Distal ulnar neuropathy from carpal ganglia: a clinical and electrophysiologic study. Neurosurgery 1998; 22(5):902–905.

52. Masear VR, Hill JJ Jr, Cohen SM. Ulnar compression neuropathy secondary to the anconeus epitrochlearis muscle. J Hand Surg [Am] 1988; 13(5):720–724.

53. Ruocco MJ, Walsh JJ, Jackson JP. MR imaging of ulnar nerve entrapment secondary to an anomalous wrist muscle. Skeletal Radiol 1998; 27(4):218–221.

54. Sheppard JE, Prebble TB, Rahn K. Ulnar neuropathy caused by an accessory abductor digiti minimi muscle. Wis Med J 1991; 90(11):628–631.

55. Shank CP, Friedman WA. Ulnar neuropathy in a patient with multiple schwannomas of the ulnar nerve. Surg Neurol 1987; 28(2):153–157.

56. Spinner RJ, Tiel RL. High ulnar nerve compression by a triceps branch schwannoma. J South Orthop Assoc 2003; 12(1):41–42.

57. Bhushan C. Solitary tuberculoid Hansen lesion of the ulnar nerve. J Neurosurg 2000; 93(5):898.

58. Chick G, Alnot JY, Silbermann-Hoffman O. Intraneural mucoid pseudocysts. A report of ten cases. J Bone Joint Surg Br 2001; 83(7):1020–1022.

59. Spinner RJ, Davids JR, Goldner RD. Dislocating medial triceps and ulnar neuropathy in three generations of one family. J Hand Surg [Am] 1997; 22(1):132–137.

60. Spinner RJ, O'Driscoll SW, Jupiter JB, Goldner RD. Unrecognized dislocation of the medial portion of the triceps: another cause of failed ulnar nerve transposition. J Neurosurg 2000; 92(1):52–57.

61. Harway RA. Ulnar neuropathy due to intraneural cyst. Orthopedics 1997; 20(4):354–355.

62. Inhofe PD, Moneim MS. Compression of the ulnar nerve at the elbow by an intraneural cyst: a case report. J Hand Surg [Am] 1996; 21(6):1094–1096.

63. Aoyama T, Takahashi S. Cubital tunnel syndrome caused by tumoral deposition of calcium pyrophosphate dihydrate crystals: a case report. J Shoulder Elbow Surg 2001; 10(2):194–196.

64. Cofan F, Garcia S, Campistol JM, Combalia A, Oppenheimer F, Ramon R. Ulnar nerve compression—a case of giant uremic tumoral calcinosis. Acta Orthop Scand 1997; 68(3):302–304.

65. Nakamichi K, Tachibana S. Cubital tunnel syndrome caused by tophaceous gout. J Hand Surg [Br] 1996; 21(4):559–560.

66. Wang HC, Tsai MD. Compressive ulnar neuropathy in the proximal forearm caused by gouty tophus. Muscle Nerve 1996; 19(4):525–527.

67. Griswold W, Piza-Katzer H, Jahn R, Herczeg E. Intraneural nerve metastasis with multiple mononeuropathies. J Peripher Nerv Syst 2000; 5(3):163–167.

68. Vijayakumar R, Ncsathurai S, Abbott KM, Eustace S. Ulnar neuropathy from diffuse intramuscular hemorrhage: a case report. Arch Phys Med Rehabil 2000; 81(8):1127–1130.

69. Yoshii S, Ikeda K, Murakami H. Ulnar nerve compression secondary to ulnar artery true aneurysm at Guyon's canal. J Neurosurg Sci 1999; 43(4):295–297.

70. Grossman JA, Becker GA. Ulnar neuropathy caused by a thrombosed ulnar vein. Case report and literature review. Ann Chir Main Memb Super 1996; 15(4):244–247.

71. Scelsa SN. Syringomyelia presenting as ulnar neuropathy at the elbow. Clin Neurophysiol 2000; 111(9):1527–1530.

72. Hochman MS, DePrima SJ, Leon BJ. Pseudoulnar palsy from a small infarct of the precentral knob. Neurology 2000; 55(12):1939–1941.

73. Escobar PL, Ballesteros J. Teres minor. Source of symptoms resembling ulnar neuropathy or C8 radiculopathy. Am J Phys Med Rehabil 1988; 67(3):120–122.

74. Husain S, Mishra B, Prakash V, Malaviya GN. Results of surgical decompression of ulnar nerve in leprosy. Acta Leprol 1998; 11(1):17–20.

75. Dellon AL, Hament W, Gittelshon A. Non-operative management of cubital tunnel syndrome: an 8 year prospective study. Neurology 1993; 43:1673–1677.

76. Friedman RJ, Cochran TP. A clinical and electrophysiological investigation of anterior transposition for ulnar neuropathy at the elbow. Arch Orthop Trauma Surg 1987; 106:375–380.

77. Black BT, Barron OA, Townsend PF, Glickel SZ, Eaton RG. Stabilized subcutaneous ulnar nerve transposition with immediate range of motion. J Bone Joint Surg 2000; 82-A(11):1544–1551.

29
Other Upper Extremity Neuropathies

J. Steven Schultz

University of Michigan Health System, Ann Arbor, Michigan, USA

ABSTRACT

Focal neuropathy of the shoulder girdle is often unrecognized as a cause of upper extremity pain and disability. Proximal mononeuropathy is a diagnostic consideration in patients with pain and weakness of the shoulder girdle. Isolated lesions of the long thoracic, spinal accessory, suprascapular, axillary, or musculocutaneous nerves may be difficult to distinguish from more commonly encountered neurologic and musculoskeletal conditions, such as cervical radiculopathy, brachial plexopathy, neuralgic amyotrophy, and rotator cuff tendinopathy. Compromise of peripheral nerves occurs as a result of direct trauma, compression or traction. In many cases, the mechanism of injury is unique to a specific nerve. A carefully history and physical examination, and an electrodiagnostic evaluation can identify these neuropathies, facilitating appropriate and timely treatment. Patients with mild or incomplete lesions usually improve with relative rest and physical therapy. Surgical management is often necessary in severe axon loss injuries.

1. INTRODUCTION

Proximal mononeuropathies constitute a relatively small cause of shoulder pain and weakness. These lesions are often obscured by other soft tissue injuries and may masquerade as myriad other musculoskeletal or neurologic conditions. Injuries to peripheral nerves occur in isolation or in combination with root, plexus, and other nerve lesions, further complicating the clinical diagnosis. Accordingly, it is important to maintain an awareness of these injuries to insure prompt diagnosis and effective treatment. The clinical and electrophysiologic features of isolated injuries to the long thoracic, spinal accessory, suprascapular, axillary, and musculocutaneous nerves are reviewed in this chapter. Etiologies of these lesions are presented, emphasizing anatomic risk factors and unique mechanisms of injury for each nerve. Finally, conservative and surgical management of these conditions are described.

2. LONG THORACIC NEUROPATHY

2.1. Anatomy

The long thoracic nerve is a purely motor nerve that supplies the serratus anterior muscle. It usually arises from branches of the fifth, sixth, and seventh cervical nerve roots shortly after they exit the intervertebral foramina, proximal to the formation of the brachial plexus (Fig. 29.1). The largest and most consistent contribution comes from the sixth nerve

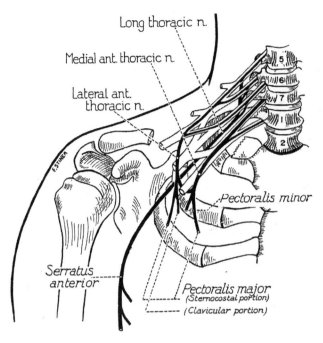

Long thoracic n.

Medial ant. thoracic n.

Lateral ant. thoracic n.

Pectoralis minor

Serratus anterior

Pectoralis major
(Sternocostal portion)
(Clavicular portion)

Figure 29.1 Long thoracic nerve. [From Haymaker and Woodhall (24).]

root. The branch from the seventh nerve root is absent in ~8% of patients and the nerve occasionally receives a contribution from the eighth cervical root (1). The branches from the fifth and sixth roots unite immediately after piercing the scalenus medius muscle. The branch arising from the seventh root joins the nerve as it travels across the scalenus posterior. The nerve then courses downward and laterally just posterior to the midaxillary line, supplying each digitation of the serratus anterior as it progresses. The lower portion of the serratus is innervated by intercostal nerves in ~20% of individuals (1).

2.2. Clinical Features

Patients with a long thoracic neuropathy typically present with a dull, aching sensation in the periscapular area, and difficulty reaching overhead. The distinguishing clinical feature of serratus anterior weakness is scapular winging. Sitting in a hard-backed chair is often uncomfortable, owing to scapular prominence. In many cases, patients are unaware of the winging until it is brought to their attention. Scapular winging from serratus anterior weakness has characteristic findings on physical examination. At rest, there is often a slight outward flaring of the inferior angle of the scapula (Fig. 29.2). Flexion of the arms forward produces winging of the entire medial scapular border (Fig. 29.3). The serratus functions primarily as a scapular stabilizer and is unique in its ability to maintain the medial border of the scapula against the thorax as the arms are thrust forward. This movement results in a posteriorly directed force upon the scapula that cannot be counterbalanced if the serratus is weak. Winging of this type is accentuated by resisted scapular protraction, pressing against a wall, or performing a push-up. There is little if any translocation of the scapula laterally because of the stabilizing action of the middle trapezius. The serratus anterior also functions as an upward rotator of the scapula; consequently, active abduction of the affected arm is often limited. However, abduction may be full due to compensatory action of the upper trapezius (2,3). Scapulohumeral rhythm is

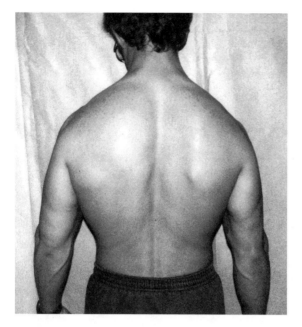

Figure 29.2   Winging of the right scapula at rest. Note prominence of the inferior scapular angle.

uniformly abnormal in these patients. The comparative features of serratus and trapezius winging are listed in Table 29.1.

2.3.   Laboratory Evaluation

Although injury to the long thoracic nerve is usually apparent on clinical evaluation, the diagnosis is confirmed by electrodiagnostic studies demonstrating isolated involvement of the nerve and excluding other causes of scapular winging, such as brachial plexopathy,

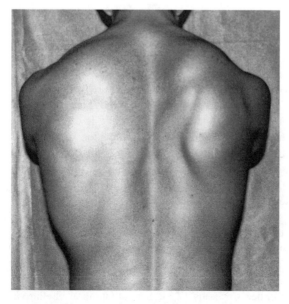

Figure 29.3   Winging of the right scapula with the arms thrust forward.

Table 29.1 Comparative Features of Serratus Anterior and Trapezius Scapular Winging

	Serratus anterior winging	Trapezius scapular winging
Muscle atrophy	Minimal	Often prominent in upper trapezius
Appearance at rest	Flaring of the inferior scapular angle	Drooped shoulder on affected side
Winging accentuated by	Forward flexion and resisted protraction	Abduction
Winging minimized by	Abduction	Forward flexion
Lateral translocation of scapula	Minimal	Often pronounced

spinal accessory neuropathy, and neuralgic amyotrophy. The degree of axon damage can be determined, which assists in prognostication.

The long thoracic nerve is readily accessible to nerve conduction studies. The superficial location of the serratus anterior muscle allows surface electrode recording, although may be technically difficult in obese individuals (4). The most common finding is a decreased or absent compound motor action potential (CMAP) when recording from the serratus anterior muscle. The distal latency is prolonged in some cases. As most laboratories do not have established normal values for long thoracic conduction studies, it is important to obtain comparative data from the uninvolved side. It is essential to establish that the spinal accessory nerve conduction studies are normal, as injury to this nerve may also cause scapular winging. Median, radial, and lateral antebrachial cutaneous sensory conduction studies are useful in excluding upper trunk brachial plexopathy.

Needle EMG demonstrates isolated denervation of the serratus anterior muscle. Sampling of the upper and middle portions of the muscle is recommended because the lower digitations are often innervated by the intercostal nerves and a false negative examination may be recorded if only inferior portions are studied. Examination of the trapezius and other limb muscles excludes lesions of the spinal accessory nerve and brachial plexus.

2.4. Differential Diagnosis

The differential diagnosis of long thoracic neuropathy is listed in Table 29.2. Among nerve injuries, spinal accessory neuropathies cause scapular winging, but with a different clinical picture from serratus anterior winging (Table 29.1). Traction injuries to the brachial plexus with root avulsion or involvement of preganglionic fibers may also result in scapular

Table 29.2 Differential Diagnosis of Long Thoracic Neuropathy

Spinal accessory neuropathy
Dorsal scapular neuropathy
Brachial plexopathy
C7 radiculopathy
Neuralgic amyotrophy
Fascioscapulohumeral dystrophy
Scapuloperoneal dystrophy
Limb-girdle dystrophy
Hypermobility syndromes

winging, but clinical and electrophysiologic abnormalities are not limited to the long thoracic nerve. Winging is occasionally seen as a manifestation of C7 radiculopathy (5).

Neuralgic amyotrophy should be considered with winging of the scapula, especially when preceded by acute severe and sharp pain in the shoulder girdle unassociated with a specific event or activity or a symptom free interval following trauma. This condition is characterized by single or multiple upper extremity mononeuropathies and patchy involvement of the brachial plexus. The most common nerves affected are the long thoracic, axillary, and suprascapular (6). When needle EMG abnormalities are isolated to the long thoracic nerve, a careful history will distinguish between neuralgic amyotrophy and other etiologies.

Various types of muscular dystrophy are associated with scapular winging, notably fascioscapulohumeral (FSH), scapuloperoneal, and limb-girdle types. These disorders are easily distinguished from long thoracic nerve injury by family history, other associated findings, and histopathologic features. Rarely, winging not associated with pain is seen as a normal variant in patients with hypermobility syndromes.

2.5. Management

Initial treatment includes relative rest and avoidance of activities that cause overstretching of the serratus anterior muscle, especially those that require the arm to assume a forward flexed position. A properly designed scapular orthotic device may be helpful (7–9). Active range of motion exercises are performed in the supine position, utilizing the weight of the body to stabilize the scapula and prevent serratus overstretch (10). Much of the pain results from biomechanical overload and contracture of periscapular and antagonist muscles. Accordingly, attention is given to stretching the latissimus dorsi, levator scapulae pectoralis minor, and rhomboid muscles. Serratus strengthening is initiated as pain and range of motion improve. Other stabilizers of the scapula, especially the upper and lower trapezius must also be strengthened. Exercising these muscles in their capacity as scapular rotators, such as raising the arm overhead while supine is recommended in the early stages of recovery (7). As strength improves, more advanced closed chain exercises such as push-ups are prescribed to enhance dynamic stability of the shoulder girdle (11).

Surgical exploration and neurolysis is considered with severe axon loss. Neurolysis of the supraclavicular portion of the nerve has been successful in patients with compressive lesions in the scalene muscles (12). Different surgical procedures have been proposed to substitute for the weak serratus anterior and stabilize the scapula against the thorax. The optimal procedure is transfer of the sternal head of the pectoralis major to the inferior angle of the scapula (13,14). Transposition of the pectoralis minor, rhomboid, or teres major muscles has also been performed (15–17). Scapular fixation to the chest wall utilizing fascial slings is less successful, as it fails to provide dynamic stability to the shoulder (14).

Prognosis is largely dependent upon the mechanism of injury. Traction injuries have a favorable outcome, with recovery rates of 90–100% (2,10,11,18). Although patients typically regain full functional use, and a mild degree of scapular winging may persist (2,11,19). Prognosis in traumatic axon loss lesions is generally poor, with maximum recovery 6 months–2 years, (average time, 9 months) (2,10,11). If there is no electrophysiologic evidence of nerve function at 2 years, the prognosis for spontaneous recovery is poor and surgical stabilization of the scapula is recommended (11).

2.6. Pathogenesis

Long thoracic mononeuropathy has been attributed to many causes (Table 29.3). The superficial location of the nerve in the lateral thorax renders it susceptible to direct

Table 29.3 Causes of Long
Thoracic Neuropathy

Direct trauma
  Motor vehicle crashes
  Falls
  Carrying knapsack
Post surgical
  Thoracotomy
  First rib resection
  Radical mastectomy
  Axillary lymph node
  dissection
Indirect trauma
  Electrocution
  Chopping wood
  Sleeping on outstretched arm
  Carrying tray overhead
Sports-related
  Tennis
  Weightlifting
  Football
  Hockey
  Golf
  Baseball
  Basketball
  Gymnastics
  Wrestling
  Archery
  Discus
  Bowling
  Ballet
  Target shooting
Nontraumatic
  Post infectious
  Post immunization
  Post partum
  Familial
  Neuralgic amyotrophy
  Idiopathic

---

trauma, including motor vehicle accidents (3,20), carrying a knapsack (21), lifting (20), sleeping on an outstretched arm (19), cervical chiropractic manipulation (22), and electric shock (14,23). Surgical procedures in the axillary region may also damage the nerve, including mastectomy (24), axillary node dissection (10), and minimally invasive mitral valve surgery (25). The proximal portion of the nerve is relatively fixed by the scalenus medius muscle and is subject to traction when the arm is raised overhead or outstretched (11,26). A tight fascial band extending from the middle scalene to the first rib has been described such that abduction and external rotation of the arm may cause the long thoracic nerve to "bow string" over the fascial band, resulting in a stretch injury to the nerve (27). Thus, stretch-induced injury, including cases involving a single strenuous exertion, appears to play a significant causative role and may be the primary mechanism of injury in patients without a history of direct trauma (2,11,19). However, when there is shoulder pain in the setting of minor trauma, neuralgic amyotrophy should be considered (28).

Athletic activities have been associated with long thoracic neuropathy. The most common is tennis, especially with serving (2,11,28–30). Other sports include weightlifting (2,11), baseball (2), football (31,32), wrestling (3), basketball (32), golf (2), archery (28), shooting a rifle (33), gymnastics, bowling, hockey, and soccer (11).

Isolated injuries to the long thoracic nerve have been reported to occur after infection (3,7,19,28), immunization (3,7,31), childbirth, and cold exposure (31). Occasionally, a causative agent cannot be identified, and most likely represent a variant of neuralgic amyotrophy (6,7,19,28,30,31,34). There is a familial neuralgic amyotrophy that includes recurrent long thoracic neuropathies (35).

3. SPINAL ACCESSORY NEUROPATHY

3.1. Anatomy

The spinal accessory, or eleventh cranial nerve, is a motor nerve that supplies the sternocleidomastoid and trapezius muscles. The spinal portion of the nerve is formed by efferent branches of the first five cervical nerve roots which ascend and enter the skull through the foramen magnum, where they briefly unite with the bulbar portion of the nerve. The spinal portion then exits the skull through the jugular foramen together with the glossopharygeal and vagus nerves. Initially, the nerve lies in close proximity to the internal carotid artery and inferior jugular vein, then descends obliquely in the posterolateral neck to innervate the sternocleidomastoid muscle. The nerve continues deep to this muscle and crosses the posterior triangle of the neck. Here, the nerve lies in a superficial location, rendering it susceptible to trauma. It first supplies the upper trapezius and then runs on the deep surface of this muscle to innervate the middle and lower portions.

Although the spinal accessory nerve does not contain sensory fibers, the ventral rami of C3 and C4 from the cervical plexus often provide proprioceptive innervation from the upper trapezius (36). C2 and occasionally C3 give off sensory branches to the sternocleidomastoid. The trapezius may also receive an efferent contribution from C3 and C4 (37,38).

3.2. Clinical Features

Shoulder pain and weakness are the presenting complaints. Pain is variable and results from contracture and overload on other musculotendinous structures in the neck and shoulder girdle. Shoulder weakness is usually pronounced and typically causes more disability than that seen in serratus anterior paresis due to the trapezius' greater role in scapular stabilization. Weakness manifests primarily as inability to fully abduct the arm, and patients have significant difficulty performing overhead activities. Intracranial or intraspinal involvement of the nerve also results in weakness and atrophy of the sternocleidomastoid resulting in difficulty turning the head to the opposite side.

Atrophy of the trapezius is most noticeable in the relatively thick upper portion of the muscle, resulting in a loss of normal contour of the top of the shoulder. When atrophy is severe, the superior border of the scapula is visible above the shoulder when viewed from the front, which has been termed "moonrise scapula" (39). The upper fibers of the trapezius are the only muscle capable of elevating the point of the shoulder. When this muscle is nonfunctional, the lateral angle of the scapula is left unsupported and pulled downward by the weight of the limb. Clinically, this results in a drooped shoulder on the affected side. The most consistent feature of spinal accessory neuropathy is scapular winging which differs from that associated with long thoracic nerve injury. With trapezius weakness, abduction of the involved shoulder results in winging of the entire medial border of the scapula (Fig. 29.4). This is in contrast to serratus anterior winging which is most prominent at the inferior angle and is precipitated upon forward flexion. The trapezius as a whole, acts to retract the scapula, and weakness of this muscle together with unopposed action of the serratus and pectoralis muscles results in lateral translocation of the scapula during the act of abduction. Additionally, active abduction is limited to $\leq 90°$ due to the pivotal role played by the upper and lower fibers of the trapezius in upward rotation of the scapula. Shoulder shrug is minimally affected because of the action of the levator scapulae.

3.3. Differential Diagnosis

Scapular winging is also a prominent clinical feature of long thoracic neuropathy; however, this results in a different clinical picture that should not be confused with spinal accessory neuropathy (Table 29.1). Other conditions that can cause winging of the scapula are listed in Table 29.2. Scapular winging that occurs following surgical procedures in the neck is far more likely to be due to spinal accessory nerve damage.

3.4. Laboratory Evaluation

The diagnosis of spinal accessory neuropathy is confirmed by electrodiagnostic studies. A CMAP can be obtained by stimulating the nerve along the posterior border of the sternocleidomastoid with recording over the upper, middle, or lower portions of the trapezius (4,37,40). As most injuries are axonal, the most constant finding is a reduced CMAP (41). A prolonged distal latency is occasionally observed in focal compression of the nerve. Comparative values from the uninvolved side are necessary to determine the significance of any abnormalities seen.

Needle EMG demonstrates denervation in the trapezius. Examination of all three portions of the muscle is helpful when looking for signs of recovery following a complete

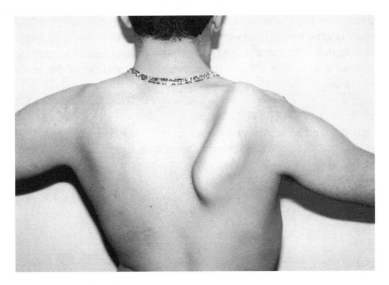

Figure 29.4 Winging of the right scapula with abduction.

injury. Involvement of the sternocleidomastoid indicates an intracranial or intraspinal lesion. It is important to examine the serratus anterior and other scapular muscles to confirm that the abnormalities are isolated to the trapezius. In cases where intracranial involvement is suspected, cranial computerized tomography (CT) or magnetic resonance imaging (MRI) is recommended (42).

3.5. Management

Early treatment consists of stretching of the rhomboids, levator scapulae, latissimus dorsi, and pectoralis minor, which have a tendency to become contracted and painful. Bracing may offer pain relief in some patients by stabilizing the scapula. Exercises to strengthen the serratus anterior, the other primary upward rotator of the scapula are given in an effort to compensate for the nonfunctional trapezius. Specific strengthening of the trapezius can begin once reinnervation is evident on electrodiagnostic studies.

Surgical exploration and neurolysis is considered in severe closed injuries if no recovery is seen after several months. Exploration is occasionally done earlier when the nerve is injured as a result of a surgical complication. Cable grafting utilizing the greater auricular nerve is often performed when the nerve is unavoidably sacrificed during radical neck dissection (38,43). Muscle transfer utilizing the levator scapulae and rhomboid muscles is successful in decreasing pain and improving function in many patients who fail or are not candidates for nerve repair (44–46).

3.6. Pathogenesis

Causes of spinal accessory neuropathy are listed in Table 29.4. The majority of injuries involve the peripheral portion of the nerve as it courses through the neck. Lesions of the intracranial portion are rare and typically result from meningioma, schwanoma, or metastases to the base of the skull (47–49). In the Vernet syndrome, the spinal accessory, glossopharygeal and vagus nerves are damaged as they pass through the jugular foramen. Patients with carotid body tumors may also present with accessory neuropathy (50).

The majority of spinal accessory neuropathies are iatrogenic, resulting from surgical procedures in the posterior triangle of the neck. Injury to the nerve can occur as a complication of lymph node biopsy (51–53), carotid endarterectomy (54–56), facelift (57), coronary artery bypass grafting (58), and internal jugular vein cannulation (59,60). The spinal accessory nerve is deliberately sacrificed during radical neck dissection, and may be injured during modified neck dissection (61,62). Intraoperative monitoring of the nerve can decrease the risk of injury (63). Blunt trauma to the neck, such as slashing in hockey or lacrosse can damage the nerve. Acute and chronic stretch injuries to the nerve have also been reported (64–66). Whiplash-type injury may also damage the nerve (67). Uncommon etiologies include suicide attempts by hanging (52), radiation (68), and penetrating trauma (42). Spinal accessory neuropathy is a rare manifestation of neuralgic amyotrophy.

4. SUPRASCAPULAR NEUROPATHY

4.1. Anatomy

The suprascapular nerve is derived from the fifth and sixth cervical nerve roots and usually arises directly from the upper trunk of the brachial plexus (Fig. 29.5). It may also arise directly from the fifth cervical root and occasionally receives a contribution from C4.

Table 29.4 Causes of Spinal
Accessory Neuropathy

Intracranial
  Meningioma
  Schwannoma
  Sarcoidosis
  Vernet syndrome
  Metastases to base of skull
Intraspinal
  Tumor
  Syringomyelia
  Motor neuron disease
  Poliomyelitis
Peripheral
  Idiopathic
    Neck dissection
    Lymph node biopsy
    Facelift
    Carotid endarterectomy
    Coronary artery bypass grafting
    Internal jugular vein cannulation
  Blunt Trauma
    Slashing in hockey
    Lacrosse
    Attempted suicide by hanging
  Traction
    Rowing
    Backpack
    Shoulder dislocation
  Radiation
  Idiopathic

It courses behind the brachial plexus between the fascia of the middle and the anterior scalene muscles, then travels deep to the omohyoid and trapezius to reach the superior border of the scapula. Here, it passes through the suprascapular foramen, a true fibro-osseous tunnel, formed by the scapular notch and overlying superior transverse scapular ligament. It first gives off a motor branch to the supraspinatus then two small sensory twigs to the acromioclavicular and glenohumeral joints. It also supplies sensory and sympathetic fibers to the spinatii and periarticular tissues. The nerve then continues downward and laterally in the supraspinatus fossa, then makes a sharp turn to pass through the spino-glenoid notch of the scapular spine, which may be covered by an inferior transverse scapular (spinoglenoid) ligament. It terminates in the infraspinatus muscle.

4.2. Clinical Features

The diagnosis of suprascapular neuropathy is often delayed or unrecognized due to the diffuse and insidious nature of symptoms. Posterior shoulder pain and weakness are the primary presenting complaints. Pain ranges from mild to severe, depending on the degree of afferent branch involvement. Pain is typically aggravated with overhead activities. Athletes engaged in throwing or overhead sports, such as baseball pitchers, volleyball, and tennis players, complain of increased pain in the cocking and release phases.

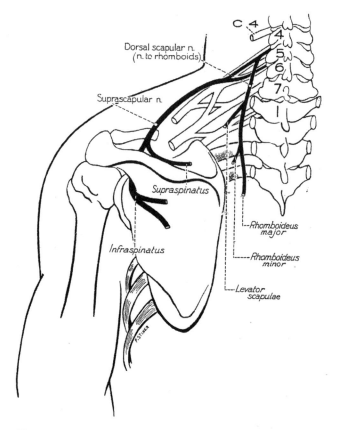

Figure 29.5 Suprascapular nerve. [From Haymaker and Woodhall (24).]

Weakness and atrophy of the infraspinatus are the principal physical findings, and the majority of patients will demonstrates weakness of external rotation of the shoulder. Supraspinatus atrophy is often masked by the overlying upper fibers of the trapezius. Weakness of the supraspinatus can be overlooked with a normally functioning deltoid, as the latter muscle is a much more powerful abductor of the arm. Sensory examination is normal, as the nerve has no cutaneous distribution. Forced adduction of the arm places the nerve on stretch and elicits pain in some patients (69,70). Tenderness over the suprascapular notch is a common finding in many patients with entrapment at this site (69). Occasionally, patients demonstrate tenderness over the spinoglenoid notch. Scapular winging is notably absent in these individuals.

4.3. Laboratory Evaluation

Suprascapular nerve conduction studies are generally less helpful than needle electromyography. Conduction studies to the supraspinatus and infraspinatus are obtained by stimulating the nerve at Erb's point, but because of the overlying trapezius muscle, surface electrode recording is not reliable (71). Consequently, nerve conduction studies using an intramuscular needle recording electrode can be used. CMAP amplitude obtained in this manner is of little diagnostic utility, owing to the limited recording area of a needle electrode. Conduction velocities are likewise of doubtful validity, due to difficulties obtaining accurate measurements in the shoulder. Thus, distal latency is the most useful parameter. The latency to the infraspinatus may be prolonged, although there is no consensus as to what constitutes a clinically significant delay or side-to-side difference. A difference of >0.4 ms correlates with denervation on needle EMG (72). Median, radial, and lateral antebrachial cutaneous sensory nerve action potential (SNAP) amplitudes are helpful in excluding upper trunk brachial plexopathy.

Needle EMG can confirm the diagnosis and differentiate from other neurologic conditions that may mimic suprascapular neuropathy (73). Abnormalities are found in the infraspinatus when the lesion is localized to either the suprascapular notch or spinoglenoid notch, whereas the supraspinatus is involved in most suprascapular notch injuries but is spared in spinoglenoid entrapment. The supraspinatus is occasionally spared in proven lesions at the scapular notch, presumably because the branch to the supraspinatus was given off proximal to the scapular notch (74). Alternatively, partial lesions of the nerve may selectively affect those fascicles that supply the infraspinatus while sparing those that supply the supraspinatus (73,75). Examination of other shoulder girdle muscles, serratus anterior, and paraspinals will distinguish isolated suprascapular neuropathy from C5 or C6 radiculopathy, upper trunk brachial plexopathy, and neuralgic amyotrophy.

Radiographs of the scapula may reveal fractures or excessive callus formation in traumatic cases. MRI is the study of choice for the evaluation of cystic lesions or other compressive etiologies, and is particularly useful when no apparent cause can be identified. Additionally, MRI can assess denervation atrophy of the spinati muscles, and therefore be of value when electrophysiologic studies are normal (76).

4.4. Differential Diagnosis

Injury to the suprascapular nerve should be considered in the differential diagnosis of rotator cuff tendinopathies, glenohumeral disorders, and myofascial pain syndrome (Table 29.5). Supraspinatus tendinosis also causes shoulder pain and weakness and is exceedingly common in athletes. Complete avulsion of the rotator cuff at its insertion typically results in disuse atrophy of the supraspinatus and infraspinatus and profound shoulder weakness. Patients with chronic adhesive capsulitis will also manifest scapular atrophy with restricted external rotation and abduction.

Patients with C5 or C6 radiculopathy or upper trunk plexopathy have a similar clinical picture; however, sensory and reflex abnormalities should differentiate these lesions from suprascapular neuropathy. Spinal accessory neuropathy causes scapular winging, while suprascapular nerve injury does not. Abrupt onset of severe sharp pain followed by weakness without a clear inciting event should raise concern for neuralgic amyotrophy.

Table 29.5 Differential
Diagnosis of Suprascapular
Neuropathy

C5, C6 radiculopathy
Upper trunk brachial plexopathy
Spinal accessory neuropathy
Neuralgic amyotrophy
Rotator cuff tendinopathy/tear
Glenohumeral disorders
Myofascial pain syndrome

4.5. Management

Conservative treatment is successful in most patients without a compressive lesion. Relative rest and range of motion exercises are prescribed in the early stage following suprascapular nerve injury. Activities that cause increased traction on the nerve, such as repetitive or sustained adduction or external rotation should be limited. Physical therapy is recommended for strengthening and to address other painful biomechanical dysfunctions of the shoulder. Suprascapular nerve block at the suprascapular notch is helpful in alleviating pain in some patients. Patients with a documented axon loss lesion in the absence of a space-occupying lesion who fail to improve with conservative measures should be referred for surgical exploration and decompression of the scapular or spinoglenoid notch (77–80). Sectioning of the transverse scapular ligament and widening of the notch has results in a favorable outcome in the majority of patients (69,70,81). Ganglion cysts may be aspirated under CT guidance or resected arthroscopically, however, large or invasive lesions usually require open excision (82,83).

4.6. Pathogenesis

A variety of causes of suprascapular neuropathy have been reported (Table 29.6). Blunt trauma, such as scapular fractures, acromioclavicular separation, and rotator cuff tears are believed to cause acute traction injury to the nerve (84–88). The suprascapular

Table 29.6   Causes of Suprascapular Neuropathy

Blunt trauma
   Scapular fracture
   Shoulder dislocation
   Acromioclavicular separation
   Fracture of proximal humerus
Post surgical
   Rotator cuff repair
   Radical neck dissection
   Supraclavicular lymph node biopsy
   Distal clavicle resection
Traction
   Sustained shoulder adduction
   Forcible shoulder depression
   Repetitive external rotation
   Anabolic steroid use
Sports-related
   Volleyball
   Baseball
   Tennis
   Football
   Weightlifting
   Wrestling
Mass lesions
   Ganglion cysts
   Chondrosarcoma
   Synovialsarcoma
   Ewing's sarcoma
   Metastatic disease

nerve is damaged with surprising frequency in anterior dislocation of the shoulder (86,89,90). Suprascapular neuropathy occurs as an infrequent complication of surgical procedures involving the neck and shoulder girdle (91,92).

Chronic repetitive traction, especially in athletes, is one mechanism. Sustained shoulder adduction is thought to cause a stretch injury to the proximal portion of the nerve, which is tethered at the suprascapular notch (84). Suprascapular neuropathy isolated to the infraspinatus muscle has been described in throwing and overhead athletes. Most of these have been reported to occur in the dominant arm of elite volleyball players (93–96), baseball pitchers (74,77,97), tennis players (87,98), weightlifters (69,81,97–100), a dancer (101), a fencer (102), and a skeet shooter (97). Many of these injuries were postulated to occur from repetitive stretch to the terminal portion of the nerve as it makes a sharp turn around the lateral aspect of the scapular spine and the relative fixation of the nerve at the spinoglenoid notch (78,102). Alternatively, repetitive throwing may cause intimal damage to the suprascapular or axillary arteries, leading to microembolization of the vaso nervorum and ultimately nerve damage (74). One case was attributed to intramuscular compression of the terminal branches from rapid hypertrophy associated with anabolic steroid use (100).

True entrapment of the suprascapular nerve can occur at the suprascapular and spinoglenoid foramina. On the basis of the relative dimensions and shape of the notch and foramen, six distinct types of suprascapular notches have been described (103). Patients with a deep, V-shaped notch are at higher risk of developing entrapment at the suprascapular notch (103). Other anatomic risk factors include hypertrophy or ossification of the superior and inferior transverse scapular ligaments and a small diameter foramen (79,102–105). Entrapment of the nerve has also been found to occur proximally between the fascia of the anterior and middle scalene muscles, between the omyhyoid and sub clavius fascia and distally within the suprascapular fossa, and between the suprascapular fascia and base of the coracoid process (74).

Compression of the suprascapular nerve also occurs from space-occupying lesions, such as a ganglion cyst, which are being identified with increasing frequency, due in large part to the routine use of MRI in the evaluation of shoulder pain (82,83,106–108). Cysts are also seen in asymptomatic patients and rarely become clinically significant unless they compress the suprascapular nerve (109). The etiology of these cysts is controversial. The proximity of many ganglion cysts to the glenohumeral joint has led some investigators to theorize that the cysts are formed by the leakage of joint fluid from glenoid labral tears (110). Additionally, ganglia are typically located in the posterior superior aspect of the joint space, corresponding to the relative weakness of the capsule above the posterior band of the inferior glenohumeral ligament, thereby allowing extravasation of joint fluid into the suprascapular and spinoglenoid foramina (110). Other malignant masses reported to cause suprascapular nerve compression include chondrosarcoma, synoviosarcoma, Ewing's sarcoma, and metastatic renal cell carcinoma, although these are quite rare (82).

5. AXILLARY NEUROPATHY

5.1. Anatomy

The axillary nerve is a mixed nerve that carries fibers from the fifth and sixth cervical roots and arises directly from the posterior cord of the brachial plexus at the level of the coracoid process (Fig. 29.6). It courses under the coracoid along the anterior surface of the subscapularis then passes through the quadrilateral space accompanied by the posterior circumflex humeral artery. The quadrilateral space is bounded superiorly by the teres minor and

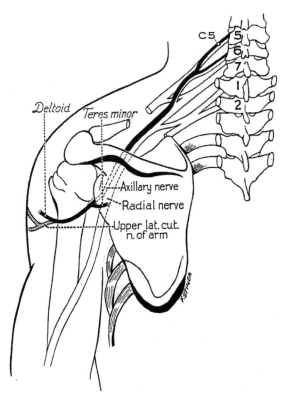

Figure 29.6   Axillary nerve. [From Haymaker and Woodhall (24).]

subscapularis, laterally by the surgical neck of the humerus, inferiorly by the teres major and medial by the long head of the triceps tendon. Here, the nerve divides into posterior and anterior branches. The posterior branch innervates the posterior deltoid and teres minor, then continues as the lateral brachial cutaneous nerve which supplies cutaneous sensation to the lateral aspect of the shoulder. The anterior branch wraps around the surgical neck of the humerus to supply the middle and anterior deltoid and provides sensory branches to the glenohumeral joint.

5.2.   Clinical Features

The principal findings are atrophy and weakness of the deltoid. Wasting of the deltoid results in loss of the normal contour of the shoulder and upper arm. In some cases, the acromion and humeral head are visible, giving the shoulder a "squared" appearance (24). Abduction weakness is the major functional deficit. Full abduction is possible with complete paralysis of the deltoid due to the action of the supraspinatus muscle. The teres minor externally rotates the arm; however, weakness of this muscle is difficult to detect clinically as the infraspinatus is much more efficient in performing this action. Sensory loss over the lateral shoulder is present in many but not all patients.

5.3.   Laboratory Evaluation

Electrophysiologic studies are valuable in confirming the diagnosis and assessing the extent of axon loss. Axillary CMAP latencies and amplitudes are reliably obtained by stimulating at Erb's point and surface electrode recording over the lateral deltoid (71). A decreased CMAP amplitude and prolonged latency are the expected abnormalities. Comparative values from the contralateral side should be obtained. No reliable technique for obtaining an axillary SNAP has been described. Median, radial, and lateral ante-brachial cutaneous SNAPs are helpful in excluding an upper trunk or posterior cord lesion.

Needle EMG abnormalities are found in the deltoid and teres minor. Examination of all three portions of the deltoid is beneficial when performing serial studies of severe axonal injuries, as reinnervation typically proceeds in a posterior to anterior fashion. It is important to study the paraspinal muscles and other shoulder girdle muscles to rule out a C5 radiculopathy or upper trunk brachial plexopathy. The rhomboids receive their innervation exclusively from C5 prior to the formation of the upper trunk, therefore are particularly useful in excluding both of these diagnoses. Additionally, sampling of the latissimus dorsi and radial innervated muscles allow an isolated axillary nerve injury to be distinguished from a posterior cord lesion.

5.4. Differential Diagnosis

Axillary neuropathy can mimic other neurologic conditions that cause shoulder pain and weakness (Table 29.7). These disorders are often difficult to distinguish solely on clinical grounds, highlighting the importance of the electrodiagnostic examination in the evaluation of these patients. Moreover, axillary nerve lesions commonly occur in combination with injuries of the brachial plexus and other peripheral nerve, further complicating the clinical diagnosis.

An important diagnostic consideration in patients with deltoid weakness is C5 radiculopathy. In contrast to isolated axillary nerve injury, weakness, and atrophy are rarely severe in radiculopathy. Additionally, neck pain and a diminished biceps reflex are typically associated with C5 root lesions. Patients with upper trunk lesions demonstrate more widespread weakness of the shoulder girdle and biceps as well as sensory loss in the thumb. As noted above, lesions of the posterior cord also result in deltoid weakness; however, involvement of radial innervated muscles is also a feature of this disorder. As it the case with other nerves arising from the brachial plexus, the axillary nerve is commonly involved in neuralgic amyotrophy. This diagnosis is considered when pain is severe and no distinct injury has occurred. Shoulder pain and abduction weakness are seen in patients with rotator cuff tears and adhesive capsulitis, although these disorders do not result in isolated atrophy and weakness of the deltoid.

5.5. Management

Treatment is guided by the severity of injury as determined by clinical and electrophysiologic examination (42). If the injury is mild, then physical therapy is appropriate for range

Table 29.7 Differential Diagnosis of Axillary Neuropathy

C5, C6 radiculopathy
Upper trunk brachial plexopathy
Posterior cord plexopathy
Neuralgic amyotrophy
Rotator cuff tendinopathy
Adhesive capsulitis of shoulder

of motion and strengthening. The prognosis for spontaneous recovery in these cases is good (111). Patients with severe axonal damage should be assessed monthly for signs of improvement (42). If there is no evidence of recovery by 3–4 months, surgical exploration is recommended (112–115). Given the short distance between the site of injury and the deltoid, the prognosis for spontaneous recovery beyond this time is poor. Surgical options include neurolysis, neurotization, and nerve grafting, which result in a good outcome in the majority of patients (112,113,115).

5.6. Pathogenesis

Causes of axillary neuropathy are listed in Table 29.8. Injury to the nerve is most likely to result from shoulder dislocation and fracture of the surgical neck of the humerus (86,89,116). In one large series, the incidence of axillary nerve injuries in patients with these conditions was 37% (89). Isolated damage to the axillary nerve was found in 8%; the remaining injuries occurred in various combinations with the suprascapular, musculocutaneous and radial nerves (89). Elderly patients and those with hematoma formation after shoulder trauma appear to be at higher risk of injuring the axillary nerve (89). Reduction of a shoulder dislocation has been reported to damage the nerve (117). Blunt trauma to the deltoid without dislocation can also damage the axillary nerve (118). Various sports have been reported to injure the nerve in this manner, including football, hockey, wrestling, boxing, and basketball (119,120). The nerve is also injured from penetrating trauma to the shoulder girdle. Injury to the anterior branch of the axillary nerve has been reported in a paraplegic patient following vigorous exercise (121). Hypertrophy of the muscles of the quadrilateral space were theorized to compress the nerve in this patient, thus this may represent the first reported case of quadrilateral space syndrome

Table 29.8   Causes of Axillary Neuropathy

Traumatic
   Shoulder dislocation
   Proximal humerus fracture
   Shoulder contusion
   Vigorous exercise
   Sleeping on a firm mattress
   Penetrating injuries
Iatrogenic
   Intramuscular injection
   Reduction of shoulder dislocation
   Shoulder arthroscopy
   Anterior shoulder surgery
   Radiofrequency capsulorrhaphy
Sports-related
   Football
   Hockey
   Basketball
   Wrestling
   Boxing
Quadrilateral space syndrome
Neuralgic amyotrophy

(discussed subsequently). Compression of the anterior branch from sleeping on a firm mattress has also been described in a patient with hereditary neuropathy with liability to pressure palsies (122).

Iatrogenic causes have also been described, including complication of shoulder arthroscopy (123), anterior shoulder surgery (124), and intramuscular injection into the deltoid (125). Axillary neuropathy is occasionally seen following radiofrequency capsular shrinkage of the shoulder (126). Indirect thermal injury to the nerve from heating of surrounding tissues was believed to be the cause in these cases.

A controversial cause of axillary neuropathy has been reported to occur in the quadrilateral space. In this syndrome, it is hypothesized that muscle hypertrophy and repeated external rotation and abduction of the arm common in throwing athletes results in a decrease in the size of the quadrilateral space, thereby compressing the axillary nerve and posterior circumflex humeral artery between surrounding muscle and proximal humerus (127). Fibrous bands have also been found to compress the nerve in the space (128). Clinically, patients with this syndrome present with localized tenderness in the quadrilateral space and provocation of symptoms with sustained abduction and external rotation of the affected limb. In initial reports of the syndrome, all patients had abnormal dynamic subclavian arteriograms, demonstrating occlusion of the posterior circumflex humeral artery with the arm abducted and externally rotated (128–130). Neurologic and electromyographic examinations were normal in all cases. Nevertheless, injury to the axillary nerve as felt to be a defining characteristic of the disorder (128). Most of these patients underwent decompression of the quadrilateral space with axillary neurolysis being performed in onc case (128,130). In another series, EMG abnormalities were found in 3 of 5 patients presumed to have the syndrome; however, other associated peripheral nerve lesions were also observed (131). It is probable that these patients actually had neuralgic amyotrophy rather than axillary nerve compression (42). Evidence for isolated involvement of the axillary nerve in the quadrilateral space was provided in a report of two elite volleyball players who presented with painless weakness and atrophy of the deltoid muscle (127). Both had decreased axillary CMAP amplitudes and isolated denervation of the deltoid on electrophysiologic studies. Complete recovery occurred with rest and conservative measures. This suggests that the quadrilateral space syndrome is a vascular phenomenon in the majority of patients and compression of the axillary nerve in the quadrilateral space is exceedingly rare.

6. MUSCULOCUTANEOUS NEUROPATHY

6.1. Anatomy

The musculocutaneous nerve usually originates from the lateral cord of the brachial plexus and carries fibers from the C5, C6, and occasionally C7 nerve roots (Fig. 29.7). Rarely, it comes off directly from the median nerve or posterior cord. Immediately after supplying the coracobracialis muscle, the nerve pierces this muscle and comes to lie between the biceps and the brachialis muscles. It innervates both heads of the biceps and brachialis then continues distally as the lateral antebrachial cutaneous nerve. The brachialis often receives an additional branch from the radial nerve. The musculocutaneous nerve occasionally gives off a branch to the pronator teres and flexor carpi radialis. The lateral antebrachial cutaneous nerve travels lateral to the biceps tendon in the antecubital fossa, then pierces the brachial fascia. It divides into anterior and posterior branches supplying sensation to the radial aspect of the forearm.

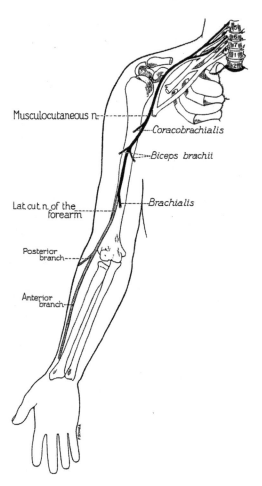

Musculocutaneous n.

Coracobrachialis

Biceps brachii

Lat.cut.n. of the forearm

Brachialis

Posterior branch

Anterior branch

Figure 29.7   Musculocutaneous nerve. [From Haymaker and Woodhall (24).]

6.2.   Clinical Features

The typical presentation is painless weakness of the arm flexors (132), although severe pain can occur in some patients (133). Sensory abnormalities in the radial forearm are commonly found. Atrophy of the biceps and brachialis can be impressive in chronic injuries. Weakness of the arm flexion and supination are the most prominent deficits; however, elbow flexion is usually preserved even in complete paralysis of these muscles owing to the actions of the brachioradialis and pronator teres. Weakness of the coracobrachialis is difficult to detect clinically. It assists in flexion of the arm at the shoulder; however, the anterior deltoid is the chief mover and can effectively mask a paralyzed coracobrachialis muscle. Similarly, the coracobrachialis is a weak adductor of the arm, although this action is brought about primarily by the pectoralis major, latissimus dorsi, and teres major. A diminished biceps reflex is frequently seen.

6.3.   Laboratory Evaluation

Electrodiagnostic examination will confirm involvement of the musculocutaneous nerve, provide information regarding extent of injury and exclude other neurologic conditions that produce a similar clinical picture. A musculocutaneous SNAP can reliably be obtained from the lateral antebrachial cutaneous nerve (134,135). A reduced or absent SNAP amplitude is expected in musculocutaneous neuropathy and upper trunk plexopathy. Radial and median SNAPs recording from the thumb are useful in excluding the latter possibility. The lateral antebrachial cutaneous SNAP will be normal in patients with C6 radiculopathy. The musculocutaneous CMAP amplitude, obtained by surface recording over the biceps and stimulating at Erb's point (71), or axilla (134), is decreased in axon loss injuries to the nerve.

Needle EMG findings are found in the coracobrachialis, biceps, and brachialis, although sparing of the coracobrachialis is seen in distal lesions. Examination of other shoulder girdle and paraspinal muscles will discriminate isolated musculocutaneous neuropathy from C6 radiculopathy and upper trunk plexopathy. Sampling of the pronator teres and flexor carpi radialis is useful in excluding a lesion of the lateral cord.

6.4. Differential Diagnosis

The differential diagnosis of musculocutaneous neuropathy is listed in Table 29.9. Weakness of arm flexion and a decreased biceps reflex are commonly seen in patients with C6 radiculopathy; however associated weakness of the deltoid and brachioradialis should differentiate this from musculocutaneous neuropathy. Upper trunk and lateral cord injuries are ruled out by electrodiagnostic studies. The musculocutaneous nerve is commonly involved in neuralgic amyotrophy in association with other peripheral nerves. The clinical presentation of neuralgic amyotrophy is distinctive and contrasts with isolated musculocutaneous injury, in which pain is generally not a prominent feature. Spontaneous rupture of the long head of the biceps tendon also produces painless weakness of arm flexion and loss of the biceps reflex. In this disorder, attempted arm flexion at the elbow causes the biceps to bunch up into a spherical shape distally, producing a very characteristic appearance. Because the brachialis and other arm flexors remain functional, rupture of the tendon results in less weakness than does musculocutaneous neuropathy. Additionally, sensation in the radial forearm is normal in patients with a ruptured biceps tendon.

6.5. Management

Patients with partial lesions of the musculocutaneous nerve benefit from relative rest and physical therapy. Emphasis is placed on maintaining range of motion and strengthening of the involved muscles. The prognosis for recovery is good (132,136–140). In severe closed injuries, serial physical and electrodiagnostic examinations should be performed to monitor for recovery. If no electrophysiologic evidence of recovery is seen in 3–4 months, surgical exploration is warranted, and neurolysis or nerve grafting considered,

Table 29.9 Differential Diagnosis of Musculocutaneous Neuropathy

---

C6 radiculopathy
Upper trunk plexopathy
Lateral cord plexopathy
Neuralgic amyotrophy
Rupture of biceps tendon

---

with good results reported with grafting (141). Initial treatment of patients with isolated injury to the lateral antebrachial cutaneous nerve consists of analgesics, splinting, and corticosteroid injections. Surgical decompression of the biceps aponeurosis in the antecubital fossa is indicated when conservative measures fail, with a favorable outcome reported in most patients (142,143).

6.6. Pathogenesis

Most injuries to the musculocutaneous nerve result from traction, compression, or a combination of both (Table 29.10). It is more common for the nerve to be injured in conjunction with the upper trunk and lateral cord than in isolation. Blunt trauma to the anterior shoulder resulting in contusions, proximal humeral, or clavicular fractures can cause direct injury to the nerve (137,144,145). Penetrating trauma such as stab or bullet wounds may also damage the nerve (42,146). Musculocutaneous neuropathy occurs in association with shoulder dislocation (89,116). Strenuous physical activity and violent elbow extension have been reported to injure the nerve (132–134,138,146). The coracobrachialis was spared in these cases, indicating compression of the nerve within this muscle, possibly due to forceful contraction or hypertrophy (132). An additional case of intramuscular compression has been reported in a weightlifter, which was believed to be due to rapid hypertrophy from anabolic steroid use (100). An unusual case of musculocutaneous neuropathy from carrying rolls of carpet has been reported (139).

Iatrogenic musculocutaneous neuropathy occurs as a complication of surgical procedures of the shoulder (123,124,140). The musculocutaneous nerve is at risk during shoulder arthroscopy (123). Three mechanisms of injury unique to this procedure have been described, including excessive glenohumeral distraction from longitudinal traction on the arm, massive extravasation of fluid in the anterior shoulder, and direct injury to the nerve via the anterior portal (123). Prolonged positioning of the arm in hyperextension, external rotation, or abduction during surgical procedures has been reported to damage the musculocutaneous nerve (136,147–149). Compression from a blood pressure cuff was hypothesized to be a contributing factor in one case (149). Musculocutaneous neuropathy occurs in association with neuralgic amyotrophy but rarely as an isolated finding.

Isolated lateral antebrachial cutaneous nerve injury is most commonly seen from compression or direct trauma in the antecubital fossa. Many of these are iatrogenic, including venipuncture of the cephalic vein and radial artery bypass in coronary artery bypass operations (150–154). Compression of the nerve by the biceps tendon and aponeurosis has been described (142,143,155,156). Lateral antebrachial nerve compression has been reported in quadriplegics (157), and from carrying a heavy handbag (158), or food tray

Table 29.10 Causes of
Musculocutaneous Neuropathy

Blunt trauma to shoulder
Shoulder dislocation
Strenuous physical activity
Violent elbow extension
Anabolic steroid use
Shoulder surgery
Shoulder arthroscopy
General anesthesia
Blood pressure cuff

(159) across the forearm. Vigorous extension and pronation of the forearm (160) and cryotherapy (161) may also damage the nerve.

7. CONCLUSIONS

Focal neuropathy of the shoulder is a frequently overlooked cause of upper extremity pain and dysfunction. These lesions often mimic other soft tissue and neurologic disorders, highlighting the critical role of EMG in establishing the diagnosis. Additionally, EMG is unique in its ability to assess pathophysiology and severity of injury, providing valuable information to guide clinical decision-making. As many of these conditions occur in distinctive settings or as a result of specific activities, it is important to obtain an accurate injury history. With prompt recognition, most proximal neuropathies respond favorably to conservative measures, although surgical management is necessary in some cases.

REFERENCES

1. Horwitz MT, Tocantins LM. An anatomic study of the role of the long thoracic nerve and the related scapular bursae in the pathogenesis of local paralysis of the serratus anterior muscle. Anat Rec 1938; 71:375–385.
2. Schultz JS, Leonard JA. Long thoracic neuropathy from athletic activity. Arch Phys Med Rehabil 1992; 73:87–90.
3. Goodman CE, Kenrick MM, Blum MV. Long thoracic nerve palsy: a follow-up study. Arch Phys Med Rehabil 1975; 56:352–355.
4. Liveson JA, Ma DM. Laboratory Reference for Clinical Neurophysiology. Philadelphia: FA Davis, 1992:48–52.
5. Makin GV, Brown WF, Ebers GC. C7 radiculopathy: importance of scapular winging in clinical diagnosis. J Neurol Neurosurg Psychiatry 1986; 49:640–644.
6. Parsonage MJ, Turner JA. Neuralgic amyotrophy: the shoulder-girdle syndrome. Lancet 1948; 1:973–978.
7. Johnson JH, Kendall HO. Isolated paralysis of the serratus anterior muscle. J Bone Joint Surg (Am) 1955; 37:567–574.
8. Truong XT, Rippel DV. Orthotic devices for serratus anterior palsy: some biomechanical considerations. Arch Phys Med Rehabil 1979; 60:66–69.
9. Marin R. Scapula winger's brace: a case series on the management of long thoracic nerve palsy. Arch Phys Med Rehabil 1998; 79:1226–1230.
10. Duncan MA, Lotze MT, Gerber LH, Rosenberg SA. Incidence, recover, and management of serratus anterior muscle palsy after axilary node dissection. Phys Ther 1983; 63:1243–1247.
11. Gregg JR, Labosky D. Harty M, Lotke, P, Ecker M, DiStefano V, Das M. Serratus anterior paralysis in the young athlete. J Bone Joint Surg (Am) 1979; 61:825–832.
12. Disa JJ, Wang B, Dellon AL. Correction of scapular winging by supraclavicular neurolysis of the long thoracic nerve. J Reconstr Microsurg 2001; 17(2):79–84.
13. Wiater JM, Flatow EL. Long thoracic nerve injury. Clin Orthop 1999; 368:17–27.
14. Marmor L, Bechtol CO. Paralysis of the serratus anterior due to electric shock relieved by transplantation of the pectoralis major muscle. J Bone Joint Surg (Am) 1963; 45:156–160.
15. Rapp IH. Seratus anterior paralysis treated by transplantation of the pectoralis minor. J Bone Joint Surg (Am) 1954; 36:852–854.
16. Herzmark MH. Traumatic paralysis of the serratus anterior relieved by transplantation of the rhomboidei. J Bone Joint Surg (Am) 1951; 33:235–238.
17. Harmon PH. Surgical reconstruction of the paralytic shoulder by multiple muscle transplantations. J Bone Joint Surg (Am) 1950; 32:583–595.

18. Fardin P, Negrin P, Dainese R. The isolated paralysis of the serratus anterior muscle: clinical and electromyographical follow-up of 10 cases. Electromyogr Clin Neurophysiol 1978; 18:379–386.

19. Overpeck DO, Ghormley RK. Paralysis of the serratus magnus muscle caused by lesions of the long thoracic nerve. J Am Med Assoc 1940; 114:1994–1996.

20. Hauser CU, Martin WF. Two additional cases of traumatic winged scapula occurring in the armed forces. J Am Med Assoc 1943; 121:667–668.

21. Ilfeld FW, Holder HG. Winged scapula: case occurring in a soldier from a knapsack. J Am Med Assoc 1942; 120:448–449.

22. Oware A, Herskovitz S. Berger AR. Long thoracic nerve palsy following cervical chiropractic manipulation. Muscle Nerve 1995; 18:1351.

23. Still JM, Law EJ, Duncan JW, Hughes HF. Long thoracic nerve injury due to an electric burn. J Burn Care Rehabil 1996; 17:562–564.

24. Haymaker W, Woodhall B. Peripheral Nerve Injuries: Principles of Diagnosis. 2nd ed. Philadelphia: WB Saunders, 1953:222–238.

25. Chaney MA, Morales M, Bakhos M. Severe incisional pain and long thoracic nerve injury after port-access minimally invasive mitral valve surgery. Anesth Analg 2000; 91:288–290.

26. Ebraheim NA, Lu J, Porshinsky B, Heck BE, Yeasting RA. Vulnerability of long thoracic nerve: an anatomic study. J Shoulder Elbow Surg 1998; 7:458–461.

27. Hester P, Caborn DN, Nyland J. Cause of long thoracic nerve palsy: a possible dynamic fascial sling cause. J Shoulder Elbow Surg 2000; 9:31–35.

28. Foo CL, Swann M. Isolated paralysis of the serratus anterior. J Bone Joint Surg (Br) 1983; 65:552–556.

29. Foucar HO. The "clover leaf" sling in paralysis of the serratus magnus. Br Med J 1933; 2:865–866.

30. Goodman CE. Unusual nerve injuries in recreational activities. Am J Sports Med 1983; 11:224–227.

31. Hannson KG. Serratus magnus paralysis. Arch Phys Med Rehabil 1948; 29:156–161.

32. Kaplan PE. Electrodiagnostic confirmation of long thoracic nerve palsy. J Neurol Neurosurg Psychiatry 1980; 43:50–52.

33. Woodhead AB III. Paralysis of the serratus anterior in a world class marksman: a case study. Am J Sports Med 1985; 13:359–362.

34. Lederman RJ. Long thoracic neuropathy in instrumental musicians: an often unrecognized cause of shoulder pain. Med Probl Perform Art 1996; 11:116–119.

35. Phillips LH. Familial long thoracic nerve palsy: a manifestation of brachial plexus neuropathy. Neurology 1986; 36:1251–1253.

36. Jenkins DB. Hollinshead's Functional Anatomy of the Limbs and Back. 6th ed. Philadelphia: WB Saunders, 1991:91.

37. Fahrer J, Ludin HP, Mumenthaler M, Neiger M. The innervation of the trapezius muscle: an electrophysiologic study. J Neurol 1974; 207:183–188.

38. Weisberger EC. The efferent supply of the trapezius muscle: a neuroanatomic basis for the preservation of shoulder function during neck dissection. Laryngoscope 1987; 97:435–445.

39. Nelson KR, Bicknell JM. Oblique pectoral crease and moonrise scapula as signs of trapezius muscle weakness. Neurology 1985; 35(suppl 1):334.

40. Green RF, Brien M. Accessory nerve latency to the middle and lower trapezius. Arch Phys Med Rehabil 1985; 66:23–24.

41. Dimitru D, Zwarts M, Amato A. Electrodiagnostic Medicine. 2nd ed. Philadelphia: Hanley and Belfus, 2002:692.

42. Stewart JD. Focal Peripheral Neuropathies. 3rd ed. Philadelphia: Lippincott, 2000:88–91, 157–181.

43. Anderson R, Flowers RS. Free grafts of the spinal accessory nerve during radical neck dissection. Am J Surg 1969; 118:796–799.

44. Bigliani LU, Compito CA, Duralde XA, Wolfe IN. Transfer of the levator scapulae, rhomboid major and rhomboid minor for paralysis of the trapezius. J Bone Joint Surg 1996; 78:1534–1540.

45. Coessens BC, Wood MB. Levator scapulae transfer and fascia lata fasciodesis for chronic spinal accessory nerve palsy. J Reconstr Microsurg 1995; 11:277–280.
46. Wiater JM, Bigliani LU. Spinal accessory nerve injury. Clin Orthop 1999; 368:5–16.
47. Greenberg HS. Metastasis to the base of the skull: clinical findings in 43 patients. Neurology 1981; 31:530–537.
48. Kaye AH. Jugular foramen schwannomas. J Neurosurg 1984; 60:1045–1053.
49. Ortiz O, Reed L. Spinal accessory nerve schwannoma involving the jugular foramen. Am J Neuroradiol 1995; 16(suppl 4):986–989.
50. Clark AJ, Chalmers RT. Bilateral carotid body tumours presenting with accessory nerve palsy. Eur J Vas Endovasc Surg 2002; 23:87–88.
51. Norden A. Peripheral injuries to the spinal accessory nerve. Acta Chir Scand 1946; 94:515–531.
52. Berry H, MacDonald EA, Mrazek AC. Accessory nerve palsy: a review of 23 cases. Can J Neurol Sci 1991; 18:337–341.
53. King RJ, Motta G. Iatrogenic spinal accessory nerve palsy. Ann R Coll Surg Engl 1983; 65:35–37.
54. Sweeney PJ, Wilbourn AJ. Spinal accessory (11th) nerve palsy following carotid endarterectomy. Neurology 1992; 42:674–675.
55. Yagnik PM, Chong PS. Spinal accessory nerve injury: a complication of carotid endarterectomy. Muscle Nerve 1996; 19:907–909.
56. Swann KW, Heros RC. Accessory nerve palsy following carotid endarterectomy: report of two cases. J Neurosurg 1985; 63:630–632.
57. Blackwell KE, Landman MD, Calceterra TC. Spinal accessory nerve palsy: an unusual complication of rhytidectomy. Head Neck 1994; 16:181–185.
58. Marini SG, Rook JL, Green RF, Nagler W. Spinal accessory nerve palsy: an unusual complication of coronary artery bypass. Arch Phys Med Rehabil 1991; 72:247–249.
59. Hoffman JC. Permanent paralysis of the accessory nerve after cannulation of the internal jugular vein. Anesthesiology 1984; 58:583–584.
60. Burns S, Herbison GJ. Spinal accessory nerve injury as a complication of internal jugular vein cannulation. Ann Int Med 1996; 125:700.
61. Ewing MR, Martin H. Disability following "radical neck dissection": an assessment based on the postoperative evaluation of 100 patients. Cancer 1952; 5:873–883.
62. Remmler D, Byers R, Scheetz J, Shell B, White G, Zimmerman S, Goepfert H. A prospective study of shoulder disability resulting from radical and modified neck dissections. Head Neck Surg 1986; 8:280–286.
63. Midwinter K, Willatt D. Accessory nerve monitoring and stimulation during neck surgery. J Laryngol Otol 2002; 116:272–274.
64. Logigian EL, McInnes JM, Berger AR, Busis NA, Lehrich JR, Shahani BT. Stretch-induced spinal accessory nerve palsy. Muscle Nerve 1988; 11:146–150.
65. Dellon AL, Campbell JN, Cornblath D. Stretch palsy of the spinal accessory nerve: case report. J Neurosurg 1990; 72:500–502.
66. Cohn BT, Brahms MA, Cohn M. Injury to the eleventh cranial nerve in a high school wrestler. Orthop Rev 1986; 15:590–595.
67. Bodack MP, Tunkel RS, Marini SG, Nagler W. Spinal accessory nerve palsy as a cause of pain after whiplash injury: case report. J Pain Symptom Manage 1998; 15:321–328.
68. Berger PS, Bataini JP. Radiation-induced cranial nerve palsy. Cancer 1977; 40:152–155.
69. Callahan JD, Scully TB, Shapiro SA, Worth RM. Suprascapular nerve entrapment: a series of 27 cases. J Neurosurg 1991; 74:893–896.
70. Antoniadis G, Richter HP, Rath S, Braun V, Moese G. Suprascapular nerve entrapment: experience with 28 cases. J Neurosurg 1996; 85:1020–1025.
71. Kraft GH. Axillary, musculocutaneous and suprascapular nerve latency studies. Arch Phys Med Rehabil 1972; 53:383–387.
72. Edgar TS, Lotz BP. A nerve conduction technique for the evaluation of suprascapular neuropathies. Muscle Nerve 1998; 21:1580.

73. Bird SJ, Williams GR, Iannotti JP. Clinical and EMG features of suprascapular neuropathy. Muscle Nerve 1997; 20:1063.

74. Ringel SP, Treihaft M, Carry M, Fisher R, Jacobs P. Suprascapular neuropathy in pitchers. Am J Sports Med 1990; 18:80–86.

75. Stewart JD. Suprascapular neuropathies. 2000 AAEM Course C: Unusual Mononeuropathies. Philadelphia, PA: American Association of Electrodiagnostic Medicine 47th Annual Scientific Meeting, 2000.

76. Zeiss J, Woldenberg LS, Saddemi SR, Ebraheim NA. MRI of suprascapular neuropathy in a weight lifter. J Comput Assist Tomogr 1993; 17:303–308.

77. Cummins CA, Bowen M, Anderson K, Messer T. Suprascapular nerve entrapment at the spinogelnoid notch in a professional baseball pitcher. Am J Sports Med 1999; 27:810–812.

78. Rengarchary SS, Neff J, Singer PA, Brackett CE. Suprascapular entrapment neuropathy: a clinical, anatomical, and comparative study. Part 1: clinical study. Neurosurgery 1979; 5:441–446.

79. Garcia G, McQueen D. Bilateral suprascapular-nerve entrapment syndrome. Case report and review of the literature. J Bone Joint Surg 1981; 63A:491–492.

80. Clein LJ. Suprascapular entrapment neuropathy. J Neurosurg 1975; 43:337–342.

81. Berry H, Kong K, Hudson AR, Moulton RJ. Isolated suprascapular nerve palsy: a review of nine cases. Can J Neurol Sci 1995; 22:301–304.

82. Fritz RC, Helms CA, Steinbach LS, Genant HK. Suprascapular nerve entrapment: evaluation with MR imaging. Radiology 1992; 182:437–444.

83. Iannotti JP, Ramsey ML. Arthroscopic decompression of a ganglion cyst causing suprascapular nerve compression. Arthroscopy 1996; 12:739–745.

84. Kopell HP, Thompson WA. Peripheral Entrapment Neuropathies. 2nd ed. Huntington, New York: Krieger, 1976:147–159.

85. Kaplan PE, Kernahan WT. Rotator cuff rupture: management with suprascapular neuropathy. Arch Phys Med Rehabil 1984; 65:273–275.

86. Wardner JM, Leonard JA, Schultz JS, Jackson MD. Concurrent suprascapular and axillary mononeuropathies. Arch Phys Med Rehabil 1989; 70.

87. Yoon TN, Grabois M, Guillen M. Suprascapular nerve injury following trauma to the shoulder. J Trauma 1981; 21:652–655.

88. Brown TD, Newton PM, Steinman SP, Levine WN, Bigliani LU. Rotator cuff tears and associated nerve injuries. Orthopedics 2000; 23:329–332.

89. DeLaat ET, Visser CJ, Coene LM, Pahlplatz PM, Tavy DJ. Nerve lesions in primary shoulder dislocations and humeral neck fractures. J Bone Joint Surg 1994; 76-B:381–383.

90. Zoltan JD. Injury to the suprascapular nerve associated with anterior dislocation of the shoulder: case report and review of the literature. J Trauma 1979; 19:203–206.

91. Zanotti RM, Carpenter JE, Blaiser RB, Greenfield ML, Adler RS, Bromberg MB. The low incidence of suprascapular nerve injury after primary repair of massive rotator cuff tears. J Shoulder Elbow Surg 1997; 6:258–264.

92. Mallon WJ, Bronec PR, Spinner RJ, Levin LS. Suprascapular neuropathy after distal clavicle excision. Clin Orthop 1996; 207–211.

93. Ferretti A, Cerullo G, Russo G. Suprascapular neuropathy in volleyball players. J Bone Joint Surg 1987; 69-A:260–263.

94. Montagna P, Colonna S. Suprascapular neuropathy restricted to the infraspinatus muscle in volleyball players. Acta Neurol Scand 1993; 87:248–250.

95. Holzgraefe M, Kukowski B, Eggert S. Prevalence of latent and manifest suprascapular neuropathy in high-performance volleyball players. Br J Sport Med 1994; 28:177–179.

96. Mittal S, Turcinovic M, Gould ES, Vishnubhakat SM. Acute isolated suprascapular nerve palsy limited to the infraspinatus muscle: a case report. Arch Phys Med Rehabil 2002; 83:565–567.

97. Liveson JA, Bronson MJ, Pollack MA. Suprascapular nerve lesions at the spinoglenoid notch: report of three cases and review of the literature. J Neurol Neurosurg Psychiatry 1991; 54:241–243.

98. Black KP, Lombardo JA. Suprascapular nerve injuries with isolated paralysis of the infraspinatus. Am J Sports Med 1990; 18:225–228.

99. Agree JC, Ash N, Cameron MC, House J. Suprascapular neuropathy after intensive progressive resistive exercise: case report. Arch Phys Med Rehabil 1986; 68:236–238.

100. Bird SJ, Brown MJ. Acute focal neuropathy in male weightlifters. Muscle Nerve 1996; 19:897–899.

101. Kukowski B. Suprascapular nerve lesion as an occupational neuropathy in a semiprofessional dancer. Arch Phys Med Rehabil 1993; 74:768–769.

102. Aiello I, Serra G, Traina GC, Tugnoli V. Entrapment of the suprascapular nerve at the spinoglenoid notch. Ann Neurol 1982; 12:314–316.

103. Rengachary SS, Burr D, Lucas S, Hassanein KM, Mohn MP, Matzke H. Suprascapular entrapment neuropathy: a clinical, anatomical, and comparative study. Part 2: anatomical study. Neurosurgery 1979; 5:447–451.

104. Kiss G, Komar J. Suprascapular nerve compression at the spinogelnoid notch. Muscle Nerve 1990; 13:556–557.

105. Kapsi A, Yanai J, Pick CG et al. Entrapment of the distal suprascapular nerve. An anatomical study. Int Orthop 1988; 12:273–275.

106. Ganzhorn RW, Hocker JT, Horowitz M, Switzer HE. Suprascapular nerve entrapment. A case report. J Bone Joint Surg 1981; 63-A:492–494.

107. McCluskey L, Feinberg D, Dolinskas C. Suprascapular neuropathy related to a glenohumeral joint cyst. Muscle Nerve 1999; 22:772–777.

108. Fehrman DA, Orwin JF, Jennings RM. Suprascapular nerve entrapment by ganglion cysts: a report of six cases with arthroscopic findings and review of the literature. Arthroscopy 1995; 1:727–734.

109. Catalono JB, Fenlin JM. Ganglion cysts about the shoulder girdle in the absence of suprascapular nerve involvement. J Shoulder Elbow Surg 1995; 3:34–41.

110. Tirman PF, Feller JF, Janzen DL, Peterfy CG, Bergman AG. Association of glenoid labral cysts with labral tears and glenohumeral instability: radiologic findings and clinical significance. Radiology 1994; 190:653–658.

111. Quan K, Iannotti JP, Williams GR, Bird SJ. Clinical and prognostic features of isolated axillary neuropathy. Muscle Nerve 1998; 21:1572.

112. Petrucci FS, Morelli A, Raimondi PL. Axillary nerve injuries-21 cases treated by nerve graft and neurolysis. J Hand Surg 1982; 7:271–278.

113. Steinman SP, Moran EA. Axillary nerve injury: diagnosis and treatment. J Amer Acad Orthop Surg 2001; 9:328–335.

114. Perlmutter GS, Apruzzese W. Axillary nerve injuries in contact sports: recommendations for treatment and rehabilitation. Sports Med 1998; 26:351–361.

115. Bonnard C, Anastakis DJ, VanMelle G, Narakas AO. Isolated and combined lesions of the axillary nerve. A review of 146 cases. J Bone Joint Surg 1999; 81-B:212–217.

116. Liveson JA. Nerve lesions associated with shoulder dislocation; an electrodiagnostic study of 11 cases. J Neurol Neurosurg Psychiatry 1984; 47:742–744.

117. Wilbourn A, Lederman R, Sweeney P. Brachial plexopathy: a complication of closed reduction of shoulder dislocation. Can J Neurol Sci 1992; 19:300.

118. Berry J, Bril V. Axillary nerve palsy following blunt trauma to the shoulder region: a clinical and electrophysiological review. J Neurol Neurosurg Psychiatry 1982; 45:1027–1032.

119. Wilbourn AJ. Electrodiagnostic testing of neurologic injuries in athletes. Clin Sports Med 1990; 9:229–245.

120. Perlmutter GS, Leffert RD, Zarins B. Direct injury to the axillary nerve in athletes playing contact sports. Am J Sports Med 1997; 25:65–68.

121. Kirby JF, Kraft GH. Entrapment neuropathy of anterior branch of axillary nerve: report of a case. Arch Phys Med Rehabil 1972; 53:338–340.

122. Simonetti S. Lesion of the anterior branch of axillary nerve in a patient with hereditary neuropathy with liability to pressure palsies. Eur J Neurol 2000; 7:577–579.

123. Stanish WD. Peterson DC. Shoulder arthroscopy and nerve injury: pitfalls and prevention. Arthroscopy 1995; 11:458–466.

124. Richard RR, Hudson AR, Bertoia JT, Urbaniak JR, Waddell JP. Injury to the brachial plexus during Putti-platt and Bristow procedures. Am J Sports Med 1987; 15:374–380.

125. Choi HR, Kondo S, Mishima S, Shimizu T, Hasegawa Y, Hirayama M, Iwata H. Axillary nerve injury caused by intradeltoid muscular injection: a case report. J Shoulder Elbow Surg 2001; 10:493–495.

126. Gries PE, Burks RT, Schickendantz MS, Sandmeier R. Axillary nerve injury after thermal capsular shrinkage of the shoulder. J Shoulder Elbow Surg 2001; 10:231–235.

127. Paladini D, Dellantonio R, Cinti A, Angeleri F. Axillary neuropathy in volleyball players: report of two cases and literature review. J Neurol Neurosurg Psychiatry 1996; 60:345–347.

128. Cahill BR, Palmer RE. Quadrilateral space syndrome. J Hand Surg 1983; 8:65–69.

129. Redler MR, Ruland LJ, McCue FC. Quadrilateral space syndrome in a throwing athlete. Am J Sports Med 1986; 14:511–513.

130. McKowen HC, Voories RM. Axillary nerve entrapment in the quadrilateral space. Case report. J Neurosurg 1987; 66:932–934.

131. Francel TJ, Dellon AL, Campbell JN. Quadrilateral space syndrome: diagnosis and operative decompression technique. Plast Reconst Surg 1991; 87:911–916.

132. Braddom RL, Wolfe C. Musculocutaneous nerve injury after heavy exercise. Arch Phys Med Rehabil 1978; 59:290–293.

133. Kim SM, Goodrich JA. Isolated musculocutaneous nerve palsy: case report. Arch Phys Med Rehabil 1984; 65:735–736.

134. Trojaborg W. Motor and senory conduction in musculocutaneous nerve. J Neurol Neurosurg Psychiatry 1976; 39:890–899.

135. Izzo KL, Aravabhumi S, Jafri A, Sobel E, Demopoulos JT. Medial and lateral antebrachial cutaneous nerves: standardization of technique, reliability and age effect on healthy subjects. Arch Phys Med Rehabil 1985; 66:592–597.

136. Karakousis CP, Hena MA, Emrich LJ, Driscoll DL. Axillary node dissection in malignant melanoma: results and complications. Surgery 1990; 108:10–17.

137. Bateman JE. Nerve injuries about the shoulder in sports. J Bone Joint Surg 1967; 49-A:785–792.

138. Simonetti S. Musculocutaneous nerve lesion after strenuous physical activity. Muscle Nerve 1999; 22:647–649.

139. Sander HW, Quinto CM, Elinzano H, Chokroverty S. Carpet carrier's palsy: musculocutaneous neuropathy. Neurology 1997; 48:1731–1732.

140. Capsi I, Ezra E, Nerubay J, Horoszovski H. Musculocutaneous nerve injury after coracoid process transfer for clavicle instability. Report of three cases. Acta Orthop Scand 1987; 294–295.

141. Osborne AW, Birch RM, Munshi P, Bonney G. The musculocutaneous nerve. J Bone Joint Surg 2000; 82-B:1140–1142.

142. Bassett FH, Nunley JA. Compression of the musculocutaneous nerve at the elbow. J Bone Joint Surg 1982; 64-A:1050–1052.

143. Davidson JJ, Bassett FH, Nunley JA. Musculocutaneous nerve entrapment revisited. J Shoulder Elbow Surg 1998; 7:250–255.

144. Kuhlman KA, Batley RJ. Bilateral musculocutaneous nerve palsy. A case report. Am J Phys Med Rehabil 1996; 75:227–231.

145. Bartosh RA, Dugdale TW, Nielsen R. Isolated musculocutaneous nerve injury complicating closed fracture of the clavicle. A case report. Am J Sports Med 1992; 20:356–359.

146. Mumenthaler M, Schliack H. Peripheral Nerve Lesions. Diagnosis and Therapy. New York: Thieme, 1991:223–224.

147. Dundore DE, DeLisa JA. Musculocutaneous nerve palsy: an isolated complication of surgery. Arch Phys Med Rehabil 1979; 60:130–133.

148. Lachman E, Rosenberg P, Gino G, Levine S, Goldberg S, Borstein M. Axonal damage to the left musculocutaneous nerve of the left biceps muscle during laparoscopic surgery. J Am Assoc Gyn Laparoscop 2001; 8:453–455.

149. Heitzner J, Miller TA. Infrequently reported vulnerability of the musculocutaneous nerve to routine activities. Muscle Nerve 1998; 21:1571.

150. Yuan RT, Cohen MJ. Lateral antebrachial cutaneous nerve injury as a complication of phlebotomy. Plast Reconstr Surg 1985; 76:299–300.

151. Stitik TP, Foye PM, Nadler SF, Brachman GO. Phlebotomy-related lateral antebrachial cutaneous nerve injury. Am J Phys Med Rehabil 2001; 80:230–234.

152. Berry PR, Walls WE. Venipuncture nerve injuries. Lancet 1977; 1:1236–1237.

153. Horowitz SH. Peripheral nerve injury and causalgia secondary to routine venipuncture. Neurology 1994; 44:962–964.

154. Brodman RF, Frame R, Camacho M, Hu E, Chen A, Hollinger I. Routine use of unilateral and bilateral radial arteries for coronary artery bypass graft surgery. J Am Coll Cardiology 1996; 28:959–963.

155. Gillingham BL, Mack GR. Compression of the lateral antebrachial cutaneous nerve by the biceps tendon. J Shoulder Elbow Surg 1996; 5:330–332.

156. Dailiana ZH, Roulot E, Le Viet D. Surgical treatment of compression of the lateral antebrachial cutaneous nerve. J Bone Joint Surg 2000; 82-B:420–423.

157. Farrage JR, Salcido R, Atchison JW, Haglund BL. Compression syndrome involving the lateral antebrachial cutaneous nerve in high level quadriplegia. J Am Paraplegia Soc 1994; 17:12–14.

158. Hale BR. Handbag paresthesia. Lancet 1976; 2:470.

159. Young AW, Redmond D, Belandres PV. Isolated lesion of the lateral cutaneous nerve of the forearm. Arch Phys Med Rehabil 1990; 71:251–252.

160. Felsenthal G, Mondell DL, Reischer MA, Mack RH. Forearm pain secondary to compression of the lateral cutaneous nerve of the forearm. Arch Phys Med Rehabil 1984; 65:139–141.

161. Bassett FH, Kirkpatrick JS, Engelhardt DL, Malone TR. Cryotherapy-induced nerve injury. Am J Sports Med 1992; 20:516–518.

30
Sciatic Neuropathy

A. Mouaz Sbei
University of Utah, Salt Lake City, Utah, USA

ABSTRACT

The sciatic nerve is the largest nerve in the lower extremity and receives fibers from L4 to S3 nerve roots. It is composed of tibial and peroneal components, and each division can be involved in a number of mononeuropathies. Knowledge of nerve anatomy and pathophysiology are aided by electrodiagnostic evaluation to localize lesion site, which guides further diagnostic testing and leads to accurate prognosis.

1. SCIATIC NERVE ANATOMY

The sciatic nerve composes the major portion of the lumbosacral plexus and leaves the pelvis through the sciatic notch (the greater sciatic foramen). The nerve consists of two trunks in a common sheath, the lateral or peroneal division and the medial or tibial division. The nerve is covered by the piriformis muscle in the pelvis (and occasionally runs through it), by the gluteus maximus muscle in the buttock, and then passes over the obturator internus muscle. After exiting from the gluteal compartment, the sciatic nerve runs posterior and medial to the hip joint and courses deeply through the thigh. At the mid-thigh level, it branches into the common peroneal and tibial nerves (Fig. 30.1).

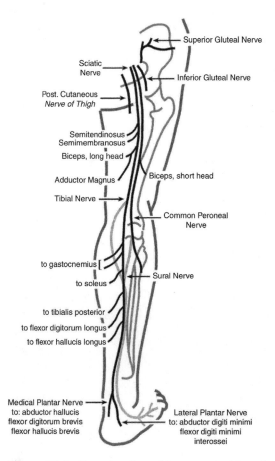

Figure 30.1   Posterior view of the course and branches of the sciatic and tibial nerves.

The sciatic nerve has no sensory branches above the popliteal area. It is responsible for the sensory innervation below the knee, except for the medial aspect of the leg and foot supplied by the saphenous nerve, a terminal branch of the femoral nerve. The sciatic nerve is responsible for the motor innervation of the hamstring muscles and all the muscles below the knee. All the hamstring muscles are innervated by the medial trunk (tibial nerve) except for the short head of the biceps femoris muscle, which is supplied by the lateral trunk (common peroneal nerve). The adductor magnus muscle is mainly innervated by the obturator nerve, but also receives some innervation from the medial trunk of the sciatic nerve.

1.1. Sciatic Mononeuropathies

Sciatic nerve injuries can be divided into three regions: (1) intrapelvic, (2) at the sciatic notch, and (3) in the thigh. In some cases, localization is uncertain despite appropriate diagnostic testing.

1.1.1. Intrapelvic Region

Trauma is the most frequent cause of sciatic nerve damage in this region. Motor vehicle accidents result in fractures and/or posterior dislocations of the hip or the sacroiliac joint and are felt to represent stretch injuries. A less common cause is a post-traumatic osseous tunnel (7).

The frequency of sciatic neuropathy associated with total hip arthroplasty is 0.7–3.7% (17,18). Specific surgical procedures are acetabular reconstruction in congenital dysplasia and revision arthroplasties. Other nerves that can also be injured after total hip arthroplasty are the superior gluteal, femoral, and obturator nerves (14). The mechanism of injury is unknown, but stretch and direct nerve trauma appear to have roles. Although sciatic neuropathies usually develop days to weeks after arthroplastic surgeries, they can be delayed by months or years after surgery (19,1). Operations that do not involve the hip joint or the nerve itself, but that are done in the lithotomy position with prolonged hip flexion, may infrequently cause stretch and compression of the sciatic nerve in the gluteal region resulting in sciatic neuropathy (16).

Tumors, including neurofibromas, lymphomas, and lipomas, can compress the sciatic nerve in the pelvis and elsewhere along its course. Less common compressive sciatic nerve injuries result from intramuscular hematomas in the gluteal muscles (surgical, spontaneous, traumatic, or anticoagulant related) and iliac arteries aneurysms.

The piriformis syndrome is a very rare and vaguely defined syndrome, and is over-diagnosed. It is thought to be due to proximal sciatic nerve compression by the piriformis muscle as the nerve passes under it or between its tendons (5). However, these anatomic findings are noted in 20% of people at autopsy (11). Moreover, some patients given a diagnosis of a piriformis syndrome based on piriformis muscle hypertrophy by imaging studies are subsequently found to have lumbosacral radiculopathies or sacral plexopathies on surgical exploration (13). Pain is the most common presentation ascribed to this syndrome. Tenderness of the sciatic nerve on deep palpation in the buttock area is often found in patients with lumbosacral radiculopathies or tumors and does not necessarily define a piriformis syndrome. If weakness and parasthesia in the sciatic nerve distribution are present at all, they are usually very mild. The Freiberg and Pace maneuvers have been advocated as having diagnostic value (8). The Freiberg maneuver is performed by passive internal rotation and adduction of the thigh (stretching of the piriformis muscle against the sciatic nerve) (10). The Pace test is active external rotation and abduction of the thigh against resistance (active contraction of the piriformis muscle) (10). The best method has yet to be clearly established, and it is prudent, therefore, to exclude all other well-defined causes of sciatic neuropathy and posterior leg pain. Surgical intervention should only be pursued if aggressive conservative therapy fails.

1.1.2. Compromise at the Sciatic Notch

Injection palsy of the sciatic nerve can result from intramusclar injections in the buttock, but is now rare (4). Nerve damage can result from a direct toxic effect of the injected drug or the sequelae of repeated injections at the same site with resultant muscle fibrosis (delayed compressive injection palsy). Injuries to other notch nerves, the gluteal nerve or posterior cutaneous nerve of the thigh, may also be seen with buttock injections (3). Causalgia usually appears immediately after the injection and most patients recover poorly (2). Endometriosis is an infrequent cause of sciatic neuropathy most commonly by nerve compression at the sciatic notch (7). The accompanying radiating posterior leg pain may vary with the menstrual cycle (catamenial sciatica). Other reported causes include delayed effect from pelvic irradiation and nerve infarction due to vasulitis, diabetes mellitus, or atherosclerosis of the iliac artery (6,7,16).

1.1.3. Focal Involvement in the Thigh

Traumatic lacerations (open femur fracture or knife wounds) and compression (hematomas) are frequent causes (20). Treatment of open femur fractures may lead to nerve entrapment by slow encapsulation by fibrosis (21). Less commonly, the nerve can become damaged from external compression from the use of a thigh tourniquet. External compression of the sciatic nerve with prolonged immobilization in comatose patients may result in sciatic neuropathy from mechanical or ischemic disruption or, less commonly, as a result of muscle necrosis as seen in the posterior compartment syndrome (7). Other causes of external compression include prolonged operations with the patient in a sitting or supine position and prolonged sitting on a hard edge seat (27). The sciatic nerve can be injured as a result of the hemodynamic instability and hypotension with reduced capillary perfusion as seen in prolonged surgeries (cardiac surgeries) (9). Entrapment by a myofascial band and tumors are also rare etiologies (16,22).

1.1.4. Symptoms

The lateral trunk of the sciatic nerve, which eventually constitutes the common peroneal nerve, is more susceptible to damage (especially when associated with hip replacement) than the medial trunk (the tibial portion). Explanations for this greater susceptibility include: (1) the lateral trunk has larger and fewer fascicles with less supportive connective tissue, (2) it is more securely fixed and angulated at the sciatic notch and the fibular neck and more likely to be compressed by stretch injury, and (3) the peroneal division lies superficial to the tibial division in the hip region.

   The clinical presentation of sciatic neuropathy includes pain, numbness, and weakness. Almost, all patients with sciatic neuropathies complain of pain at some point during the course. The pain may be felt immediately or within weeks to months after the injury. This dysesthetic pain (burning sensation or sharp pain) is usually in the posterior aspect of the thigh and leg and extends to the foot. Less commonly, pain is predominantly in the foot. There may be associated low back pain. In patients with tumors, pain may be prominently nocturnal. Numbness or paresthesia may be present along the sciatic cutaneous distribution. Foot drop is usually the most prominent motor symptom because of tibialis anterior muscle weakness. Complete isolated injury of the proximal sciatic nerve is very rare and may result in severe paralysis (flail lower leg) and sensory loss.

1.1.5.   Examination Findings

Physical findings vary depending on the lesion site. The straight leg raising test, although not specific, may intensify pain. Weakness (most commonly toe flexion/extension weakness followed by ankle plantar/dorsiflexion), diminished or absent ankle reflexes, and varying sensory deficits may be found. Hamstring muscles are relatively spared owing to the fact that they are the most proximal innervated muscles by the sciatic nerve and will be involved only with proximal lesions, and the medial trunk of the sciatic nerve (which innervates most of the hamstring muscles) is less susceptible to injury than the lateral trunk. Tenderness along the sciatic nerve may be seen in infiltrative tumors.

1.1.6.   Differential Diagnosis

The differential diagnosis of sciatic mononeuropathies includes: (1) lumbosacral radiculopathies, (2) lumbosacral plexopathy, (3) common peroneal mononeuropathy, and (4) tibial mononeuropathy. The clinical distinction between the earlier entities and a sciatic mononeuropathy is not always readily apparent. As a result, electrodiagnostic tests and imaging studies are often required to distinguish between these conditions.

Electrodiagnostic Tests.   Motor conduction studies of the common peroneal nerve are helpful for detecting conduction block across the fibular head. Sensory conduction studies of the sural and superficial peroneal sensory nerve may show post-ganglionic axonal damage with reduced amplitudes in sciatic mononeuropathy and lumbosacral plexopathy. An attempt to establish an objective method for the diagnosis of the piriformis syndrome is based on the H-reflex. Prolongation of the latency with hip flexion, adduction, and internal rotation (FAIR test) has been reported to have a sensitivity of 0.88 and a specificity of 0.83 (13). Another electrodiagnostic method is based on showing an increased latency of cauda equina action potentials recorded with epidural electrodes at L3–4 after stimulation of the peroneal nerve at the fibular head (12).

Needle electromyography (EMG) is most helpful in localizing the site of the nerve lesion by recording abnormal spontaneous activity (positive waves and fibrillation potentials), reflecting denervation, and motor units with reduced recruitment, increased amplitude, and greater complexity, reflecting collateral reinnervation. Gluteal muscle involvement indicates either a very proximal sciatic nerve injury at the sciatic notch level (where coexisting gluteal nerves lesions could occur as they emerge from the notch) or a lesion proximal to the origin of the sciatic nerve (L5–S1 radiculopathy or a lumbosacral plexopathy). Involvement of the short head of the biceps femoris muscle confirms that the lateral trunk of the sciatic nerve is injured, rather than the common peroneal nerve, a distinction that is sometimes difficult to make clinically. The needle EMG examination should also include the femoral nerve-innervated muscles and lumbosacral paraspinal muscles (to exclude a radiculopathy or more diffuse process) (23).

Imaging Studies.   Magnetic resonance (MR) neurogram provides the best resolution in investigating sciatic neuropathy and lumbosacral plexopathy and can be particularly helpful in identifying masses and infiltrating lesions such as tumors and neurosarcoidosis. Computed tomography (CT) may be helpful in investigating compressive lesions associated with surgery or coagulopathic hematomas and bony abnormalities. If an arterial aneurysm or thrombosis is suspected, interventional angiography is indicated.

Laboratory Tests.   Laboratory tests should be selected on the basis of the history, physical examination, and electrodiagnostic testing. If noncompressive nerve lesions, such as vasculitis (a rare cause of sciatic neuropathy), are possible, appropriate serologic and pathologic evaluation should be pursued.

1.1.7. Management and Prognosis

Dysesthetic sciatic neuropathy pain, regardless of etiology, is usually responsive to pharmacological therapy (tricyclic antidepressants, carbamazepine, or gabapentin) or topical medications (lidocaine patch). Foot drop can be compensated for by an ankle-foot orthoses (AFO). Additional treatment depends on the type of the lesion, the etiology, and needle EMG findings. Evidence of re-enervation suggests that spontaneous recovery is expected and, as such, a waiting approach is recommended. Early surgical exploration of the sciatic nerve should be carried out for resection of any compressive lesions such as hematoma, tumor, osseous or fibrosis formation, or endometriosis. Full recovery of a complete sciatic nerve palsy occurring after an open femur fracture was reported with neurolysis of scars around the sciatic nerve (21). The appropriate medical management should be focused on the suspected predisposing factors such as diabetes mellitus.

Treatment of the piriformis syndrome includes steroid and botulinum toxin injections of the piriformis muscle (15). Results are variable, and conservative and surgical outcomes are similar in a 10 year study with two-thirds of patients diagnosed with piriformis syndrome clinically or using the FAIR test.

The prognosis of sciatic mononeuropathy is largely dependent on the etiology, the severity of the nerve injury, and the ability to remove any triggering factors. In general, sciatic neuropathy as a complication of total hip arthroplasty carries a relatively good prognosis, and a nearly full recovery is expected to 2–3 years after the injury. The worst prognosis is seen in patients with complete motor and sensory deficits and in patients with causalgic pain. A favorable prognosis can be predicted when a compound motor action potential can be recorded from the extensor digitorum brevis muscle 3 weeks after injury, because it signifies the presence of uninterrupted axons.

2. PERONEAL NERVE ANATOMY

The lateral trunk of the sciatic nerve becomes the common peroneal nerve at the level of the upper popliteal fossa. Two sensory nerves branches form at the upper popliteal fossa: (1) a sural communicating branch joins the main sural nerve from the tibial nerve and (2) the lateral cutaneous nerve of the calf. The common peroneal nerve then winds around the fibular neck, where it is covered mainly by skin. It then pierces the superficial head of the peroneus longus muscle, through a tendinous tunnel between the edge of the peroneus longus muscle and the fibula (the fibular tunnel), to reach the anterior compartment of the leg. The nerve divides into two main branches as it exits from the fibular tunnel, the superficial peroneal nerve and the deep peroneal nerve (Fig. 30.2).

The superficial peroneal nerve passes through the lateral compartment of the leg along the shaft of the fibula to the lateral malleolus, where it pierces the deep fascia and divides into: (1) sensory branches to the skin of the anterolateral aspect of the lower leg; (2) motor supply to the peroneus longus and brevis muscle; (3) accessory deep peroneal nerve, an anomalous branch found as a normal variant in ~30% of people, that supplies all or part of the extensor digitorum brevis muscle (which usually receives innervation from the deep peroneal nerve only); and (4) medial and lateral

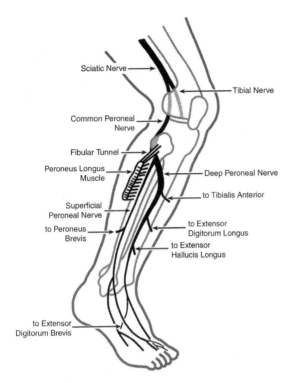

Sciatic Nerve

Tibial Nerve

Common Peroneal
Nerve

Fibular Tunnel

Peroneus Longus
Muscle

Deep Peroneal Nerve

to Tibialis Anterior

Superficial
Peroneal Nerve

to Peroneus
Brevis

to Extensor
Digitorum Longus

to Extensor
Hallucis Longus

to Extensor
Digitorum Brevis

Figure 30.2 Anterolateral view of the course and branches of the common peroneal nerve.

terminal cutaneous branches that supply the dorsal aspect of the foot, except for a web between the first and the second toes.

The deep peroneal nerve passes through the anterior compartment of the leg to the ankle where it passes under a thin extensor retinaculum and gives rise to lateral and medial branches which supply: (1) motor innervation of the anterior tibialis, extensor hallucis longus, extensor digitorum longus, and peroneus tertius muscles; (2) lateral motor terminal branch to the extensor digitorum brevis muscle; and (3) medial sensory branch, which passes under the tendon of the extensor hallucis brevis muscle, which supplies the web space between the first and the second toe.

2.1. Common Peroneal Mononeuropathies

2.1.1. Compressive Neuropathies

Compressive neuropathy of the common peroneal occurs more commonly at the fibular head (where it is covered with skin for ~10 cm) or rarely at the fibular tunnel. Symptoms include acute or subacute foot drop, ankle instability, and paresthesias over the antero-lateral leg and the dorsum of the foot. Pain is uncommon, and when present, is vague and deeply aching at the knee. Physical findings include weakness restricted to the ankle dorsiflexion and toe extension and to a lesser degree foot eversion due to innervation from the superficial branch. The superficial peroneal nerve is usually less involved than the deep peroneal nerve due to the topographical anatomical arrangement of the common peroneal nerve. At the fibular head, the deep peroneal nerve fascicles are placed medially and in direct contact with the fibular bone, whereas the superficial peroneal branch is located laterally away from direct pressure. Testing foot inversion in the setting of a complete foot drop should be done with the ankle passively dorsiflexed to 90° to avoid apparent but false ankle inversion weakness. Deep tendon reflexes in the lower extremity are usually normal. A sensory deficit over the anterolateral leg and the dorsum of the foot is commonly elicited.

External compression at the fibular head occurs in a number of situations, including prolonged bed positioning (comatose patients), long operations with side positioning or when the leg is held to the table by a support beside the knee, below-the-knee casts or orthotic devices, and use of knee supports during labor and delivery. It is also observed in patients who are unaware of parasthesias, as occurs during sleep or as a result of excessive alcohol or drugs, and crossing of the legs for prolonged periods of time. Leg crossing causing subacute peroneal mononeuropathy is frequently associated with marked weight loss, which presumably reduces the thin protective tissues over the nerve at the fibular head. Observing a slight depression in the soft tissues over the fibular head supports the diagnosis of leg crossing as a possible cause of peroneal neuropathy (16).

Internal pressure and entrapment of the peroneal nerve (within the fibular tunnel or between tendons of anterior compartment muscles and the head of the fibula) is a rare cause.

Factors that may predispose to the external and internal compressive etiologies are the presence of underlying peripheral neuropathy, diabetes, dieting resulting in marked weight loss, and squatting for long periods of time.

2.1.2. Trauma

Direct blows and lacerations, dislocation of the knee, fracture of the head or neck of the fibula, and surgical and arthroscopic knee procedures are common causes. Acute plantar flexion–inversion injuries at the ankle due to excessive stretching of the peroneus longus muscle or the common peroneal nerve itself (e.g., while skiing) have been described (24).

2.1.3. Popliteal Masses

Baker's cysts arising from the gastrocnemius-semimembranosus bursa are common causes, whereas nerve sheath tumors, lipomas, callus from old bone fractures, and hematomas are rare.

2.1.4. Mononeuropathy Multiplex Syndrome

The common peroneal nerve is the most frequently involved nerve in vasculitis and other causes including diabetes and leprosy.

2.1.5. Anterior Compartment Syndrome

Acute compartmental syndromes usually result from bleeding, trauma, post-ischemia, or spontaneously after excessive exercise and represent an emergency syndrome that requires rapid diagnosis and treatment. Clinical findings are (1) severe spontaneous pain and tenderness to palpation over the anterior leg compartment, (2) pain with passive foot plantar flexion and toe flexion, and (3) weakness of the anterior compartment muscles (tibialis anterior, extensor hallicis longus, and extensor digitorum longus) manifesting by foot drop or less commonly, an isolated "toe drop." The deep peroneal nerve may or may not be involved, and the extensor digitorum brevis muscle (located distal to the compartment) becomes weakened only when the deep peroneal nerve is involved by ischemia as a result of the syndrome. As ischemia of the deep peroneal nerve evolves, a sensory deficit manifests itself in the web between the first and the second toes.

2.1.6. Lateral Compartment Syndrome

The superficial peroneal nerve is primarily involved in this rather uncommon syndrome. Clinical findings include pain and tenderness over the lateral aspect of the leg, pain with passive foot inversion, and ankle eversion weakness (due to involvement of the peronei muscles). When the superficial peroneal nerve becomes involved, sensory loss over develops over the dorsum of the foot.

2.1.7. Anterior Tarsal Tunnel Syndrome

This extremely rare syndrome is observed when there is involvement of the distal portion of the deep peroneal nerve at the ankle and results from ankle injuries associated with swelling. Predisposing factors are tight boots or high-heeled shoes with a tight strap or a high top. The most common symptoms are pain and dysesthesia in the ankle and dorsum of the foot with nocturnal exacerbation. Walking usually provides a partial relief. Weakness is often restricted to the extensor digitorum brevis (24,25,27).

2.1.8. Differential Diagnosis

The differential diagnosis includes: (1) common peroneal nerve mononeuropathy (and less commonly, isolated deep peroneal mononeuropathy), (2) sciatic mononeuropathy, (3) lumbosacral plexopathy, and (4) lumbar radiculopathy (L5 and rarely L4). Less common causes are motor neuron disease (ALS), peripheral polyneuropathy (especially hereditary types), muscular dystrophies with distal involvement and distal myopathies, upper motor neuron weakness (parasagital cerebral or thoraco-lumbar lesions), and focal foot dystonia.

Electrodiagnostic Tests. In peroneal mononeuropathies, the sural response should be normal, but the superficial peroneal sensory response will be absent or reduced in amplitude. Peroneal motor nerve conduction studies across the fibular head are informative in localizing the site of a lesion. Recordings should be made from the anterior tibialis muscle, if the response from the extensor digitorum muscle is absent.

Needle EMG is very sensitive to denervation and can localize lesions when nerve conduction studies are normal. Muscles that distinguish among radiculopathies, proximal sciatic neuropathies, and peroneal neuropathies are anterior tibialis muscle (L4–5 radiculopathy, deep peroneal nerve injury), peroneal muscles (L5–S1 radiculopathy, superficial peroneal nerve), short head of the biceps femoris (injury to the lateral trunk of the sciatic nerve—common peroneal above knee), posterior tibialis muscle (L4–5 radiculopathy, tibial nerve injury), gluteal muscles, tensor facia lata (L5–S1 radiculopathy, nonperoneal, and nontibial nerves injured), and lumbosacral paraspinal muscles (lumbosacral radiculopathy) (25,26).

Imaging Studies. Magnetic resonance imaging (MRI) and MR neurograms can detect compressing or infiltrative masses (cysts, bony lesions, ganglia, and tumors), hematomas, or vascular lesions.

2.1.9. Management and Prognosis

Conduction slowing or block across the fibular head indicates a compressive neuropathy at that site. These lesions are caused by segmental demyelination and, with removal of the causative compression, prognosis is excellent and usually, recovery is expected in 2–3 months (16,26). The prognosis with axonal damage depends upon the degree of axonal loss and may result in a degree of permanent ankle dorsiflexion weakness. AFOs or high boots are helpful. If no improvement is observed >4–6 months (no evidence of re-innervation in tibialis anterior or peroneus longus muscles by needle EMG), surgical exploration should be considered even in the absence of structural lesions on imaging studies. An immediate surgical intervention is warranted if a complete transection is suggested by lacerating trauma and in the setting of acute compartment syndrome. When the transection is incomplete or in the case of blunt trauma, the likely injury is neurapraxia or axonotmesis and a waiting approach for spontaneous improvement is recommended.

3. TIBIAL NERVE ANATOMY

The tibial nerve is the continuation of the medial trunk of the sciatic nerve (L5, S1, and S2 roots). This nerve separates from the sciatic nerve above the popliteal fossa, passes through the fossa, and then runs deep to the calf muscles. At the foot, the nerve runs under the flexor retinaculum (the roof of the tarsal tunnel) before giving off the calcaneal branch and the two plantar nerves (medial and lateral). In ~30% of people, these branches come off within the tarsal tunnel itself. The flexor retinaculum, unlike the thick volar carpal tunnel ligament, is a thin fibrous band. The plantar nerves end by dividing into the interdigital nerves that pass between the distal heads of the metatarsal bones, crossing the deep transverse metatarsal ligaments (Fig. 30.1). The tibial nerve innervates the following: (1) *Popliteal fossa*. The sural nerve (which also receives a communicating branch from the common peroneal nerve) descends in the midline of the calf and passes behind the lateral malleolus to supply the skin over the lateral aspect of the ankle and the foot up to the base of the fifth toe. (2) *Calf*. Motor branches supply the plantaris, popliteus, gastrocnemius, soleus, tibialis posterior, flexor digitorum longus, and flexor hallucis longus muscles. (3) *Tarsal tunnel*. (a) The calcaneal branch provides sensation to the medial portion of the heel and part of the calcaneus. (b) The medial plantar nerve supplies sensory branches (the interdigital nerves and the medial plantar proper digital nerve) to the anterior two-thirds of the medial aspect of the sole of the foot, and to the first three toes, plus half of the fourth toe. It also supplies the abductor hallucis, flexor digitorum brevis, and flexor hallicus brevis muscles. (c) The lateral plantar nerve supplies sensation to the anterior two-thirds of the lateral aspect of the sole of the foot and to the fifth toe and lateral half of the fourth toe. It also supplies abductor digiti quinti, abductor hallucis, flexor digiti quinti, interossei, and quadratous plantae muscles.

3.1. Tibial Mononeuropathies

Tibial nerve entrapment neuropathies are relatively rare compared with sciatic and peroneal neuropathies, in part because it lies deep in the leg. Tibial entrapment neuropathies can be divided by lesion site.

3.1.1. Above the Ankle

Deep posterior compartment syndromes are characterized by pain localizing to the distal posteromedial leg, tenderness over the distal posteromedial leg, pain with passive foot dorsiflexion and toe extension, and weakness of plantar flexion/foot inversion/toes flexion and intrinsic foot muscles weakness. Other etiologies are external trauma to the knee and leg or fracture, localized hypertrophic mononeuropathy, and stretching injury from ankle sprains.

3.1.2. Tarsal Tunnel Syndrome

Although frequently linked to ankle and foot paresethias and pain, true tibial nerve injury within the tarsal tunnel is uncommon. The tarsal tunnel is located behind and below the medial malleolus. Any space occupying or narrowing lesions within this fibro-osseous tunnel can compress the tibial nerve and result in the tarsal tunnel syndrome (TTS). Trauma is the most common etiology and includes ankle fractures and dislocations, severe ankle twisting, and post-traumatic fibrosis. Vessel abnormalities in the form of dilated or varicose veins constricting the tibial nerve branches, account for 17% of the TTS cases. Other causes include external compression (tight shoes or casts), idiopathic thickening of the flexor retinaculum, tendon cysts "ganglia," the presence of an accessory or hypertrophied abductor hallucis muscle, rheumatoid arthritis of the foot joints, teno- . synovitis, and, more rarely, nerve sheath tumors.

Common symptoms include burning pain and paresthesias in the toes and the sole of the foot with occasional radiation to the calf. Symptoms may be exacerbated at night (15–42% of cases), aggravated by ambulation, and relieved by rest and removal of the shoes. Examination may reveal tenderness to palpation over the flexor retinaculum and sensory deficit over the cutaneous distribution of the tibial nerve or its branches. A positive Tinel's sign over the tibial nerve (percussion behind the medial malleolus) is positive in nearly all cases. Although weakness is almost never elicited, atrophy of the abductor hallucis muscle may be detected (30,31).

Most patients with a presumptive diagnosis of TTS are found to have distal sensory neuropathy, especially when symptoms are bilateral. In true TTS, there should be no objective sensory loss over the dorsum of the foot. Additional diagnostic considerations are plantar fascitis, in which pain tends to occur in the morning and improves with activity, calcaneal bursitis, and tenosynovitis.

3.1.3. Morton's Neuroma

Plantar interdigital nerves may be damaged between the heads of adjacent metatarsal bones before they divide into two digital nerves. Although it is referred to as a neuroma, it is mostly made up of fibrous nodule rather than neural tissue. The most commonly involved interdigital nerve is between the third and the fourth metatarsal bones. Women are more frequently affected than men, possible related to narrow shoes. Repeated trauma, resulting in a fixed hyperextended metatarsophalangeal joint, is the most common accepted mechanism. Predisposing factors include barefoot running on a hard surface, shortened heel cord, rheumatoid arthritis, high-heeled shoes, work related stooping, interphalangeal fracture, and finally, gait disturbances with fanning and hyperextension of the toes at the metatarsophalangeal joints. Another mechanism is entrapment of the interdigital nerve by the deep transverse metatarsal ligament.

The presenting symptom is localized pain on the plantar aspect between two metatarsal heads (typically third and fourth). Pain often radiates to the toes and may also extend proximally. Pain is first triggered by walking and relived by removing the shoes, but then progresses to nocturnal pain. There may be an associated numbness of one or two toes. The diagnosis is mainly by clinical examination. The web-space compression test is compression of the web space with the thumb and the index fingers which produces severe pain. The "Mulder sign" (palpable click on compression) is characteristic.

3.1.4. Sural Neuropathy

Sural neuropathies are associated with lateral ankle pain and concomitant loss of sensation in the sural nerve distribution (the lateral aspect of the ankle and foot) (29). The most common cause is iatrogenic from sural nerve biopsy, and the area of sensory loss diminishes in size over few weeks. The most common noniatrogenic etiology is trauma from prolonged resting of the leg against a hard surface or by repeated job-related blunt trauma. Occasionally, a Baker's cyst in the popliteal fossa may press on the nerve.

3.1.5. Diagnosis

Electrodiagnostic Tests. Nerve conduction studies of the sural nerve may reveal a reduced or absent response. Studies of the medial and the lateral plantar nerves can be helpful in confirming true plantar neuropathies, either within or distal to the tarsal tunnel with either absence of the response or a slowed conduction (25,30).

Needle EMG study can be used to determine the distribution of involvement, and should include peroneal innervated muscles, the hamstrings, gluteal, and lumbosacral paraspinal muscles. Needle EMG is of a limited value in confirming the diagnosis of TTS, because mild dennervation in the intrinsic foot muscles is not an infrequent observation in normal individuals.

Imaging Studies. MRI and CT are useful to detect structural lesions proximal to the ankle and to detect the majority of Morton's neuromas. Imaging studies are rarely helpful in cases of TTS (32,33).

3.1.6. Management and Prognosis

In true TTS, conservative management is appropriate before surgery (16,30,34). This includes changing from high-heeled to flat and wider shoes, and the use of shoes pads. Nonsteroidal anti-inflammatory medications and local injections of corticosteroids and/ or anesthetics at the tarsal tunnel may relieve symptoms and may also be a supportive diagnostic test. Immobilizing the ankle with a lightweight plastic orthosis may help some patients (31). However, even when the cause of TTS is unknown, 75% of patients will report improvement in their symptoms with surgical decompression (28). Conservative therapy is less effective for Morton's neuromas and surgical decompression by incising the deep transverse metatarsal ligament without excising the neuroma.

REFERENCES

1. Glover MG, Convery FR. Migration of fractured greater trochanteric osteotomy wire with resultant sciatica. A report of two cases. Orthopedics 1989; 12:743–744.
2. Gilles FH, Matson DD. Sciatic nerve injury following misplaced gluteal injection. J Pediatr 1970; 76:247–254.
3. Bergeson PS, Singer SA, Kaplan AM. Intramuscular injections in children. Pediatrics 1982; 70(6):944–948.
4. Napiontek M, Ruszkowski K. Paralytic drop foot and gluteal fibrosis after intramuscular injections. J Bone Joint Surg 1993; 75B:83–85.
5. Hughes SS, Goldstein MN, Hicks DG et al. Extrapelvic compression of the sciatic nerve. An unusual cause of pain about the hip: report of five cases. J Bone Joint Surg 1992; 74A:1553–1559.
6. Jones HR, Gianturco LE, Gross PT et al. Sciatic neuropathies in childhood: a report of ten cases and review of the literature. J Child Neurol 1988; 3:193–199.

7. Yuen EC, Yuen TS. Sciatic neuropathy. Neurol Clin 1999; 17(3):617–631.

8. Kline DG. Comment to the piriformis muscle syndrome: a simple diagnostic maneuver. Neurosurgery 1994; 34:514.

9. McManis PG. Sciatic nerve lesions during cardiac surgery. Neurology 1994; 44:684–687.

10. Parziale JR, Hudgins TH, Fishman LM. The piriformis syndrome. Am J Orthop 1996; 25:819–823.

11. Pecina M. Contribution to the etiological explanation of the piriformis syndrome. Acta Anta (Basel) 1979; 105:181–187.

12. Nakamura H et al. Piriformis syndrome diagnosed by cauda equina action potentials: report of two cases. Spine 2003; 15:28(2):E37–E40.

13. Fishman LM et al. Piriformis syndrome: diagnosis, treatment, and outcone-a 10-year study. Arch Phys Med Rehabil 2002; 83(3):295–301.

14. McCrory P, Bell S. Nerve entrapment syndromes as a cause of pain in the hip, groin, and buttock. Sports Med 1999; 27(4):261–274.

15. Fishman LM, Anderson C, Rosner B. BOTOX and physical therapy in the treatment of piriformis syndrome. Am J Phys Med Rehabil 2002; 81(2):936–942.

16. Stewart JD. Focal Peripheral Neuropathies, Lippencott Williams & Wilkins, 3rd ed. 2000.

17. Schmaizried TP, Amstutz HC, Dorey FJ. Nerve palsy associated with total hip replacement. Risk factors and prognosis. J Bone Joint Surg 1991; 73A:1074–1080.

18. DeHart MM, Riley LH Jr. Nerve injuries in total hip arthroplast. J Am Acad Ortho Surg 1999; 7(2):101–111.

19. Katsimihas M, Hutchinson et al. Delayed transient sciatic nerve palsy after total hip arthroplasty. J Arthroplasy 2002; 17(3):379–381.

20. Aboulafia AJ et al. Neuropathy secondary to pigmented villondular synovitis of the hip. Clin Ortho 1996; 325:174–180.

21. Tomaino MM. Complete sciatic nerve palsy after open femur fracture: successful treatment with neurolysis 6 months after injury. Am J Orthop 2002; 31(10):585–588.

22. Venna N, Bielawski M, Spatz EM. Sciatic nerve entrapment in a child. Case report. J Neurosurg 1991; 75:652–654.

23. Yuen EC, So YT, Oiney RK. The electrophysiologic features of sciatic neuropathy in 100 patients. Muscle Nerve 1995; 18:414–420.

24. Katirji B. Peroneal neuropathy. Neurol Clin 1999; 17(3):567–591.

25. Preston DC, Shapiro BE. Electromyography and neuromuscular disorders. Clinical-electrophysiologic correlations. Boston: Butterworth-Heinemann, 1998.

26. Sourkes M, Stewart JD. Common peroneal neuropathy: a study of selective motor and sensory involvement. Neurology 1991; 41:1029–1033.

27. Howard JF. Syllabus of Muscle and Nerve Disease. University of North Carolina at Chapel Hill, 2002.

28. Oh SJ, Meyer RD. Entrapment neuropathy of the tibial (posterior tibial) nerve. Neurol Clin 1999; 17(3):593–615.

29. Refaeian M et al. Isolated sural neuropathy presenting as lateral ankle pain. Am J Phys Med Rehabil 2001; 80(7):543–546.

30. Lau JT, Daniels TR. Tarsal tunnel syndrome: a review of the literature. Foot Ankle Int 1999; 20(3):201–209.

31. Reade BM et al. Tarsal tunnel syndrome. Clin Podiat Med Surg 2001; 18(3):395–408.

32. Erickson SJ, Quinn SF, Kneeland JB et al. MR imaging of the tarsal tunnel and related spaces: normal and abnormal findings with anatomic correlation. Am J Roentgenol 1990; 155:323–328.

33. Shapiro PP, Shapiro SL. Sonographic evaluation of interdigital neuroma. Foot Ankle Int 1995; 16:604–605.

34. Hammerschlag WA, Goldner JL, Bassett FH. Posterior tibial nerve entrapment: a thirty-three year review. Am Orthop Foot Ankle Soc 1998; July.

31

Focal Neuropathies of the Femoral, Obturator, Lateral Femoral Cutaneous Nerve, and Other Nerves of the Thigh and Pelvis

Kevin J. Felice
University of Connecticut Health Center, Farmington, Connecticut, USA

ABSTRACT

Mononeuropathies in proximal lower extremities are rare, with the exception of the lateral femoral cutaneous nerve of the thigh (meralgia paresthetica). Electrodiagnosis has a prominent role in confirming which nerve is involved, localizing the site of the lesion and understanding the type and extent of nerve injury. The major nerves of the lower extremity are reviewed.

1. FOCAL NEUROPATHIES OF THE FEMORAL NERVE

1.1. Anatomy

The femoral nerve is a mixed nerve, containing both motor and sensory fibers. It originates from the posterior divisions of the ventral rami of L2-4 spinal nerves. As it emerges from the lumbar plexus, it runs between psosas and iliacus muscles (L2-3), innervating both of them (Fig. 31.1) (1,2). It then descends beneath the inguinal ligament, lateral to the femoral artery, and enters the thigh. The femoral nerve then divides into anterior and posterior divisions within the femoral triangle. The anterior division divides into a muscular branch, which supplies the sartorius muscle (L2-3), and a sensory branch, the medial cutaneous nerve of the thigh (Fig. 31.2). The posterior division divides into muscular branches supplying the pectineus (L2-3) and the quadriceps femoris complex (rectus femoris, vastus interomedialis, vastus lateralis, and vastus medialis—L2-4), and a sensory branch, the saphenous nerve. The saphenous nerve descends with the femoral artery along the medial thigh through Hunter's canal. The nerve gives off the infrapatellar branch and then descends along the lower leg to innervate the skin of the medial foreleg.

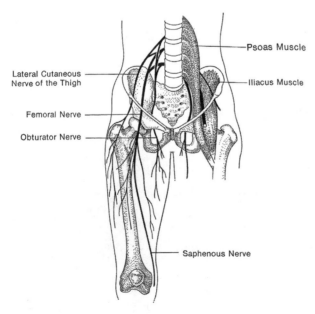

Figure 31.1 Origin and course of the femoral, obturator, and lateral femoral cutaneous nerves. [From Stewart (2), p. 458, with permission.]

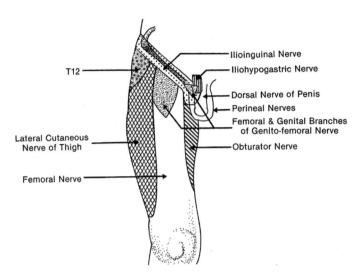

Figure 31.2 Innervation of the skin of the inguinal area and upper thigh. [From Stewart (2), p. 491, with permission.]

1.2. Clinical Features and Differential Diagnosis

The clinical features of femoral mononeuropathy depend on the site of injury (1,2). Lesions of the proximal segment in the lumbar plexus or within the pelvis are associated with weakness of hip flexion (psoas, iliacus, and rectus femoris involvement), knee extension (quadriceps involvement), and lateral thigh rotation (sartorius involvement). Sensory loss and paresthesias occur along the anteromedial thigh and inner foreleg. The patellar reflex is hypoactive or absent. Quadriceps muscle atrophy may occur within weeks, especially with axonal nerve injuries. Lesions at or near the ilioinguinal ligament spare hip flexion because motor branches to the psoas and the iliacus come off more proximally. Lesions within the femoral triangle or upper thigh may cause selective motor or sensory symptoms. Sensory symptoms limited to the medial knee and foreleg may result from isolated lesions of the saphenous nerve in thigh or knee. Damage to the infrapatellar branch of the saphenous nerve results in numbness and paresthesias in the skin over the patella (gonyalgia paresthetica) (3). Other localization considerations in patients with weakness or sensory symptoms in the distribution of the femoral nerve include lesions of the lumbar plexus, L2-4 spinal roots or segments, and lateral femoral cutaneous nerve.

1.3. Etiologies

Trauma is the most common cause (Table 31.1) (1,2,4). Many traumatic cases are iatrogenic from nerve injury sustained during surgical procedures (5–7). The mechanisms of femoral nerve injury in these cases include compression, blunt trauma, stretch, and laceration. Other causes include noniatrogenic trauma (compression from hematoma, abscess, tumors, or pseudoaneurysm), diabetes mellitus, localized hypertrophic neuropathy, vasculitis, radiation-induced neuropathy, and idiopathic neuropathy (1,2,8–13). Unilateral or bilateral femoral mononeuropathies may occur in surgical or obstetric patients while in the lithotomy position, presumedly due to nerve compression against the inguinal ligament or excessive stretch of the nerve (14). Isolated injury of the saphenous nerve may occur in thigh, knee, or foreleg (Table 31.2). Iatrogenic trauma caused by

Table 31.1 Causes of Femoral Neuropathy

Trauma
  Iatrogenic
    Inguinal herniorrhaphy
    Total hip replacement
    Intraabdominal surgeries
    Gynecological surgeries
    Lumbar sympathectomy
    Laparoscopic procedures
  Other trauma
    Bullet and stab wounds
    Blunt trauma
    Hip and pelvic fractures
    Stretch injuries
Lithotomy position
  Childbirth
  Surgical procedures
Compression
  Hematoma
  Abscess
  Tumors
  Pseudoaneurysm
Diabetes mellitus
Localized hypertrophic neuropathy
Vasculitis
Radiation-induced
Idiopathic

knee surgeries, arthroscopy, and saphenous vein harvesting are the most common causes of saphenous mononeuropathy (1,2,15–18).

1.4. Diagnostic Studies

The clinical examination is most informative for localization of femoral nerve lesions. Electrodiagnostic studies are useful to verify the clinical diagnosis and exclude other sites of injury (e.g., femoral neuropathy vs. L2-4 radiculopathy), to provide more precise localization (e.g., femoral neuropathy proximal vs. distal to the innervation of the iliacus), to determine the type of nerve injury (e.g., axonal, demyelinating, or mixed), to determine whether or not surgical intervention is necessary, and to predict recovery and prognosis. Routine electrodiagnostic studies include nerve conduction studies (NCS) and needle electromyography (EMG). General knowledge of the pathophysiology and electrodiagnostic features of focal demyelinating injury, Wallerian degeneration, and reinnervation via both collateral sprouting and axonal regeneration is necessary in order to accurately interpret these studies (19,20). Saphenous sensory and femoral motor NCS are optimally performed 10 days following an acute nerve injury. Techniques for performing these studies have been reported (21–23). As Wallerian degeneration is complete at this point, such studies are better able to distinguish among focal demyelinating, axonal, and mixed nerve injuries. A preserved saphenous sensory nerve action potential (SNAP) at day 10 post-injury in a patient with a suspected

Table 31.2 Causes of Saphenous Neuropathy

Thigh
  Compression
    Fibrous bands
    Branches of femoral vessels
  Entrapment at subsartorial canal exit
  Lacerations
  Arterial surgery
  Nerve tumors
Knee
  Knee surgery and arthroscopy
  External compression (e.g., surfer's neuropathy)
  Meniscal cyst
Foreleg
  Saphenous vein harvest for coronary artery bypass surgery
  Saphenous vein cannulation
  Ankle injuries
  Trauma
  Lacerations
Infrapatellar branch
  Blunt trauma, compression, and lacerations
  Knee surgery and arthroscopy
  Entrapment at the sartorius tendon

femoral neuropathy suggests either selective injury to the femoral nerve without involvement of saphenous sensory fibers, or proximal focal demyelinating injury to the femoral nerve, or nerve injury proximal to the dorsal root ganglion cells (e.g., L2-4 radiculopathy). At day 10 post-injury, a preserved femoral compound muscle action potential (CMAP) from a paralyzed rectus femoris muscle also attests to a primary demyelinating injury, and predicts a good recovery and prognosis. Attenuated or absent saphenous SNAP and femoral CMAP responses are consistent with axonal or mixed injuries, and predict a prolonged recovery. EMG provides information about active axonal injury (e.g., presence of fibrillations and positive sharp waves) and extent of nerve repair (e.g., nascent motor unit action potentials suggest repair via axonal regeneration).

Neuroimaging, including ultrasound computed tomography and magnetic resonance imaging (MRI), may be used to assess for compressive or infiltrative nerve lesions (e.g., hemorrhage and metastases), nerve sheath tumors, focal edema, and sources of nerve entrapment (24). In general, MRI provides the best soft tissue contrast and anatomical detail among imaging modalities. In addition, the recent technique of magnetic imaging neurography can identify small focal areas of nerve edema, entrapment, or compression (24–26).

1.5. Management

Initial management of femoral nerve injuries is depends on the suspected type of injury (2). With mild to moderate nerve injuries (e.g., blunt trauma and stretch), restitution by remyelination, collateral sprouting, or both may be evident within weeks to months. Severe axonal injuries require reinnervation by axonal regeneration and repair may not be evident for 6–12 months. If complete disruption (e.g., laceration) of the nerve is suspected, early exploration and surgical repair is indicated. EMG studies can document nerve continuity or discontinuity, and serial studies can assess early (subclinical) axonal regeneration. Management of iliacus hematomas includes reversal of anticoagulation and treatment of pain (2). Surgical evacuation should be considered in patients with large hematomas and substantial clinical deficits (9,11).

2. FOCAL NEUROPATHIES OF THE OBTURATOR NERVE

2.1. Anatomy

The obturator nerve is a mixed nerve that originates from the anterior divisions of the ventral rami of the L2-4 spinal nerves and traverses the lumbar plexus (Fig. 31.1) (1,2). The nerve passes through the pelvis via the obturator canal, and within the canal supplies the obturator externus muscle (L2-4). Outside of the canal, it divides into the anterior and posterior divisions which descend along the medial thigh. The anterior division supplies the pectineus (L2-4), adductor longus (L2-4), adductor brevis (L2-4), and gracilis (L2-4). The anterior division terminates in a sensory branch that innervates the skin along the medial thigh (Fig. 31.2). The posterior division supplies the obturator externus (L2-4), adductor magnus (L2-4) (which also receives innervation from the sciatic nerve), and adductor brevis muscle (L2-4).

2.2. Clinical Features and Differential Diagnosis

Lesions of the obturator nerve cause weakness of thigh adduction, wasting of the medial thigh muscles (with axonal injuries), and sensory loss or paresthesias affecting the medial thigh. Patients usually note difficulties with hip and thigh stabilization, especially during certain activities (e.g., squatting and sexual intercourse). Other localization sites to consider in patients with weakness or sensory symptoms in the distribution of the obturator nerve include lesions of the lumbar plexus, or L2-4 spinal roots or segments.

2.3. Etiologies

Causes of obturator mononeuropathy include trauma, compression, nerve tumors, entrapment within the obturator foramen, diabetes mellitus, myositis ossificans, and idiopathic injury (Table 31.3) (1,2,4,27–32). Within the lumbar plexus, the obturator nerve may be damaged during pelvic surgical or laparoscopic procedures, and by compression or infiltration from metastatic disease or endometriosis (28,32). Damage may result from obturator hernias, following cancer surgery in the pelvis, iliopsoas hemorrhage, pelvic fractures, or during hip surgery. Prolonged hip flexion during certain urological surgical procedures may stretch the nerve at the bony obturator foramen. Obturator mononeuropathy may result from prolonged labor or difficult childbirth due to compression of the nerve between the fetal head and the bony pelvis (30). Nerve entrapment by thickened fascia overlying the adductor brevis muscle has been described in athletes (31). We recently evaluated a unilateral obturator mononeuropathy attributed to stretch or compression during an endoscopic hysterectomy.

2.4. Diagnostic Studies

There are no NCS techniques for evaluating the obturator nerve (21) and electrodiagnostic evaluation is limited to needle EMG of hip adductor muscles. Focal demyelinating lesions or neurapraxic injury of the obturator nerve can be inferred by reduced recruitment (higher

Table 31.3 Causes of
Obturator Neuropathy

Trauma
   Iatrogenic
      Pelvic surgery
      Hip surgery
      Laparoscopic surgery
      Femoral artery procedures
   Pelvic fractures
Compression
   Tumors
   Endometriosis
   Obturator hernias
   Fibrous bands
Childbirth
Nerve tumors
Entrapment in obturator foramen
Diabetes mellitus
Myositis ossificans
Idiopathic

discharge rates) and from normal-appearing motor unit action potentials in hip adductor muscles. In distinction, mixed and axonal injuries from noniatrogenic trauma would be associated with fibrillation potentials and positive sharp waves during the subacute to early chronic phase of injury, and motor unit action potentials (nascent units) reflecting reinnervation during the chronic phase. MRI of the thigh may provide additional information in selected situations. For example, prominent atrophy of the hip adductor muscles would be consistent with severe axonal or mixed nerve injury, whereas normal-appearing or mildly atrophic muscles assessed several months post-injury would be more consistent with neuropraxic nerve injury.

2.5. Management

Good clinical outcome is reported in most patients regardless of etiology (27). Patients with partial injuries should be observed because recovery by remyelination or collateral reinnervation occurs over a period of several months. Severe or complete injuries may require early surgical exploration and nerve grafting (34). Obturator neuropathy following hip arthroplasty may be caused by nerve encasement in surgical cement, early surgical exploration is indicated. Surgical exploration for possible nerve entrapment within the obturator canal, nerve infiltration by metastatic disease, or endometriosis should be considered in patients with progressive and unexplained symptoms.

3. FOCAL NEUROPATHIES OF THE LATERAL FEMORAL CUTANEOUS NERVE

3.1. Anatomy

The lateral femoral cutaneous nerve of the thigh (LFCN) originates from the anterior primary rami of the L2-3 spinal roots within the psoas muscle (Fig. 31.1) (1,2).

The nerve emerges from the lateral border of the psoas muscle, crosses the iliacus muscle, passes under the lateral part of the inguinal ligament medial to the anterior superior iliac spine, and enters the upper thigh beneath the fascia lata. In the upper thigh, the LFCN divides into anterior and posterior divisions. The anterior division innervates the skin of the anterior thigh to the knee whereas the posterior division supplies the skin along the upper and lateral aspects of the thigh (Fig. 31.2).

3.2. Clinical Features and Differential Diagnosis

LFCN lesions cause sensory loss, paresthesias, or pain involving the anterolateral thigh (meralgia paresthetica). Symptoms are worsened when standing or walking, especially in obese patients, presumably due to compression of the nerve along the anterior superior iliac spine by the protuberant abdomen. Other localization considerations in patients with symptoms of meralgia paresthetica include lesions of the femoral nerve, lumbar plexus, or L2-4 spinal roots or segments.

3.3. Etiologies

There are multiple sites for nerve injury, including the abdomen, pelvis, inguinal ligament, and thigh (Table 31.4). In the abdomen, the LFCN may be compressed by psoas hemorrhage, abscess, or tumor (2,4,35). Surgical trauma may result from renal transplants, hysterectomies, or other surgeries (36–38). Procurement of iliac bone for grafting may injure the LFCN in the pelvis (39). Obesity and constricting garments or belts are potential causes of external compression of the nerve near the anterior superior iliac spine or the inguinal ligament, and can be associated with bilateral meralgia paresthetica (2,4,40,41).

Table 31.4 Causes of Lateral Femoral Cutaneous Neuropathy

Abdomen
   Iliopsoas hemorrhage
   Psoas tumor
   Surgery (e.g., renal transplants and abdominal hysterectomy)
Pelvis
   Iliac bone procurement for grafting
   Surgery in the iliac fossa
Inguinal ligament
   External compression and angulation
      Corsets, belts, and other constricting garments
      Prolonged sitting in the lotus position
      Protuberant abdomen in obese patient
      Seat-belt trauma
   Entrapment
   Trauma
   Surgical Injury
   Idiopathic
Thigh
   External compression
   Trauma
   Lacerations
   Injections
   Surgical injury

Other causes are trauma, compression, lacerations, injection injuries, and surgical injuries (42,43).

3.4. Diagnostic Studies

Several techniques are available for recording the LFCN sensory nerve action potentials (21,44,45). The nerve is stimulated with either surface or needle electrodes just medial to the anterior superior iliac spine and the SNAP is recorded along the anterolateral thigh. However, NCS of the LFCN are technically difficult to perform in normal subjects, and particularly in obese subjects. A major limitation is that the SNAP is of low amplitude (2–10 μV) and usually requires signal averaging. Comparative studies on the asymptomatic side are required in an patient found to have an absent LFCN response in the symptomatic limb. Given these limitations, lateral femoral cutaneous mononeuropathy remains primarily a clinical diagnosis. When appropriate, imaging studies of the retroperitoneal space and pelvis are needed to assess for metastatic disease or hemorrhage.

3.5. Management

In most patients, symptoms resolve spontaneously within weeks to months (2,46), and conservative management of idiopathic meralgia paresthetica is appropriate. Patients should be educated on potential causes (e.g., obesity and constricting garments or belts) of meralgia paresthetica and instructed on appropriate modifications. Analgesics and medications for neuropathic pain may be appropriate for patients with especially bothersome symptoms. Local anesthetics and corticosteroids may provide pain relief and can be repeated at intervals (46,47). Surgical decompression of the nerve at the inguinal ligament may be appropriate for patients with recalcitrant pain symptoms (46). Nerve transection is preferred over decompression by some surgeons; however, the paucity of reported cases hampers comparative analyses (48).

4. FOCAL NEUROPATHIES OF OTHER NERVES OF THIGH AND PELVIS

4.1. Posterior Femoral Cutaneous Nerve of the Thigh

Sensory nerve fibers of the posterior femoral cutaneous nerve of the thigh (PFCN) originate from the anterior primary rami of S1-3 spinal roots (Fig. 31.3) (1,2). The PFCN exits the pelvis via the greater sciatic notch and descends the posterior thigh. The nerve is initially deep to the gluteus maximus muscle, but descends superficially down the back of the thigh to the knee. The PFCN innervates the skin of lower buttock, posterior thigh, and popliteal fossa, and lesions cause paresthesias or sensory loss in these areas. The PFCN may be damaged in sacral plexus, greater sciatic foramen, buttocks, or upper thigh (Table 31.5). Posterior femoral cutaneous neuropathy may be due to compression or infiltration (malignancies), trauma (falls on the buttock), injection injuries, compression from bicycle seat, and lacerations (1,2,49–52).

4.2. Iliohypogastric Nerve

The iliohypogastric nerve is a mixed nerve originating from the anterior primary rami of T12-L1 spinal roots. It emerges from the lateral border of the psoas muscle (Fig. 31.4) (1,2) and traverses with the ilioinguinal nerve around the abdominal wall and along the

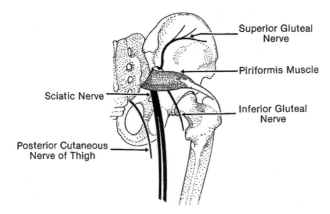

Figure 31.3 Course of the posterior femoral cutaneous nerve. [From Stewart (2), p. 377, with permission.]

upper border of the iliac crest. In the abdomen, the iliohypogastric and ilioinguinal nerves provide motor branches to the internal oblique and transversus abdominis muscles. The terminal branches of the iliohypogastric nerve are the lateral and anterior cutaneous sensory branches. The lateral branch supplies the skin along the upper aspect of the buttock and the anterior branch supplies a small patch of skin over the pubis (Fig. 31.2). Lesions of the iliohypogastric nerve are associated with sensory loss, paresthesias, or pain in the distribution of the lateral and anterior branches. Iliohypogastric neuropathies may result from lesions in the lumbar plexus or abdomen (Table 31.6). Damage may be caused by compression or infiltration by tumors, surgical incisions, trauma, or compression (1,2).

4.3. Ilioinguinal Nerve

The ilioinguinal nerve is a mixed nerve originating from the anterior primary rami of the L1 spinal root (Fig. 31.4) (1,2), and travels just below and parallel to the iliohypogastric nerve in the abdomen. The nerve pierces the internal oblique and transversus abdominis muscles, and supplies motor branches to these muscles, and then enters the inguinal canal and passes through the superficial inguinal ring together with the spermatic cord in men or round ligament in woman. Sensory fibers emerge from the canal to supply the skin along the medial thigh below the inguinal ligament, symphysis pubis and external genitalia (Fig. 31.2). Lesions of the ilioinguinal nerve are associated with lower abdominal

Table 31.5 Causes of Posterior Femoral Cutaneous Neuropathy

Sacral plexus
  Malignancy
Buttocks
  Falls on to the buttocks
  Injections
  Prolonged sitting (e.g., bicycle riding)
  Trauma
  Lacerations

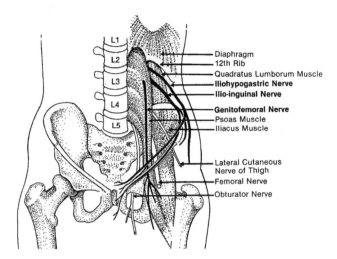

Figure 31.4   Course of the iliohypogastric, ilioinguinal, and genitofemoral nerves. [From Stewart (2), p. 490, with permission.]

pain, sensory loss or paresthesias in this distribution, and tenderness below the anterior superior iliac spine. The ilioinguinal nerve may be injured in the lumbar plexus, abdomen, and inguinal canal (Table 31.7) (1,2). In the lumbar plexus or retroperitoneal space, the ilioinguinal nerve may be damaged by tumor compression, infiltration, or surgical injuries (53,54). Along the anterior abdominal wall, the nerve may be damaged by surgical incisions, trauma, or entrapment within abdominal muscles (55). The inguinal canal is a potential site for injury due to hernia surgery, or compression by endometriosis, lipoma, or leiomyoma. Neuropathy may occur after childbirth due to stretching of the nerve (2,56). Ilioinguinal neuropathy or neuralgia may be idiopathic.

4.4. Genitofemoral Nerve

Mixed nerve fibers of the genitofemoral nerve originate from the anterior primary rami of L1-2 spinal roots (Fig. 31.4) (1,2). The nerve passes through the psoas muscle and travels downward to the inguinal ligament where is divides into the external spermatic (genital) and lumboinguinal (femoral) branches. The genital branch enters the deep inguinal ring and traverses the inguinal canal where it terminates in a motor branch innervating the cremaster muscle and sensory branch supplying the skin along the scrotum (or labia majoris)

Table 31.6   Causes of Iliohypogastric Neuropathy

Lumbar plexus or retroperitoneal space
   Tumors
   Surgical incisions (e.g., nephrectomy)
Abdomen
   Surgical incisions (e.g., appendectomy)
   Trauma
   Compression

Table 31.7 Causes of Ilioinguinal Neuropathy

Lumbar plexus or retroperitoneal space
   Tumors
   Surgery
Anterior abdominal wall
   Surgical incisions
   Entrapment within the abdominal layers
   Lower abdominal surgeries (e.g., appendectomy)
Inguinal canal
   Herniorrhaphy
   Endometriosis
   Lipoma
   Leiomyoma
Unknown site
   After childbirth
   Idiopathic

and adjacent medial thigh (Fig. 31.2). The femoral branch passes under the inguinal ligament and supplies the skin along the upper thigh and the femoral triangle. Lesions of the genitofemoral nerve are associated with sensory loss, paresthesias, or pain along the medial inguinal area, upper thigh, and lateral aspect of scrotum or labia. Standing or extending the hip may worsen the symptoms. There is often tenderness along the inguinal canal. The cremaster reflex is an unreliable sign of nerve function. The genitofemoral nerve may be damaged in the lumbar plexus, abdomen, or inguinal area (Table 31.8) (1,2,57,58). In the lumbar plexus or retroperitoneal space, the genitofemoral nerve may be injured by tumor compression, infiltration, or surgical trauma. Surgical incisions and trauma are causes of injury in the abdomen and inguinal area.

4.5. Pudendal Nerve

Mixed nerve fibers of the pudendal nerve originate from the anterior primary rami of S1-4 spinal roots (Fig. 31.5) (1,2). The nerve exits the pelvis through the greater sciatic notch to reach the perineum. The three major branches of the pudendal nerve include the inferior rectal nerve, perineal nerve, and dorsal nerve of the penis (or clitoris) (Fig. 31.6). The inferior rectal nerve innervates the external anal sphincter and provides sensory branches to the lower anal canal and perianal skin. The perineal nerve innervates the perineum,

Table 31.8 Causes of Genitofemoral Neuropathy

Lumbar plexus or retroperitoneal space
   Tumors
   Surgery
Abdomen
   Surgical incisions
Inguinal area
   Inguinal herniorrhaphy
   Appendectomy
   Cesarean section

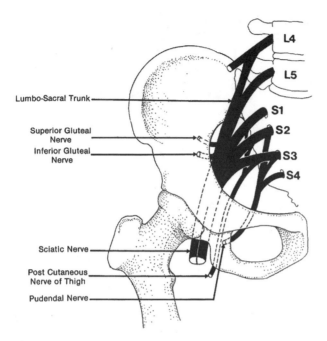

Figure 31.5 Origin of the pudendal nerve. [From Stewart (2), p. 376, with permission.]

erectile tissue of the penis, external urethral sphincter, and skin of the perineum, scrotum (or labia). The dorsal nerve supplies sensation to the penis (or clitoris). Lesions of the pudendal nerve are associated with sensory loss or paresthesias in the distribution of the nerve, difficulty with bladder and bowel control, and erectile impotence. Causes of pudendal neuropathy include pelvic and hip fractures, hip surgeries, buttock injections, surgical compressions, entrapment from surgical sutures, and compression from long distance bicycle riding (Table 31.9) (1,2,59–62).

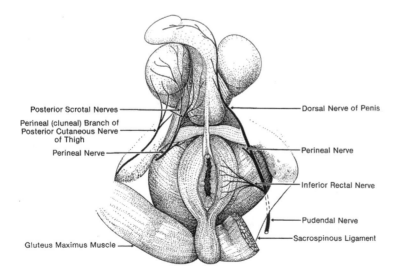

Figure 31.6 View of the perineum showing the course and branches of the pudendal nerve. [From Stewart (2), p. 378, with permission.]

Table 31.9 Causes of Pudendal Neuropathy

Pelvic and hip fractures
Hip surgery
Buttock injections
Surgical compression (e.g., perineal post)
Entrapment by surgical suture
Compression from long bicycle rides

4.6. Diagnostic Studies

Neurophysiology techniques are available for the PFCN, ilioinguinal nerve, and pudendal nerve (63–71). These studies are technically challenging, however, as they either require specialized equipment (e.g., pudendal nerve conduction study) or the compound nerve action potentials are of low-amplitude and difficult to discern. Computed tomographic or MRI scans are warranted when hemorrhage or tumor infiltration are suspected causes of nerve injury.

4.7. Management

Management of these uncommon focal neuropathies includes etiologic identification, surgical exploration or decompression if applicable, resection of painful neuromas, and symptomatic management. Local anesthetic or corticosteroid nerve blocks may be especially helpful to alleviate the neuropathic pain associated with ilioinguinal, iliohypogastric, and genitofemoral neuropathies (2). Carbamazepine and other medications for neuropathic pain have also been used successfully for symptomatic treatment (2,72).

REFERENCES

1. Brazis PW, Masdeu JC, Biller J. Localization in Clinical Neurology. 4th ed. Philadelphia: Lippincott Williams and Wilkins, 2001.
2. Stewart JD. Focal Peripheral Neuropathies. 3rd ed. Philadelphia: Lippincott Williams and Wilkins, 2000.
3. Massey EW. Gonyalgia paresthetica. Muscle Nerve 1981; 4:80–81.
4. Busis NA. Femoral and obturator neuropathies. Neurol Clinics 1999; 3:633–653.
5. Jog MS, Turley JE, Berry H. Femoral neuropathy in renal transplantation. Can J Neurol Sci 1994; 21:38–42.
6. Sharma KR, Cross J, Santiago F, Ayyar R, Burke G. Incidence of femoral neuropathy following renal transplantation. Arch Neurol 2002; 59:541–545.
7. Kuntzer T, van Melle G, Regli F. Clinical and prognostic features in unilateral femoral neuropathies. Muscle Nerve 1997; 20:205–211.
8. Takao M, Fukuuchi Y, Koto A, Tanaka K, Momoshima S, Kuramochi S, Takeda T. Localized hypertrophic mononeuropathy involving the femoral nerve. Neurology 1999; 52:389–392.
9. Ahuja R, Venkatesh P. Femoral neuropathy following anticoagulant therapy: a case report and discussion. Conn Med 1999; 63:69–71.
10. Mendes DG, Nawalkar RR, Eldar S. Post-irradiation femoral neuropathy: a case report. J Bone Joint Surg 1991; 73A:137–140.
11. Young MR, Norris JW. Femoral neuropathy during anticoagulant therapy. Neurology 1976; 26:1173–1175.

12. Cranberg L. Femoral neuropathy from iliac hematoma: report of a case. Neurology 1979; 29:1071–1072.

13. Taragin DL, Scelsa SN, Pyburn DD. Bilateral femoral neuropathies following femoral artery puncture. Muscle Nerve 1996; 19:1641–1642.

14. Hakim MA, Katirji MB. Femoral neuropathy induced by the lithotomy position: a report of 5 cases with a review of the literature. Muscle Nerve 1993; 16:891–895.

15. Senegor M. Iatrogenic saphenous neuralgia: successful therapy with neuroma resection. Neurosurgery 1991; 28:295–298.

16. Murayama K, Takeuchi T, Yuyama T. Entrapment of the saphenous nerve by branches of the femoral vessels: a report of two cases. J Bone Joint Surg 1991; 73A:770–772.

17. Adar R, Meyer E, Zweig A. Saphenous neuralgia: a complication of vascular reconstructions below the inguinal ligament. Ann Surg 1979; 190:609–613.

18. Luerssen TG, Campbell RL, Defalque RJ, Worth RM. Spontaneous saphenous neuralgia. Neurosurgery 1983; 13:238–241.

19. Robinson L. Traumatic injury to peripheral nerves. Muscle Nerve 2000; 23:863–873.

20. Chaudhry V, Cornblath DR. Wallerian degeneration in human nerves: serial electrophysiological studies. Muscle Nerve 1992; 687–693.

21. Oh SJ. Clinical Electromyography: Nerve Conduction Studies. 2nd ed. Philadelphia: Williams and Wilkins, 1993.

22. Stohr M, Shumm F, Ballier R. Normal sensory conduction in the saphenous nerve in man. EEG Clin Neurophysiol 1978; 44:172–178.

23. Ertekin C. Saphenous nerve conduction in man. J Neurol Neurosurg Psychiatry 1969; 31:28–33.

24. Halford H, Graves A. Imaging techniques. In: Bertorini TE, ed. Clinical Evaluation and Diagnostic Tests for Neuromuscular Disorders. Boston: Butterworth and Heinemann, 2002:565–593.

25. Filler AG, Howe FA, Hayes CE et al. Magnetic resonance neurography. Lancet 1993; 341:659–661.

26. Filler AG, Kliot M, Howe FA et al. Application of magnetic resonance neurography in the evaluation of patients with peripheral nerve pathology. J Neurosurg 1996; 85:299–309.

27. Sorenson EJ, Chen JJ, Daube JR. Obturator neuropathy: causes and outcome. Muscle Nerve 2002; 25:605–607.

28. Rogers LR, Borkowski GP, Albers JW, Levin KH, Barohn RJ, Mitsumoto H. Obturator mononeuropathy caused by pelvic cancer: six cases. Neurology 1993; 43:1489–1492.

29. Pellegrino MJ, Johnson EW. Bilateral obturator nerve injuries during urologic surgery. Arch Phys Med Rehabil 1988; 69:46–47.

30. Warfield CA. Obturator neuropathy after forceps delivery. Obstet Gynecol 1984; 64:47S–48S.

31. Bradshaw C, McCory P, Bell S, Brukner P. Obturator nerve entrapment: a cause of groin pain in athletes. Am J Sports Med 1997; 25:402–408.

32. Redwine DB, Sharpe DR. Endometriosis of the obturator nerve: a case report. J Reprod Med 1990; 35:434–435.

33. Scotto V, Rosica G, Valeri B et al. Benign schwannoma of the obturator nerve: a case report. Am J Obstet Gynecol 1998; 179:816–817.

34. Vasilev SA. Obturator nerve injury: a review of management options. Gynecol Oncol 1994; 53:152–155.

35. Amoiridis G, Wöhrle J, Grunwald I, Przuntek. Malignant tumour of the psoas: another cause of meralgia paresthetica. Electromyogr Clin Neurophysiol 1993; 33:109–112.

36. Jablecki CK. Postoperative lateral femoral cutaneous neuropathy. Muscle Nerve 1999; 1129–1131.

37. Yamout B, Tayyim A, Farhat W. Meralgia paresthetica as a complication of laparoscopic cholecystectomy. Clin Neurol Neurosurg 1994; 96:143–144.

38. Rao T, Kim H, Mathrubhutham M, Lee KN. Meralgia paresthetica: unusual complication of inguinal herniorrhaphy. J Am Med Assoc 1977; 237:2525.

39. Weikel AM, Habal MB. Meralgia paresthetica: a complication of iliac bone procurement. Plast Reconstr Surg 1977; 60:572–574.

40. Jefferson D, Eames RA. Subclinical entrapment of the lateral femoral cutaneous nerve: an autopsy study. Muscle Nerve 1979; 2:145–154.

41. Richer LP, Shevell MI, Stewart J, Poulin C. Pediatric meralgia paresthetica. Pediatr Neurol 2002; 26:321–323.

42. Ecker AD, Woltman HW. Meralgia paresthetica: a report of one hundred and fifty cases. J Am Med Assoc 1938; 110:1650–1652.

43. Beresford HR. Meralgia paresthetica after seat-belt trauma. J Trauma 1971; 11:629–630.

44. Butler ET, Johnson EW, Kaye AZ. Normal conduction velocity in the lateral femoral cutaneous nerve. Arch Phys Med Rehabil 1974; 55:31–32.

45. Sarala PK, Nishihira T, Oh SJ. Meralgia paresthetica: electrophysiological study. Arch Phys Med Rehabil 1979; 60:30–31.

46. Williams PH, Trzil KP. Management of meralgia paresthetica. J Neurosurg 1991; 74:76–80.

47. Dureja GP, Gulaya V, Jayalakshmi TS, Mandal P. Management of meralgia paresthetica: a multimodality regimen. Anesth Analg 1995; 80:1060–1061.

48. van Eerten PV, Polder TW, Broere CA. Operative treatment of meralgia paresthetica: transection versus neurolysis. Neurosurgery 1995; 37:63–65.

49. McKain CW, Urban BJ. Pain and cluneal neuropathy following intragluteal injection. Anesth Analg 1978; 57:138–141.

50. Arnoldussen WJ, Korten JJ. Pressure neuropathy of the posterior femoral cutaneous nerve. Clin Neurol Neurosurg 1980; 82:57–60.

51. Chutkow JG. Posterior femoral cutaneous neurolagia. Muscle Nerve 1988; 11:1146–1148.

52. Iyer VG, Shields CB. Isolated injection injury to the posterior femoral cutaneous nerve. Neurosurgery 1989; 25:835–838.

53. Stultz P, Pfeiffer KM. Peripheral nerve injuries resulting from common surgical procedures in the lower portion of the abdomen. Arch Surg 1982; 117:324–327.

54. Sippo WC, Gomez AC. Nerve entrapment syndromes from lower abdominal surgery. J Fam Pract 1987; 25:585–587.

55. Kanai H, Hirakawa M, Arimura Y, Taniguchi M, Tsuruya K, Masutani K, Ninomiya T, Sugawara K, Koga Y, Hirakata H. Ilioinguinal neuralgia complicating percutaneous renal biopsy. J Neurol 2001; 248:708–709.

56. Hahn L. Clinical findings and results of operative treatment in ilioinguinal nerve entrapment syndrome. Br J Obstet Gynaecol 1989; 96:1080–1083.

57. Laha RK, Rao S, Pidgeon CN. Genito-femoral neuralgia. Surg Neurol 1977; 8:280–282.

58. Obrien MD. Genito-femoral neuropathy. Br Med J 1979; 1:1052.

59. Hofmann A, Jones RE, Schoenvogel R. Pudendal-nerve neuropraxia as a result of traction on the fracture table: a report of four cases. J Bone Joint Surg Am 1982; 64:136–138.

60. Goodson JD. Pudendal neuritis from biking. N Engl J Med 1981; 304:365.

61. Gibson GR. Impotence following fractured pelvis and ruptured urethra. Br J Urol 1970; 42:86–88.

62. Allen RE, Hosker GL, Smith ARB, Warrell DW. Pelvic floor damage and childbirth: a neurophysiological study. Br J Obstet Gynecol 1990; 97:770–779.

63. Dumitru D, Nelson MR. Posterior femoral cutaneous nerve conduction. Arch Phys Med Rehabil 1990; 71:979–982.

64. Ellis RJ, Geisse H, Holub BA, Swenson MR. Ilioinguinal nerve conduction. Muscle Nerve 1992; 15:1194.

65. Kiff ES, Swash M. Slowed conduction in the pudendal nerves in idiopathic faecal incontinence. Br J Surg 1984; 71:614–616.

66. Snooks SJ, Swash M. Perineal nerve and transcutaneous spinal stimulation: new method for investigation of the urethral striated musculature. Br J Urol 1984; 56:406–409.

67. Clawson D, Cardenas D. Dorsal nerve of the penis nerve conduction velocity: a new technique. Muscle Nerve 1991; 14:845–849.

68. Kaneko S, Bradley WE. Penile electrodiagnosis. Value of bulbocavernosus reflex latency versus conduction velocity of the dorsal nerve of the penis in diagnosis of diabetic impotence. J Urol 1986; 137:933–935.

69. Kothari MJ, Bauer SB. Urodynamic and neurophysiologic evaluation of patients with diastematomyelia. J Child Neurol 1997; 12:97–100.
70. Kothari MJ, Kelly M, Darbey M, Bauer S, Scott RM. Neurophysiologic assessment of urinary dysfunction in children with thoracic syringomyelia. J Child Neurol 1995; 10:451–454.
71. Fowler CJ. Pelvic floor neurophysiology. Methods Clin Neurophysiol 1991; 2:1–24.
72. Rizzo MA. Successful treatment of painful traumatic mononeuropathy with carbamazepine: insights into a possible molecular pain mechanism. J Neurol Sci 1997; 152:103–106.

32

Management of Traumatic Mononeuropathies

Lisa DiPonio, James A. Leonard Jr, and John E. McGillicuddy
University of Michigan Medical Center, Ann Arbor, Michigan, USA

ABSTRACT

The management of traumatic mononeuropathies begins with recognition of nerve injury, which can be difficult in the setting of multiple traumatic injuries and fractures, particularly if there is poor patient cooperation due to brain injury. Knowledge of regional anatomy increases the suspicion of nerve injuries associated with various fractures, lacerations, or dislocations as well as iatrogenic causes. When nerve injury is suspected, clinical, electrodiagnostic evaluation or imaging studies can confirm nerves involved and determine severity. A decision for operative intervention in the form of exploration and repair or grafting procedures must be made. Nonoperative lesions can be managed with rehabilitation.

1. CLINICAL FEATURES/DIFFERENTIAL DIAGNOSIS

1.1. Clinical Findings and Classification System of Nerve Injuries

Nerves may be damaged primarily during the initial injury or secondarily as a result of edema, infection, ischemia, or scar formation (Table 32.1). Nerve root avulsion occurs when traction is placed on a nerve root sufficient to separate it from the spinal cord. Stretch injuries to peripheral segments are associated with open and closed fractures as well as soft tissue injuries. Nerve transections are associated with open injuries and sometimes with displacement of fracture fragments. Crush injuries are caused by acute or prolonged pressure. Nerves can also be damaged by ischemia as part of compartment syndrome or by vascular compromise.

The response of nerves to injury is limited, regardless of the mechanism of injury. Crush and angulation injuries preferentially affect myelin, and the predominant mechanism of tissue damage is localized ischemia. If ischemia is severe or prolonged, axons can be affected. In laceration or stretch injuries, axons and structural components are injured and Wallerian degeneration results.

Table 32.1 Orthopedic Injuries and Commonly Associated Peripheral Nerve Injuries

Orthopedic injury	Commonly associated nerve injury
Shoulder dislocation	Axillary
Humerus fracture	Radial
Elbow dislocation	Median
Monteggia fracture	Radial
Wrist	Median, ulnar, or radial
Pelvis	Cauda equina, radicular, plexus
Acetabular fracture	Sciatic
Hip dislocation	Femoral, sciatic
Femur fracture	Sciatic, tibial/peroneal components
Distal femur fracture	Tibial (medial), peroneal (lateral)
Tibial fracture	Tibial, deep peroneal
Fibular fracture	Common or superficial peroneal
Medial malleolus (tibia)	Tibial
Lateral malleolus (fibula)	Sural
Metatarsals	Interdigital nerves

Wallerian degeneration is the hallmark of axonal injury regardless of the mechanism. Seddon's classification of nerve injury describes three degrees of severity of nerve injury (1). Neurapraxia refers to focal demyelination that is sufficient to interrupt saltatory nerve conduction. The clinical result is sensory or motor loss despite axonal continuity. Symptoms in the acute phase are as severe as those from nerve transection, but prognosis for spontaneous recovery is excellent. Axonotmesis refers to loss of axonal continuity with preservation of structural and supportive neural tubules. It also carries a good prognosis for spontaneous recovery, although not as quickly as neurapraxia. Neurotmesis refers to discontinuity of the axons as well as their supporting structures. This carries a worse prognosis and is the only injury benefiting from surgical repair or grafting.

An updated classification proposed by Sunderland has five degrees of injury (2). Sunderland's first-degree injury is identical to Seddon's neurapraxia. Sunderland's second, third, and fourth-degree injuries correspond to different severities of Seddon's axonotmesis. A second-degree injury is axonal disruption but sparing of endoneurium, perineurium, and epineurium. A third-degree injury is sparing of perineurium and epineurium, and a fourth-degree injury is sparing of epineurium only. Sunderland's fifth-degree of injury is identical to Seddon's neurotmesis.

1.2. Anatomic Correlates

1.2.1. Spinal Accessory Nerve

This is the sole motor innervation to the trapezius muscle, and also innervates the sternocleidomastoid muscle. It has a superficial location in the subcutaneous tissue on the floor of the posterior cervical triangle which is bordered by the trapezius posteriorly, the sternocleidomastoid anteriorly, and the clavicle inferiorly. It is most commonly injured during surgical procedures, but is susceptible to trauma by blunt or penetrating injuries to the neck or by traction injury from dislocations of the sternoclavicular or acromioclavicular joints. The trapezius muscle serves to elevate, retract, and rotate the scapula, and disruption leads to lateral winging of the scapula and weakness of arm abduction past 90°. This nerve has no cutaneous innervation (Table 32.2).

1.2.2. Suprascapular Nerve

This nerve originates from the upper trunk of the brachial plexus and carries fibers from C5 and C6. It travels behind the plexus, under the trapezius muscle, to the scapula, where it passes through the suprascapular notch and innervates the supraspinatus muscle, and then around the lateral edge of the scapular spine to innervate the infraspinatus muscle. The nerve can be injured by scapular fracture, blunt trauma to the shoulder girdle, or traction through the nerve by a longitudinal pull on the upper extremity. The supraspinatus muscle helps elevate the arm over the first 90° and the infraspinatus muscle assists in external rotation of the arm. It has no cutaneous sensory innervation.

1.2.3. Axillary Nerve

This is a branch of the posterior cord and contains fibers from C5 and C6. It branches from the posterior cord near the lateral scapular border and sends a branch to teres minor. It then bifurcates into cutaneous and motor branches and courses posteriorly around the proximal humerus, supplies the posterior, middle, and anterior deltoid muscle. The sensory branch goes on to supply a small cutaneous segment in the lateral upper arm.

Axillary mononeuropathy results in weakness of shoulder abduction or sensory loss on the lateral upper arm. Injury occurs with proximal humeral fractures and, less commonly, with scapular fractures. The nerve is susceptible to traction injury of the plexus because it is tethered to the deltoid muscle close to the shoulder. The nerve can also be injured from scar tissue formation in the quadrilateral space (formed by the teres major muscle, triceps, humerus, and teres minor) through which the nerve passes or when other injuries occur, which require the use of axillary crutches (crutch paralysis).

1.2.4. Radial Nerve

This is the continuation of the posterior cord and carries fibers from C5, C6, C7, and C8. After leaving the plexus, the nerve travels posterior to the axillary artery and gives branches to the posterior cutaneous nerve of the arm and the triceps and anconeus muscles. At this level the nerve may be damaged by traction or tourniquet application. It then travels in the spiral groove of the humerus where it is vulnerable to damage related to humeral fractures or compression. Distal to the spiral groove, it pierces the lateral intermuscular septum and travels anterior to the lateral condyle of the humerus, giving branches to the brachialis, brachioradialis, and extensor carpi radialis longus muscles. At this point, it bifurcates into the posterior interosseous nerve (PIN) and the superficial branch. The PIN passes through the arcade of Frohse and then travels along the posterior interosseous membrane, where it innervates the other extensors muscles of the forearm. It travels along with the posterior interosseous artery and may be compressed by a traumatic aneurysm. It may also be injured by proximal radial fractures or penetrating injuries. The superficial branch continues superficially along the lateral border of the forearm where it is vulnerable to injuries associated with fractures of the distal and proximal radius or forced wrist hyperpronation.

Lesions in the axilla or proximal to the spiral groove may lead to sensory loss on the posterior arm above the elbow (posterior cutaneous nerve of arm) and weakness and dropped triceps reflex. Lesions within the spiral groove lead to sensory loss on the extensor surface of the forearm (posterior cutaneous nerve of forearm) and complete wrist drop.

Table 32.2 Summary of Nerve Injuries and Associated Muscles, Functional Deficits, and Functional Interventions

Nerve	Suprascapular	Axillary	Radial	Musculo-cutaneous	Median	Ulnar
Major muscles innervated	Spinati	Deltoid	Triceps, forearm extensors	Biceps brachii	Pronator teres, flexor digitorum profundus 1 and 2, thumb opposition	Flexor digitorum profundus 1 and 2, hand, and intrinsics
Functional deficit	Weakness of internal and external rotation	Weakness of arm abduction beyond 30°	Weakness of arm extension, wrist drop, loss of power grasp	Weakness of arm flexion, supination	Weakness of arm pronation, distal index and middle finger flexion, thumb opposition	Weakness of grip, hand function
Functional intervention	Shoulder support sling	Shoulder support sling	Splinting wrist fusion muscle tendon transfer	Functional arm support sling, elbow fusion, muscle tendon transfer	Splinting, muscle tendon transfer	Splinting, muscle tendon transfer

Nerve	Gluteals: superior and inferior	Femoral	Sciatic	Peroneal	Tibial
Major muscles innervated	Superior: gluteus medius and minimus, tensor fascia lata. Inferior: gluteus maximus	Quadriceps	Hamstrings, ankle dorsiflexors, plantarflexors, everters, and inverters	Ankle dorsiflexors and everters	Ankle plantarflexors and inverters
Major functional deficit	Superior: Trendelenberg gait. Inferior: weakness of hip extension	Weakness of knee extension	Flail foot	Foot drop	Weakness of toe-off
Functional intervention	Superior: cane in contralateral hand. Inferior: use hand rail or cane for stairs	KAFO with locking knee joint or knee extension assist, or ground reaction AFO	Double action or solid ankle AFO	AFO with dorsiflexion assist	AFO with dorsiflexion stop

Lesions distal to the spiral groove, but proximal to the elbow, such as can be seen with a distal fracture of the humerus, may lead to wrist drop with radial deviation and sparing of the forearm sensation and the brachioradialis reflex. Lesions involving the PIN give a purely motor syndrome of finger drop with radial deviation (due to the sparing of the extensor carpi radialis branch located proximal to the elbow). Lesions involving the superficial branch of the radial nerve would give a purely sensory syndrome affecting the dorsal radial hand, also known as cheiralgia paresthetica.

1.2.5. Musculocutaneous Nerve

The musculocutaneous nerve is a branch of the lateral cord containing fibers from C5 and C6. It travels between the axillary artery and median nerve, enters the coracobrachialis muscle which it supplies, and descends between the biceps and brachialis muscles which it also supplies. As it travels past the shoulder, it is relatively protected from injury related to humeral fractures because of its location between these muscles. Sensory fibers of the nerve continue distally past the elbow in the antecubital fossa where it could be injured by venipuncture or cutdown procedures due to its location directly under the median cubital vein. The nerve continues as the lateral antebrachial cutaneous nerve where it supplies cutaneous sensation to the lateral forearm.

The musculocutaneous nerve is often damaged in plexus injuries involving the lateral cord. Diagnosis of musculocutaneous mononeuropathy is suspected when there is a penetrating injury to the arm. A lesion in the upper arm leads to weakness of elbow flexion, especially with the forearm supinated. The brachioradialis is a strong flexor of the elbow, which is innervated by the radial nerve, and can mask biceps weakness. Lesions of the musculocutaneous nerve also produce sensory loss in the lateral forearm. Lesions located closer to the elbow, such as in the cubital fossa, produce a purely sensory syndrome with loss at the lateral forearm.

1.2.6. Median Nerve

This nerve forms in the axilla from branches of the lateral cord (containing C6 and C7 fibers) and the medial cord (containing C8 and T1 fibers). The nerve travels down the medial side of the arm in close proximity to the brachial artery into the cubital fossa. It is vulnerable to injury from penetrating injuries or sheath hemorrhage. No branches are given off proximal to the elbow, making it impossible to determine the location of a nerve injury in the shoulder or upper arm based on the sensorimotor findings alone. After crossing into the forearm between the two heads of the pronator teres muscle, it sends a branch, the anterior interosseous nerve (AIN). The AIN travels along the interosseous membrane and gives branches to the flexor digitorum profundus, flexor pollicis longus, and pronator quadratus muscles. Pseudo-AIN syndrome is a condition where median nerve injuries at the elbow preferentially affect the fibers of the AIN. This occurs with supracondylar humeral fractures, proximal radial fractures, and trauma from venipuncture or cut down at the cubital fossa. The symptoms of pseudo-AIN syndrome are similar to AIN syndrome (discussed subsequently), with relative sparing of the other motor branches, but there may be subtle median sensory changes in the hand.

The AIN travels along the interosseous membrane and is susceptible to injury from penetrating injuries or secondarily due to scar tissue formation in the anterior forearm. After the AIN branch, the median nerve continues in the volar forearm. Proximal to the flexor retinaculum, it gives off the palmar cutaneous branch, and then passes through the flexor retinaculum into the hand where it divides into the terminal sensory and motor branches. The palmar cutaneous branch can be damaged by lacerations in the forearm. In ∼15% of individuals, anomalous innervation between the median and ulnar nerves occurs in the forearm (Martin–Gruber anastamosis). Most cases involve motor branches from the median to the ulnar nerve that innervate hand muscles that are normally median innervated. In this case, a median nerve injury in the forearm distal to the anastamosis would spare some of the median innervated muscles in the hand. Martin–Gruber anastamosis can also involve motor branches sent from the median to the ulnar nerve that go on to innervate hand muscles that are normally ulnar innervated. In this case, a median nerve injury proximal to the anastamosis would involve ulnar innervated muscles in the hand. Less commonly, fibers can be sent from the ulnar to the median nerve that sometimes innervate median and sometimes ulnar muscles. Anomalous innervations involving the median and ulnar nerves also occur in the hand. In as many as 2% of individuals, the abductor pollicis brevis and flexor pollicis brevis are innervated by the ulnar nerve, and in as many individuals, the adductor pollicis is innervated by the median nerve. In 1% of individuals, the first dorsal interosseous muscle is innervated by the median nerve. Awareness of common anomalous innervations can help avoid mistaken diagnosis.

Median mononeuropathy is suspected when there is sensory loss in the thenar aspect of the palm and the volar first through third digits, together with weakness of wrist pronation, flexion of the distal phalanges of the thumb, index and middle finger, and abduction and opposition of the thumb. These latter two movements are relatively easily substituted for by other ulnar innervated muscles of the hand, and to exclude a median neuropathy, careful examination, including palpation for contractions of the muscles in question, is required. Lesions at or proximal to the elbow produce all of the symptoms described. Lesions of the AIN produce weakness of flexion of the distal phalanges and thumb, making it difficult for the patient to form the "OK" sign. Lesions in the distal forearm will produce weakness of thenar opposition and abduction. Palmar sensation is spared if the lesion is distal to the palmar cutaneous branch in the forearm. Lesions of the digital sensory branches in the hand commonly occur from lacerations in the palm or fingers. Digital nerve lacerations in the palm cause sensory loss of the adjacent sides of two fingers, or if distal, the side of one finger.

1.2.7. Ulnar Nerve

The ulnar nerve is a branch of the medial cord of the brachial plexus and carries fibers from C7, C8, and T1. It leaves the axilla and travels in the upper arm medial to the brachial artery. At the elbow, it enters the cubital tunnel formed by the medial ligament of the elbow joint and the aponeurosis between the olecranon and medial epicondyle of the humerus. In the arm, the nerve is vulnerable to traction injuries. At the elbow, it is vulnerable to injury related to distal humeral fractures or fracture or dislocation of the elbow. Distal to the elbow, it sends motor branches to the flexor carpi ulnaris and flexor digitorum profundus muscles. The former muscle is a wrist flexor with ulnar deviation and the latter flexes the distal phalanges of the fourth and fifth digits. In the forearm, it is vulnerable to injuries from forearm fractures (Colles' fracture). In the mid to distal forearm, two sensory branches are given off, the palmar cutaneous and the dorsal cutaneous, which supply sensory innervation to the palmar and dorsal hand, respectively. The nerve then passes through a tunnel formed by the pisiform and hamate bones of the wrist (Guyon's Canal) and enters the hand. There it divides into a superficial sensory branch which supplies the fourth and fifth digits and a deep motor branch which innervates the muscles of the hand.

Ulnar nerve lesions are suspected when there is sensory loss on the lateral hand and weakness of finger abduction and adduction. Ulnar nerve lesions can be confused with C8 radiculopathies because of similar sensory distributions, but are differentiated by lack of weakness of distal index and middle finger flexors (median nerve) and extension of the index finger (radial nerve), or the presence of Froment's sign (discussed subsequently). Lesions at or proximal to the elbow cannot be localized based on sensorimotor physical examination findings alone because the nerve gives no branches proximal to the elbow. Lesions just distal to mid forearm spare the flexor carpi ulnaris and flexor digitorum profundus muscles but may involve the palmar or dorsal cutaneous branches, depending on the location. Lesions at or distal to the wrist spare cutaneous sensation on the hypothenar aspects of the palm and dorsal hand. Froment's prehensile test is a test for weakness of ulnar muscles in the hand. To demonstrate, the patient is given a sheet of paper and told to hold it between the thumbs and index fingers of both hands and pull laterally. Because of weakness of the first dorsal interosseous muscle, the median innervated flexor pollicis longus muscle will substitute for it. The result is extension of the proximal phalynx of the thumb and flexion of the distal phalynx, which is known clinically as Froment's sign.

1.2.8. Femoral Nerve

The femoral nerve arises from the posterior rami of L2, L3, and L4. It forms within the psoas and travels between the psoas and iliacus muscles, both of which it supplies. It then descends underneath the inguinal ligament, lateral to the femoral artery, into the thigh. After passing the inguinal ligament it bifurcates into anterior and posterior divisions. The anterior division supplies the sartorius muscle (a thigh flexor and external rotator) and continues as the medial cutaneous nerve of the thigh. The posterior division divides in the proximal thigh into the saphenous sensory nerve, which travels posteriomedial to the knee and provides sensory innervation to the medial leg, and motor branches which supply the pectineus and quadriceps muscles (knee extensors). The most common cause of femoral neuropathy is trauma, usually iatrogenic from hip replacement or attempts at femoral artery cannulation. The nerve is vulnerable to injury from traction placed for pelvic, acetabular or femoral fractures. It can also be damaged or compressed from iliopsoas hemorrhage. Femoral mononeuropathy is diagnosed by weakness of knee extension and loss of the patellar reflex. It is accompanied by sensory loss on the medial leg as far as the ankle.

1.2.9. Obturator Nerve

The obturator nerve arises from the anterior rami of L2, L3, and L4. It travels near the midline of the pelvis through the obturator canal, where it is vulnerable to injury from pelvic fractures or iliopsoas hemorrhage. Obturator mononeuropathy causes weakness of thigh adduction with the leg extended and sensory loss of the distal medial thigh.

1.2.10. Gluteal Nerves

The superior gluteal nerve arises from L4, L5, and S1, leaves the pelvis via the sciatic notch, and supplies the tensor fascia lata, the gluteus minimus, and the gluteus medius muscles, all of which abduct and internally rotate the thigh. This nerve is vulnerable to injury from posterior pelvic fractures and with hip fracture and dislocation. A lesion of this nerve produces a Trendelenberg sign during gait, which is a drop of the contralateral side of the pelvis while the contralateral leg is elevated. The inferior gluteal nerve arises from L5, S1, and S2 and travels under the piriformis muscle, after which it innervates the gluteus maximus muscle. It can be injured by pelvic fractures especially near the sciatic foramen. A lesion to the inferior gluteal nerve causes weakness of hip extension that may not become apparent until the patient attempts to get up from a low chair or climb stairs.

1.2.11. Sciatic Nerve

The sciatic nerve arises from L4, L5, S1, and S2 roots. After leaving the sacral plexus, it exits the pelvis under the piriformis muscle and enters the thigh. It travels through the posterior thigh, where it sends branches to the hamstring muscles (semimembranosis, semitendonosis, and biceps femoris, which are knee flexors). Proximal to the popliteal fossa, it bifurcates into the tibial nerve (posterolaterally) and the peroneal nerve (medially). The sciatic nerve in the proximal thigh is vulnerable to injury from hip fracture dislocation, gluteal hemorrhage, or blunt trauma. In the mid or distal thigh, the nerve is vulnerable to injury from femur fractures or penetrating injuries. Sciatic nerve lesions in the proximal thigh lead to weakness of knee flexion, sensory loss on the medial leg and the entire foot, and a flail foot.

1.2.12. Tibial Nerve

The tibial nerve leaves the sciatic nerve just above the popliteal fossa. As it passes through the popliteal fossa, it is vulnerable to trauma from popliteal hemorrhage or knee dislocation. The tibial nerve gives off the medial sural cutaneous nerve, which supplies the posterolateral proximal calf and later joins the lateral sural cutaneous nerve (branch of the common peroneal nerve) to form the sural nerve. Distal to the popliteal fossa, the tibial nerve supplies the gastrocnemius and soleus, popliteus and plantaris muscles. It then travels distally between the gastroc-soleus and posterior tibialis muscles in the deep posterior compartment of the leg. There it supplies the posterior tibialis, flexor digitorum longus, and flexor hallicis longus muscles. Then, along with the tendons of these muscles and the posterior tibial artery, it enters the tarsal tunnel, an irregularly shaped, fibroosseous tunnel formed by the medial malleolus, calcaneous, deltoid ligaments, and flexor retinaculum of the medial ankle. Here, the nerve is vulnerable to compression or damage from hyperpronation, inversion injuries, fractures, or dislocations. It can also be compressed secondarily by an ill-fitting cast. In the distal tunnel, the nerve divides into medial and lateral plantar branches and also sends a small, medial calcaneal branch which supplies the medial heel. The medial plantar nerve supplies the skin on the medial two-thirds of the sole of the foot and the first and second lumbricals, abductor hallicis, flexor digitorum brevis, and flexor hallicis brevis muscles. The lateral plantar nerve supplies the skin on the lateral one-third of the sole, the abductor digiti minimi, flexor digiti minimi, adductor hallicis, interossei, and third and fourth lumbrical muscles. The medial and lateral plantar nerves are vulnerable to damage by tarsal and metatarsal fractures.

Tibial mononeuropathy is suspected when there is weakness of ankle plantarflexion and inversion with sparing of dorsiflexion and eversion. Sensory changes occur on the sole of the foot and medial heel. Tibial mononeuropathy at the tarsal tunnel leads to sensory loss or burning paresthesias of the sole of the foot and weakness of foot intrinsics, with sparing of plantarflexion and inversion strength. Tibial compression at the tarsal tunnel may preferentially affect the medial or lateral plantar nerve branches within the tunnel. Compression of the medial or lateral plantar nerves in the foot leads to weakness of foot intrinsics medially or laterally and sensory loss or paresthesias on the medial or lateral sole of the foot.

1.2.13. Peroneal Nerve

The common peroneal nerve leaves the sciatic nerve just proximal to the popliteal fossa. It travels in the lateral part of the fossa where it gives off a sensory branch, the lateral sural cutaneous nerve, and subsequently the lateral cutaneous nerve of the calf. The common peroneal nerve continues to move laterally and hooks around the fibular head, where it is vulnerable to external compression because of its superficial position. From there, it enters the lateral compartment peroneus longus muscle where it bifurcates into superficial and deep branches.

The superficial branch continues through the lateral compartment of the leg, where it is vulnerable to damage from fibular fractures or compartment pressures and supplies the peroneus longus and brevis muscles. It then exits the lateral compartment and forms two terminal sensory branches, the intermediate and medial dorsal cutaneous branches which supply the dorsum of the foot, excepting the lateral most portion and the web space between the first and second toes. In about one-fourth of individuals, an accessory peroneal nerve branches from the superficial peroneal nerve to innervate the extensor digitorum brevis muscle.

The deep peroneal nerve enters the anterior compartment where it travels along the interosseous membrane with the anterior tibial artery and veins. It shares the anterior compartment with the tibialis anterior, extensor hallicis longus, and extensor digitorum longus muscles, which it supplies. It is vulnerable to injury from tibial fractures or compartment syndrome. It continues under the extensor retinaculum where it then innervates the extensor hallicis brevis and extensor digitorum brevis muscles, then continues as a sensory nerve to supply the web space between the first and second toes.

Peroneal mononeuropathy is suspected when there is foot drop with sensory loss on the dorsum of the foot. Common peroneal mononeuropathies produce loss of sensation and weakness in the entire peroneal distribution and weakness of dorsiflexion and eversion. Lesions of the superficial branch would eversion weakness and sensory loss on the dorsum of the foot. Damage to the terminal superficial branch, vulnerable to laceration on the anterior lower leg, causes sensory loss on the dorsum (sparing the web space between the first and second toes) without eversion weakness. A lesion of the deep peroneal nerve, as seen in anterior compartment syndrome, causes weakness of ankle dorsiflexion with sparing of eversion and sensory loss confined to the web space between the first and second toes.

Peroneal mononeuropathy can be difficult to differentiate from L5 radiculopathy because of the high representation of L5 fibers in the peroneal nerve. It is helpful to know certain anatomical tests. A peroneal mononeuropathy affects ankle eversion and not inversion, whereas an L5 radiculopathy affects both. This may be difficult to differentiate, however, because of the ability of the medial gastrocnemius to substitute for the action of the posterior tibialis. A peroneal mononeuropathy does not affect knee flexion or hip abduction, which may be affected by an L5 radiculopathy. A peroneal mononeuropathy may produce a Tinel's sign at the fibular head. Ultimately, further laboratory evaluation including an electrodiagnostic study is helpful.

1.3. Screening Tests

Simple screening tests for peripheral nerve injuries can be administrated in the field. In the upper extremity, the ability to make the "OK sign" (thumb and index finger form a circle) and intact sensation on the volar index finger suggests neuronal continuity of the median nerve and medial cord of the plexus. However, thumb opposition can often be accomplished with a median nerve lesion by substitution, and is therefore not a reliable indicator of median nerve continuity unless contraction of the opponens pollicis is palpated. Abduction of the fifth and index fingers (especially including palpation of first dorsal interosseous muscle contraction) indicates continuity of the ulnar nerve and lower trunk of the plexus. Distal phalanx extension or the "hitchhiker's sign" (extension of the thumb) indicates continuity of the radial nerve and posterior cord. In the lower extremity, extension and flexion of the great toe indicates continuity of the peroneal and tibial branches of the sciatic nerve. Intact sensation on the medial ankle, or the ability to extend the knee actively, indicates continuity of the femoral nerve.

2. PATHOGENESIS AND NERVE RESPONSE TO INJURY

2.1. Neural Injury in Neurotmesis or Sunderland's Fifth-Degree Lesion

Following a complete nerve transection, the nerve ends retract due to the elasticity of endoneurium. All components of the axon, including the epineurium, perineurium, and endoneurial tubes, are disrupted. Within hours, the fragment distal to the site of injury shows disintegration of neurofibrils, and within 24–48 h the axons begin to fragment, beginning at the nodes of Ranvier and progressing to the internodal segments. Schwann cells are also affected, and myelin is retracted beginning at the nodes of Ranvier, first at the portion just distal to the site of injury, and progressing further distally over the next 24–36 h. Schwann cells show an increase in size of the cell's nucleus. By 72 h, the myelin sheath forms segmented myelin ovoids and an increase in the Schwann cell nucleus mitotic activity occurs. Over the next several days, Schwann cells continue to proliferate, engulfing and breaking down the residual components of the axons within the endoneurial tubes. There is profound proliferation at the proximal end of the severed nerve, perhaps attempting to bridge the gap that was formed by the transection and retraction. By the 10th day postinjury, the entire axon distal to the transection consists of a series of myelin ovoids and by the 35th day, all axonal material has been removed and digested by these myelin ovoids. The residual endoneurial tubes shrink in diameter but can remain intact throughout the nerve distal to the injury for several months, waiting for some axonal regrowth from a proximal segment of the nerve.

Proximal to the site of injury, axonal degeneration takes place as well. If the endoneurial tube is disrupted, axonal degeneration can progress several centimeters proximally. In addition, if the nerve is severely injured, reactions affecting the cell body may occur. Proximal and sensory nerves are more likely than distal and motor nerves to experience axonal reaction. When this reaction occurs, the first phase is known as the reactive phase. During this period, the cell body and the nucleus become swollen and begin producing substances needed for regeneration. Most peripheral nerve cells then enter a recovery phase over the next 10–20 weeks, during which the cell body returns to normal. Full recovery is dependent upon the ability of the proximal severed nerve ending to bridge the gap and establish axonal continuity with the end organ. If axonal continuity does not occur, the cell body is more likely to enter a degenerative phase and eventually disintegrate over weeks to several months.

2.2. Neural Regeneration After Sunderland's Neurotmesis or Fifth-Degree Lesions

In some cases, within days proliferating Schwann cells and fibroblasts at the proximal end of the severed nerve are able to close the gap. This bridge of Schwann cells, debris, and fibroblasts is referred to as the bands of Bunger. The proximal axons send out collateral sprouts which penetrate the bands of Bunger in a disorganized fashion. If a sprout encounters scar tissue, blood clot, and so on, it may change direction, double back, bifurcate, or form a terminal bulb. If an axonal sprout is able to reach an endoneurial tube, the Schwann cells align about the advancing axon and the myelin sheath is reformed from the myelin ovoids. The formation of the myelin sheath takes several days longer than the advancement of the axon, and therefore remyelination lags behind axonal regrowth. Full maturation can take a year or more.

The success of the regeneration process has several factors. These include patient age, length of the gap, length of time since the injury, amount and severity of bleeding and scar tissue formation in the area, and location of the nerve injury. The closer the injury is to the cell body, the faster the rate of axonal sprout advancement. Therefore, injuries that are more proximal have faster rates of axonal regrowth. In true neurotmesis, however, functional recovery in the absence of surgical intervention is rare. The axonal reaction limits the number of surviving cell bodies capable of supporting any axons. The axons that do survive have limited chance of locating an endoneurial tube to enter, particularly if there is a true separation of nerve ends or significant clot or scarring. Even if axons do find endoneurial tubes to enter, many will enter an inappropriate type of tube, that is, a motor axon entering sensory nerve endoneurial tube, resulting in a nerve that is in continuity but not functional.

If a nerve is surgically grafted, the regeneration process takes place at the proximal end of the graft and the proximal end of the distal nerve stump. Thus, there is twice the opportunity for advancing neurites both to get lost in clot or scar tissue and to enter inappropriate endoneurial tubes. For successful recovery to take place after a graft, a neurite must find and enter an endoneurial tube in the graft, and the same axon from the distal end of the graft needs to enter the endoneurial tube of the same type of axon at the distal nerve stump. Studies suggest that inappropriate regeneration (neurites entering the wrong type of endoneurial tube) is more of a problem than lack of regeneration (3).

2.3. Neural Injury and Regeneration in Sunderland's Fourth- and Third-Degree Lesions

In fourth- and third-degree lesions, the endoneurium remains intact. In third-degree lesions, perineurium and epineurium are spared, and in fourth-degree lesions, epineurium is spared. Response to injury is similar to that in neurotmesis, but with continuity of perineurium and/or epineurium, some of the funincular organization of the nerve is spared. This may improve the chance of advancing neurites for successful regeneration. Particularly in fourth-degree lesions, advancing neurites can be blocked by scar or clot and form a tangle of disorganized neurites (neurofibrillar brush) and form a neuroma in continuity. This is histologically similar to a neuroma at a severed nerve end, but the presence of intact epineurial and/or perineurial structures cause the nerve to appear to be in continuity. Palpation of the nerve at this location during surgical exploration reveals a focal increase in nerve diameter, raising the suspicion of a neuroma in continuity.

2.4. Neural Injury and Regeneration in Axonotmesis or Sunderland's Second-Degree Lesion

With axonotmesis, endoneurial tubes are intact. The previously described events of Wallerian degeneration occur proximally and distally to the site of injury. However, when entering the regeneration phase, the advancing neuritis simply follow the intact endoneurial tubes to reinnervate the distal segments and eventually reach the appropriate end organs with no chance of aberrant innervation.

2.5. Neural Injury and Regeneration in Neurapraxia

In Neurapraxia, segmental demyelination occurs but axons and their supporting structures are intact. The electrophysiologic correlate of neurapraxia is conduction block, or the loss of saltatory conduction across a segment of nerve, resulting in loss of motor and/sensory function. In the mildest cases, neurapraxia involves only focal nerve ischemia which is reversible within minutes to hours. More severe cases of neurapraxia involve moderate or severe demyelination, and remyelination occurs spontaneously. Moderate cases will resolve within 4 weeks, but more severe cases may take 3–6 months. When remyelination is prolonged, secondary axonal loss can occur at the site of demyelination. Overall, however, the prognosis for recovery in neurapraxia is excellent.

3. LABORATORY EVALUATION

3.1. Blood and Serum Testing

Blood and serum testing is minimally helpful in diagnosing traumatic mononeuropathies. Evidence for a superimposed neuropathy might be detected from fasting glucose, hemoglobin A_{1C}, and vitamin B_{12}.

3.2. Imaging Studies

Radiographs are useful in the initial workup in the setting of multiple trauma when nerve damage is suspected. Soft tissues and other structures are not adequately visualized on plain radiographs, and nerve or other soft tissue trauma certainly cannot be excluded based on normal radiographs. A chest radiograph may be helpful to look for a clavicle fracture (which may lead to lateral divisional brachial plexopathy), diaphragmatic paralysis (suggesting pathology of proximal roots of C3, C4, or C5), or fracture of the first or second rib. Myelography is useful if root avulsion is suspected. Magnetic resonance neurography can visualize peripheral nerves and demonstrate nerve discontinuity, abnormal enlargement, and abnormal signal in peripheral nerves (4). It is not, however, a substitute for a clinical examination. Traditional magnetic resonance imaging techniques can also be used to demonstrate soft tissue swelling or injury in the vicinity of peripheral nerves.

High resolution ultrasound can detect abnormalities in soft tissue and nerves, and can identify nerve compression, entrapment, and discontinuity of nerves (Fig. 32.1).

3.3. Electrodiagnostic Evaluation

Electrodiagnostic studies are valuable because they assess the continuity of nerves. The major limitation in the setting of acute traumatic mononeuropathies is that electrodiagnosis cannot provide information about the pathology of the lesion, and full characterization of the severity of a nerve injury is not possible until 3 weeks have elapsed.

Electrodiagnostic studies are divided into nerve conduction studies (NCS) and needle electromyography (EMG). NCS can document nerve damage, but during the first several days may not be able to differentiate between neurapraxia (conduction block), axonotmesis, and neurotmesis. They can be useful at localizing a site of injury using the "inching" technique. With a complete nerve transection, this technique is less useful, because after the first 24–48 h, Wallerian degeneration makes it impossible to stimulate the nerve at or distal to the injury to allow for localization.

Serial electrodiagnostic evaluations performed every 1–3 months following the injury can provide information pertinent to management. With neurapraxia, an EMG study several weeks after injury will reveal no abnormal spontaneous activity in the affected nerve's distribution, supporting an excellent prognosis of spontaneous recovery. With axonotmesis, abnormal spontaneous activity will be seen, and the presence of

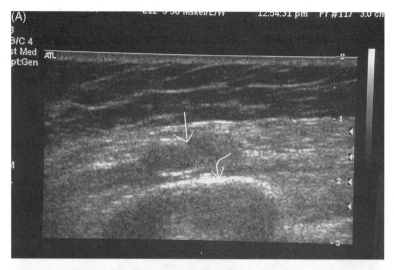

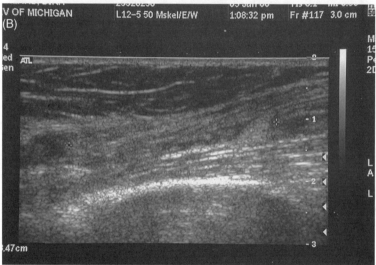

Figure 32.1 A 28-year-old female with radial nerve transection after humeral fracture. (A) Sonogram longitudinal to the radial nerve shows the retracted, enlarged, and abnormally hypoechoic stump of the radial nerve (arrow) at the site of the humerus fracture (curved arrow). (B) Sonogram distal to (A) shows the separation of the proximal and distal stump radial nerve stumps (between crosshairs). Ultrasound images courtesy of Jon Jacobson, University of Michigan Medical Center, Department of Radiology.

recruited motor units with voluntary activation signifies axonal regrowth into the muscle. With neurotmesis, the continued presence of abnormal spontaneous activity and absence of recruitable motor unit potentials suggests no active regrowth and surgical repair or nerve graft (or other intervention) should be considered.

Intraoperative electrodiagnostic studies provide information about axonal continuity that cannot be determined from surface recording. Intraoperative recording is useful in the acute setting to determine if axonal continuity is present, and in the subacute setting to see if axonal regrowth has begun to take place. Because the nerves can be studied at a very proximal location, axonal regrowth can be detected before there are clinical signs of recovery. Surgically exposed nerves are directly stimulated and responses recorded across a suspected lesion before and after neurolysis. This technique is useful in all but Sunderland's fifth-degree lesions. A nerve that has the external appearance of continuity may have endoneurial or perineurial disruption and may not regenerate. Conversely, a nerve that appears unhealthy on direct inspection may have regenerated. The intraoperative study can also be used to detect the proximal margin of a nerve lesion. Often hemorrhage, ischemia, or infection may lead to fibrosis that may extend a considerable distance proximal to the obvious lesion. Moving the electrodes proximally until a normal section of nerve is located will allow the identification of the distal-most segment of undamaged nerve. Unfortunately, Wallerian degeneration prevents the distal margin of injury from being similarly identified electrodiagnostically.

4. SURGICAL AND NONSURGICAL MANAGEMENT

4.1. Open Injuries

Traumatic nerve injury in the setting of an open wound requires immediate surgical exploration, provided there are no contraindications from other injuries or the patient's overall status. If the nerve is transected, and the two ends identified, immediate end-to-end repair offers the best opportunity for nerve recovery. If the transection resulted in jagged nerve endings, they must be trimmed back to a clean normal appearing nerve before anastamosis can be attempted. With retraction and trimming of a damaged nerve end, it may not be possible to approximate the ends for a repair, and a nerve graft will be required. Sural nerve is typically used as the graft donor. Grafting a gap of >14 cm will not likely result in good recovery of nerve function. Repair of transected nerve, even delayed repair, at the earliest surgically appropriate time will yield the best recovery results. A 2–4 week delay after transection results in the loss of nerve elasticity with greater difficulty approximating the ends for primary repair without putting significant tension on the sutures (5).

If the wound is contaminated or the patient's overall status does not permit, the nerve cannot be repaired acutely. In this case, the ends of the transected nerve, if identified, can be marked with surgical clips to facilitate repair at a later date. It is also possible that during surgery, the suspect peripheral nerve may appear to be in continuity and even normal in appearance. In this situation, the nerve injury may represent neurapraxia or axonotmesis, and should be left alone.

Later exploration and repair is often made complex by retraction of the transected nerve endings and scar formation at the previous operative field/injury site. If the nerve was cleanly transected, but the ends have retracted, dissection of the nerve endings from surrounding scar as well as along the course of the nerve proximally and distally will likely be required to free up the sufficient nerve to allow approximation and suturing with as little tension at the suture line as possible.

4.2. Closed Injuries

Closed peripheral nerve injuries present more diagnostic and management challenges than open injuries. Examination at presentation in the emergency room may identify a nerve injury and even the likely anatomic location, but the mechanism or degree of injury may be uncertain. Electrodiagnostic studies and somatosensory evoked potential studies are useful to help assess the degree of nerve injury, whether neurapraxia, axonotmesis, or neurotmesis. They can determine whether there is continuity of the nerve and to what degree. Serial studies can also determine evidence of early recovery. They can also provide some information about prognosis for functional recovery that will help guide decisions to pursue nonoperative or operative treatment strategies. Imaging techniques are able to provide additional information about the anatomy of the peripheral nerve complementing the functional and physiologic information of the clinical and electrodiagnostic examination.

Neurapraxic lesions have an excellent functional recovery. Management is directed toward avoiding complications such as contracture and additional trauma to insensate or unstable body parts. If there is incomplete axon loss, the amplitudes of the motor and sensory evoked responses on NCS provide an approximation percentage of preserved nerve function. The time course of recovery depends upon the site of the lesion and the distance to the various motor branches of the involved nerve distal to the site of the lesion. Generally, recovery of motor and sensory function occurs in a sequential order from proximal to distal if complete reinnervation/recovery occurs. Regenerating axons are said to grow approximately one millimeter per day. An additional factor in motor recovery is terminal collateral sprouting from the remaining intact axons. This process typically takes 6–12 weeks and is documented during EMG by an increase in motor unit potential complexity amplitude. Treatment interventions will be required for longer periods of time and the need for splinting or orthotics is more likely to compensate for altered function or to prevent additional complications while awaiting recovery. After a sufficient period of time, generally 6 months (depending on the nerve and site of injury), if there has been little or no evidence of recovery or improvement in function, surgical exploration should be considered to determine if scar, neuroma in continuity, or surgically improvable lesion is present.

A complete lesion, based on clinical examination and electrodiagnostic testing, should be followed for evidence of recovery with serial examinations. In the absence of any recovery >3 months, surgical exploration of the nerve to look for a repairable lesion should be considered. External neurolysis and direct visual evaluation of the nerve fascicle-by-fascicle, further assisted by direct intraoperative electrophysiologic evaluation of the individual nerve bundles, can identify functioning and nonfunctioning fascicles. An increase in the diameter of a nerve suggests a neuroma in continuity. Those which demonstrate the presence of recordable nerve action potentials need not be repaired or grafted and those that demonstrate no response can be repaired in the hopes of improving recovery and function.

When considering delayed repair and grafting procedures, appropriate timing can maximize a patient's chances of functional recovery. Surgery and grafting performed too early, before it is determined that neurotmesis is truly present, can negate the opportunity for spontaneous recovery. If done too late, axonal stenosis can affect distal segments before the axonal regeneration reaches them, making it difficult for regenerating axons to reach their end organs. Contraindications to surgical repair include neurapraxia or axonotmesis, nerve root avulsion, spinal cord injury or other lesion that would impede functional recovery, and if >2 years have passed since the initial injury.

Poor functional outcome following nerve grafting is more likely to be from aberrant regeneration rather than from a lack of regeneration. This is why it is appropriate to allow time for axonotmetic lesions to show signs of recovery. If there is any chance that there is axonotmesis and not neurotmesis, graft should not be attempted because the aberrant regeneration will cause significant functional loss.

4.3. Physical and Occupational Therapy

The same therapies are appropriate for both open and closed injuries. Physical and occupational therapy may be necessary to maintain range of motion and strength, or provide strategies to deal with altered mobility or activities of daily living. Splinting in the upper extremities or bracing in the lower extremities may be required for protection or stabilization, especially if there are other associated injuries such as fractures in the involved extremity.

4.4. Compensatory Surgical Options

When functional recovery does not occur, with or without surgical interventions, consideration can be given to reconstructive surgery such as muscle or tendon transfer or joint stabilization. This is especially appropriate in the upper extremity.

4.5. Compensatory Orthotic Options

4.5.1. Axillary Neuropathy

A deltoid aid, Swedish sling, overhead sling, or counterbalance arm sling can help position the arm for exercise activities in therapy. Elbow and wrist straps can be suspended from overhead support that can be freestanding or attached to a wheelchair or table which allows the arm to swing as a pendulum to support a weak deltoid. The bulk of this system makes its use outside of an institutional setting impractical. To reduce pain from a chronically distracted shoulder, an arm sling such as a figure of eight or universal sling can be considered.

4.5.2. Musculocutaneous Neuropathy

A circumferential humeral proximal forearm cuffs suspended from a shoulder saddle by straps and/or a Bowden cable can compensate for elbow flexion weakness. The elbow locking and unlocking mechanism can be operated via a chest strap [Fig. 32.2(A and B)].

4.5.3. Radial Neuropathy

Compensation for triceps muscle weakness is usually not indicated for everyday function. The major problem is lack of forearm and finger extensors causes a weak grip. A forearm-wrist extension assist orthosis can compensate by assisting with extensor strength of the

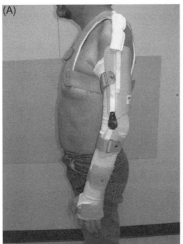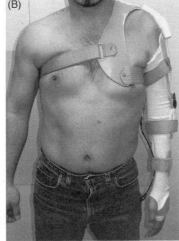

Figure 32.2 The elbow locking and unlocking mechanism: (A) side view; (B) frontal view.

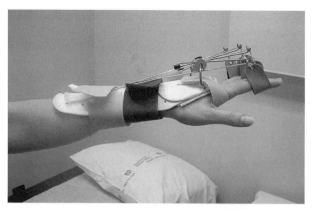

Figure 32.3 Forearm-wrist extension assist orthosis.

fingers (Fig. 32.3). Neutral resting hand splints are helpful in preventing or reducing flexion contractures and overstretching of the extensors of the wrist and fingers.

4.5.4. Median and Ulnar Neuropathies

A tenodesis orthosis can use the strength of the radial wrist extensors to create opposition of the thumb and index fingers to compensate for loss of grip and fine motor control (Figs. 32.4 and 32.5). In median neuropathies, a hand-based thumb opponens splint (Figs. 32.6 and 32.7) assists thenar opposition. In ulnar neuropathies, a metatarsophalangeal (MP)-blocking figure eight splint [Fig. 32.8(A and B)] which blocks the MP joints at 70–90° of flexion, can allow extension of the proximal and distal interphalangeal joints in the absence of ulnar intrinsic hand muscles. If ulnar nerve repair in the forearm is performed, an ulnar gutter splint to digits 4 and 5 positions the forearm, wrist, and hand for prevention of contractures.

4.5.5. Gluteal Neuropathy

Orthotic compensation for hip abduction weakness and a Trendelenberg gait, or drop of the contralateral buttock during stance phase would involve a bulky and uncomfortable brace that is not commonly accepted by patients. Less cumbersome is a cane in the contralateral hand with placement during heel strike on the weak side. Only a few pounds of pressure placed on the cane is able to correct the drop. Inferior gluteal mononeuropathy

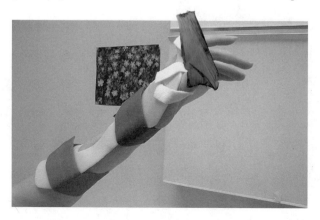

Figure 32.4 Tenodesis orthosis using radial wrist extensors.

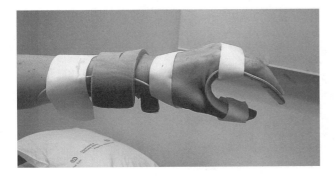

Figure 32.5   Tenodesis orthosis using radial wrist extensors.

leads to weakness of hip extension which may not become apparent until the patient tries to climb stairs or a steep hill. The most useful intervention is a handrail to allow the patient to use the upper extremities to assist with ascending the stairs.

4.5.6.   Femoral Neuropathy

Without intervention, the patient will compensate by snapping the knee straight during late swing phase (genu recurvatum) and will begin heel strike with a straight knee. A ground reaction ankle foot orthosis (AFO) is an AFO with plantarflexion assist. During heel strike, this device will apply an extension moment to the knee to stabilize it during heel strike and stance phases. The ground reaction AFO is useful with mild or moderate knee extension weakness such as with incomplete nerve injuries. In severe or complete femoral neuropathies, the knee will need to be stabilized with a knee ankle foot orthosis (KAFO) with either an extension assist or a knee locking mechanism.

4.5.7.   Sciatic Neuropathy

An insensate and flail foot with weakness of both dorsiflexion and plantarflexion can be helped by a double action AFO which will assist with both dorsiflexion and plantarflexion. Usually, these devices consist of a calf cuff and double metal upright sides with spring loaded ankle joints and stirrups to attach the device to the outside of a shoe. If the patient has a strong preference for a lower profile polypropylene device, the orthosis should be custom molded and covered with a soft material to protect the insensate foot from skin breakdown.

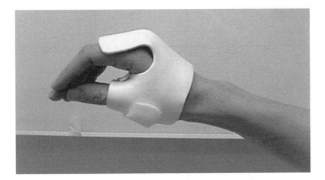

Figure 32.6   A hand-based thumb opponens splint.

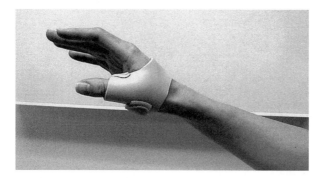

Figure 32.7   Hand-based thumb opponens splint.

4.5.8.   Tibial Neuropathy

An AFO in neutral position assists with toe-off will assist with weakness of ankle plantar-flexion and inversion. If a polypropylene device is selected, it should be custom molded and have a soft cover to protect the insensate sole against skin breakdown.

4.5.9.   Peroneal Neuropathy

An AFO with dorsiflexion assistance prevents foot drop and tripping, and the compensatory hip-hike gait that may lead to hip and knee pathology over time. When fitting the AFO, the orthotist must be careful not to fit a calf cuff that puts excessive pressure at

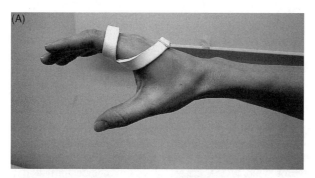

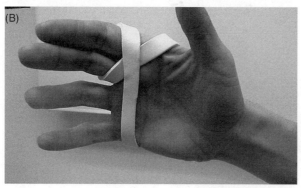

Figure 32.8   Metatarsophalongeal-blocking figure light splint.

the fibular neck, as this could further compress the peroneal nerve and prevent functional recovery that would otherwise happen.

5. PROGNOSIS

Prognosis varies according to the mechanism and location of injury. The most important prognosticating factor is the severity of nerve injury, and few reports include the severities of nerve injuries according to the Seddon or Sunderland classifications. When taking into account all the injuries, however, spontaneous recovery is the rule rather than the exception (7). Closed injuries have better prognosis for spontaneous recovery than do open injuries. Seddon (8) reported 83.5% spontaneous recovery in cases of neuropathy associated with closed upper extremity fracture, but only 17% in those associated with open fracture. Nerve injuries associated with joint dislocations have poorer prognosis than those associated with fractures, because the tight fascial envelopes that hold nerves close to joints cause excessive traction on nerves when the joints dislocate. The radial nerve is the most commonly injured nerve (9). Omer (10) reported a 70% rate of spontaneous recovery after radial nerve paralysis associated with humeral fractures. Shaw and Sakellarides (11) reported spontaneous recovery in radial nerve palsies in 40% of cases of primary injury and in 100% of cases of secondary injury where the paralysis resulted from manipulation or open reduction. Hunter (12) reported 83% spontaneous recovery of sciatic nerve lesions, and Seddon (9) reported 73% recovery. Peroneal nerve injuries have been reported to have lower incidences of spontaneous recovery. Meyers et al. (13) reported functional recovery of only 2 of 14 cases of peroneal palsies that occurred after traumatic dislocation of knee joints. Ottolenghi and Traversa (14) described recovery in 12 of 22 cases of common peroneal nerve injury.

Less is known about the long-term results following operative nerve repair or grafting. Gaul (15) reported that recovery can continue for 24 or even >50 months. However, several factors can be useful in predicting the chances of recovery after peripheral nerve repair. The most important is patient age. Patients younger than 12 have a good chance of functional recovery, and this chance diminishes in patients >50 years of age, and very old patients experience poorer functional recovery (7). Another factor is the type of nerve involved. Nerves that contain a single type of fiber have higher incidence of recovery than mixed nerves, explained by the high incidence of aberrant regeneration possible in mixed nerves. Other factors include the type of trauma that caused the neuropathy. Crush injuries that include injury to neural vascular support, contaminated or infected wounds do worse than cleanly transected nerves. The time of repair of a primary laceration will also affect recovery, as nerve retraction will affect the amount of tension placed on the sutures. When jagged nerve endings have to be trimmed back to allow for end-to-end repair, the resulting end-to-end gap will result in increased tension on the sutures and more chance of fibrous scarring at the site. When a gap is present that is greater than a few centimeters, nerve grafting will achieve better results than end-to-end repair due to the necessary tension to close such a gap.

The ultimate prognosis for both conservatively and operatively managed nerve injuries will be improved by a rehabilitative program designed to increase the patient's ability to use new or altered patterns of activation. Prognosis is dependent not only on neural regeneration and correct reinnervation, but also on the patient's age, health, social support, motivation, beliefs, perseverance, and activity level. Nerve regeneration and collateral sprouting can occur up to 3 years after an injury. However, reorganization and refinement of central neural pathways and coordination of movement can continue for at least 5 years and longer in the young patient.

APPENDIX: TREATMENT ALGORITHM FOR TRAUMATIC MONONEUROPATHIES

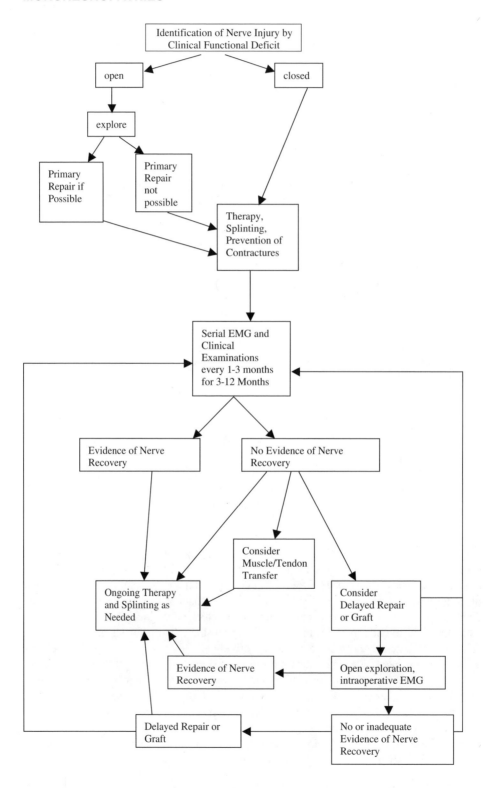

REFERENCES

1. Seddon HJ. Three types of nerve injury. Brain 1943; 66:237–288.
2. Sunderland S. A classification of peripheral nerve injuries producing loss of function. Brain 1951; 74:491–516.
3. Toby et al. Changes in the structural properties of peripheral nerves after transection. J Hand Surg 1996; 21A:1086–1090.
4. Aagaard BD. Magnetic resonance neurography: magnetic resonance imaging of peripheral nerves. Neuroimaging Clin N Am 2001; 11(1):131–146.
5. Martinoli C. Tendon and nerve sonography. Radiol Clin North Am 1999; 37(4):691–711.
6. Kline, DG. Nerve Injuries: Operative results for major nerve injuries, entrapmentz, and tumors. WB Saunders 1995.
7. Omer G, Spinner M, van Beek A, eds. Management of Peripheral Nerve Problems. 2nd ed. WB Saunders Co., 1998.
8. Seddon HJ. Nerve lesions complicating certain closed bone injuries. J Am Med Assoc 1947; 135:691–694.
9. Seddon HJ. Surgical Disorders of the Peripheral Nerves. 2nd ed. Edinburgh: Churchill Livinstone, 1975:691–694.
10. Omer GE, Results of untreated peripheral nerve injuries. Clin Orthop 1982; 163:15–19.
11. Shaw J, Sakellarides H. Radial-nerve paralysis associated with fractures of the humerus. A review of forty-five cases. J Bone Joint Surg 1967; 49A:899–902.
12. Hunter GA. Posterior dislocation and fracture dislocation of the hip, a review of fifty-seven patients. J Bone Joint Surg 1969; 51B:38–44.
13. Meyers MH, Moore TM, Harvey JP. Follow-up notes on articles previously published in the Journal: traumatic dislocation of the knee joint. J Bone Joint Surg 1975; 57A:430–433.
14. Ottolenghi CE. Traversa CH. Vascular and nervous complications in injuries of the knee joint. [Journal Article]. Reconstr Surg Traumatol 1974; 14:114–135.
15. Gaul S. Intrinsic motor recovery: a long term study of ulnar nerve repair. J Hand Surg 1982; 7:502–508.

33

Cranial Mononeuropathies

Mark B. Bromberg
University of Utah, Salt Lake City, Utah, USA

ABSTRACT

Cranial nerve (CN) mononeuropathies are an uncommon form of peripheral neuropathy. When symptoms occur suddenly there is concern for a stroke, which often leads to an extensive workup. However, isolated cranial mononeuropathies are distinct clinical entities. Although a cause can be identified in many patients, in a large number the cause remains unknown and is considered to be idiopathic. This chapter reviews acute onset acquired mononeuropathies affecting the peripheral component of CN III–XII. Paroxysmal cranial neuropathies will not be considered in detail.

1. CN III, IV, AND VI (OCULOMOTOR, TROCHLEAR, AND ABDUCENS)

1.1. Anatomy

The extramedullary course of CN III (oculomotor) begins as rootlets along the ventral surface of the mesencephalon, merging into a nerve trunk of about 15,000 large myelinated fibers (two-thirds from the ipsilateral nuclear complex and one-third from the contralateral complex) and a lesser number of small myelinated parasympathetic fibers from the Edinger–Westphal nucleus. The nerve passes between the posterior cerebral and superior cerebellar arteries, and travels forward and passes through the cavernous sinus. The nerve then enters the orbit through the superior orbital fissure and divides into superior and inferior divisions. The superior division innervates the superior rectus and the levator palpebare muscles, whereas the inferior division innervates the inferior rectus, medial rectus, and superior oblique muscles.

CN IV (trochlear) includes about 2500 fibers from the contralateral nucleus and leaves the dorsal brainstem below the inferior cerebellar peducles and curves around the brainstem. It passes between the posterior cerebral and superior cerebellar arteries. It also passes through the cavernous sinus and enters the orbit through the superior orbital fissure to innervate the superior oblique muscle.

CN VI (abducens) rootlets arise from the pontomedullary junction and join to form a nerve trunk of about 7000 fibers. It passes through the cavernous sinus and enters the orbit through the superior orbital fissure to innervate the lateral rectus muscle.

Within the cavernous sinus, CN III, IV, and VI and the ophthalmic and maxillary divisions of CN V are in close proximity.

1.2. Symptoms and Signs

Neuropathies of these nerves result in diplopia and ptosis ipsilateral to the lesion. Note, lesions of CN IV may rarely be associated with contralateral ptosis. Lesions of CN III lead to diplopia with inability to adduct or look down and up, and as a consequence, the eye assumes a position of downward abduction. There is also ptosis and a dilated pupil. Lesions of CN IV lead to diplopia with inability to rotate the eye down and out, and the eye assumes a slightly elevated position. The patient can easily compensate for weakness of the superior oblique muscle by rotating (tilting) the head to the opposite side. Lesions of CN VI lead to diplopia because of inability to abduct the eye.

1.3. Causes

Head trauma is the cause of double vision in 15% of cases, affecting CN VI most commonly, followed by CN III, with CN IV being the least affected (1,2). There is controversy whether CN VI's greater susceptibility to injury is solely due to its greater intracranial length (3).

Tumors are the cause of another 15% of diplopia, and most commonly affect CN VI, alone or in combination (1,2). Primary brainstem tumors and metastatic tumors are equally represented, and affect intramedullary nerve tracts. Pituitary tumors affect these nerves as they pass through the cavernous sinus, and pituitary apoplexy causes loss of vision as well as diplopia. Isolated tumors of CN III, IV, and VI are rare. Disorders affecting the cavernous sinus may involve multiple CNs, and are discussed with CN V.

Vascular disease is felt to be the cause in 15% of neuropathies affecting CN III, IV, and VI (1,2). The collateral blood supply is relatively poor, and atherosclerosis associated with hypertension and hyperlipidemia is felt to lead to nerve ischemia, and ocular palsies are therefore more common in the elderly. Diabetic-based ocular palsies are perhaps the most common cause, and have a classic presentation of sudden onset associated with severe retro-orbital pain and weakness attributed to CN III and VI and less frequently to CN IV (1). Pupillary function is spared in three-quarters of patients. Clinical features are similar for patients with impaired glucose tolerance (4). The lesion appears to be primary demyelinating, with lesser axonal damage (5).

An aneurysm is a classic cause of CN III palsy, and is usually associated with pupillary dysfunction; however, with normal pupillary function minimal palsy has also been described (1,6). The aneurysm is most commonly in the internal carotid artery, in the region of the posterior communicating artery. Nerve palsy may result from direct mass effects in unruptured aneurysms or the effects of the hemorrhage in ruptured aneurysms.

Historically, syphilis was a common cause of ocular palsies (7). Lyme borreliosis may involve CN III, IV, and VI as the only neurologic manifestation of infection (8).

The Tolosa–Hunt syndrome includes recurrent unilateral retro-orbital pain followed by paresis of CN III, IV, VI, and the ophthalmic division of CN V with spontaneous resolution (9). Pathologic investigation indicates granulomatous tissue in the cavernous sinus. Neurosarcoidosis less commonly involves CN III, IV, and VII than CN VII (10).

Approximately 25% of neuropathies involving CN III, IV, and VI are of undetermined cause (1,2). There is also a benign CN VI palsy described in children (11).

1.4. Diagnostic Testing

Clinical assessment of eye movements is the most useful test to distinguish among nerves causing diplopia, and the diagnostic palsies are described earlier. Imaging studies (MRI, CT, and ultrasound) can help isolate the site of the lesion and suggest causes (12,13). Among patients with known vascular risks, imaging studies identify an alternative cause in 15% (13).

1.5. Treatment and Prognosis

In the setting of trauma, the nature of the injuries determines the degree of CN damage. Complete nerve avulsion has a poor prognosis. Lesser injuries lead to spontaneous recovery within weeks, and axonal injuries take 4–6 months. Neuropathies attributed to vascular causes improve without treatment, and those due to diabetes have a good recovery because of the demyelinating nature of the lesion. For the same reasons, idiopathic neuropathies also have a favorable prognosis.

Associated movements are those that are outside of the intended activation pattern. This can lead to chronic diplopia in certain directions of gaze. One explanation is aberrant (anomalous) regeneration from axonal damage leading to inappropriate re-innervation of muscles, whereas another is based on central (nuclear) reorganization or release (14). With neuropathies due to tumor, the nature and treatment of the underlying tumor are the most important prognostic factors.

2. CN V (TRIGEMINAL)

2.1. Anatomy

CN V has prominent sensory and motor functions. The sensory component supplies the face and is organized into three divisions: ophthalmic, maxillary, and mandibular. The pathways from the receptors mainly are as follows. The ophthalmic division (CN V1) supplies sensation to the forehead, cornea, and sinuses. The nerve passes through the superior orbital fissure and cavernous sinus. The maxillary division (CN V2) supplies sensation to the middle portion of the face. The nerve passes through the cavernous sinus and the foramen rotundum. The mandibular division (CN V3) provides sensation from the jaw, teeth, and anterior two-thirds of the tongue. It passes through the foramen ovale. All three divisions join at the trigeminal ganglion, which enters the brainstem at the pons.

The motor division is much smaller, and supplies primarily the muscles of mastication. It arises from the lateral portion of the pons, where it joins the sensory fibers of the mandibular division and passes through the foramen ovale to innervate the tensor palatini and tensor tympani, the medial pterygoid, the masseter, the lateral pterygoid, and finally the temporalis muscle.

2.2. Symptoms and Signs

Numbness, and less so pain, in the distribution of one or more branches is the most common presenting symptom, whereas weakness of mastication is less common (15). There may be an alteration in taste (16,17). The rate of progression of symptoms is largely dependent upon the pathophysiologic process and its location along the three pathways of CN V. In progressive conditions, numbness may begin in one division and spread to others. The maxillary and mandibular divisions appear to be more commonly affected than the ophthalmic division. Symptoms may also start on one side and spread to the other side.

2.3. Causes

There is an association with connective tissue diseases, including undifferentiated scleroderma and Sjögren syndrome (16,18). Because only sensory function is involved with connective tissue diseases, a ganglionopathy is postulated. Primary neoplasms include cerebellopontine angle neuromas and meningiomas. An interesting presentation of metastatic neoplasms is initial involvement of the mental nerve branch, giving rise to a numb chin. Chin numbness may herald the diagnosis of cancer, and primary tumor types cover a wide spectrum (19). Undiagnosed or idiopathic trigeminal neuropathies frequently develop suddenly with facial numbness, which may spread from one division to another.

2.4. Diagnostic Testing

Initial diagnosis is by clinical examination. Electrophysiologic testing with blink reflexes can help define CN V involvement of the ophthalmic division, but the reflex may be normal (16). MRI is appropriate because of the high frequency of underlying neoplasms.

2.5. Treatment and Prognosis

For patients with connective tissue diseases, treatment of the underlying disease does not reliably result in lessening of symptoms (18). Among those with no identifiable cause, half experienced a clinical remission without treatment (17). Corticosteroids have been tried with variable success, but there are no controlled trials.

2.6. Cavernous Sinus Syndrome

CN III, IV, V1 and V2, and VI pass through the cavernous sinus, and all but CN V2 also pass through the superior orbital fissure. Thus, it is difficult to precisely localize a lesion to either of these two structures by clinical examination. Symptoms include ptosis, diplopia, and small and poorly reactive pupils. There is also frequent retro-orbital pain, conjunctival rubor, and proptosis. Causes of cavernous sinus syndrome include aneurysms, meningiomas, pituitary tumors, and infectious and inflammatory processes. Diagnostic evaluation includes MRI or CT to further localize the lesion and help determine pathology type. Treatment is based on the pathological processes.

3. CN VII (FACIAL)

3.1. Anatomy

CN VII leaves the brainstem at the cerebellopontine angle and enters the internal auditory meatus with CN VIII. It follows a tortuous pathway in the temporal bone. Initially, it lies in the internal auditory canal for 7–8 mm, and then enters the facial canal for 3–4 mm. It makes a sharp turn and travels 12–13 mm close to the middle ear. The geniculate ganglion is in this segment and supplies fibers to mucus membranes and lacrimal glands via the greater superficial petrosal nerve. There follows a 10–14 mm mastoid segment where the motor nerve to the stapedius muscle branches off. The chorda tympani conveys taste from the anterior two-thirds of the tongue and joins CN VII in this segment. The nerve leaves the skull at the stylomastoid foramen, and the first motor branches are to the posterior belly of the stylohyoid, digastric, and occipital muscles. The nerve then travels through the parotid gland, and terminal motor branches are the temporal, zygomatic, buccal, mandibular and cervical to innervate muscles of facial expression.

3.2. Symptoms and Signs

The primary symptom is facial weakness. This condition was first written about by Sir Charles Bell in 1829, when he described a benign condition that was already familiar to contemporary clinicians. Clinical features are an acute onset, or progression over several hours, of unilateral weakness of facial muscles that is complete in 70% and partial in 30% of patients. There are also manifestations of loss of other functions subserved by CN VII, such as decreased lacrimation, and altered taste (20). Abnormal sensation also occurs, including dysesthesias in the trigeminal and glossopharyngeal nerve distributions. There may be pain on the affected side of the face and temporary alterations in hearing (21). The incidence of Bell palsy is ~20/100,000 in the general population, affecting adults more than children (22). It appears to be three times more common in pregnant women (23).

CN VII weakness may occur in the setting of a rash involving the external auditory meatus, the Ramsay Hunt syndrome (24). Slow progressive facial weakness (over days) is less consistent with Bell palsy.

3.3. Causes

The majority of cases of CN VII palsies, which include Bell palsy, are classified as idiopathic, and nerve damage probably occurs secondary to compression from edema within the confines of the boney canal. There are data implicating an underlying viral infection as the cause for these cases (25). Evidence for herpes simplex virus in association with 80% of idiopathic Bell palsy is from DNA analysis by polymerase chain reaction followed by hybridization with Southern blot analysis of endoneurial fluid at the time of decompression surgery (26). The most clearly defined viral cause of CN VII neuropathy is the Ramsay Hunt syndrome, facial weakness with erythematous vesicular rash in the ear (24).

An associated underlying condition or cause is found in the minority of patients. The incidence of diabetes mellitus is high, leading to the conclusion that Bell palsy may represent a diabetic mononeuropathy in these patients (27). Otitis media is a rare cause. Bell palsy occurs more frequently in the setting of Lyme disease, and Borellia burgdorferi may account for 25% of cases in endemic areas, many without other clinical features of Lyme disease (28). Neurosarcoid presenting as an isolated CN VII palsy is less common than in association with other cranial neuropathies (10). Surgical trauma to CN VII may occur during procedures on the temporal bone. Close head trauma resulting in fractures of the temporal bone is another cause.

The degree of nerve fiber damage ranges from neurapraxia to axonotemesis. Within a patient there may be varying proportions of each process, which probably account for the range of clinical outcomes (20).

3.4. Diagnostic Testing

Functional tests include measurement of submandibular salivary flow and electrodiagnostic testing. Measurements of salivary flow require cannulation of Wharton ducts and is technically difficult. Nerve conduction measurements focus on the nerve segment distal to the site of nerve damage in the temporal bone. The evoked response to activation of the nerve at the level of the parotid gland will be within the normal range for the first 2 days after acute onset of weakness, even if there is complete axonal damage (29). After the third day, if there is significant axonal damage (axotemesis lesion), the evoked motor response will fall in proportion to the number of viable axons. Nerve fibers affected by conduction block (neurapraxic lesion) will contribute to the evoked potential, but not to voluntary activation. If the evoked response is >10% of the contralateral (normal) side, prognosis is favorable because this indicates that there are a significant number of viable fibers. Needle EMG assesses the distribution of denervation in the form of abnormal spontaneous activity (positive sharp waves and fibrillation potentials). However, it takes ≥5 days for abnormal spontaneous activity to appear. Imaging studies using quantitative MRI suggest some degree of prognostication, with poorer results among patients with greater signal abnormalities (30).

3.5. Treatment and Prognosis

The proposed inflammatory pathology has led to the use of corticosteroids, and the proposed viral pathogenesis has led to the use of anti-viral agents. Although some reports have favored these agents, the Cochrane Database Systematic Review has analyzed data for corticosteroids and acyclovir or valaciclovir. The Cochrane Review selects randomized or quasirandomized trials for the various agents, as sole agent or in combination. Appropriately conducted trials are reviewed and meta-analyses are preformed. Improved outcome has not been demonstrated for any of the agents, either alone or in combination (31,32). A Cochrane Review of acupuncture indicated that acupuncture alone might be more associated with a better outcome than medications or the combination, but methodological differences among trials prevented a meta-analysis (33).

The inaccessible site of pathology means that a clinical determination of the degree of neurapraxia and axonotemesis by electrodiagnostic testing cannot be determined until after the fourth day of onset. The full extent of nerve damage has probably occurred by this time, and surgical intervention is unwarranted (20,29).

Overall prognosis from retrospective reviews indicates that 80–85% of patients have a full or satisfactory return of strength (22). There may be residual symptoms that include crocodile tears and other forms of aberrant re-innervation such as lower facial muscle twitching with eye blinking (synkensis) (14,34). Prognostic factors have been challenging to identify, but age >55 years, complete paralysis, and hypertension are negative factors.

4. CN VIII (ACOUSTIC AND VESTIBULAR)

4.1. Anatomy

There are two divisions, one serving the vestibular system and the other the auditory system. The vestibular division originates from the hair cells in the semicircular canals and the macula of the utricle and saccule, whereas the cochlear division originates from hair cells in the organ of Corti. The vestibular nerve contains about 20,000 fibers and the cochlear nerve about 30,000 fibers. Both divisions lie in the temporal bone in close association with CN VII. CN VIII leaves the skull through the internal auditory meatus and joins the brainstem at the pontomedullary junction in the cerebellopontine angle. The intracranial portion of the nerve includes a junctional zone between the proximal segment, which is a central fiber tract with neuroglial support cells and a more distal segment, which is a peripheral nerve with Schwann cell support cells.

4.2. Symptoms and Signs

Damage to the nerve can result in both hearing loss and tinnitus and vertigo in various proportions. Acute causes tend to include symptoms in both divisions, whereas slow progressive causes tend to present with hearing loss. The Ramsay Hunt syndrome begins with deep ear pain, followed in several days by vesicular eruptions in the external auditory canal eventually leading to hearing loss and vertigo (24). CN VII is frequently involved. Acute labrynthitis is associated with vertigo with spontaneous nystagmus (35). Vestibular symptoms may be associated with other cranial neuropathies (CN V, VII, X, XI) (36).

4.3. Causes

Trauma involving the temporal bone can damage both CN VIII and CN VII. The injury can be a stretching of the nerve on a complete severance. Acoustic nerve Schwannomas tend to arise within the internal auditor meatus because the junction between the proximal extension of the neuroglial investment of the nerve and the distal Schwann cell investment is close to the meatus. Up to 10% of unilateral tumors are associated with neurofibromatosis.

 Viral infections may affect the labrynth (labrynthitis) or the nerve, although direct evidence for this etiology is often lacking because of the isolated location of the nerve. The Ramsay Hunt syndrome is due to herpes zoster (24).

 The consensus is that diabetes mellitus does not contribute to acute hearing loss (15). Sarcoidosis uncommonly affects CN VII in isolation (10). Evidence for borrelia infection has been found in patients with vertigo (37).

4.4. Diagnostic Testing

Batteries of tests for cochlear and vestibular functions require special equipment and include audiograms, tone decay, evoked responses, and electronystagrams with provocative tests (vestibulo-ocular, caloric) (38). Imaging tests are important to exclude tumors.

4.5. Treatment and Prognosis

Surgical and radiation treatments of tumors are appropriate with outcome dependent upon many variables (39). Vertigo associated with presumed viral etiology resolve spontaneously (36).

5. CN IX (GLOSSOPHARYNGEAL)

5.1. Anatomy

The nerve arises from a line of rootlets in a sulcus along the lateral border of the medulla. The nerve is associated with CN X, and both pass through the jugular foramen and into the neck. Motor fibers innervate the stylopharyngeus muscle. Sensory fibers subserve taste along the posterior two-thirds of the tongue and sensation of the soft palate and related structures, and a branch supplies sensation to part of the external ear and the tympanic membrane. There are parasympathetic fibers in the lesser superficial petrosal nerve that controls secretions of the parotid gland. The carotid sinus nerve is a branch of CN IX.

5.2. Symptoms and Signs

Because of its close proximity with CN X, lesions usually involve both nerves, and symptoms are more often related to that nerve. There may be difficulties in swallowing and impaired taste from posterior portions of the tongue. Glosspharyngeal neuralgia refers to episodes of sudden onset of lancinating unilateral pain at the base of the tongue and faucial region with similarities to trigeminal neuralgia.

5.3. Causes

Cerebropontine angle tumors may also affect CN IX. Lesions in the jugular foramen may affect both CN IX and X, giving rise to a jugular foramen syndrome (Vernet syndrome). Causes include glomus tumors and other neoplasms.

5.4. Diagnostic Testing

Assessment of taste perception of the posterior portion of the tongue can be performed. Cutaneous stimulation for the gag reflex is supplied by this nerve, and can be tested by lightly stroking the posterior pharynx.

5.5. Treatment and Prognosis

These are dependent upon underlying causes, especially in the setting of tumors. Crocodile tears (paroxysmal lacrimation with gustatory stimuli) may occur after injury or surgery on the ear or after CN VII neuropathies. This is due to the close proximity of fibers in the inner ear and cross-innervation of sprouting fibers that involve the lesser superficial petrosal nerve which supplies the parotid gland (34).

6. CN X (VAGUS)

6.1. Anatomy

The nerve is formed from rootlets emerging from a lateral sulcus of the medulla. The nerve is joined by fibers from CN XI that have ascended through the foramen magnum, although they remain as a discrete fascicle. The combined nerve passes through the jugular foramen. In the neck, the pharyngeal nerve supplies all pharyngeal constrictor muscles except the stylopharynegeus and tensor palati, as well as the palatoglossus muscle of the tongue. The superior laryngeal nerve also innervates constrictor muscles and the cricothyroid muscle. The recurrent laryngeal nerve follows an asymmetric course to supply the remaining muscles of the larynx. Visceral afferent fibers supply sensation from the pharynx, larynx, trachea, esophagus, and viscera. Visceral efferent fibers supply the heart and visceral organs.

6.2. Symptoms and Signs

Unilateral lesions usually include both CN IX and X and result in voice hoarseness and difficulty swallowing and nasal regurgitation due to weakness of soft palate elevation which normally closes off the nasopharynx during swallowing. Lesions of the recurrent laryngeal nerve also cause voice hoarseness.

6.3. Causes

Isolated lesions may result from tumors affecting the base of the skull and the jugular vein. Recurrent laryngeal nerve lesions occur most commonly in association with surgery of the carotid artery, the thyroid, and thoracic cavity (40). One-quarter to one-third of cases are thought to be idiopathic (40,41). Men are more often affected than women, and the left recurrent laryngeal nerve more than the right, perhaps because of its greater length. Concurrent diabetes may be a contributing factor in a small percentage (41). Idiopathic superior laryngeal nerve palsies are felt to be common and are due to reactivation of herpes simplex infection (42).

6.4. Diagnostic Testing

Inspection reveals asymmetry of the soft palate, lower on the affected side, and deviation of the uvula to the opposite side. Indirect laryngoscopy can detect abnormal vocal cord function. Needle EMG can distinguish between superior laryngeal and recurrent laryngeal lesions (41). Testing of cardiac autonomic function will not be discussed.

6.5. Treatment and Prognosis

Lesions associated with cancers have a variable prognosis (43). Lesions associated with carotid and thyroid surgery may recover spontaneously, and are thus presumed to be due to tissue swelling. With idiopathic recurrent laryngeal neuropathies, 85% show some degree of spontaneous recovery and 35% resolve completely (43,44).

7. CN XI (SPINAL ACCESSORY)

7.1. Anatomy

Rootlets contributing to CN IX include the most caudal region of the mesencephalon and the first five to seven cervical segments. The cervical rootlets form a nerve that ascends through the foramen magnum and joins with the cranial rootlets and CN X. The combined nerves pass through the jugular foramen. CN XI descends in the carotid sheath, but leaves it and penetrates the sternocleidomastoid muscle which it supplies. The nerve then crosses the posterior triangle of the neck to reach the trapezius muscle and supplies the upper one-third.

7.2. Symptoms and Signs

Lesions of the deep, proximal portion, result in weakness of the sternocleidomastoid muscle affecting head rotation to the opposite side and weakness of the upper trapezius with poor shoulder and arm elevation above the horizontal axis on the same side. Lesions of the superficial, distal portion in the posterior triangle result in weakness only of the trapezius muscle. There may be mild winging of the scapula.

7.3. Causes

The portion of the nerve in the jugular foramen and carotid sheath may be affected by tumors. The most common causes of nerve injury in the neck are from surgical procedures, notably radical neck dissections and cervical lymph node biopsy, but neuropathies can also occur when the nerve is in continuity (45). Delayed weakness after surgical procedures suggests lesions from scar tissue (45). Less common causes are carotid endarterectomy and central line placement. Weakness attributed to focal radiation for cancer may occur years after treatment (46). Idiopathic lesions occur and may be heralded by pain along the posterior border of the sternocleidomastoid muscle (47).

7.4. Diagnostic Testing

Needle EMG can document denervation of the sternocleidomastoid and upper trapezius muscles.

7.5. Treatment and Prognosis

Varying degrees of spontaneous improvement may occur when damage is due to surgery, but some patients accept a certain degree of weakness (45). Surgical grafting following injury from radical neck surgery has been reported to be successful (48). Spontaneous neuropathies may or may not show improvement with time (47).

8. CN XII (HYPOGLOSSAL)

8.1. Anatomy

The nerve arises from rootlets along the medulla, merging to form two bundles that pass through the hypoglossal foramen. It passes down from the angle of the jaw and innervates the thyrohyoid muscle and intrinsic muscles of the tongue (hyoglossus, styloglossus, genioglossus, and geniohyoid muscles).

8.2. Symptoms and Signs

Unilateral lesions result in tongue deviation to the side of the lesion. Atrophy of the affected half may occur. Swallowing is affected to a greater degree than speech. Glosso-dynia is a syndrome with burning pain in the tongue or the oral cavity, which may be similar to trigeminal neuralgia.

8.3. Causes

Tumors in the region of the hypoglossal foramen or neck are rare causes as are also trauma and dental extractions. Idiopathic mononeuropathies are described (49).

8.4. Diagnostic Testing

Needle EMG demonstrates denervation.

8.5. Treatment and Prognosis

Prognosis depends upon underlying causes. Idiopathic forms frequently resolve without specific treatment (49).

9. SUMMARY

CN mononeuropathies are due to many causes, but two are noteworthy. A progressive mononeuropathy may be related to cancer and predate the diagnosis. Accordingly, an imaging study is appropriate even when there is an apparent cause. Idiopathic CN mononeuropathies, those without identifiable cause, are common and the prognosis is generally favorable without specific treatment.

REFERENCES

1.   Rucker C. The causes of paralysis of the third, fourth, and sixth cranial nerves. Am J Ophthalmol 1966; 61:1293–1298.
2.   Rucker C. Paralysis of the third, fourth, and sixth cranial nerves. Am J Ophthalmol 1958; 46:787–794.
3.   Hanson R, Ghosh S, Gonzalez-Gomez I, Levy M, Gilles F. Abducens length and vulnerability? Neurology 2004; 62:33–36.
4.   Teuscher A, Meienberg O. Ischaemic oculomotor nerve palsy. Clinical features and fascular risk factors in 23 patients. J Neurol 1985; 232:144–149.
5.   Asbury A, Aldredge H, Hershberg R, Fisher C. Oculomotor palsy in diabetes mellitus: a clinico-pathological study. Brain 1970; 93:555–566.
6.   Bartleston J, Trautmann J, Sundt T. Minimal oculomotor nerve paresis secondary to unruptured intracranial aneurysm. Arch Neurol 1986; 43:1015–1020.
7.   Green W, Hackett E, Schlezinger N. Neuro-ophthalmologic evaluatioin of oculomotor nerve paralysis. Arch Ophthalmol 1961; 72:154–167.
8.   Lesser R, Kornmehl E, Pachner A et al. Neuro-ophthalmologic manifestations of Lyme disease. Ophthalmology 1990; 97:699–706.
9.   Hunt W, Meagher J, LeFever H, Zeman W. Painful ophthalmoplegia: its relation to indolent inflammation of the cavernous sinus. Neurology 1961; 11:56–62.
10. Delany P. Neurologic manifestations in sarcoidosis. Review of the literature, with a report of 23 cases. Ann Intern Med 1977; 87:336–345.
11. Knox D, Clark D, Schuster F. Benign VI nerve palsies in children. Pediatrics 1967; 40:560–564.
12. Eisenkraft B, Oritz A. Imaging evaluation of cranial nerves 3, 4, and 6. Semin Ultrasound CT MR 2001; 6:488–501.
13. Chou K, Galetta S, Liu G et al. Acute ocular motor mononeuropathies: prospective study of roles of neuroimaging and clinical assessment. J Neurol Sci 2004; 219:35–39.
14. Wartenberg R. Associated movements in the oculomotor and facial muscles. Arch Neurol Psychiatry 1946; 55:439–488.
15. Spillane J, Wells C. Isolated trigeminal neuropathy: a report of 16 cases. Brain 1959; 82:391–416.
16. Lecky B, Hughes R, Murray N. Trigeminal sensory neuropathy. Brain 1987; 110:1463–1485.
17. Blau J, Harris M, Kennett S. Trigeminal sensory neuropathy. N Engl J Med 1969; 281:873–876.
18. Hagen N, Stevens J, Michet C. Trigeminal sensory neuropathy associated with connective tissue diseases. Neurology 1990; 40:891–896.
19. Harris C, Baringer J. The numb chin in metastatic cancer. West J Med 1991; 155:528–531.
20. Adour K, Byl F, Hilsinger R, Kahn Z, Sheldon M. The true nature of Bell's palsy: analysis of 1,000 consecutive patients. Laryngoscope 1978; 88:787–820.
21. Abour K. Diagnosis and management of facial paralysis. N Engl J Med 1982; 307:348–354.

22. Katausic S, Beard C, Wiederholt W, Bergstralh E, Kurland L. Incidence, clinical features, and prognosis in Bell's palsy, Rochester, Minnesota, 1968–1982. Ann Neurol 1986; 20:622–627.

23. Gillman G, Schaitkin B, May M, Klein S. Bell's palsy in pregnancy: a study of recovery outcomes. Otolaryngol Head Neck Surg 2002; 126:26–30.

24. Sweeney C, Gliden D. Ramsay Hunt syndrome. J Neurol Neurosurg Psychiatry 2001; 71:149–154.

25. Baringer J. Herpes simplex virus and Bell palsy. Ann Intern Med 1996; 124:63–65.

26. Murakami S, Mizobuchi M, Nakashiro Y, Doi T, Hato N, Yanagihara N. Bell palsy and herpes simplex virus: identification of viral DNA in endoneurial fluid and muscle. Ann Intern Med 1996; 124:27–30.

27. Pecket P, Schattner A. Concurrent Bell's palsy and diabetes mellitus: a diabetic mononeuropathy? J Neurol Neurosurg Psychiatry 1982; 45:652–655.

28. Halpern J, Golightly M. Long Island Neuroborreliosis Collaborative Study Group. Lyme borreliosis in Bell's palsy. Neurology 1992; 42:1268–1270.

29. Albers J, Bromberg M. Bell's palsy. In: Johnson R, ed. Current Therapy in Neurologic Disease. 3rd ed. Philadelphia: Dekker, 1990:376.

30. Kress B, Griesbeck R, Stippich C, Bahren W, Sartor K. Bell palsy: quantitative analysis of MR imaging data as a method of predicting outcome. Radiology 2004; 230:504–509.

31. Allen D, Dunn L. Aciclovir or valaciclovir for Bell's palsy (idiopathic facial paralysis). Cochrane Database Syst Rev 2004; (3):CD001869.

32. Salinas R, Alvarez G, Alvarez M, Ferreira J. Corticosteroids for Bell's palsy (idiopathic facial paralysis). Cochrane Database Syst Rev 2002; (1):CD001942.

33. He L, Zhou D, Wu B, Li N, Zhou M. Acupuncture for Bell's palsy. Cochrane Database Syst Rev 2004; (1):CD002914.

34. Boyer F, Gardner W. Paroxysmal lacrimation (syndrome of crocodile tears) and its surgical treatment. Arch Neurol Psychiatry 1949; 61:56–64.

35. Dix M, Hallpike C. The pathology, symptomatology and diagnosis of certain common disorders of the vestibular system. Ann Otol Rinol Laryngol 1952; 61:987–1016.

36. Adour K, Sprague M, Hilsinger R. Vestibular vertigo. A form of polyneuritis? J Am Med Assoc 1981; 246:1564–1567.

37. Rosenhall U, Hanner P, Kaijser B. Borrelia infection and vertigo. Acta Otolaryngol 1988; 106:111–116.

38. Luxon L. Diseases of the eighth cranial nerve. In: Dyck P, Thomas P, Griffin J, Low P, Poduslo J, eds. Peripheral Neuropathy. 3rd ed. Philadelphia: WB Saunders Co, 1993:837–868.

39. Chakrabarti I, Apuzzo M, Giannota S. Acoustic neuroma: decision making with all the tools. Clin Neurosurg 2003; 50:293–312.

40. Williams R. Idiopathic recurrent laryngeal nerve paralysis. J Laryngol Otol 1959; 73:161–166.

41. Berry H, Blair R. Isolated vagus nerve palsy and vagal mononeuritis. Arch Otolaryngol 1980; 106:333–338.

42. Abour K, Schneider G, Hilsinger R. Acute superior laryngeal nerve palsy: Analysis of 78 cases. Otolaryngol Head Neck Surg 1980; 88:418–424.

43. Huppler E, Schmidt H, Devine K, Gage R. Ultimate outcome of patients with vocal-cord paralysis of undetermined cause. Am Rev Tuberc 1956; 72:52–60.

44. Blau J, Kapadia R. Idiopathic palsy of the recurrent laryngeal nerve: a transient cranial mononeuropathy. BMJ 1972; 4:259–261.

45. Gordon S, Graham W, Black J, Miller S. Accessory nerve function after surgical procedures in the posterior trangle. Arch Surg 1977; 112:264–268.

46. Berger P, Bataini J. Radiation-induced cranial nerve palsy. Cancer 1977; 40:152–155.

47. Eisen A, Bertrand G. Isolated accessory nerve palsy of spontaneous origin. Arch Neurol 1972; 27:496–502.

48. Ballantyne A, Guinn G. Reduction of shoulder disability after neck dissections. Am J Surg 1962; 112:662–665.

49. Afifi A, Rifai Z, Faris K. Isolated, reversible, hypoglossal nerve palsy. Arch Neurol 1984; 41:1218.

Treatment of Peripheral Neuropathy

34
A Diagnostic and Treatment Approach to Painful Neuropathy

Hiroyuki Nodera and David N. Herrmann
University of Rochester Medical Center, Rochester, New York, USA

ABSTRACT

Painful neuropathies are a common and heterogeneous group of disorders. Although many patients with neuropathies experience pain, for some it is the cardinal symptom and contributes substantially toward their disability. The presence and quality of neuropathic pain cannot predict the etiology of the peripheral neuropathy, but consideration of the severity, distribution, temporal profile, and other neurologic factors can help diagnostically. This chapter discusses the clinical features, pathophysiology, and management of neuropathic pain. A diagnostic approach is presented, and therapeutic options for treatment are included.

1. WHAT IS NEUROPATHIC PAIN?

The term denotes pain that originates from a primary lesion or injury to neural pathways (1–3). It may originate in either the central nervous system (CNS) or the peripheral nervous system (PNS). Neuropathic pain is contrasted with adaptive or physiologic pain and inflammatory pain. In health, physiologic pain occurs when peripheral nociceptors and intact sensory pathways are transiently stimulated by noxious stimuli. Inflammatory pain originates from tissue injury or inflammatory mediators stimulating peripheral nociceptors. In contrast, peripheral neuropathic pain evolves from combinations of stimulus independent (spontaneous) and stimulus dependent pain. Patients with painful neuropathies may use several descriptors of pain simultaneously, and the terms and quality of pain symptoms may evolve over time. Spontaneous manifestations of neuropathic pain include intermittent or persistent "burning," "aching," "jabbing," and "lancinating" pains. Stimulus-evoked neuropathic pain comprises hyperalgesia (an exaggerated pain response to a normally noxious stimulus), allodynia (pain to innocuous stimuli, such as touch or temperature), and temporal summation (repetitive application of a single noxious stimulus is perceived as increasing pain sensation). Hyperalgesia and allodynia may be mechanical, thermal, or chemical in type (4). Pain and sensory loss in a known peripheral nerve distribution is a clue to a peripheral neuropathic origin. Although neuropathic and inflammatory pain are conceptually distinct entities, they may be difficult to distinguish clinically, and may coexist in the same patient (e.g., in acute radiculopathies).

Neuropathic pain descriptors may also resemble those associated with musculoskeletal disorders (e.g., "cramping" or "deep aching" pain). Inflammatory pain, like neuropathic pain may manifest with regional hypersensitivity, and the pain response may extend beyond the primary area of tissue injury (5). Nonetheless, the distinction between inflammatory and neuropathic pain components is important, as they may show differential responses to treatment. Nonsteroidal anti-inflammatory agents are very effective in controlling inflammatory pain, but have a limited effect upon neuropathic pain.

2. PATHOPHYSIOLOGY OF NEUROPATHIC PAIN

The mechanisms of neuropathic pain include both central and peripheral nerves (1–3). Pain is a feature of predominantly small fiber peripheral neuropathies, reflecting the unique role of damaged, small diameter unmyelinated nociceptive afferents (C-fibers) in mediating neuropathic pain (6). The role of small diameter sensory fibers is supported by associations of neuropathic pain intensity with the degree of loss of unmyelinated intra-epidermal nerve endings on punch skin biopsy (7). However, the diameter of sensory fiber involvement is not tightly linked to the presence of neuropathic pain (8). Some small fiber neuropathies may be painless, whereas large fiber axonal neuropathies may be painful (8). Primary axonal neuropathies are more likely to be painful than primary demyelinating ones (8), but this is not always the case, as in radicular pain in Guillain–Barré syndrome (GBS). Axonal regeneration appears to be a factor for the development of neuropathic pain (8), and neuropathic pain may persist despite resolution of sensory deficits.

Animals models of neuropathic pain and micro-neurography have shown that after peripheral nerve injury, a complex series of morphological and chemical changes occur in the PNS and CNS that underlie the development and maintenance of neuropathic pain.

2.1. Peripheral Nervous System Alterations

"Sensitization" of primary sensory afferents (unmyelinated, high threshold polymodal C-fibers, and lightly myelinated A-δ fibers) is a key occurrence. This results in enhanced nerve excitability with increased spontaneous discharges, and ectopic discharges from the dorsal root ganglia (DRG), damaged sensory terminals, and neuromas of injured nerves. Ephaptic transmission may also occur between adjacent regions of damaged or demyelinated sensory afferents. Alterations in ion channel expression, in particular Na-channels, are a major contributor to peripheral sensitization (9). There are at least six distinct voltage-gated Na-channels expressed on primary sensory neurons within the DRG. They may be divided into tetrodotoxin (TTX)-resistant and TTX-sensitive groups. After peripheral nerve injury, expression of two subtypes of TTX-resistant Na^+-channels (Nav 1.9 and Nav 1.8) in the DRG decreases with a concomitant redistribution of the Nav 1.8 channel to neuromas and axon terminals of injured small diameter DRG neurons. There is also *de novo* expression of TTX-sensitive type III channels on small diameter nociceptive neurons that do not normally express type III channels (9). These changes are thought to contribute to neuronal/axonal hyperexcitability and neuropathic pain (2,9). Other factors for sensitization of peripheral nociceptors include release of inflammatory mediators (e.g., PGE2, bradykinin, epinephrine) and cytokines [e.g., tumor necrosis factor (TNF)-α], even in noninflammatory painful human neuropathies (10).

Enhanced peripheral nociceptive input to dorsal horn neurons induces a series of functional alterations in the CNS, including sustained increase in the excitability of second order dorsal horn neurons (central sensitization), and suppression of CNS anti-nociceptive pathways.

2.2. Central Nervous System Alterations

Central sensitization reflects a persistent state of hyperexcitability of dorsal horn neurons induced through activation of peripheral nociceptive neurons and a concomitant inhibition of anti-nociceptive GABA-ergic, opiate and glycine pathways in the spinal cord. One aspect of central sensitization, demonstrated in animal models of neuropathic pain, is the phenomenon of "wind up". This is a state of increasing responsiveness of nociceptive DRG neurons to ongoing or repeated peripheral nociceptive C-fiber firing (1). Central sensitization contributes to an enhanced pain response to noxious stimuli and a pain response to ordinarily innocuous stimuli in neuropathic pain states (allodynia). Further, receptive fields of dorsal horn pain neurons increase in size, and the repertoire of stimuli that induces their activation also increases.

Central sensitization is mediated through activation of N-methyl-D-aspartate (NMDA) and alpha-amino-3-hydroxy-5-methyl-4-isoxazolepropionic acid (AMPA) receptors on dorsal horn pain neurons by glutamate. Further, substance P, acting at the G protein-coupled postsynaptic neurokinin-1 receptor with signaling through protein kinase C activates NMDA receptors, facilitates excitatory synaptic responses (4). Sensitization of dorsal horn pain neurons also increases intracellular calcium through AMPA receptors (4). Another factor enhancing central sensitization is the inhibition of antinociceptive CNS pathways by a number of mechanisms. NMDA receptor activation mediates depression of inhibitory GABA-ergic and glycinergic neurons in lamina II of the dorsal horn (4). Expression of micro-opioid receptors on the presynaptic terminal of primary nociceptive afferents in the dorsal horn is down-regulated in most neuropathic pain models, whereas there is up-regulation of the endogenous opioid antagonist cholecystokinin (CCK) in peripheral nerve and increased staining of CCK-B receptors in the dorsal horn.

2.3. Dorsal Horn Alterations

There is controversial evidence that central terminals of axotomized DRG neurons undergo aberrant sprouting into lamina II of the dorsal horn, an area that normally only receives C-fiber nociceptive input. It is hypothesized that the development of synaptic connections between low threshold ordinarily nonnociceptive A-β-fibers with lamina II cells that ordinarily receive nociceptive fiber input promotes painful responses to nonnoxious stimuli (11,12). It is also believed that injury to and ectopic activity within first order nociceptive neurons results in death of some inhibitory interneurons in the dorsal horn and down-regulation of neurotransmitters and receptors critical to antinociceptive responses.

2.4. Sympathetic Nervous System Alterations

Sympathetic neurons are believed to sprout into the DRG (13). Functional linkage between the sympathetic and the sensory nervous systems also occurs through expression of alpha-adrenergic receptors on injured sensory neurons, and the sensitization of nociceptive C-terminals by release of inflammatory mediators from sympathetic nerve terminals (1) contributing to sympathetically maintained neuropathic pain (14). An immunohistochemical study of sural nerve reported an increased density of surviving sympathetic fibers when compared with somatic sensory fibers in painful neuropathies (15).

3. CLINICAL ASPECTS OF PAINFUL NEUROPATHIES

The clinical aspects of painful neuropathies can be used to guide the choice of test, and an algorithm is outlined in Fig. 34.1.

3.1. Clinical Characterization

Symptoms of a painful neuropathy can be characterized by spatial distribution [focal, multifocal, or diffuse (symmetric)] (Table 34.1) and temporal profile (acute, subacute or chronic, progressive, relapsing, or monophasic courses) (Table 34.2). Other helpful features include: (i) pattern of nerve fiber (sensory small fiber, large fiber predominant, small and large fibers, motor fiber involvement, autonomic involvement), (ii) pathophysiology (primarily axonal or primarily demyelinating), (iii) sporadic or familial, and (iv) associated comorbidity (medical conditions, medications, toxins) (16). Painful neuropathies that are markedly asymmetric in distribution (either focal or multifocal) are almost always acquired and have a limited differential diagnosis, which includes vasculitis (mononeuritis multiplex), compressive, infiltrative (neoplasms) infectious, or traumatic etiologies. Symmetric painful neuropathies are more common and raise a broader set of differential diagnoses. Most symmetric painful neuropathies predominantly affect sensory axons, but predominantly demyelinative and motor neuropathies (e.g., acquired inflammatory demyelinating polyneuropathy, anti-MAG neuropathy, and perhexiline toxicity) may also be painful. Although the primary pathophysiology (axonal or demyelinative) may be inferred to some extent from the clinical findings, electrodiagnostic studies are essential in most instances to clarify the likely primary pathophysiology and to assess the symmetry of the neuropathy.

Consideration of the pattern of nerve fiber class involvement is used diagnostically (Table 34.3). Relatively pure small fiber sensory involvement, as suggested by a presentation comprising burning and lancinating pain (with or without demonstrable abnormalities on pinprick or thermal testing), and normal reflexes, position sense and strength testing, suggests a very narrow list of possibilities, most commonly, impaired glucose tolerance (IGT) or mild diabetes associated distal polyneuropathy, idiopathic small fiber sensory neuropathy and rarely connective tissue disease or toxin exposure. Painful sensory neuropathies with prominent cardiac dysautonomia (e.g., orthostatic hypotension) suggest diabetes mellitus, acquired or familial amyloidosis, paraneoplasia, or a toxic neuropathy (e.g., cisplatin). In some instances, specialized tests of small fiber function are helpful to characterize the pattern of nerve fiber class involvement.

The medical and family history, and inquiry regarding potentially neurotoxic prescription and nonprescription medications, toxin exposure, and alcohol abuse is critical. Although inherited neuropathies are traditionally regarded as not associated with positive sensory phenomena or pain, pain may be a prominent feature of hereditary sensory and autonomic neuropathy (HSAN) type I, familial burning feet syndrome, Fabry disease, familial amyloidosis, and is an under recognized component (but not the dominant feature) of Charcot–Marie–Tooth disease (17). The clinical examination should include assessment for foot deformity (suggestive of a genetically determined neuropathy), signs of connective tissue disease (rash, arthropathy/joint deformity, sicca, Raynaud's phenomenon), stigmata of toxic neuropathy (Mees lines in arsenic and thallium poisoning), hair loss (thallium poisoning), hyperlipidemia, and adenopathy (HIV infection). Patients rarely volunteer a detailed drug exposure history, and questioning should be specific and direct in this regard.

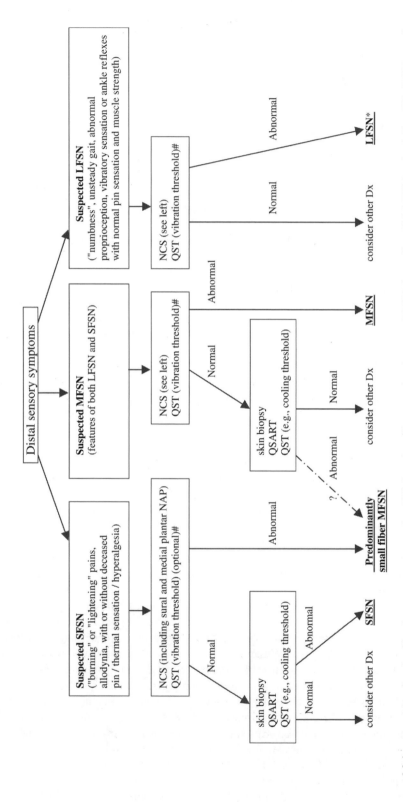

Figure 34.1   Algorithm for classificating sensory neuropathy (SN) based on fiber type involvement. LFSN, large fiber SN; MFSN, mixed fiber SN; SFSN, small fiber SN; Dx, diagnosis; NAP, nerve action potential; QST, quantitative sensory testing; QSART, quantitative sudomotor autonomic reflex testing. *May require skin biopsy/QSART to further classify as predominantly large fiber MFSN if these are abnormal. #vibrometry is optional if NCS is indeterminate.

Table 34.1 Spatial Pattern of Peripheral Neuropathies

Focal (asymmetric)	Multifocal (asymmetric)	Diffuse (symmetric)
Mononeuropathy	Multiple mononeuropathies	Polyneuropathy
Monoradiculopathy	Polyradiculopathy	Dorsal root ganglionopathy
Brachial plexopathy	Motor neuropathy	Motor neuronopathy
Lumbosacral plexopathy	Motor neuronopathy	
Motor neuronopathy		
Dorsal root ganglionopathy		

Source: Modified with permission from Herrmann and Logigian (22).

3.2. Diagnostic Testing

Electrodiagnostic testing consists of nerve conduction studies (NCS) and needle EMG and is largely limited to assessment of large fibers. It can confirm the presence of a neuropathy and evaluate the symmetry, pattern of nerve fiber class involvement, pathophysiology (axonal or demyelinative), severity, and distribution. Electrodiagnostic testing may fail to disclose the presence of a neuropathy when small diameter sensory or autonomic fibers are exclusively involved. However, the majority of painful neuropathies include some large fiber involvement, and electrodiagnostic testing is useful (16,18,19). For patients with suspected pure small fiber neuropathy, specific tests of small fiber function include quantitative sensory testing (QST) (cooling and heat-pain detection thresholds), quantitative sudomotor axon reflex testing, thermoregulatory sweat testing, and punch skin biopsy with assessment of epidermal nerve fiber density and morphology (16,19). Assessments of epidermal innervation at the distal leg and thigh are objective, minimally invasive, and more sensitive than sural nerve biopsy in the detection of somatic unmyelinated C-fiber loss (6,20). As not all instances of burning feet are due to small fiber neuropathy, and normal epidermal innervation warrants consideration of alternative etiologies (CNS demyelinating disease). The major limitation of skin biopsy testing is that it does not offer an etiologic diagnosis.

Cutaneous nerve biopsy (sural nerve) is useful to confirm suspected PNS vasculitis. A simultaneous muscle and nerve biopsy is advocated in the evaluation of PNS vasculitis and increases diagnostic sensitivity by 25% (21). A pattern of focal perineurial inflammation (perineuritis) may also be seen in this group of patients and, while often, idiopathic may be associated with underlying sarcoidosis, cryoglobulinemia, or occult malignancy (22).

3.3. Laboratory Testing

The choice of laboratory studies should be based on a considered approach (22). When the history and physical examination do not provide a clue to the presence of a systemic disease associated with neuropathy, screening tests designed to detect their presence is usually negative (22). Screening antibody panels without regard for the type of neuropathy is not cost effective (18,22). Reasonable studies include: a complete blood count, serum electrolytes, creatinine and BUN, liver enzymes, vitamin B12 deficiency, and an oral glucose tolerance test (OGTT). Patients with chronic painful sensorimotor polyneuropathies should be screened for paraproteinemia with serum immunofixation, as standard serum protein electrophoresis may not identify small monoclonal spikes. Testing for paraneoplastic antibodies (Anti-Hu) and imaging (chest CT) for an occult neoplasm in the setting of a sensory neuronopathy should be considered in patients with a history of

Table 34.2 Classification of Painful Neuropathies

Axonal	Demyelinating
Symmetric painful neuropathies	
Acute	
Alcoholic/nutritional	GBS
Vasculitis	
Arsenic (rarely demyelinating)	
Idiopathic sensory neuronopathy	
(can also be asymmetric)	
Thallium	
Subacute/chronic	
Idiopathic sensory neuropathy	CIDP (rarely with axonal abnormality)
Amyloidosis	Perhexiline
Uremia (mixed axonal/demyelinative)	Suramin
Diabetes mellitus	Paraprotein-associated
(mixed axonal/demyelinative)	
Sarcoidosis	
PNS vasculitis	
Lyme disease	
Fabry disease	
Tangier disease	
HIV-associated	
HSAN	
Familial burning feet syndrome	
Paraneoplastic	
Medication	
HMG-CoA reductase inhibitor (?)	
Taxol	
Cisplatin	
Isoniazid	
Gold (mixed axonal/demyelinating)	
Disulfiram	
Antiretroviral (stavudine, didanosine,	
zalcitabine)	
Metronidazole	
Thalidomide	
Vincristine	
n-Hexane (mixed axonal/demyelinating)	
Asymmetric painful neuropathies	
Acute	
Vasculitis	GBS (rarely asymmetric)
Lyme disease	
Perineuritis	
Diabetes (truncal neuropathy)	
Carcinomatous	
Trigeminal neuropathy	
Subacute/chronic	
Vasculitis, isolated PNS	CIDP (rare)
Vasculitis, systemic	
Vasculitis, connective tissue disease	
Vasculitis with infection	
Diabetes mellitus	
Sarcoidosis	

Table 34.3 Painful Small Fiber Neuropathy

Acute
   Diabetes mellitus (e.g., insulin initiation)
   Acute idiopathic small-fiber sensory neuropathy
Chronic
   Impaired glucose tolerance (?)
   HIV-associated neuropathy
   Chronic idiopathic small-fiber sensory neuropathy
   Primary amyloidosis
   Familial amyloidosis
   Fabry's disease
   Tangier disease
   Familial burning feet syndrome
   Hereditary sensory and autonomic neuropathies (types I, III, IV, V)

smoking and in those who develop unexplained painful progressive sensorimotor polyneuropathies >3–5 years.

4. CAUSES OF PAINFUL NEUROPATHIES

4.1. Drugs

Pain is a prominent feature of the toxic neuropathies associated with metronidazole, thalidomide, taxol, cisplatin, perhexiline, isoniazid, gold, disulfiram, suramin, and antiretroviral di-deoxynucleoside inhibitors (stavudine, didanosine, zalcitabine). Statins have received recent attention as possibly being associated with peripheral neuropathies (23).

4.2. Alcoholic/Nutritional Neuropathy

Painful distally dominant axonal neuropathy with degeneration of myelinated and unmyelinated fibers and segmental demyelination on nerve biopsy is associated with alcohol (24). However, alcohol-associated neuropathy is often clinically indistinguishable from that attributed to malnutrition (thiamine and niacin deficiencies). There has been a longstanding controversy as to whether the pathophysiology of alcohol-associated neuropathy is a direct toxic effect of alcohol or whether it is referable to malnutrition and hypovitaminosis. The occurrence of painful alcoholic polyneuropathy with predominantly small-fiber loss and normal thiamine status has been reported, and contrasted with the polyneuropathy due to thiamine deficiency states in which diffuse axon loss occurs (25).

4.3. Arsenic

Acute exposure manifests as nausea, vomiting, diarrhea, mental status change, and potentially death within 24 h. If the patient survives, chronic manifestations appear within 7–10 days such as gray discoloration of the skin, and peripheral neuropathy. Mee's lines may appear up to weeks or months following exposure. The peripheral neuropathy may resemble GBS clinically and electrophysiologically at the outset. Pain and paresthesias in the distal legs are a hallmark and are followed by an ascending sensorimotor polyneuropathy (26).

4.4. Thallium

Acute poisoning causes abdominal pain, nausea, vomiting, and diarrhea. Neurologic symptoms of mental status changes and polyneuropathy typically develop within several days. Painful distal lower extremity dysesthesias predominate initially, followed by the progression of sensory symptoms to more proximal portions of the limbs and even to cranial nerves. Motor manifestations develop somewhat later. Other chronic manifestations include scalp alopecia, visual, and cardiac dysfunction (26).

4.5. Diabetes

Pain is often the dominant symptom of diabetic neuropathy (27,28). Painful asymmetric diabetic neuropathies include acute opthalmoplegia, thoracic (truncal) neuropathy, and lumbosacral radiculo-plexo-neuropathy (diabetic amyotrophy). Painful symmetric diabetic neuropathies range from pure acute or chronic small fiber involvement to sensorimotor polyneuropathies. Up to one-third of diabetic neuropathy patients develop pain in the feet and legs. Pain is a less frequent feature of type 1 diabetes than of type 2 diabetes. The mechanisms of pain in diabetic neuropathy are unclear. Electrodiagnostic, QST, and sural nerve biopsy fails to differentiate patients with painful and painless diabetic distal polyneuropathies (29). There is growing evidence that patients with IGT detected by OGTT may also develop painful predominantly small fiber sensory neuropathies (30). It has yet to be determined whether intervention with diet or with oral hypoglycemic agents affects the natural history of this entity.

4.6. Hyperlipidemia

There are conflicting data that marked hypertriglyceridemia may be associated with mild slowly progressive polyneuropathies with foot pain (31–33).

4.7. Uremic Neuropathy

Painful dysesthesias and burning feet may herald the development of symptomatic distal sensory neuropathies in patients with endstage renal disease. The neuropathic pain usually resolves with dialysis, however, electrophysiologic abnormalities often persist.

4.8. HIV

Painful distal symmetrical polyneuropathy (DSP) is now the most prevalent neurological complication of HIV infection, occurring in 20% to 35% of patients with HIV (34). HIV DSP is a predominantly small fiber sensory disorder characterized by debilitating length-dependent pain, decreased pinprick and temperature sensations chiefly in the distal aspects of the lower extremities, diminished reflexes, and sparse motor involvement (e.g., weak intrinsic foot muscles). The pathophysiology of painful HIV DSP remains uncertain, but evidence favors HIV-triggered immune dysregulation, macrophage infiltration, and cytokine neurotoxicity within the DRG and peripheral nerves (35,36).

4.9. Hereditary Sensory and Autonomic Neuropathy

Among the six major types of HSAN, pain is most often associated with type 1. This autosomal dominant disorder is characterized by distal sensory loss in the legs, skin ulcers,

Charcot joint formation, and foot deformities. Despite a severe loss of sensation, patients in some kindreds report lancinating pain in the feet. The clinical expression of HSAN I may be restricted to lancinating pains in some affected individuals.

4.10. Fabry Disease

Fabry disease is an X-linked recessive lysosomal storage disease caused by deficiency of α-galactosidase. Patients develop angiokeratomas, corneal opacities, acral burning, dysautonomia, strokes, and subsequently renal failure. It is a painful small fiber sensory neuropathy with sparse or no sensory deficits on examination that may manifest as young as 5 years of age, and in female carriers (37). Patients experience intermittent bouts of burning and aching pain in the hands and feet. Pain may be accompanied by an elevation of body temperature. Anticonvulsants, in particular, often relieve the neuropathic pain, and there has been recent report of the efficacy of enzyme replacement therapy in treating the small fiber neuropathy (37,38).

4.11. Amyloid Neuropathies

Primary and various forms of familial amyloid polyneuropathies are associated with neuropathic pain. Clinically and pathologically, small diameter sensory fibers are most affected at the outset, and manifestations include painful, distal symmetric sensorimotor polyneuropathy with prominent pain, and temperature sensation loss (39). Other prominent neurologic manifestations include carpal tunnel syndrome and autonomic dysfunction.

4.12. Inherited Burning Feet Syndrome

An autosomal dominant burning feet syndrome has been reported in two German families characterized by burning, tingling, and a dull ache in the feet and legs (40). Onset of symptoms ranged between 12 and 40 years of age. Affected individuals had a normal neurological examination and normal or only mildly abnormal finding on electrodiagnostic tests, but a marked loss of unmyelinated nerve fibers on sural nerve biopsy. No linkage to any HSAN genetic locus has been found. Twenty-six percent of patients had foot deformities, and 26% of the patients had an affected first-degree relative, suggesting an inherited basis (41).

4.13. Tangier Disease

Tangier disease is characterized by large orange-yellow tonsils, adenopathy, hepatosplenomegaly, and an increased risk of developing coronary artery disease with absent or very low HDL levels. One-third express signs of polyneuropathy, including a slowly progressive, symmetric, predominantly upper extremity neuropathy with symptoms similar to those of syringomyelia (42).

4.14. Guillain–Barré Syndrome

Pain may be a presenting symptom of GBS. In a prospective series, 86% described pain on admission, and half reported sensory symptoms preceding weakness by approximately one week (43). The quality of pain varies, and is most commonly described as a "radicular type" back and leg pain; however, patients may complain of painful dysesthesias, myalgias, and joint pain. Almost 50% of patients in this study reported moderate-severe pain requiring oral and parenteral analgesics. The etiology of the pain is multifactorial, and includes inflammatory responses to roots and peripheral nerves, immobility, poor posture due to paraspinal weakness.

4.15. Chronic Inflammatory Demyelinating Polyneuropathy

Chronic inflammatory demyelinating polyneuropathy (CIDP) causes pain in up to 40% of patients. Pain is occasionally an initial and disabling symptom (44). The quality of pain varies, and includes burning dysesthesias, radicular pain, aching or cramping muscle pain, and lancinating pain. Rarely, CIDP patients may develop low back and radicular pain due to compression of hypertrophic nerve roots (45).

4.16. Paraproteins

A minority of patients with monoclonal gammopathy associated neuropathies, especially multiple myeloma, cryoglobulinemia, and macroglobulinemia, develop painful dysesthesias (46). An association between polyclonal antibodies to sulfatide moieties and a distal painful predominantly sensory polyneuropathy has been suggested (47), but the strength of the association is not sufficiently strong to warrant screening for anti-sulfatide antibodies (18,19).

4.17. Sensory Ganglionopathies

Idiopathic and secondary ganglionopathies (e.g., paraneoplastic, toxic, Sjögrens syndrome), while often painless, may manifest with numbness, painful dysesthesias, and lancinating pains in one limb with progression to involve all limbs, the trunk and face (48). Rarely, in idiopathic cases patients do develop an acute, patchy cutaneous burning and hyperalgesia syndrome that is believed to represent a purely small fiber sensory ganglionopathy (6)

4.18. Peripheral Nervous System Vasculitis

Vasculitic neuropathies are traditionally associated with focal or multifocal neuropathic pain (49). The origin of pain appears to be multifactorial and may be explained by dysregulation of neurotrophic factors in vasculitic nerve tissues leading to changes in pain perception (50), as well as an inflammatory reaction to necrotic tissue.

4.19. Cryptogenic or Idiopathic Polyneuropathies

Despite an exhaustive work-up, an etiologic diagnosis is not established in 10–35% of patients with sensory-predominantly polyneuropathies (18). Cryptogenic sensory polyneuropathies typically manifest in mid-to-late adulthood as a slowly progressive, distal painful polyneuropathy. Pain is often disabling. A subset of patients with cryptogenic sensory polyneuropathies, have a relatively pure small fiber sensory presentation, with burning, throbbing, and lancinating pains in the feet and hands, but normal strength, deep tendon reflexes, proprioception, and normal or only mild vibratory loss (6,18,19). Such patients, because of the paucity of abnormalities on examination and NCS, are occasionally misdiagnosed and inappropriately managed as having a musculoskeletal (e.g., plantar fasciitis) or psychiatric disorder.

5. TREATMENT OF NEUROPATHIC PAIN

The effective management of painful neuropathies consists of disease modifying interventions (e.g., immunotherapy) removal of exacerbating or provocative factors (e.g., alcohol, toxins, malnutrition) and symptomatic therapies (pharmacologic and nonpharmacologic). A list of pain-relieving agents is included in Table 34.4, and an algorithm in Table 34.5.

5.1. Tricyclic Antidepressants

Tricyclic antidepressants (TCAs) are the most widely studied agents for neuropathic pain (51–53) and include imipramine and nortriptyline, which are serotonin/norepinephrine reuptake inhibitors, and desipramine which is a relatively selective norepinephrine reuptake inhibitor. TCAs have pleiotropic effects on neuropathic pain, including Na-channel blockade of ectopic discharges in the PNS, and alteration of 5-hydroxytryptamine (5-HT) and norepinephrine activity in the CNS nociceptive-modulation system (52). Differences in efficacy among the various TCAs are minimal, despite varying pharmacology, and efficacy in terms of number needed to treat (NNT) to have one patient with a >50% reduction in pain intensity is comparable to that of various anticonvulsant agents (Fig. 34.2) (53). TCAs are limited by their adverse effects including constipation, dry mouth, cognitive change, urinary hesitancy, somnolence, orthostatic hypotension, and weight gain. Nortryptiline and desipramine are less sedating and have fewer anticholinergic side effects. Amitryptiline remains an excellent choice where sleep disruption is present and cost is an issue. TCAs are contraindicated in patients with closed-angle glaucoma, prostatic hypertrophy, and acute myocardial infarction. Slow titration is a key to their successful application.

Several newer antidepressants show promise as adjunctive therapy. Venlafaxine is a 5-HT and norepinephrine reuptake inhibitor, and animal and uncontrolled human studies have shown therapeutic potential for neuropathic pain (54). Bupropion, a nontricyclic antidepressant is a specific inhibitor of neuronal norepinephrine reuptake and a weak inhibitor of dopamine reuptake. A controlled trial using a sustained-release preparation (Bupropion SR 150–300 mg/day) showed a therapeutic effect in neuropathic pain (55). Selective serotonin reuptake inhibitors (SSRIs) have generally been disappointing (52,56,57). Fluoxetine has shown little efficacy in neuropathic pain, whereas more consistent efficacy has been suggested for paroxetene.

5.2. Anticonvulsants

Anticonvulsant drugs have been used for the treatment of neuropathic pain with an efficacy similar to the TCAs (53). Carbamazepine and phenytoin nonspecifically block Na^+-channels. Sodium valproate's therapeutic effect is thought to be mediated through potentiation of GABA-ergic neurons by increasing GABA synthesis and release. An uncontrolled study in patients with cancer-related neuropathic pain reported efficacy for sodium valproate (58). Sodium valproate is well tolerated, but adverse effects include hair loss, gastrointestinal distress, skin rash, hepatic dysfunction, bone marrow suppression, weight gain, tremor, and parkinsonism. Gabapentin has a more favorable side effect profile and does not require laboratory monitoring for toxicity. Several double-blind randomized controlled studies (mostly in diabetic neuropathy) confirm gabapentin's efficacy for neuropathic pain (59,60). Although its mechanism of action is uncertain, it may act in part by binding to the $\alpha2\delta$ subunit of N-type Ca^{2+}-channels and stabilized neuronal excitability (61). Overall, the efficacy of gabapentin appears to be slightly less than that of the TCAs (53), but because of its favorable side effect profile and a lack of drug

Table 34.4 Summary of Therapeutic Agents Used for Painful Neuropathies

Drug	Mechanism of action	Daily dose (mg)	Major side effects	Note
Antidepressant				
Tricyclics/tetracyclic	Na-channel inhibition		Anticholinergic effects	
	5-HT/Nor inhibition		Cardiac effects	
Amitriptyline		10–150		Useful with concurrent insomnia
Nortriptyline		10–150		Least cardiac effects
Desipramine		25–200		Least anticholinergic side effects
Bupropion	Nor/DA reuptake inhibition	150–300	CNS stimulation	Each dose should be ≤150 mg
Venlafaxine	5-HT/Nor reuptake inhibition	75–225	Seizure	Relatively short half-life
SSRI	5-HT reuptake inhibition		Hypertension	
			Diarrhea, insomnia, headache	
Paroxetine		20–60	Sedation	High protein binding
Sertraline		50–200	Milder side effects	
Anticonvulsants				
Phenytoin	Na-channel blocking	200–400	Bone marrow suppression	
Carbamazepine	Na-channel blocking	50–900	Hyponatremia, ataxia, hepatic failure	
Sodium valproate	GABAergic potentiation	500–1500	Rash, hepatic failure, anemia	
Gabapentin	Ca-channel agonist	200–3600	Sedation	Generally well tolerated
Lamotrigine	Na-channel stabilization glutamate release inhibition	25–500	Stevens–Jones syndrome	To be slowly titrated
Topiramate	Na-channel blocking	50–400	Kidney stone, CNS dysfunction	
Oxcarbazepine	Na-channel blocking	600–2400	Hyponatremia, sedation,	
Tiagabine	GABA reuptake inhibition	4–56	Sedation	
Levetiracetam	Unknown	1000–3000	Sedation, transient psychosis	
Ion channel blockers				
Mexiletine	Na-channel blocking	300–750	Arrhythmia	EKG monitoring
Opiates/Opioids				
Tramadol	Micro-opioid receptors agonist	200–400	Seizure	Less frequent addiction
Topicals				
Lidocaine patch (5%)	Na-channel blocking	May use up to three patches/24 h only use for 12 h in a 24 h period	Local irritation CNS effect (rare)	Suitable for localized pain

Note: 5-HT, 5-hydroxytryptamine; Nor, noradrenaline; DA, dopamine.

Table 34.5 Algorithm for Management of Neuropathic Pain

	Comments
First-line therapy	
Gabapentin	Generally well-tolerated if titrated properly, more expensive than tricyclics.
Amitriptyline	Suitable for patients with limited budget, with insomnia, with no contraindications (e.g., cardiac conduction block, closed-angle glaucoma, concurrent autonomic neuropathy). Anticholinergic effects may limit its use.
Nortriptyline/ Desipramine	Suitable for patients with therapeutic effect by amitriptyline, but limited tolerance due to its anticholinergic side effects. May have weaker therapeutic effect than amitriptyline.
Second-line therapy	
Tramadol	To be avoided to patients with potential for abuse.
Lidocaine patch	Suitable for patients with focal areas of neuropathic pain, with severe nocturnal pain or daily fluctuation.
	Randomized clinical trials are lacking.
Third-line therapy	
Lamotrigine	Requires slow titration.
Oxcarbazepine	Generally considered to be safe. Double blind study is lacking.
Topiramate	Especially suitable for obese patients with pain due to its effect on losing weight.
Phenytoin ⎫ Carbamazepine ⎬	Potential for toxicity. Side effect profiles less favorable than those of "newer" anticonvulsants.
Duloxetine	Effective in depressive patients with pain. Also effective in stress urinary incontinence.
Pregabalin	Also effective on sleep.
Mexiletine	Contraindicated to patients with cardiac conduction abnormality. Periodic EKG required.
SSRI	Suitable for patients with depression.
TENS unit ⎫ Biofeedback/ ⎬ coping skills ⎭	Evidence mostly anecdotal. Should be individualized.
Fourth-line therapy	
Long-acting narcotics (e.g., MScontin)	Consider in combination with other agents.

interactions, gabapentin is a first-line agent in the treatment of neuropathic pain. An initial dose of 100–300 mg at bedtime, with slow titration by 300 mg every 5–7 days to a TID schedule is appropriate. Most patients show a response between 300 and 900 mg TID, and there is little evidence that supports use of doses >3000 mg/day for neuropathic pain (59). Drowsiness or dizziness may occur if titration is too rapid. Occasional patients develop unacceptable pedal edema, and the agent requires a dose reduction in those with moderate renal dysfunction (GFR <50 mL/min). A drawback of gabapentin is its cost and three times/day dosing.

Lamotrigine stabilizes the slow inactivated conformation of a subtype of an Na-channel and inhibits glutamate release as well as modulating calcium and potassium currents. Randomized controlled trials show a therapeutic effect of lamotrigine in painful diabetic and HIV-associated neuropathies (62,63). In most studies, lamotrigine has been well tolerated, although its application is limited by a need for slow titration.

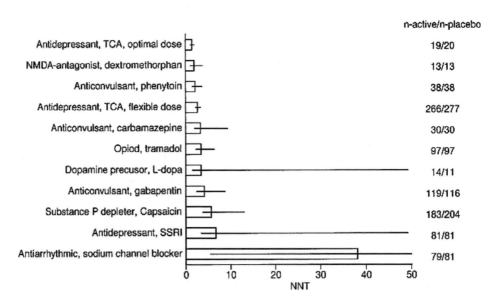

n-active/n-placebo

Antidepressant, TCA, optimal dose	19/20
NMDA-antagonist, dextromethorphan	13/13
Anticonvulsant, phenytoin	38/38
Antidepressant, TCA, flexible dose	266/277
Anticonvulsant, carbamazepine	30/30
Opiod, tramadol	97/97
Dopamine precusor, L-dopa	14/11
Anticonvulsant, gabapentin	119/116
Substance P depleter, Capsaicin	183/204
Antidepressant, SSRI	81/81
Antiarrhythmic, sodium channel blocker	79/81

Figure 34.2   NNT to obtain one patient with >50% pain relief calculated for combined data. [With permission from Sindrup and Jensen (53).]

5.3. Local Anesthetics

Transdermal drug delivery has several advantages in the treatment of neuropathic pain in that it limits systemic side effects and directs therapy to the symptomatic sites. Lidocaine, a local anesthetic and antiarrhythmic drug exerts effects on neuropathic pain by nonspecific stabilization of Na-channels. An open-label studies of a topical 5% lidocaine-impregnated patch demonstrated significant pain relief in the majority of subjects (64). The lidocaine patch is approved by the FDA in the treatment of post herpetic neuralgia (65).

5.4. Systemic Anti-Arrhythmic Agents/Na-Channel Blockers

Mexiletine is an anti-arrhythmic Na^+-channel blocker that has been tried in painful diabetic polyneuropathy with mixed results (66–68). The largest study showed significant pain relief only at high dose (675 mg/day) therapy (68).

5.5. Opioids

Tramadol is a centrally acting, synthetic, nonnarcotic analgesic with low-affinity binding to micro-opioid receptors and weak inhibition of norepinephrine and serotonin reuptake. It has been found to be efficacious in several double-blind randomized controlled trials in painful neuropathy (69,70). It has a relatively low addictive potential, particularly in patients with chronic neuropathic pain, and is a useful and well tolerated second-line agent for treatment of painful neuropathy, alone or in combination with an antidepressant or anticonvulsant. Tramadol is started in a dose of 50 mg at bedtime and titrated in 50 mg increments to a maximum of 400 mg in 3–4 divided doses. A lowered threshold for seizures is a consideration when higher doses of tramadol are used in combination with TCAs or SSRIs. Tramadol use may be accompanied by constipation, drowsiness, or rarely respiratory depression.

Stronger opiates have historically been felt to be relatively ineffective for neuropathic pain, and there has been reluctance to prescribe them for chronic neuropathic pain. There is a lack of randomized controlled studies in the setting of severe painful polyneuropathy. They are used in combination with first line agents, for severe and intractable neuropathic pain (52). Longer acting opiates (extended-release morphine, methadone) are preferred because of lower addictive potential.

5.6. NMDA Antagonists

NMDA antagonists may have a role in modulating the effect of excitatory amino acids on neuropathic pain (1,2). A controlled trial of dextromethorphan showed a modest beneficial effect in painful diabetic neuropathy and post herpetic neuralgia (71). Side effects of sedation, ataxia, nausea, and vomiting may limit its use. Riluzole has anticonvulsive, neuroprotective, and antinociceptive effects in animal studies, but a small, controlled study did not find efficacy in painful peripheral poly- and mono-neuropathies of various etiologies (72).

5.7. Other Agents

Capsaicin is a topical natural alkaloid derived from chillies, and exhibits antinociceptive effects chiefly by depletion of substance P at sensory nerve terminals. Although approved for the management of postherpetic neuralgia, studies have been contradictory in terms of its efficacy in painful polyneuropathies (73,74). Its use is limited by skin irritation during the first few weeks of topical application, often requiring pretreatment with an anesthetic spray. Moreover, recent animal and human studies have demonstrated that topical capsaicin activation produces profound reversible, epidermal denervation in normal individuals with concurrent loss of thermal and of pain sensation (75).

5.8. Psychological and Behavioral Approaches

Pain perception is modified by a patient's psychological state and coping skills, and patients with painful neuropathies report significantly more anxiety and depression (76,77). There have been case series of successful treatment of neuropathic pain with biofeedback (77). Multidisciplinary approaches, including biofeedback, operant-behavioral, and cognitive-behavioral interventions, may be considered as an adjunct to pharmacological options (76).

5.9. Acupuncture and Electrical Nerve Stimulation

Acupuncture, transcutaneous electrical nerve stimulation and its variants [percutaneous electrical nerve stimulation (PENS)] are based on the gate-control theory of Melzack and Wall (78,79). Despite several smaller studies claiming a therapeutic effect of acupuncture in neuropathic pain syndromes, a recent large-scale randomized trial in HIV-associated painful neuropathy failed to confirm efficacy (80). There have been therapeutic effects of electrical nerve stimulation reported by smaller studies (81,82).

5.10. Future Therapeutic Directions

As cellular and molecular mechanisms of neuropathic pain are elucidated, novel therapeutic approaches directly targeting molecules that modulate pain are being considered. Candidate molecules include, TNF-α, bradykinin, nerve growth factor (NGF), selective

Na$^+$-channel blockade (e.g., Nav 1.8 channel blockade), and endogenous opioids. Clinical trials of subcutaneous NGF, in diabetic and HIV-related neuropathies failed to confirm an effect of NGF upon progression of these neuropathies, however, an effect upon pain was evident in HIV neuropathy (83–85).

6. FOLLOW-UP OF NEUROPATHIC PAIN IN THE CLINIC

The quality and intensity of neuropathic pain should ideally be assessed and followed using validated measures to determine adequacy of pain management. Pain intensity is readily assessed by a 0–10 Likert visual analog scale. The McGill pain scale, neuropathic pain scale, and Gracely pain scales are among those that may be used to more rigorously assess both the intensity and the quality of neuropathic pain.

REFERENCES

1. Bridges D, Thompson SWN, Rice ASC. Mechanisms of neuropathic pain. Br J Anaesth 2001; 87:12–26.
2. Suzuki R, Dickenson AH. Neuropathic pain: nerves bursting with excitement. Neuroreport 2000; 11:R17–R21.
3. Baron R. Peripheral neuropathic pain: from mechanisms to symptoms. Clin J Pain 2000; 16:S12–S20.
4. Woolf CJ, Mannion RJ. Neuropathic pain: aetiology, symptoms, mechanisms, and management. Lancet 1999; 353:1959–1964.
5. Kidd BL, Urban LA. Mechanisms of inflammatory pain. Br J Anaesth 2001; 87:3–11.
6. Holland NR, Crawford TO, Hauer P, Cornblath DR, Griffin JW, McArthur JC. Small-fiber sensory neuropathies: clinical course and neuropathology of idiopathic cases. Ann Neurol 1998; 44:47–59.
7. Polydefkis M, Yiannoutsos CT, Cohen BA, Hollander H, Schifitto G, Clifford DB, Simpson DM, Katzenstein D, Shriver S, Hauer P, Brown A, Haidich AB, Moo L, McArthur JC. Reduced intraepidermal nerve fiber density in HIV-associated sensory neuropathy. Neurology 2002; 58:115–119.
8. Dyck PJ, Thomas PK, eds. Peripheral Neuropathy. 3rd ed. Philadelphia: W.B. Saunders, 1993.
9. Waxman SG, Dib-Hajj S, Cummins TR, Black JA. Sodium channels and their genes: dynamic expression in the normal nervous system, dysregulation in disease states. Brain Res 2000; 886:5–14.
10. Empl M, Renaud S, Erne PF, Straube A, Schaeren-Wiemers N, Steck AJ. TNF-alpha expression in painful and nonpainful neuropathies. Neurology 2001; 56:1371–1377.
11. Woolf CJ, Shortland P, Coggeshall RE. Peripheral nerve injury triggers central sprouting of myelinated afferents. Nature 1992; 355:75–78.
12. Tong YG, Wang HF, Ju G, Grant G, Hokfelt T, Zhang X. Increased uptake and transport of cholera toxin B-subunit in dorsal root ganglion neurons after peripheral axotomy: possible implications for sensory sprouting. J Comp Neurol 1999; 404:143–158.
13. Chung K, Kim HJ, Na HS, Park MJ, Chung JM. Abnormalities of sympathetic innervation of the area of injured peripheral nerve in a rat model of neuropathic pain. Neurosci Lett 1993; 162:85–88.
14. Ramer MS, Thompson SW, McMahon SB. Causes and consequences of sympathetic basket formation in dorsal root ganglia. Pain 1999; 82(Suppl 1):S111–S120.
15. Bickel A, Butz M, Schmelz M, Handwerker HO, Neundorfer B. Density of sympathetic axons in sural nerve biopsies of neuropathy patients is related to painfulness. Pain 2000; 84:413–419.

16. Nodera H, Logigian EL, Herrmann DN. Class of nerve fiber involvement in sensory neuropathies: clinical characterization and utility of the plantar nerve action potential. Muscle Nerve 2002; 26:212–217.

17. Carter GT, Jensen MP, Galer BS, Kraft GH, Crabtree LD, Beardsley RM, Abresch RT, Bird TD. Neuropathic pain in Charcot–Marie–Tooth disease. Arch Phys Med Rehab 1998; 79:1560–1564.

18. Wolfe GI, Baker NS, Amato AA, Jackson CE, Nations SP, Saperstein DS, Cha CH, Katz JS, Bryan WW, Barohn RJ. Chronic cryptogenic sensory polyneuropathy: clinical and laboratory characteristics. Arch Neurol 1999; 56:540–547.

19. Periquet MI, Novak V, Collins MP, Nagaraja HN, Erdem S, Nash SM, Freimer ML, Sahenk Z, Kissel JT, Mendell JR. Painful sensory neuropathy: prospective evaluation using skin biopsy. Neurology 1999; 53:1641–1647.

20. Herrmann DN, Griffin JW, Hauer P, Cornblath DR, McArthur JC. Epidermal nerve fiber density and sural nerve morphometry in peripheral neuropathies. Neurology 1999; 53:1634–1640.

21. Said G, Lacroix-Ciaudo C, Fujimura H, Blas C, Faux N. The peripheral neuropathy of necrotizing arteritis: a clinicopathological study. Ann Neurol 1998; 23:461–465.

22. Herrmann DN, Logigian EL. Approach to peripheral nerve disorders. In: Katirji B, Kaminski HJ, Preston DC, Ruff RL, Shapiro BE, eds. Neuromuscular Disorders—in Clinical Practice. Boston: Butterworth Heinemann, 2002:501–512.

23. Gaist D, Jeppesen U, Andersen M, García Rodríguez LA, Hallas J, Sindrup SH. Statins and risk of polyneuropathy: a case–control study. Neurology 2002; 58:1333–1337.

24. Behse F, Buchthal F. Alcoholic neuropathy: clinical, electrophysiological, and biopsy findings. Ann Neurol 1977; 2:95–110.

25. Koike H, Mori K, Misu K, Hattori N, Ito H, Hirayama M, Sobue G. Painful alcoholic polyneuropathy with predominant small-fiber loss and normal thiamine status. Neurology 2001; 56:1727–1732.

26. Spencer PS, Schaumberg HH, eds. Experimental and Clinical Neurotoxicology. 2nd ed. New York: Oxford University Press, 2000.

27. Archer AG, Watkins PJ, Thomas PK, Sharma AK, Payan J. The natural history of acute painful neuropathy in diabetes mellitus. J Neurol Neurosurg Psychiatry 1983; 46:491–499.

28. Galer BS, Gianas A, Jensen MP. Painful diabetic polyneuropathy: epidemiology, pain description, and quality of life. Diabetes Res Clin Prac 2000; 47:123–128.

29. Malik RA, Veves A, Walker D, Siddique I, Lye RH, Schady W, Boulton AJ. Sural nerve fibre pathology in diabetic patients with mild neuropathy: relationship to pain, quantitative sensory testing and peripheral nerve electrophysiology. Acta Neuropathol 2001; 101:367–374.

30. Singleton JR, Smith AG, Bromberg MB. Painful sensory polyneuropathy associated with impaired glucose tolerance. Muscle Nerve 2001; 24:1225–1228.

31. McManis PG, Windebank AJ, Kiziltan M. Neuropathy associated with hyperlipidemia. Neurology 1994; 45:2119–2120.

32. David WS, Mahdavi Z, Nance M, Khan M. Hyperlipidemia and neuropathy. Electromyogr Clin Neurophysiol 1999; 39:227–230.

33. Drory VE, Groozman GB, Rubinstein A, Korczyn AD. Hyperlipidemia may cause a subclinical peripheral neuropathy. Electromyogr Clin Neurophysiol 1999; 39:39–41.

34. So YT, Holtzman DM, Abrams DI, Olney RK. Peripheral neuropathy associated with acquired immunodeficiency syndrome. Prevalence and clinical features from a population-based survey. Arch Neurol 1988; 45:945–948.

35. Brannagan TH, Nuovo GJ, Hays AP, Latov N. Human immunodeficiency virus infection of dorsal root ganglion neurons detected by polymerase chain reaction in situ hybridization. Ann Neurol 1997; 42:368–372.

36. Glass JD, Wesselingh SL. Microglia in HIV-associated neurological diseases. Microsc Res Tech 2001; 54:95–105.

37. Brady R, Schiffmann R. Clinical features of and recent advances in therapy for Fabry disease. JAMA 2000; 284:2771–2775.

38. Filling-Katz MR, Merrick HF, Fink JK, Miles RB, Sokol J, Barton NW. Carbamazepine in Fabry's disease: effective analgesia with dose-dependent exacerbation of autonomic dysfunction. Neurology 1989; 39:598–600.

39. Kelly JJ, Kyle RA, O'Brien PC, Dyck PJ. The natural history of peripheral neuropathy in primary systemic amyloidosis. Ann Neurol 1979; 6:1–7.

40. Kuhlenbäumer G, Young P, Kiefer R, Timmerman V, Wang JF, Schroeder JM, Weis J, Ringelstein EB, Van Broeckhoven C, Stoegbauer F. A second family with autosomal dominant burning feet syndrome. Ann NY Acad Sci 1999; 883:445–448.

41. Novak V, Freimer ML, Kissel JT, Sahenk Z, Periquet IM, Nash SM, Collins MP, Mendell JR. Autonomic impairment in painful neuropathy. Neurology 2001; 56:861–868.

42. Gibbels E, Shaefer HE, Runne U, Schröder JM, Haupt WF, Assmann G. Severe polyneuropathy in Tangier disease mimicking syringomyelia or leprosy. J Neurol 1985; 232:283–294.

43. Moulin DE, Hagen N, Feasby TE, Amireh R, Hahn A. Pain in Guillain–Barré syndrome. Neurology 1997; 48:328–331.

44. McCombe PA, Pollard JD, McLeod JG. Chronic inflammatory demyelinating polyradiculoneuropathy. A clinical and electrophysiological study of 92 cases. Brain 1987; 110:1617–1630.

45. Di Guglielmo G, Di Muzio A, Torrieri F, Repaci M, De Angelis MV, Uncini A. Low back pain due to hypertrophic roots as presenting symptom of CIDP. Ital J Neurol Sci 1997; 18:297–299.

46. Vrethem M, Cruz M, Wen-Xin H, Malm C, Holmgren H, Ernerudh J. Clinical, neurophysiological and immunological evidence of polyneuropathy in patients with monoclonal gammopathies. J Neurol Sci 1993; 114:193–199.

47. Dabby R, Weimer LH, Hays AP, Olarte M, Latov N. Antisulfatide antibodies in neuropathy: clinical and electrophysiologic correlates. Neurology 2000; 54:1448–1452.

48. Sterman AB, Schaumburg HH, Asbury AK. The acute sensory neuronopathy syndrome: a distinct clinical entity. Ann Neurol 1980; 7:354–358.

49. Hawke SH, Davies L, Pamphlett R, Guo YP, Pollard JD, McLeod JG. Vasculitic neuropathy. A clinical and pathological study. Brain 1991; 114:2175–2190.

50. Yamamoto M, Ito Y, Mitsuma N, Li M, Hattori N, Sobue G. Pathology-related differential expression regulation of NGF, GDNF, CNTF, and IL-6 mRNAs in human vasculitic neuropathy. Muscle Nerve 2001; 24:830–833.

51. McQuay HJ, Tramèr M, Nye BA, Carroll D, Wiffen PJ, Moore RA. A systematic review of antidepressants in neuropathic pain. Pain 1996; 68:217–227.

52. Galer BS. Painful neuropathy. Neurol Clin 1998; 16:791–811.

53. Sindrup SH, Jensen TS. Pharmacologic treatment of pain in polyneuropathy. Neurology 2000; 55:915–920.

54. Kiayias JA, Vlachou ED, Lakka-Papadodima E. Venlafaxine HCl in the treatment of painful peripheral diabetic neuropathy. Diabetes Care 2000; 23:699.

55. Semenchuk MR, Sherman S, Davis B. Double-blind, randomized trial of bupropion SR for the treatment of neuropathic pain. Neurology 2001; 57:1583–1588.

56. Sindrup SH, Gram LF, Brosen K, Eshoj O, Mogensen EF. The selective serotonin reuptake inhibitor paroxetine is effective in the treatment of diabetic neuropathy symptoms. Pain 1990; 42:135–144.

57. Sindrup SH, Bjerre U, Dejgaard A, Brosen K, Aaes-Jorgensen T, Gram LF. The selective serotonin reuptake inhibitor citalopram relieves the symptoms of diabetic neuropathy. Clin Pharmacol Ther 1992; 52:547–552.

58. Hardy JR, Rees EA, Gwilliam B, Ling J, Broadley K, A'Hern R. A phase II study to establish the efficacy and toxicity of sodium valproate in patients with cancer-related neuropathic pain. J Pain Symptom Manage 2001; 21:204–209.

59. Backonja M, Beydoun A, Edwards KR, Schwartz SL, Fonseca V, Hes M, LaMoreaux L, Garofalo E. Gabapentin for the symptomatic treatment of painful neuropathy in patients with diabetes mellitus: a randomized controlled trial. J Am Med Assoc 1998; 280:1831–1836.

60. Gorson KC, Schott C, Herman R, Ropper AH, Rand WM. Gabapentin in the treatment of painful diabetic neuropathy: a placebo controlled, double blind, crossover trial. J Neurol Neurosurg Psychiatry 1999; 66:251–252.

61. Gee NS, Brown JP, Dissanayake VU, Offord J, Thurlow R, Woodruff GN. The novel anti-convulsant drug, gabapentin (Neurontin), binds to the alpha2delta subunit of a calcium channel. J Biol Chem 1996; 271:5768–5776.

62. Eisenberg E, Lurie Y, Braker C, Daoud D, Ishay A. Lamotrigine reduces painful diabetic neuropathy: a randomized, controlled study. Neurology 2001; 57:505–509.

63. Simpson DM, Olnery R, McArthur JC, Khan A, Godbold J, Ebel-Frommer K. A placebo-controlled trial of lamotrigine for painful HIV-associated neuropathy. Neurology 2000; 54:2115–2119.

64. Devers A, Galer BS. Topical lidocaine patch relieves a variety of neuropathic pain conditions: an open-label study. Clin J Pain 2000; 16:205–208.

65. Galer BS, Rowbotham MC, Perander J, Friedman E. Topical lidocaine patch relieves postherpetic neuralgia more effectively than a vehicle topical patch: results of an enriched enrollment study. Pain 1999; 80:533–538.

66. Dejgard A, Petersen P, Kastrup J. Mexiletine for treatment of chronic painful neuropathy. Lancet 1988; 1(8575–8576):1550–1555.

67. Stracke H, Meyer UE, Schumacher HE, Federlin K. Mexiletine in the treatment of diabetic neuropathy. Diabetes Care 1992; 15:1550–1555.

68. Oskarsson P, Ljunggren JG, Lins PE. Efficacy and safety of mexiletine in the treatment of painful diabetic neuropathy. The Mexiletine Study Group. Diabetes Care 1997; 20:1594–1597.

69. Sindrup SH, Andersen G, Madsen C, Smith T, Brosen K, Jensen TS. Tramadol relieves pain and allodynia in polyneuropathy: a randomised, double-blind, controlled trial. Pain 1999; 83:85–90.

70. Harati Y, Gooch C, Swenson M, Edelman S, Greene D, Raskin P, Donofrio P, Cornblath D, Sachdeo R, Siu CO, Kamin M. Double-blind randomized trial of tramadol for the treatment of the pain of diabetic neuropathy. Neurology 1998; 50:1842–1846.

71. Nelson KA, Park KM, Robinovitz E, Tsigos C, Max MB. High-dose oral dextromethorphan versus placebo in painful diabetic neuropathy and postherpetic neuralgia. Neurology 1997; 48:1212–1218.

72. Galer BS, Twilling LL, Harle J, Cluff RS, Friedman E, Rowbotham MC. Lack of efficacy of riluzole in the treatment of peripheral neuropathic pain conditions. Neurology 2000; 55:971–975.

73. Low PA, Opfer-Gehrking TL, Dyck PJ, Litchy WJ, O'Brien PC. Double-blind, placebo-controlled study of the application of capsaicin cream in chronic distal painful polyneuropathy. Pain 1995; 62:163–168.

74. Capsaicin Study Group. Treatment of painful diabetic neuropathy with topical capsaicin. A multicenter, double-blind, vehicle-controlled study. Arch Intern Med 1991; 151:2225–2229.

75. Nolano M, Simone DA, Wendelschafer-Crabb G, Johnson T, Hazen E, Kennedy WR. Topical capsaicin in humans: parallel loss of epidermal nerve fibers and pain sensation. Pain 1999; 81:135–145.

76. DePalma MT, Weisse CS. Psychological influences on pain perception and non-pharmacologic approaches to the treatment of pain. J Hand Therapy 1997; 10:183–191.

77. Haythornthwaite JA, Benrud-Larson LM. Psychological assessment and treatment of patients with neuropathic pain. Curr Pain Headache Rep 2001; 5:124–129.

78. Melzack R, Wall P. Pain mechanisms: a new theory. Science 1965; 150:171–179.

79. He LF. Involvement of endogeneous opioid peptides in acupuncture analgesia. Pain 1987; 31:99–121.

80. Shlay JC, Chaloner K, Max MB, Flaws B, Reichelderfer P, Wentworth D, Hillman S, Brizz B, Cohn DL for the Terry Beirn Community Programs for Clinical Research on AIDS. Acupuncture and for pain due to HIV-related peripheral neuropathy: a randomized controlled trial. JAMA 1998; 280:1590–1595.

81. Kumar D, Marschall HJ. Diabetic peripheral neuropathy: amelioration of pain with transcutaneous electrostimulation. Diabetes Care 1997; 20:1702–1705.

82. Hamza MA, White PF, Craig WF, Ghoname ES, Ahmed HE, Proctor TJ, Noe CE, Vakharia AS, Gajraj N. Percutaneous electrical nerve stimulation: a novel analgesic therapy for diabetic neuropathic pain. Diabetes Care 2000; 23:365–370.

83. Apfel SC, Schwartz S, Adornato BT, Freeman R, Biton V, Rendell M, Vinik A, Giuliani M, Stevens JC, Barbano R, Dyck PJ. Efficacy and safety of recombinant human nerve growth factor in patients with diabetic polyneuropathy: a randomized controlled trial. rhNGF Clinical Investigator Group. JAMA 2000; 284:2215–2221.
84. McArthur JC, Yiannoutsos C, Simpson DM, Adornato BT, Singer EJ, Hollander H, Marra C, Rubin M, Cohen BA, Tucker T, Navia BA, Schifitto G, Katzenstein D, Rask C, Zaborski L, Smith ME, Shriver S, Millar L, Clifford DB, the AIDS Clinical Trials Group Team. A phase II trial of nerve growth factor for sensory neuropathy associated with HIV infection. Neurology 2000; 54:1080–1088.
85. Schifitto G, Yiannoutsos C, Simpson DM, Adornato BT, Singer EJ, Hollander H, Marra CM, Rubin M, Cohen BA, Tucker T, Koralnik IJ, Katzenstein D, Haidich B, Smith ME, Shriver S, Millar L, Clifford DB, McArthur JC. The AIDS Clinical Trials Group Team 291. Long-term treatment with recombinant nerve growth factor for HIV-associated sensory neuropathy. Neurology 2001; 57:1313–1316.

35

Intravenous Immunoglobulin in the Treatment of Peripheral Neuropathy

Reem F. Bunyan
King Faisal University, Al-Khobar, Saudi Arabia

ABSTRACT

Intravenous immunoglobulin is used in the treatment of autoimmune disorders including peripheral neuropathies. Clinical benefit is shown in Guillain-Barré syndrome, chronic inflammatory demyelinating polyradiculoneuropathy, multifocal motor neuropathy. Other neuropathies have been less well studied. Clinical pharmacology, dosing and precautions, and clinical experience are reviewed in this chapter.

1. INTRODUCTION

Immunoglobulins (Igs) were initially administered by intramuscular injection, but later modified for intravenous administration and called intravenous immunoglobulin (IVIg). The initial use was replacement therapy for various immunodeficiency states. The first indication for autoimmune disorders was to treat elevated platelet counts in hypogammaglobulinemia and immune thyrombocytopenia (1). Subsequent clinical and experimental evidence has confirmed the immunomodulatory effects of IVIg in autoimmune disorders and its use in peripheral neuropathies.

2. IMMUNOGLOBULINS

Igs are glycoproteins synthesized by B lymphocytes and are either expressed on B cell surfaces or secreted as soluble factors. Circulating Igs are also referred to as antibodies. They constitute 25% of serum protein and represent the gamma band (or gamma globulin band) on an electrophoretic plate. Each Ig molecule is composed of two heavy (H) chains and two light (L) chains held together by covalent and noncovalent bonds. The carboxy terminal of the H chains is the Fc region of the Ig: crystallizable region. The N terminal of both H and L chains form the Fab region: antigen-binding region (Fig. 35.1). Igs are classified into five isotypes on the basis of the H chain. In order of their serum concentrations, these are IgG, IgA, IgM, IgD, and IgE. IgG and IgA are further subdivided into allotypes on the basis of specific H chain antigens: IgG_1, IgG_2, IgG_3, and IgG_4 and IgA_1 and IgA_2. There are two types of L chains: kappa and lamda. Each B cell clone produces one Ig allotype and one type of L chain. Ig idiotypes are based on the Fab region that is specific for a certain antigen.

    IgG constitutes most of the circulating Ig in the blood and cerebrospinal fluid. Its half-life is $\sim$23 days. IgA exists as a dimer and is the main Ig present in the mucous

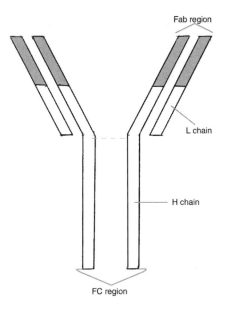

Figure 35.1   Basic antibody components.

membranes. It is also secreted in milk and tears. IgM exists as a pentamer and is mostly in blood. It has a short half-life of 2–5 days and has a role in the primary immune response. IgD functions as a surface receptor on mature B cells. IgE plays a role in allergic reactions and immune responses to parasitic infestations.

3. AUTOIMMUNITY

Autoimmunity results from reactivity of the immune system against self. It is a result of a breakdown in the normal mechanisms of self-tolerance. Most autoimmune disorders are multifactorial and result from complex interactions between genetic and environmental factors. Some of these disorders result from autoantibody production, whereas others result from abnormal self-reactive T cell responses. While most autoimmune disorders run a chronic course, some are monophasic and seldom recur (e.g., Guillain-Barré syndrome—GBS).

Myelin components are a common target of autoimmune responses. This may be partly explained by the natural sequestration of neural structures by the blood–brain and blood–nerve barriers. Antigenic components of certain infectious agents are similar to myelin. This explains post-infectious autoimmune GBS following infection by *Campylobacter jejuni* bacteria.

Treatment of autoimmune disorders is by administering immune modulating or immunosuppressive agents. Most of these agents are nonspecific and exert their effect on the entire immune system.

4. COMPARISON BETWEEN PLASMA EXCHANGE AND IVIg

Plasma exchange (PE) or plasma apheresis is a process of separating blood into cellular components and plasma. Plasma is then discarded and replaced by a suitable colloid to reconstitute blood. The mechanism of action of PE relates to discarding the humoral factors involved in the autoimmune process. Although this therapeutic modality is para-doxically the opposite of IVIg, both are often used to achieve rapid and aggressive recovery in similar immune conditions. In addition, neither is associated with long-term toxic manifestations of immunosuppressant drugs and both have similar costs. IVIg has the advantage of ease of administration via a peripheral intravenous access, whereas PE requires either large bore peripheral intravenous lines or a central vascular access. PE depends on equipment availability that is often only at larger medical centers.

5. INTRAVENOUS IMMUNE GLOBULIN

IVIg is an intravenous solution composed of heterogenous human IgG and trace amounts of IgA and IgM. IVIg is prepared by cold ethanol fractionation of Ig pooled from a number of donors ranging between 3000 and 10,000 (2). All samples undergo testing for antibodies against HIV1, HIV2, HIV p24 antigen, hepatitis B surface antigen, hepatitis C, syphilis, and liver transaminases. The amount of IgG subtypes (allotypes) parallels that in human plasma, although different products differ in titers against specific antigens.

6. IVIg PHARMACOLOGY

6.1. Route of Administration

IVIg is prepared for intravenous administration using a peripheral intravenous line. Some IVIg preparations require reconstitution prior to administration. Preparations differ in their compatibility with intravenous fluids, concentration, amount of IgA, sodium and sugar contents, pH, the need for reconstitution, and cost. The infusion is usually started at a slow rate of $\sim$50 mL/h. The rate is increased on the basis of patient tolerance and usually does not exceed 200 mL/h.

6.2. Kinetics

Ig blood concentrations peak immediately after infusion and are dose-related. Blood levels correlate with the administered dose. Sixty percent of the administered dose remains in the intravascular compartment and the rest in the extravascular compartment. Within 24 h of administration, 30% of the given dose is removed by catabolism and distribution. Serum IgG levels return to normal within 3–4 weeks (Fig. 35.2). The metabolic fate of IVIg is not known; the serum half-life varies between 21 and 29 days depending on the product, but the biological half-life is not known. IVIg crosses the placenta and is excreted in breast milk. IVIg also penetrates the blood–brain barrier, and CSF IgG levels double in the first 48 h after administration and return to baseline levels in 1 week (3).

6.3. Interactions

Manufacturers recommend that patients not receive live vaccines during the time period of 14 days prior to and 3 months after receiving IVIg. This is because IVIg contains anti-bodies that inactivate certain live vaccines such as the MMR (measles/mumps/rubella), rotavirus vaccine, and varicella live vaccine.

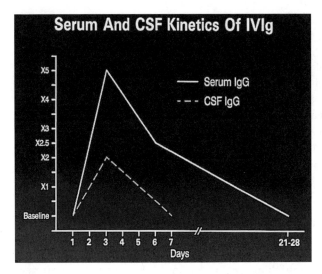

Figure 35.2 Serum and CSF IgG 3 days after infusion of IVIg. IgG increases fivefold in serum and twofold in the CSF. Rapid diffusion into the extravascular space follows (3).

6.4. Monitoring

There are no uniform guidelines for monitoring IVIg in the treatment of autoimmune disease. We recommend baseline laboratory studies to include complete blood count and renal function tests. The need to screen for IgA deficiency prior to the use of IVIg is debated because reactions to IgA are extremely rare. Serum protein electrophoresis and immunofixation results are altered after IVIg infusion and thus should be obtained either prior to administration or >4 weeks after the last dose.

7. MECHANISM OF ACTION

The mechanism of action of IVIg in autoimmune diseases is unknown, and multiple mechanisms probably play a role (Table 35.1). Some mechanisms are likely more important than others and may vary among autoimmune diseases.

7.1. Anti-idiotypes

The Fab portion of the Ig contains the variable region that determines Ig specificity. These are called idiotypes. Sera from normal individuals contain Ig against some of these

Table 35.1 Mechanisms of Action of IVIg

Fab anti-idiotypic Ab
Fc Receptor blockade
Suppression of pathogenic cytokines
Inhibition of complement
Accelerated Ab clearance
Remyelination

variable regions and are called anti-idiotypes, that is, antibodies to antibodies. In contrast to IgG from a single individual, 40% of IVIg's IgG is in the dimeric form as a result of two IgG molecules specifically binding to each other at the Fab region (2). This proportion is higher with a higher number of donors and indicates the wider variety of anti-idiotypes. Anti-idiotypic antibodies bind and neutralize circulating autoantibodies. They also down-regulate their production by B cells. This mechanism of action plays an important role in antibody-mediated disease like anti-myelin associated glycoprotein (MAG) Ab neuropathy, antiGM1 Ab neuropathy, and Lambert Eaton Myasthenic Syndrome. In a small study using IVIg to treat pemphigus foliaceus, IVIg therapy resulted in a selective drop of autoantibody titers (anti-desmoglein 1 antibodies) (4).

7.2. Fc Receptor

The Fc portions of IgG saturate surface Ig receptors on macrophages, resulting in nonspecific macrophage Fc receptor blockade. This leads to the inhibition of macrophage-mediated phagocytosis. This mechanism plays an important role in idiopathic thrombocytopenic purpura (ITP) by inhibiting platelet uptake by macrophages. It may also play a role in macrophage-mediated myelin destruction.

7.3. Complement

IgG Fc portions bind complement, resulting in inability of the available C3 molecules to further activate the remainder of the complement cascade and the formation of the membranolytic attack complex. This role of IVIg is important in dermatomyosits which includes complement-mediated vascular damage, and there is a >90% disappearance of complement from the tissue after IVIg administration in this disease (5).

7.4. Cytokines

Non-specific binding of Fc portion of IgG with macrophages inhibits the production of IL-1 and TNFα. This plays a role in controlling vascular inflammation in Kawasaki disease. Controlling the production of pro-inflammatory cytokines is an important mechanism of action in most autoimmune processes.

7.5. Accelerated Antibody Clearance

In vitro studies reveal that IVIg infusion results in a drop in the level of endogenous IgG by ~40%, 3 days after a single infusion. Computational studies to predict this effect in humans reveal a possible maximal reduction by 25% 3–4 weeks after administering a 2 g/kg dose. This prolonged and sustained effect is attributed to accelerated clearance of IgG (6).

7.6. Remyelination

In vitro experimental allergic encephalitis models show that polyclonal Ig promotes remyelination (7,8). This might explain some of the effects of IgG in demyelinating disease. The exact mechanism of enhancing remyelination is not known.

8. DOSE

The dose generally used in the treatment of autoimmune disorders is 2 g/kg divided over 2–5 days. This is the dose used in the initial trial of IVIg in ITP (1). Dose–response relationships likely vary among autoimmune disorders. The required maintenance dose and frequency is not known. Dosing schedules vary, with some clinicians using fixed dose and variable dosing intervals and others using fixed intervals and reduced doses. This variability arises from lack of knowledge of the biological half-life and the likelihood that maintenance doses vary between disease states.

9. VIRAL SAFETY

IVIg is a blood product derived from donor plasma. Donor screening includes a medical history and physical examination. Plasma processing takes place when all tests prove negative and after 60 days of quarantine (9). At that point viral inactivation and removal methods are used to eliminate possible contaminants and ensure safety. Viral inactivation methods vary among manufacturers and include physical methods (such as dry heat, pasteurization) and chemical methods (such as solvents, detergents, low pH incubation, caprylate). Viral removal takes place by using physical methods such as partitioning, chromatography, or filtration. IVIg is generally a safe product and has a good viral safety record. Apart from the outbreak of hepatitis C in 1992–1993, no other cases were identified (10,11).

10. CONTRAINDICATIONS

IVIg is contraindicated in patients with IgA deficiency. These patients carry the risk of anaphylaxis by circulating IgE antibodies against IgA. The incidence of IgA deficiency is approximately 1:700, but reported anaphylactic reactions are rare (9). Preparations devoid of IgA are available and suitable for these patients. Relative contraindications include conditions that predispose to renal toxicity or a hypercoagulable state (Table 35.2).

11. SIDE EFFECTS

Most side effects to IVIg are mild, self-limited, and easy to treat (Table 35.3). Headache is the commonest side effect and occurs more often in patients with a history of migraine headaches. Others include fever, malaise, body aches, and chills.

Renal failure is a serious adverse reaction to the use of IVIg. In most cases, this is attributed to osmolar renal tubular damage. Sucrose and maltose-containing preparations

Table 35.2 Contraindications to the Use of IVIg

Absolute	IgA deficiency
Relative	Agammaglobulinemia
	Hypogammaglobulinemia
	Dehydration
	Pregnancy
	Lactation
	Renal disease
	Cardiac disease
	Cerebrovascular disease
	Diabetes mellitus

Table 35.3   Side Effects of IVIg

Serious	Anaphylactic shock
	Renal tubular necrosis
	Osmotic nephrosis
	Stroke
	Myocardial infarction
	Stevens Johnson syndrome
	Hemolytic anemia
Less serious	Headache
	Fever
	Chills
	Diaphoresis
	Hypotension
	Nausea
	Vomiting
	Back pain
	Arthralgia
	Myalgia
	Aseptic meningitis
	Chest pain
	Rash
	Injection site reactions
	Phlebitis
	Pruritus

are associated with a higher frequency of renal impairment. It is often reversible. BUN and creatinine levels return to baseline values in ~20 days.

Vascular adverse reactions include cardiovascular and cerebrovascular thrombosis as a result of increased serum viscosity. Caution should be taken when treating patients with risk factors to thrombotic disease. The American Red Cross guidelines indicate using IVIg at concentrations of 5% or less in patients with signs of thrombosis. A low concentration and slow rate of infusion is recommended to avoid thrombotic events in high-risk patients.

Anaphylactic reactions due to IgA deficiency are rare and occur at a rate of 1.3:1,000,000 transfusions of blood or blood products in the USA. The infusion should be stopped immediately at the earliest sign of anaphylaxis. IgA depleted IVIg is a suitable alternative for these patients.

Aseptic meningitis is an uncommon reaction to IVIg. This, too, is reported to occur more frequently in patients with a history of migraine headaches. It is characterized by a severe headache and meningismus. CSF studies are those of aseptic meningitis. Treatment is symptomatic.

A number of rare reactions to IVIg are reported, such as hemolytic anemia (12) and cryoglobulinemic vasculitis (13).

12. INDICATIONS

IVIg is generally used for three purposes: as a replacement therapy, to treat immunodeficiency states, and to treat autoimmune disorders (Table 35.4).

Table 35.4 Uses of IVIg

Immunodeficiency
  Agammaglobulinemia/hypogammaglobulinemia
Bacterial infection
Bone marrow transplantation
Autoimmune disease
  Guillain–Barré syndrome
  Chronic inflammatory demyelinating polyneuropathy
  Multifocal motor neuropathy
  Graft vs. host disease
  Dermatomyositis
  Polymyositis
  Kawasaki disease
  Myasthenia gravis
  Lambert Eaton myasthenic syndrome
  Systemic lupus erythematosus
  Antiphospholipid syndrome
  Vasculitis
  Stiff person syndrome
  Multiple sclerosis
  Rasmussen's encephalitis
  Intractable epilepsy in children
  Idiopathic thrombocytopenic purpura

13. THERAPEUTIC USES OF IVIg FOR PERIPHERAL NEUROPATHY

IVIg has been shown to be effective in the treatment of autoimmune disorders of the peripheral nerve.

13.1. Guillain–Barré Syndrome

GBS is a syndrome of acute areflexic quadriparesis. The most common type is acute inflammatory demyelinating polyradiculoneuropathy (AIDP). Other types include Fisher syndrome and axonal GBS.

A number of trials of IVIg in GBS have been conducted (Table 35.5). In the 1980s, two large randomized controlled trials showed the efficacy of PE in treatment of AIDP (14,15). Several randomized double blind placebo-controlled trials comparing IVIg to PE, confirmed that IVIg (at a dose of 0.4 g/kg/day for 5 days) is equally effective as PE (16,17). Another study compared IVIg alone, PE alone, and PE followed by IVIg. Recovery rates in all groups were similar after 4 weeks, with no additional benefit in the combination group (18).

A small study compared IVIg and 500 mg of methylprednisolone (MP) intravenously with IVIg alone. Although this group was not randomized and controlled, the group receiving both IVIg and MP showed a more rapid recovery (19). Another small randomized study included PE alone, selective Ig adsorption by extracorporeal elimination, or a combination of Ig absorption and IVIg. The combination was more efficacious (20).

A double-blind placebo-controlled comparison of two doses of IVIg in AIDP patients with contraindications to PE in Ref. (21). A dose of 0.4 g/kg per day for 3 days vs. the same dose for 6 days showed a trend toward a better outcome in the group

Table 35.5 Clinical Trials of the Use of IVIg in AIDP

Principal author/ study group	n	Treatment groups	Outcome measures	Results
Dutch group/van der Meche and Schmitz (16)	147	ROCT of PE 200–250 mL/kg over 4–5 days vs. IVIg 0.4 g/kg per day for 5 days	Improvement by ≥ 1 grades on the GBS FDS	IVIg is at least as effective as PE, possibly more efficacious
PE/sandoglobulin GBS trial group (18)	383	Multicenter, RCBT of PE alone, IVIg alone, PE followed by IVIg	The GBS FDS	No difference in the three groups
Bril et al. (17)	50	ROT of IVIg 0.4 g/kg per day for 4 days vs. PE	Time to improve one disability grade, disability grade at 1 month, and time to reach FDS grade 1	Both groups did equally well
Dutch (19)	25	Pilot study of IVIg and MP 500 mg vs. IVIg	Improvement by ≥ 1 grades on GBS FDS	IVIg and MP superior to IVIg alone
Haupt et al. (20)	45	Randomized trial of PE alone, selective IA by extracorporeal elimination, Ig adsorption plus IVIg	Clinical score	Selective IA plus IVIg is superior to PE alone
Raphael et al. (21)	39	Multicenter, RDBT of IVIg 0.4 g/kg per day for 3 days vs. 0.4 g/kg per day for 6 days (3.8% albumin was given on 4th to 6th days in the group treated for 3 days)	Time needed to regain ability to walk 5 m with assistance (GBS disability grade 3)	The 6 day group did better; not statistically significant. The subgroup requiring ventilatory assistance did better; statistically significant

Note: ROCT, randomized open controlled trial; RCBT, randomized controlled blinded trial; ROT, randomized open trial; GBS, Guillain–Barré syndrome; FDS, functional disability scale; PE, plasma exchange; MP, methylprednisolone; IA, Ig adsorption.

that was treated for 6 days. This difference was statistically significant in patients requiring mechanical ventilation, which comprised approximately half of the patients.

Some patients with GBS have antiganglioside antibodies to GM1 (usually of the IgG or IgA type). The role of these antibodies remains unclear; however, their presence probably predicts quick reversibility of the demyelinating process with early therapy. In a nonrandomized uncontrolled study patients with GBS and anti-GM1 Ab were treated with either IVIg or PE. The groups treated with IVIg had a faster recovery (22). IVIg might be the treatment of choice in this subgroup of GBS.

13.1.1.   GBS Variants

Variants of GBS have been less systematically studied due to their lower incidence. The axonal form of GBS is strongly associated with exposure to *Campylobacter jejuni* infection and has a poor prognosis regardless of the modality of treatment (23).

The Fisher variant is generally considered a milder form with fewer patients requiring mechanical ventilation. A case of a 3-year-old child with a severe course improved with IVIg (24).

13.1.2.   Treatment Failure and Relapses

Patients with GBS who do not respond to IVIg or PE are considered treatment failures. The rate of treatment failure with PE and IVIg are probably similar. Though uncommon, GBS can recur months or years after the initial illness. Relapses occur with similar frequencies in patients treated with PE or IVIg (25).

13.2.   Chronic Inflammatory Demyelinating Polyradiculoneuropathy

Chronic inflammatory demyelinating polyradiculoneuropathy (CIDP) is a chronic autoimmune demyelinating polyneuropathy. Even though both AIDP and CIDP are acquired inflammatory demyelinating neuropathies, CIDP is considered a different disease and not simply a chronic form of GBS. Clinically, CIDP runs a chronic course with sensorimotor and/or autonomic symptoms lasting >8 weeks. Patients may have relapses and remissions. In distinction to GBS, CIDP is responsive to corticosteroids. CIDP is also responsive to PE, IVIg, and other immunosuppressants.

Several randomized controlled trials showed the efficacy of IVIg in CIDP (Table 35.6). Mendell et al. conducted a multicenter, randomized, double-blind placebo-controlled trial of IVIg in untreated patients with CIDP using 1 g/kg per day on days 1 and 2 then 1 g/kg on day 21 compared with 5% albumin. Seventy-six percent of patients showed improvement as early as 10 days after the first infusion (30). Another smaller crossover trial comparing oral prednisolone and IVIg showed that both arms were equally efficacious, with the IVIg limb showing slightly greater short-term efficacy (31). Long-term effects of IVIg have been studied, and two out of three responders to IVIg had benefits up to 6 and 12 months after a single treatment of 0.4 g/kg for 5 days (29).

13.2.1.   CIDP in Diabetes Mellitus

CIDP may occur at a higher frequency in patients with diabetes mellitus (DM) than in nondiabetics (32,33). There appears to be no epidemiologic or clinical differences in CIDP between diabetics and nondiabetics (34). In an uncontrolled trial of IVIg in patients with diabetic demyelinating polyneuropathy, clinically significant improvement was seen in 21 out of 26 patients (35). However, diabetics are more prone to developing

Table 35.6 Clinical Trials of the Use of IVIg in the Treatment of CIDP

Principal author/ study group	n	Treatment groups	Primary outcome measures	Results
Vermeulen et al. (26)	28	DBPCT of IVIg 0.4 g/kg per day for 5 consecutive days vs. placebo (albumin)	Six point Rankin scale, sum of MRC scale of 3 arm and 3 leg muscles	IVIg superior to placebo
Dyck et al. (27)	20	RSBCOT of PE twice weekly for 3 weeks followed by once weekly for 3 weeks vs. IVIg 0.4 g/kg once a week for 3 weeks followed by 0.2 g/kg once a week for 3 weeks. The washout period was at least 6 weeks	Neuropathy disability score (NDS), summated CMAP of ulnar, median and peroneal nerves	Both modalities resulted in statistically significant improvement. No difference between the two
Hahn et al. (28)	30	DBPCCOT of IVIg 0.4 g/kg per day for 5 consecutive days vs. placebo (10% dextrose). Variable washout periods	NDS, functional clinical grade, and grip strength	IVIg superior to placebo
Thompson et al. (29)	7	DBPCCOT of IVIg 0.4 g/kg per day for 5 days vs. placebo (albumin) followed by enrolling patients that relapsed into arm 2: IVIg 0.4 g/kg every 3 weeks vs. placebo (albumin)	Improvement in three measures of: AI, 10 m walk time, expanded MRC sum score, 9 hole peg test time, mean myometer score or two muscle groups, and HMAS	Three patients responded, two of the three responders remained stable 6 months and 1 year after infusion. The 3rd patient remained stable with the regimen in arm 2 of the study.
Mendell et al. (30)	50	Multicenter, RDBPCT of IVIg 1g/kg on day 1,2 and 21 vs. placebo (5% albumin)	Change in muscle strength from baseline to day 42 by manual muscle testing	IVIg superior to placebo
Hughes et al. (31)	24	Multicenter RDBCT of oral prednisolone followed by IVIg vs. IVIg followed by prednisolone. Doses: prednisolone: 60 mg qam for 2 weeks, 40 mg qam for 1 week, 30 mg qam for 1 week, 20 mg qam for 1 week, then 10 mg qam for 1 week, IVIg: 1 g/kg per day for 2 days or 2 g/kg in 24 h, placebo (6% albumin)	Novel disability scale: INCAT disability scale	Both treatment arms equally efficacious

Note: DBPCT, double-blind placebo-controlled trial; RDBPCT, randomised double-blind placebo-controlled trial; RSBCOT, randomized single-blinded cross-over trial; DBPCCOT, Double-blind placebo-controlled cross-over trial; NDS, neuropathy disability score; CMAP, compound muscle action potential; AI, ambulation index; HMAS, Hammersmith motor ability score.

renal impairment. Whether diabetics should receive IVIg with low sucrose or maltose to prevent renal toxicity was not confirmed by clinical studies.

13.3. Multifocal Motor Neuropathy

Multifocal motor neuropathy (MMN) is an acquired inflammatory demyelinating poly-neuropathy that has both similarities and differences from CIDP (36). Patients with MMN develop a chronic asymmetric, predominantly distal, lower motor neuron syndrome with electrodiagnostic findings of demyelination. This disorder is uncommon, but there have been four small randomized, double-blind, placebo-controlled trials confirming the efficacy of IVIg (37–40). Patients with MMN often have anti-GM1 antibody (usually IgM), but neither the presence nor the titer predict response to therapy.

13.4. Peripheral Neuropathy Associated with Monoclonal Gammopathy

Autoimmune peripheral neuropathies may be associated with monoclonal antibodies. In most situations, these neuropathies are acquired demyelinating polyneuropathies and are considered special subtypes of CIDP.

13.4.1. Anti-MAG Ab

Anti-MAG antibody neuropathy is a chronic predominantly sensory slowly progressive symmetric neuropathy. MAG is a protein essential in keeping the myelin sheath tightly wound around the axon. This neuropathy responds poorly to IVIg in no more than 18% of patients and may be less effective than PE (41,42).

13.4.2. Anti-GM1 Ab

Anti-ganglioside GM1 antibodies are present in patients with MMN (usually of the IgM type) and in some patients with GBS (usually of the IgG or IgA type). Patients with MMN respond to IVIg, but the presence of antibody does not seem to predict responsive-ness to therapy (discussed earlier). GBS associated with anti-GM1 antibodies has a good prognosis when treated with IVIg (22).

13.4.3. Monoclonal Gammopathy of Undetermined Significance

Neuropathies associated with monoclonal gammopathy of undetermined significance (MGUS) are variable in clinical and electrodiagnostic features. Patients often have a slowly progressive, distal, predominantly sensory symmetric polyneuropathy. MGUS-associated neuropathies associated with IgG and IgA are more responsive to therapy with IVIg than those associated with IgM (43).

13.4.4. Multiple Myeloma

Multiple myeloma (MM) is a plasma cell malignancy resulting in the production of large amounts of monoclonal antibody. Overall, peripheral neuropathy associated with MM is rare. Osteosclerotic myeloma (OM) is an uncommon type of MM characterized by sclero-tic bony lesions. Up to half of these patients have a demyelinating peripheral neuropathy with predominantly distal symmetric motor deficits. IVIg is not generally useful in the treatment of OM associated neuropathy; but there is a report of a rapidly progressive neuropathy that responded to IVIg (44).

Peripheral neuropathy can occur in the setting of multiple organ disorders. The POEMS syndrome includes *p*olyneuropathy, *o*rganomegaly, *e*ndocrinopathy, *M* protein, and *s*kin changes. This neuropathy often responds to treatment of the primary disease, but not to IVIg.

13.5. Paraneoplastic Neuropathy

Paraneoplastic neuropathies may be clinically isolated or in association with other neurologic manifestations, such as encephalitis or cerebellar degeneration. A few case reports indicate responsiveness to treatment with IVIg such as that reported by Mowzoon and Bradley (45).

13.6. Vasculitic Neuropathy

There are no clinical trials assessing IVIg in vasculitic neuropathy. IVIg has, however, been effective in the treatment of vasculitic disorders such as Kawasaki disease (46,47), SLE (48,49), systemic vasculitis (50) and ANCA positive Wegener's granulomatosis (51), and Churg–Strauss syndrome (52).

14. PREGNANCY

The treatment of autoimmune neuropathy during pregnancy is challenging. IVIg is used during pregnancy to treat other autoimmune disorders. As an example: weekly doses of 1–2 g/kg are used to treat alloimmune thrombocytopenia (maternal–fetal platelet Ab incompatibility) with no significant maternal or fetal adverse events (53). There is limited published experience treating GBS. Regimens have included the combinations of PE and IVIg at a dose of 5 g/day for 6 days or IVIg 0.4 g/kg per day for 5 days alone and results have varied (54,55). The disease process itself is apparently not different when complicating pregnancy than otherwise. No maternal or fetal adverse reactions were reported.

15. CHILDREN AND ELDERLY

IVIg has been used in patients from 2- to 93-year-old with no age-related side effects (56,57). In a retrospective study of patients 60 years or older that allowed a comparison between IVIg and PE, there were more side effects from PE (58).

16. SUMMARY

IVIg provides a form of immunotherapy with rapid onset of action, simple route of administration, and few significant adverse reactions. It is a first line agent in the treatment of GBS, CIDP, and MMN.

REFERENCES

1. Imbach P et al. High dose of intravenous gammaglobulin for idiopathic thrombocytopenic purpura in childhood. Lancet 1981; 1:1228–1231.

2. Dalakas MC. Mechanism of action of intravenous immunoglobulin and therapeutic considerations in the treatment of autoimmune neurologic diseases. Neurology 1998; 51(6 suppl 5): S2–S8.

3. Dalakas MC. Mechanisms of action of IVIg and therapeutic considerations in the treatment of acute and chronic demyelinating neuropathies. Neurology 2002; 59(12 suppl 6): S13–S21.

4. Sami N, Bhol KC, Ahmed AR. Influence of IVIg therapy on autoantibody titers to desmoglein 1 in patients with pemphigus foliaceus. Clin Immunol 2002; 105(2):192–198.

5. Dalakas MC et al. A controlled trial of high-dose intravenous immune globulin infusions as treatment for dermatomyositis. N Engl J Med 1993; 329(27):1993–2000.

6. Bleeker WK, Teeling JL, Hack CE. Accelerated autoantibody clearance by intravenous immunoglobulin therapy: studies in experimental models to determine the magnitude and time course of the effect. Blood 2001; 98(10):3136–3142.

7. Rodriguez M, Lennon VA. Immunoglobulins promote remyelination in the central nervous system. Ann Neurol 1990; 27(1):12–17.

8. van Engelen BG et al. Promotion of remyelination by polyclonal immunoglobulin in Theiler's virus-induced demyelination and in multiple sclerosis. J Neurol Neurosurg Psychiatry 1994; 57(suppl):65–68.

9. Gelfand E. In: Dalakas M, Spath P, eds. Safety in Intravenous Immunoglobulin Therapy, Intravenous Immunoglobulins in the Third Millenium. The Parthenon publishing groups, 2004:71–75.

10. Outbreak of hepatitis C associated with intravenous immunoglobulin administration—United States, October 1993–June 1994. Morbid Mortal Weekly Rep 1994; 43:505–509.

11. Breese J, Mast E, Coleman PJ. Hepatitis C virus infection associated with administration of intravenous immune globulin. A cohort study. J Am Med Assoc 1996; 267:1563–1567.

12. Wilson JR, Bhoopalam H, Fisher M. Hemolytic anemia associated with intravenous immunoglobulin. Muscle Nerve 1997; 20(9):1142–1145.

13. Odum J et al. Cryoglobulinaemic vasculitis caused by intravenous immunoglobulin treatment. Nephrol Dial Transplant 2001; 16(2):403–406.

14. Plasmapheresis and acute Guillain-Barre syndrome. The Guillain-Barre syndrome Study Group. Neurology 1985; 35(8):1096–1104.

15. Efficiency of plasma exchange in Guillain-Barre syndrome: role of replacement fluids. French Cooperative Group on Plasma Exchange in Guillain-Barre syndrome. Ann Neurol 1987; 22(6):753–761.

16. van der Meche FG, Schmitz PI. A randomized trial comparing intravenous immune globulin and plasma exchange in Guillain-Barre syndrome. Dutch Guillain-Barre Study Group. N Engl J Med 1992; 326(17):1123–1129.

17. Bril V et al. Pilot trial of immunoglobulin versus plasma exchange in patients with Guillain-Barre syndrome. Neurology 1996; 46(1):100–103.

18. Randomised trial of plasma exchange, intravenous immunoglobulin, and combined treatments in Guillain-Barre syndrome. Plasma Exchange/Sandoglobulin Guillain-Barre Syndrome Trial Group. Lancet 1997; 349(9047):225–230.

19. Treatment of Guillain-Barre syndrome with high-dose immune globulins combined with methylprednisolone: a pilot study. The Dutch Guillain- Barre Study Group. Ann Neurol 1994; 35(6):749–752.

20. Haupt WF et al. Sequential treatment of Guillain-Barre syndrome with extracorporeal elimination and intravenous immunoglobulin. J Neurol Sci 1996; 137(2):145–149.

21. Raphael JC et al. Intravenous immune globulins in patients with Guillain-Barre syndrome and contraindications to plasma exchange: 3 days versus 6 days. J Neurol Neurosurg Psychiatry 2001; 71(2):235–238.

22. Kuwabara S et al. Intravenous immunoglobulin therapy for Guillain-Barre syndrome with IgG anti-GM1 antibody. Muscle Nerve 2001; 24(1):54–58.

23. Chowdhury D, Arora A. Axonal Guillain-Barre syndrome: a critical review. Acta Neurol Scand 2001; 103(5):267–277.

24. Arakawa Y et al. The use of intravenous immunoglobulin in Miller Fisher syndrome. Brain
     Dev 1993; 15(3):231–233.
25. Sater RA, Rostami A. Treatment of Guillain-Barre syndrome with intravenous immuno-
     globulin. Neurology 1998; 51(6 suppl 5):S9–S15.
26. Vermeulen M. et al. Intravenous immunoglobulin treatment in patients with chronic inflamma-
     tory demyelinating polyneuropathy: a double blind, placebo controlled study. J Neurol Neuro-
     surg Psychiatry 1993; 56(1):36–39.
27. Dyck PJ et al. A plasma exchange versus immune globulin infusion trial in chronic inflamma-
     tory demyelinating polyradiculoneuropathy. Ann Neurol 1994; 36(6):838–845.
28. Hahn AF et al. Intravenous immunoglobulin treatment in chronic inflammatory demyelinating
     polyneuropathy. A double-blind, placebo-controlled, cross-over study. Brain 1996; 119(Pt 4):
     1067–1077.
29. Thompson N et al. A novel trial design to study the effect of intravenous immunoglobulin in
     chronic inflammatory demyelinating polyradiculoneuropathy. J Neurol 1996; 243(3):280–285.
30. Mendell JR et al. Randomized controlled trial of IVIg in untreated chronic inflammatory
     demyelinating polyradiculoneuropathy. Neurology 2001; 56(4):445–449.
31. Hughes R et al. Randomized controlled trial of intravenous immunoglobulin versus oral
     prednisolone in chronic inflammatory demyelinating polyradiculoneuropathy. Ann Neurol
     2001; 50(2):195–201.
32. Sharma KR et al. Demyelinating neuropathy in diabetes mellitus. Arch Neurol 2002; 59(5):
     758–765.
33. Lozeron P et al. Symptomatic diabetic and non-diabetic neuropathies in a series of 100 diabetic
     patients. J Neurol 2002; 249(5):569–575.
34. Rotta FT et al. The spectrum of chronic inflammatory demyelinating polyneuropathy. J Neurol
     Sci 2000; 173(2):129–139.
35. Sharma KR et al. Diabetic demyelinating polyneuropathy responsive to intravenous immuno-
     globulin therapy. Arch Neurol 2002; 59(5):751–757.
36. Chaudhry V. Multifocal motor neuropathy. Semin Neurol 1998; 18(1):73–81.
37. Azulay JP et al. Intravenous immunoglobulin treatment in patients with motor neuron
     syndromes associated with anti-GM1 antibodies: a double-blind, placebo-controlled study.
     Neurology 1994; 44(3 Pt 1):429–432.
38. Van den Berg LH et al. Treatment of multifocal motor neuropathy with high dose intravenous
     immunoglobulins: a double blind, placebo controlled study. J Neurol Neurosurg Psychiatry
     1995; 59(3):248–252.
39. Federico P et al. Multifocal motor neuropathy improved by IVIg: randomized, double-blind,
     placebo-controlled study. Neurology 2000; 55(9):1256–1262.
40. Leger JM et al. Intravenous immunoglobulin therapy in multifocal motor neuropathy: a
     double-blind, placebo-controlled study. Brain 2001; 124(Pt 1):145–153.
41. Dalakas MC et al. A controlled study of intravenous immunoglobulin in demyelinating neuro-
     pathy with IgM gammopathy. Ann Neurol 1996; 40(5):792–795.
42. Gorson KC et al. Treatment experience in patients with anti-myelin-associated glycoprotein
     neuropathy. Muscle Nerve 2001; 24(6):778–786.
43. Gorson K, Allam G, Ropper A. Chronic inflammatory demyelinating polyneuropathy: clinical
     features and response to treatment in 67 consecutive patients with and without a monoclonal
     gammopathy. Neurology 1997; 2(48):321–328.
44. Benito-Leon J et al. Rapidly deteriorating polyneuropathy associated with osteosclerotic
     myeloma responsive to intravenous immunoglobulin and radiotherapy. J Neurol Sci 1998;
     158(1):113–117.
45. Mowzoon N, Bradley W. Successful immunosuppressant therapy of severe progressive
     cerebellar degeneration and sensory neuropathy. J Neurol Sci 2000; 1(178):63–65.
46. Newburger JW et al. The treatment of Kawasaki syndrome with intravenous gamma globulin.
     N Engl J Med 1986; 315(6):341–347.
47. Harada K. Intravenous gamma-globulin treatment in Kawasaki disease. Acta Paediatr Jpn
     1991; 33(6):805–810.

48. Boletis JN et al. Intravenous immunoglobulin compared with cyclophosphamide for proliferative lupus nephritis. Lancet 1999; 354(9178):569–570.
49. Levy Y et al. A study of 20 SLE patients with intravenous immunoglobulin–clinical and serologic response. Lupus 1999; 8(9):705–712.
50. Levy Y et al. Serologic and clinical response to treatment of systemic vasculitis and associated autoimmune disease with intravenous immunoglobulin. Int Arch Allergy Immunol 1999; 119(3):231–238.
51. Jayne DR et al. Intravenous immunoglobulin for ANCA-associated systemic vasculitis with persistent disease activity. Q J Med 2000; 93(7):433–439.
52. Levy Y et al. Marked improvement of Churg-Strauss vasculitis with intravenous gammaglobulins. South Med J 1999; 92(4):412–414.
53. Lucas GF et al. Effect of IVIgG treatment on fetal platelet count, HPA-1a titre and clinical outcome in a case of feto-maternal alloimmune thrombocytopenia. Br J Obstet Gynaecol 2002; 109(10):1195–1198.
54. Yaginuma Y, Kawamura M, Ishikawa M. Landry-Guillain-Barre-Strohl syndrome in pregnancy. J Obstet Gynaecol Res 1996; 22(1):47–49.
55. Yamada H et al. Massive intravenous immunoglobulin treatment in pregnancy complicated by Guillain-Barre Syndrome. Eur J Obstet Gynecol Reprod Biol 2001; 97(1):101–104.
56. Zafeiriou DI et al. Single dose immunoglobulin therapy for childhood Guillain-Barre syndrome. Brain Dev 1997; 19(5):323–325.
57. Uldry PA, Bogousslavsky J, Regli F. Guillain-Barre syndrome in a 93-year-old woman: rapid improvement of neurologic function following intravenous immunoglobulin. Schweiz Arch Neurol Psychiatr 1991; 142(4):301–305.
58. Rana SS, Rana S. Intravenous immunoglobulins versus plasmapheresis in older patients with Guillain-Barre syndrome. J Am Geriatr Soc 1999; 47(11):1387–1388.

36

Treatment of Immune-Mediated Peripheral Neuropathy

Orly Vardeny and A. Gordon Smith
University of Utah, Salt Lake City, Utah, USA

ABSTRACT

Pharmacologic treatment of peripheral neuropathies is challenging and has largely been effective only for immune-mediated neuropathies. Although animal models of immune-mediated neuropathies have provided insight into pathophysiology, our understanding of initiating and perpetuating immune factors remains incomplete. Most drugs used for immune-mediated neuropathies were originally developed for connective tissue diseases. There are few randomized controlled trials for neuropathies, and most data on efficacy are from case series. Despite these limitations, there are useful empiric data on dosing, efficacy, and side effects for a range of immunomodulating and immunosuppressing agents. This chapter reviews how to use commonly prescribed agents, focusing on dosing, pharmacokinetics, and dynamics, and side effects. The indications for use are briefly reviewed; detailed discussions of specific indications are contained in the relevant chapters.

1. PREDNISONE

1.1. Efficacy

Prednisone was demonstrated to be effective in a case of a relapsing neuropathy that failed to respond to placebo (1). Subsequent open-label, and retrospective reviews, and one controlled trial have confirmed the efficacy of prednisone in chronic inflammatory demyelinating polyradiculopathy (CIDP) (2–6).

Prednisone is ineffective for acute inflammatory demyelinating polyradiculopathy (AIDP) and multifocal motor neuropathy, even though they are felt to be immune-mediated (7–11).

1.2. Dosing

There are little data on optimal dosing, duration of high dose, and taper rates for CIDP (12). Most reports start with doses of ~60 mg/day, and the only controlled trial started with 120 mg QOD. High doses are usually maintained for 4 weeks and then converted to alternate-day schedule before tapering. Taper schedules vary markedly and are commonly adjusted on the basis of patient response, with temporary increases if the patient's condition relapses (2,4,6,13).

1.3. Pharmacodynamics

The therapeutic mechanism of prednisone is poorly understood, and there are multiple possible sites of action. Corticosteroids inhibit T-cell proliferation, T-cell dependent immunity, and cytokine gene transcription (including the IL-1, IL-2, IL-6, interferon γ, and tumor necrosis factor-α genes). They prevent macrophage activation, antigen presentation, IL-1 production, and inhibit their function as effector cells. Corticosteroids inhibit the generation of cytotoxic T-cells. They have a less marked effect on B-cell function. (14–16).

1.4. Pharmacokinetics

Prednisone is a pro-drug, and equilibrium strongly favors the formation of prednisolone, the active agent (17). Conversion is achieved largely on first-pass metabolism through the liver (18). Small variations in the rate of prednisolone availability are unlikely to be of clinical significance because of its multiple sites of action and long-term immunologic effects (19,20).

Prednisolone is bound reversibly to albumin and to alpha-1 glycoprotein, a corticosteroid-binding globulin (transcortin). Protein binding is concentration-dependent and is diminished in hypoproteinemic states. Prednisolone is primarily eliminated by hydroxylation and conjugation, and only 2.5% of a dose of prednisone appears in the urine in its unmetabolized form. The mean half-life of prednisolone is 2.6–5 h (21). There is circadian variation in the clearance of prednisolone and is responsible for a greater effect per dose when taken in the morning. This is due to higher morning cortisol concentrations, resulting in a competitive decrease in the metabolism of prednisolone, leading to its decreased clearance (22). These circadian effects favor the choice of morning doses rather than evening doses (22).

Enzyme inducing drugs, including barbiturate agents, phenytoin, and rifampin, significantly increase the metabolic clearance of corticosteroid agents. The steroid dosage should be increased during concomitant administration (18,23,24).

1.5. Side Effects

The medical complications of glucocorticoid therapy are listed in Table 36.1 (12). The risks are theoretically dose- and time-dependent. Alternate-day dosing is felt to reduce side effects, but controlled trials are lacking (12,25). Doses up to 100 mg of prednisone daily may be taken for up to 3 weeks without significant risk for major adverse effects. It is not possible to stipulate a daily dose at which the risk of side effects is nonexistent. In adults, it is likely that 10 mg daily of prednisone will eventually lead to some side effects (26). Even, smaller daily doses of 7.5 mg, if taken in the long-term, are still associated with complications in the elderly (26).

1.5.1. Central Nervous System

Mild euphoria, depression, and insomnia may occur within the first 1–2 weeks of therapy. Other central nervous system side effects include insomnia, personality changes, mania, and hallucinations. A dose reduction results in abatement within 2 weeks in 50% of patients (27). Severe depression and psychosis rarely occurs at doses of >40 mg/day (5% risk) (28,29). Preexisting psychological problems increase the risk for adverse

Table 36.1   Medical Complications of Corticosteroids

Early
  Insomnia
  Emotional lability
  Enhanced appetite and weight gain
With co-morbidities
  Hypertension
  Diabetes mellitus
  Peptic ulcer disease
  Acne vulgaris
With sustained treatment
  Cushingoid habitus
  Hypothalamic-pituitary–adrenal suppression
  Infection diathesis
  Osteonecrosis
  Myopathy
  Impaired wound healing
Insidious and delayed (dose related)
  Osteoporosis
  Skin atrophy
  Cataracts
  Atherosclerosis
  Growth retardation
  Fatty liver
Rare and unpredictable
  Psychosis
  Pseudotumor cerebri
  Glaucoma
  Epidural lipomatosis
  Pancreatitis

Source: Adapted from Boumpas (14).

psychiatric reactions (30). If there is no therapeutic alternative, steroid psychosis can be managed with phenothiazines or lithium carbonate.

1.5.2. Hypertension

Fluid retention, enhancement of the vasoconstrictor effects of endogenous substances, and increased concentrations of renin substrate lead to hypertension (31).

1.5.3. Electrolyte Disturbances

Prednisone increases the distal renal tubular reabsorption of sodium in exchange for potassium, hydrogen, and ammonium ions, leading to hypernatremia and hypokalemic alkalosis in some individuals (32).

1.5.4. Osteoporosis

Osteoporosis occurs in up to 50% of patients on long-term glucocorticoid therapy and is due to decreased bone formation through direct inhibition of osteoblastic activity and increased bone resorption. Resorption is a consequence of secondary hyperparathyroidism caused by corticosteroid-induced hypercalciuria and inhibition of intestinal calcium absorption, as well as increased urinary calcium excretion (33). Trabecular bone in the spine and ribs is preferentially affected (34). Postmenopausal women and elderly or immobilized patients are at greater risk. Bone loss is more prominent in the early stages of corticosteroid therapy. Alternate-day treatment appears to have no advantage over daily use (35).

   Guidelines for preventing steroid-induced osteoporosis are similar to idiopathic osteoporosis and focus on exercise and adequate diet. Recommendations for calcium and vitamin D intake (dietary and supplemental) are 1200–1500 mg/day of calcium and 800 IU of vitamin D. Higher vitamin D doses are not recommended for routine use because of propensity for calcium urolithiasis (36). Baseline bone density scans are recommended for patients utilizing corticosteroids for long-term therapy. If osteopenia or osteoporosis is present, treatment with bisphosphanates is warranted (37–39).

1.5.5. Cutaneous Effects

Easy bruising, purpura, and ecchymoses are common in older patients on long-term corticosteroid treatment. These complications are attributed to diminished phagocytosis of extravasated blood and changes in connective tissue. Hirsutism occurs in ~10% of patients on long-term therapy (31,32).

1.5.6. Glucose Intolerance

Corticosteroids impair carbohydrate metabolism by increasing hepatic gluconeogenesis and by decreasing peripheral tissue utilization of glucose. There is also evidence for a component of insulin resistance (40). Steroid-induced diabetes is usually mild and can be managed by diet and oral hypoglycemic agents. Overt diabetes is unusual and usually resolves with discontinuance of steroid. Individuals with preexisting diabetes are at greatest risk for developing diabetes (40,41).

1.5.7. Aseptic Necrosis

Corticosteroids can cause aseptic necrosis of the femoral head. Fat microemboli are thought to occlude subchrondral end-arterioles leading to bone-cell death (42). Necrosis is heralded by pain and diagnosed by MRI showing a lucent area between the collapsed bone and the overlying cartilage (42). Hyperuricemia, alcoholism, hyperlipidemia, and polycythemia are predisposing risk factors (42).

1.5.8. Peptic Ulcer Disease

There is a small but significant association between corticosteroid therapy and peptic ulceration (43). Multivariate analysis demonstrated that risk factors for developing ulcers are previous history of peptic ulcer disease, cumulative prednisone dose of >1000 mg or therapy >30 days, and concurrent nonsteroidal anti-inflammatory drug (NSAID) therapy (43,44). Prophylaxis with a histamine H2-receptor antagonist is appropriate if two or more risk factors are present or if the patient is receiving concurrent treatment with a NSAID (44).

1.5.9. Infections

Corticosteroids impair cell-mediated immunity and inhibit monocyte responsiveness to chemotactic factors. However, the degree of increased susceptibility to infections is difficult to assess on the basis of clinical trials but is likely low (45). The risk may be higher for patients receiving corticosteroids in combination with other immunosuppressant agents.

1.5.10. Ocular Effects

The risk of posterior subcapsular cataracts increases with corticosteroid therapy >1 year or doses >10 mg of prednisone per day. Other ocular effects include increased intraocular pressure, more often in patients with myopia or diabetes mellitus (46,47).

1.5.11. Adrenal Suppression

Interruption of adrenal function occurs after a few days of high-dose corticosteroid therapy, and long-term daily therapy may suppress hypothalamic–pituitary–adrenal function for 9–12 months after cessation of treatment (48,49). However, examples of clinical adrenal suppression are rare. Traditional taper schedules appear to be reasonable, but supplemental administration of corticosteroid therapy during physiological stress is reasonable (50).

1.6. Pregnancy Issues

The risk for human teratogenesis is low with corticosteroids. This is due to inactivation of prednisolone in the placenta, allowing only 10% of the active drug to reach the fetus (51).

2. AZATHIOPRINE

2.1. Efficacy

Only one randomized controlled study comparing prednisone alone or with azathioprine in CIDP has been performed, and it did not show a benefit to additional azathioprine (52). However, there are uncontrolled trials supporting its use as a steroid-sparing agent (2,53). An uncontrolled trial in AIDP yielded inconclusive results (54).

2.2. Dosing

Doses of 1.5–3 mg/kg per day in divided doses to minimize gastrointestinal side effects are common, but optimum dosing has not been established for CIDP. A mild leukopenia has been used as a therapeutic guide, although it is not required for a beneficial effect (2,55).

2.3. Pharmacodynamics

Azathioprine, a purine analog, inhibits cellular proliferation by serving as a purine antagonist. Its greatest effect is on rapidly dividing cell lines such as the bone marrow.

2.4. Pharmacokinetics

Azathioprine has a half-life of 4.5–5 h. Inactive metabolites are excreted in the urine (56). It is metabolized by xanthine oxidase, and concomitant administration of allopurinol, a xanthine oxidase inhibitor, delays its activation, potentially causing bone marrow suppression. The dose of azathioprine should be reduced to one-fourth when administered together with allopurinol (57).

2.5. Side Effects

2.5.1. Hematologic

Bone marrow suppression can occur at any dose and time during therapy, although it is most common 7–14 days after the initiation of therapy (15).

Mild leukopenia and macrocytosis are the most commonly seen side effects, and occasionally, anemia, thrombocytopenia, and pancytopenia may be noted. Macrocytosis correlates poorly with the dose of azathioprine, and hepatic enzymes, folate, and B12 levels are usually normal (58–60).

Generally, even mild leukopenia should be monitored closely. The dose should be lowered when WBC falls below 4000/mm, and therapy should be discontinued when counts reach 2500/mm, or if the absolute neutrophil count falls below 1000/mm (61). Therapy may be re-initiated after 2–3 weeks provided the practitioner monitors therapy closely.

2.5.2. Hepatotoxicity

Elevated alkaline phosphatase and total bilirubin levels are markers of azathioprine hepatotoxicity, but elevations in AST and ALT also occur, usually early in the course of therapy. Levels more than three times the upper limit of normal should prompt discontinuation of therapy. The etiology of hepatic dysfunction has been difficult to ascertain, but enzymes return to normal with discontinuation of therapy. Severe hepatic toxicity leading to liver failure is very rare (62).

2.5.3. Gastrointestinal

Nausea and vomiting are common side effects, particularly at the onset of therapy with azathioprine. Usually, these side effects are not bothersome enough to discontinue therapy, and they generally abate with time. Increasing the number of daily doses and taking azathioprine after meals often abolishes this discomfort (63). An idiosyncratic reaction of azathioprine occurs in ~15% of patients and is heralded by nausea and vomiting. Rechallenge is rarely successful (63–65).

2.5.4. Carcinoma

The degree to which azathioprine increases the risk of malignancy remains unclear given the underlying disorder may also increase risk (63). Neoplasias reported include transitional cell carcinoma of the bladder, adrenocortical carcinoma, acute leukemia, and cervical atypia in women.

2.6. Pregnancy Issues

Active metabolites may cross the placenta (66), and there are reports of chromosomal aberrations and neonatal lymphopenia and thrombocytopenia in children born to women receiving azathioprine (67). Small amounts appear in breast, but harmful effects have not been reported (67).

3. CYCLOPHOSPHAMIDE

3.1. Efficacy

Efficacy in CIDP has been limited to open-label studies. Combinations of oral pulse cyclophosphamide and prednisone have been effective in CIDP associated with a monoclonal gammopathy of undetermined significance (68). A good response to monthly pulse IV cyclophosphamide treatment has been reported in patients refractory to other treatment modalities (69). Cyclophosphamide (both oral and intravenous) has been used with success in multifocal motor neuropathy (8) and peripheral nerve vasculitis (70).

3.2. Dosing

Doses range from 2 mg/kg orally daily for 6–12 months (71) to 1 g/m^2 intravenously monthly for 6 months (69). Another regimen is 200 mg/kg intravenously over 4 days accompanied by forced diuresis and mesna (72). Pulse dosing is better tolerated.

3.3. Pharmacodynamics

Cyclophosphamide covalently bonds with nucleophilic cellular substances (alkylation) leading to disruption of the nucleic acids of DNA and abnormal cell replication (73). Pharmacologic activity requires metabolism by hepatic microsomal enzymes to form the active derivatives including phosphoramide mustard. The effects of cyclophosphamide upon immunologically competent cells include depletion of lymphocytes and changes in function of remaining cells. It is toxic to lymphocytes and reduces B-lymphocyte function (74,75). Cyclophosphamide has immunopotentiating properties which include selective inhibition of T-suppressor cells (76). Cyclophosphamide inhibits the inflammatory response in addition to its immunosuppressant actions (77).

3.4. Pharmacokinetics

Oral cyclophosphamide is metabolized by the liver into active metabolites (phosphoramide mustard) and inactive metabolites (4-keto cyclophosphamide, carboxyphospramide, acroelein). Inactive metabolites are excreted in the urine (56). Acrolein contributes to hemorrhagic cystitis (78).

3.5. Side Effects

3.5.1. Hematologic

Cyclophosphamide causes a dose-related leukopenia, with the nadir between 7 and 14 days following treatment and recovery between 21 and 25 days (79). Thrombocytopenia may rarely occur.

3.5.2. Gastrointestinal

Nausea and vomiting are prominent, especially with intravenous therapy, due to direct stimulation of the chemoreceptor trigger zone in the medulla (80). Individual patient tolerance varies greatly with psychological preconditioning playing a large role (80). Oral cyclophosphamide is better tolerated after a meal consisting of cold food.

3.5.3. Hair

Scalp hair loss occurs in 20–50% of patients, and axillary, extremity, and pubic hair loss may occur with long-term therapy. Hair loss occurs within 1–2 weeks and is maximal at 1–2 months and may be minimized by gentle scalp care including short-term tourniquets or ice bag application. Alopecia is generally reversible with cessation of therapy. Regrowth may be preceded by unusual texture and different shade but often returns to normal after therapy ends (79).

3.5.4. Genitourinary

Hemorrhagic cystitis occurs in up to 20–30% of subjects receiving cyclophosphamide due to acrolein. Aggressive hydration prior to cyclophosphamide therapy reduces accumulation (79). Sodium-2-mercaptoethane sulfonate (mesna) has been shown to reduce the risk of hemorrhagic cystitis. There is an increased frequency of bladder fibrosis and carcinoma, which may be unrelated to cystitis (79).

3.5.5. Carcinoma

The most ominous side effect is an elevated long-term risk of cancer including transitional cell bladder cancer and lymphoma. Risk is related to the cumulative dose over time and previous exposure to cytotoxic therapy (79).

3.5.6. Pulmonary

Interstitial pneumonitis and pulmonary fibrosis are rare but can be life-threatening (81,82).

3.5.7. Infections

Leukopenia and granulocytopenia, especially during the nadir, can predispose to infections.

3.6. Pregnancy Issues

The frequency of infertility increases with the duration of therapy. In postpubertal males, cyclophosphamide causes a selective inhibition of spermatogenesis, with little or no effect on testosterone production (56,79). Postpubertal females can experience a medication-induced menopause associated with decreased serum and urinary estrogen levels and increased levels of urinary gonadotrophins. There is an absence of ova, loss of follicular maturation, and fibrosis. Although there have been reports of renewed fertility in males and females following cessation of therapy (especially after short courses of cyclophosphamide), the loss of fertility is usually permanent. If cyclophosphamide is used before the onset of puberty, testicular and ovarian tissues generally mature and function normally. Patients of childbearing age may be offered sperm or egg banking prior to initiation of therapy.

It is currently unclear whether cyclophosphamide is teratogenic. Its use during the second and third trimesters does not appear to be associated with neurologic abnormalities or birth defects, although transient infantile bone marrow suppression has been reported (51). Cytotoxic material may also appear in the breast milk and may induce leukopenia in breast-fed infants.

4. MYCOPHENOLATE MOFETIL

4.1. Efficacy

Mycophenolate mofetil is commonly used to prevent organ rejection in transplant patients. Data from neuromuscular diseases are scarce. Small case series with CIDP have shown moderate improvements in strength and the ability to reduce steroid requirements (83,84).

4.2. Dosing

In neuromuscular disease, the common starting dose is 500 mg daily, with an increase to 1 g twice daily over 2–3 weeks (83). In renal transplant patients, higher doses do not result in better outcomes and often lead to an increased incidence of adverse effects. Dosages should be interrupted or reduced in patients with an absolute neutrophil count $< 1.3 \times 10^3/mm^3$.

4.3. Pharmacodynamics

Mycophenolate mofetil inhibits the proliferation of B and T lymphocytes through non-competitive, reversible inhibition of inosine monophosphate dehydrogenase, a key enzyme in the *de novo* synthetic pathway of guanine nucleotides. There are two pathways for purine biosynthesis, a *de novo* pathway and a salvage pathway. Lymphocytes can only use the *de novo* pathway, whereas other cells use both pathways. Mycophenolate blocks the synthesis of guanosine and enhances the synthesis of adenosine, resulting in inhibition of purine synthesis only in lymphocytes (16,85–87).

4.4. Pharmacokinetics

Mycophenolate mofetil is hydrolyzed in the liver to its biologically active metabolite, mycophenolic acid (MPA). MPA subsequently undergoes glucuronidation in the liver and kidney to form an inactive metabolite which is excreted in the urine and bile. The intestinal microfloral B-glucuronidase deconjugates the inactive metabolite in the GI tract to form MPA, leading to a second plasma peak at 6–12 h. MPA is highly protein bound to albumin and displays an elimination half-life of ∼17 h. Severe renal impairment decreases binding of MPA to albumin, therefore, increasing its free fraction in serum.

Studies of drug interactions with mycophenolate mofetil are limited. The absorption of mycophenolate mofetil is decreased with administration of cholestyramine and antacids containing magnesium and aluminum; therefore, mycophenolate should not be simultaneously administered with these agents (85).

4.5. Side Effects

Adverse effects are mild and rarely require discontinuation of therapy. The most common adverse effects seen at dose of 1 g twice daily in renal transplant patients are gastrointestinal (diarrhea, abdominal pain, nausea, dyspepsia, vomiting), hematologic (leukopenia, anemia, thrombocytopenia, pancytopenia), and opportunistic infections (CMV, herpes simplex, candida). Lymphomas were rare (0.6%) and occurred less frequently compared with rates seen with azathioprine. Gastrointestinal complaints may respond to a dose division of three or four times per day. Hematologic adverse effects generally reverse within a week of discontinuation.

5. CYCLOSPORINE

5.1. Efficacy

There are no controlled studies in CIDP. The largest case series included an initial high dose of 3–10 mg/kg per day, which was tapered to a maintenance dose 2–5 mg/kg per day. Most patients had an improvement by at least one functional grade or a reduction in annual relapse rates. Side effects were common and included nephrotoxicity, hypertension, nausea, hirsutism, and edema, which are consistent with known limiting side effects of cyclosporine (88–90).

5.2. Dosing

Common starting doses are 3–5 mg/kg per day, with maintenance doses of 2 mg/kg per day with periodic serum concentration monitoring. Empiric data indicate doses >7 mg/kg per day are associated with higher incidence of side effects (89). The dose of cyclosporine should be divided to limit toxicity.

5.3. Pharmacodynamics

The mechanism of action depends on the formation of a heterodimeric complex with cyclophilin. The complex binds calcineurin and inhibits its phosphatase activity, thereby inhibiting *de novo* expression of nuclear regulatory proteins and helper T-cell activation genes encoding for IL-2. This results in inhibition of the induction phase of the immune response in a dose-related fashion by blocking gene transcription and production of IL-2 by helper T-cells, preventing IL-2-driven clonal expansion. The combination of protein kinase C activation and increased intracellular calcium ions is responsible for full T-cell activation. Cyclosporine may interfere with these calcium-mediated pathways. Reduced IL-2 expression inhibits production of a wide range of other cytokines, including gamma interferon, thus blocking recruitment and activation of macrophages (16,91).

5.4. Pharmacokinetics

Oral cyclosporine absorption exhibits large intra- and inter-patient variability. Low absorption may be due to the presence of cytochrome P-450 enzymes and P-glycoprotein (a transport protein responsible for preventing drugs from penetrating the cell) in the gastrointestinal tract. Absorption also varies with type of cyclosporine formulation. Fatty food decreases the area under the curve; therefore, cyclosporine should be taken on a consistent basis with regard to food. Cyclosporine is 90% protein bound primarily to lipoproteins. It undergoes extensive hepatic metabolism through the CYP 3A4 enzyme, with minor gut and kidney metabolism. It is widely excreted through bile and displays a serum half-life of 8 h (range 5–15 h). Cyclosporine is an inhibitor of 3A4 and P-glycoprotein, therefore, drugs that are substrates for these display altered concentrations. Both inhibitors and inducers of the CYP 3A4 enzyme and P-glycoprotein significantly alter cyclosporine levels. Increased cyclosporine concentrations occur with inhibitors of 3A4 such as antifungal agents (ketoconazole, fluconazole, itraconazole), antibiotics (clarithromycin, erythromycin), selective serotonin re-uptake inhibitors (fluvoxamine, sertraline), calcium channel blockers (diltiazem, verapamil), HMG CoA reductase inhibitors (atorvastatin, simvastatin, losartan), and grapefruit juice. Decreased cyclosporine levels occur during co-administration with inducers of 3A4 or P-glycoprotein such as carbamazepine, phenobarbital, phenytoin, rifamin, and St. John's wort (92,93).

5.5. Side Effects

Nephrotoxicity and hypertension are the most serious side effects. Patients with preexisting moderate or severe renal impairment should be excluded from therapy; serum creatinine, creatinine clearance, and cyclosporine levels should be monitored and an effort made to maintain the lowest effective dose. Nausea, edema, and hirsutism are less serious and did not lead to discontinuation of therapy in clinical studies.

5.6. Pregnancy Issues

Cyclosporine is extensively excreted in breast milk and should therefore be avoided during breastfeeding (94). Reviews of case series of pregnancies in women receiving cyclosporine after liver transplantation found no increased risk of congenital malformations or maternal complications (95,96). Development did not appear to be adversely affected in the offspring (children up to 8 years old), although longer-term consequences are not known. In several case reports, cyclosporine use after transplantation did not result in fetal anomalies (51,67).

6. RITUXIMAB

A few case series of rituximab therapy in anti-MAG and other antibody-related polyneuropathies have provided encouraging results (97–99) with few side effects. The dose of rituximab used is 375 mg/m^2 weekly for 4 weeks and may be continued once every 10 weeks thereafter (98). Pretreatment with acetaminophen and diphenhydramine limits infusion-related side effects and reactions.

Rituximab is a chimeric mouse–human monoclonal antibody that specifically binds the surface membrane protein CD20 on B-lymphocytes, thus eliminating B-cells from the circulation. It induces antibody-dependent cell and complement-mediated cytotoxicity in these cells (100). The half-life ranges from 59 h (after the first infusion) to 174 h (after the fourth infusion). Rituximab is detected in serum up to 3–6 months after completion of therapy. As its effects on the fetus and infant are unknown, it should be avoided during pregnancy and breastfeeding.

Table 36.2 Monitoring and Management of Immunosuppressant Therapies

Agent	Complication	Monitoring/management
Corticosteroids	Adrenal suppression	Taper slowly after prolonged therapy
	Fluid/electrolyte disturbances	Monitor electrolytes
	Cataracts	Regular eye exams
	Peptic ulcer	GI protection
		H2 blockers
		Proton pump inhibitors
	Osteoporosis	Periodic bone density scans
		Bisphosphanates for treatment or prevention
	Diabetes mellitus	Periodic fasting/random blood glucose monitoring
Azathioprine	Leukopenia, thrombocytopenia	Monitor WBC and adjust dose
	Liver toxicity	Monitor LFTs
		D/C if 2X upper normal limit or 3X baseline levels
Cyclosporine	Nephrotoxicity	Therapeutic drug monitoring
		Monitor serum creatinine
		Evaluate drug interactions
Cyclophosphamide	Neutropenia	Monitor WBC
		Periodic dose cycling
	Gastrointestinal	Administer at bedtime with sedative
		Administer oral therapy with food
		Utilize antiemetic therapy
	Urotoxicity	Administer with mesna
		Proper hydration
		Periodic urine cytology
Mycophenolate mofetil	Neutropenia	Monitor WBC
	Gastrointestinal	Divide oral doses

Source: Adapted from Min and Monaco (15), Matell (63), and Frasier et al. (79).

Common side effects are related to infusion and include hypotension, nausea, vomiting, rash, fever, and chills. Others include anemia and thrombocytopenia, necessitating monitoring complete blood counts with differentials at regular intervals throughout therapy.

7. OTHER IMMUNOSUPPRESSANT AGENTS

A number of other immunosuppressive agents, including methotrexate and interferons, have been given to patients who are refractory to conventional drugs. All data are from small trials and case reports. Methotrexate does not appear to be effective in immune-mediated neuropathies. Both interferon beta (101,102) and interferon alpha (103) have been used in neuropathy with some success (104).

Table 36.2 delineates appropriate monitoring parameters as well as management of common complications from immunosuppressant agents.

REFERENCES

1. Austin GH. Recurrent polyneuropathies and their corticosteroid treatment; with five-year observations of a placebo-controlled case treated with corticotrophin, cortisone, and prednisone. Brain 1958; 81(2):157–192.

2. Dalakas MC, Engel WK. Chronic relapsing (dysimmune) polyneuropathy: pathogenesis and treatment. Ann Neurol 1981; 9:134–135.

3. Wertman E, Argov Z, Abramsky O. Chronic inflammatory demyelinating polyradiculoneuropathy: features and prognostic factors with corticosteroid therapy. Eur Neurol 1988; 28(4):199–204.

4. Dyck PJ, O' Brien PC, Oviatt KF et al. Prednisone improves chronic inflammatory polyradiculoneuropathy more than no treatment. Ann Neurol 1982; 11:136–141.

5. McCombe PA, Pollard JD, McLeod JG. Chronic inflammatory demyelinating polyradiculoneuropathy. A clinical and electrophysiological study of 92 cases. Brain 1987; 110:617–630.

6. Barohn RJ, Kissel JT, Warmolts JR, Mendell JR. Chronic inflammatory demyelinating polyradiculoneuropathy: clinical characteristics, course, and recommendations for diagnostic criteria. Arch Neurol 1989; 46:878–884.

7. Pestronk A, Cornblath DR, Ilyas AA et al. A treatable multifocal motor neuropathy with antibodies to GM1 ganglioside. Ann Neurol 1988; 24:73–78.

8. Feldman EL, Bromberg MB, Albers JW, Pestronk A. Immunosuppressive treatment in multifocal motor neuropathy. Ann Neurol 1991; 30:397–401.

9. Pestronk A, Chaudhry V, Feldman EL et al. Lower motor neuron syndromes defined by patterns of weakness, nerve conduction abnormalities, and high titers of antiglycolipid antibodies. Ann Neurol 1990; 27:316–326.

10. Donaghy M, Mills KR, Boniface SJ et al. Pure motor demyelinating neuropathy: deterioration after steroid treatment and improvement with intravenous immunoglobulin. J Neurol Neurosurg Psychiatr 1994; 57:778–783.

11. Hughes RA, Van der Meche FG. Corticosteroids for treating Guillain–Barre syndrome (Cochrane review). The Cochrane Library (Issue 2) 1999.

12. Bromberg MB, Carter O. Corticosteroid use in the treatment of neuromuscular disorders: empirical and evidence-based data. Muscle Nerve. 2004; 30(1):20–37.

13. Smith A, Bromberg M. Treatment of inflammatory demyelinating neuropathies. J Clin Neuromuscul Dis 1999; 1: 21–31.

14. Boumpas DT, Chrousos GP, Wilder RL, Cupps TR, Balow JE. Glucocorticoid therapy for immune-mediated diseases: basic and clinical correlates. Ann Intern Med 1993; 119:1198–1208.

15. Min DI, Monaco AP. Complications associated with immunosuppressive therapy and their management. Pharmacotherapy 1991; 11(5):119S–125S.

16. Suthanthiran M, Morris RE, Strom TB. Immunosuppressants: cellular and molecular mechanisms of action. Am J Kidney Dis 1996; 28(2):159–172.

17. Jenkins JS, Sampson PA. Conversion of cortisone to cortisol and prednisone to prednisolone. Br Med J 1967; 1:205–207.

18. Pickup ME. Clinical pharmacokinetics of prednisone and prednisolone. Clin Pharmacokinet 1979; 4:111–128.

19. Sullivan TJ, Sakmar E, Albert KS, Blair DC, Wagner JG. In vitro and *in vivo* availability of commercial prednisone tablets. J Pharm Sci 1975; 64:1723–1725.

20. Frey BM, Frey FJ. Clinical pharmacokinetics of prednisone and prednisolone. Clin Pharmacokinet 1990; 19(2):126–146.

21. Begg EJ, Atkinson HC, Gianarakis N. The pharmacokinetics of corticosteroid agents. Med J Aus 1987; 146:37–41.

22. Meffin PJ, Brooks PM, Sallustio BC. Alterations in prednisolone disposition as a result of time of administration, gender, and dose. Br J Clinic Pharmacol 1984; 17:394–404.

23. Frey J. Kinetics and dynamics of prednisolone. Endocrine Rev 1987; 8:453–473.

24. Leger U, Benet L. Marked alterations in prednisolone elimination for women taking oral contraceptives. Clin Pharmacol Ther 1982; 31:243.

25. Frey F, Rüegsegger M, Frey B. The dose-dependent systematic availability of prednisone: one reason for the reduced biological effect of alternate-day prednisone. Br J Clin Pharmacol 1986; 21:183–189.

26. Thomas TPL. The complications of systemic corticosteroid therapy in the elderly. Gerontology 1984; 30:60–65.

27. Silva RG, Tolstunov L. Steroid-induced psychosis: report of case. J Oral Maxillofac Surg 1995; 53:183–186.

28. Peet M, Peters S. Drug-induced mania. Drug Safe 1995; 12:146–153.

29. Hall RC, Popkin MK, Stickney SK, Gardner ER. Presentation of the steroid psychoses. J Nerv Ment Dis 1979; 167:229–236.

30. Dujorne CA, Azarnoff DL. Clinical complications of corticosteroid therapy. Med Clin N Am 1973; 57:1331–1342.

31. Kida-Kimble MA, Young L, eds. Applied Therapeutics: The Clinical Use of Drugs, 5th ed. Vancouver, WA: Applied Therapeutics, Inc., 1992.

32. David DS, Greico MH, Cushman P. Adrenal glucocorticoids after 20 years: a review of their clinically relevant consequences. J Chron Dis 1970; 22:637–711.

33. Baylink DJ. Glucocorticoid-induced osteoporosis. N Engl J Med 1983; 309:306–308.

34. Lukert BP, Raisz LG. Glucocorticoid-induced osteoporosis: pathogenesis and management. Ann Intern Med 1990; 112:352–364.

35. Gluck OS, Murphy WA, Hahn TJ, Hahn B. Bone loss in adults receiving alternate day glucocorticoid therapy: a comparison with daily therapy. Arthritis Rheum 1981; 24:892–898.

36. Buckley LM, Leib ES, Cartularo KS, Vacek PM, Cooper SM. Calcium and vitamin D3 supplementation prevents bone loss in the spine secondary to low-dose corticosteroids in patients with rheumatoid arthritis: a randomized, double-blind, placebo-controlled trial. Ann Intern Med 1996; 125:961–968.

37. Adachi JD, Olszynski WP, Hanley DA et al. Semin Arthritis Rheum 2000; 29(4):228–251.

38. Saag KG, Emkey R, Schnitzer TH et al. Alendronate for the prevention and treatment of glucocorticoid-induced osteoporosis. N Engl J Med 1998; 339:292–299.

39. Homik J, Cranney A, Shea B et al. Bisphosphonates for steroid-induced osteoporosis (Cochrane Review). The Cochrane Library 2000; (Issue 2).

40. Braithwaite SS, Barr WG, Rahman A, Quddusi S. Managing diabetes during glucocorticoid therapy: how to avoid metabolic emergencies? Postgrad Med 1998; 104:163–166,171,175–177.

41. Hoogwerf B, Danese RD. Drug selection and the management of corticosteroid-related diabetes mellitus. Rheum Dis Clin N Am 1999; 25(3):489–505.

42. Richards M, Santiago M, Klaustermeyer B. Aseptic necrosis of the femoral head in corticosteroid-treated pulmonary disease. Arch Intern Med 1980; 140:1473–1475.

43. Messer J, Reitman D, Sacks HS, Smith H Jr, Chalmers TC. Association of adrenocorticosteroid therapy and peptic ulcer disease. N Engl J Med 1983; 309:21–24.

44. Twycross R. The risks and benefits of corticosteroids in advanced cancer. Drug Safe 1994; 11:163–178.

45. Dale DC, Petersdorf RG. Corticosteroids and infectious diseases. Med Clin N Am 1973; 57:1277–1287.

46. David DS, Berkowitz JS. Ocular effects of topical and systemic corticosteroids. Lancet 1969; 2:149–151.

47. Gourley DR, McKenzie C. Glaucoma. In: Herfindal ET, Gourley DR, Hart LL, eds. Clinical Pharmacy and Therapeutics. 4th ed. Baltimore, MD: Williams & Wilkins, 1988.

48. Chamberlin P, Meyer WJ. Management of pituitary–adrenal suppression secondary to corticosteroid therapy. Pediatrics 1981; 67:245–251.

49. Hodding GC, Jann M, Ackerman IP. Drug withdrawal syndromes. Western J Med 1980; 133:383–391.

50. Krasner AS: Glucocorticoid-induced adrenal insufficiency. JAMA 1999; 282(7):671–676.

51. Esplin MS, Branch DW. Immunosuppressive drugs and pregnancy. Obstet Gyn Clin N Am 1997; 24(3):601–616.

52. Dyck PJ, O'Brien P, Swanson C, Low P, Daube J. Combined azathioprine and prednisone in chronic inflammatory demyelinating polyneuropathy. Neurology 1985; 35:1173–1176.

53. Walker GL. Progressive polyradiculoneuropathy. Treatment with azathioprine. Aust NZ J Med 1989; 9:184–187.

54. Yuill BG, Win burn WR, Liversedge LA: Treatment of polyneuropathy with azathioprine. Lancet 1970; 2:854.

55. Corley CC, Lessner HE, Larsen WE. Azathioprine therapy of "autoimmune" diseases. Am J Med 1966; 41:404–412.

56. Clements PJ, Davis J. Cytotoxic drugs: their clinical application to the rheumatic diseases. Semin Arthritis Rheu 1986; 15(4): 231–254.

57. Nashel DJ. Mechanisms of action and clinical applications of cytotoxic drugs in rheumatic disorders. Med Clin N Am 1985; 69(4):817–840.

58. Klippel JH, Decker JL. Relative macrocytosis in cyclophosphamide and azathioprine therapy. JAMA 1974; 229:180–181.

59. Wickramasinghe SN, Dodsworth H, Rault RM, Hulme B. Observations on the incidence and cause of macrocytosis in patients on azathioprine therapy following renal transplantation. Transplantation 1974; 18:443–446.

60. Declerck YA, Ettenger RB, Ortega JA, Pennisi AJ. Macrocytosis and pure RBC anemia caused by azathioprine. Am J Dis Child 1980; 134:377–379.

61. Kissel JT, Levy RJ, Mendell JR, Griggs RC. Azathioprine toxicity in neuromuscular disease. Neurology 1986; 36:35–39.

62. Sparberg M, Simon N, DelGreco F. Intrahepatic cholestasis due to azathioprine. Gastroenterology 1969; 57:439–441.

63. Matell G. Immunosuppressive drugs: azathioprine in the treatment of myasthenia gravis. Ann NY Acad Sci 1987; 505:589–594.

64. Cunningham T, Barraclough D, Muirden K. Azathioprine-induced shock. Br Med J 1981; 283:823–824.

65. King JO, Laver MC, Fairley KF, Ames GA. Sensitivity to azathioprine. Med J Aust 1972; 2:939–941.

66. Saarikoski S, Seppala M. Immunosuppression during pregnancy: transmission of azathioprine and its metabolites from mother to the fetus. Am J Obstet Gynecol 1973; 115:1100–1106.

67. Little BB. Immunosuppressant therapy during gestation. Semin Perinatol 1997; 21(2):143–148.

68. Notermans NC, Lokhorst HM, Franssen H et al. Intermittent cyclophosphamide and prednisone treatment of polyneuropathy associated with monoclonal gammopathy of undetermined significance. Neurology 1996; 47:1227–1233.

69. Good JL, Chehrenama M, Mayer RF, Koski CL. Pulse cyclophosphamide therapy in chronic inflammatory demyelinating polyradiculoneuropathy. Neurology 1998; 51(6):1735–1738.

70. Collins MP, Periquet MI, Mendell JR, Sahenk Z, Nagaraja HN, Kissel JT. Nonsystemic vasculitic neuropathy: insights from a clinical cohort. Neurology 2003; 61(5):623–630.

71. Bouchard C, Lacroix C, Plante V et al. Clinicopathologic findings and prognosis of chronic inflammatory demyelinating polyneuropathy. Neurology 1999; 52:498–503.

72. Brannagan TH III, Pradhan A, Heiman-Patterson T et al. High-dose cyclophosphamide without stem-cell rescue for refractory CIDP. Neurology 2002; 58:1856–1858.

73. Fisher DS. Alkylating agents. In: Fischer DS, Marsh JC, eds. Cancer Therapy. Boston: GK Hall Medical Publishers, 1982.

74. Cupps TR, Edgar LC, Fauci AS. Suppression of human B lymphocyte function by cyclophosphamide. J Immunol 1982; 128:2453–2457.

75. Oterness IG, Chang YH. Comparative study of cyclophosphamide, 6-mercaptopurine, azathiopurine and methotrexate: relative effects on the humoral and the cellular response in the mouse. Clin Exp Immunol 1976; 26:346–354.

76. Kerckhaert JA, Hofhuis FM, Willers JM. Effects of variation in time and dose of cyclophosphamide injection on delayed hypersensitivity and antibody formation. Cell Immunol 1977; 29:232–237.

77. Stevens JE, Willoughby DA. The anti-inflammatory effect of some immunosuppressive agents. J Pathol 1969; 97:367–373.

78. Cox PJ. Cyclophosphamide cystitis—identification of acrolein as the causative agent. Biochem Pharmacol 1979; 28:2045–2049.

79. Frasier LH, Sarathchandra K, Kehrer JP. Cyclophosphamide toxicity: characterizing and avoiding the problem. Drugs 1991; 42(5):781–795.

80. Dorr RT, Fritz WL, eds. Cancer Chemotherapy Handbook. New York: Elsevier, 1980.

81. Cooper AJD, White DA, Matthay RA. Drug-induced pulmonary disease. Am Rev Respir Dis 1986; 133:321–340.

82. Maxwell I. Reversible pulmonary edema following cyclophosphamide treatment. JAMA 1974; 229:137–138.

83. Mowzoon N, Sussman A, Bradley WG. Mycophenolate (Cellcept) treatment of myasthenia gravis, chronic inflammatory polyneuropathy, and inclusion body myositis. J Neurol Sci 2001; 185:119–122.

84. Chaudhry V, Cornblath DR, Griffin JW, O'Brien R, Drachman DB. Mycophenolate mofetil: a safe and promising immunosuppressant in neuromuscular diseases. Neurology 2001; 56:94–96.

85. Sievers TM, Rossi SJ, Ghobrial RM et al. Mycophenolate mofetil. Pharmacotherapy 1997; 17(6):1178–1197.

86. Sievers TM, Simmons WD, Rayhill SC, Sollinger HW. Preliminary risk-benefit assessment of mycophenolate mofetil in transplant rejection. Drug Saf 1997; 17:75–92.

87. Allison AC, Kowalski WJ, Muller CD, Eugui EM. Mechanisms of action of mycophenolic acid. Ann NY Acad Sci 1993; 696:63–87.

88. Mahattanakul W, Crawford TO, Griffin JW, Goldstein JM, Cornblath DR. Treatment of chronic inflammatory demyelinating polyneuropathy with cyclosporine-A. J Neurol Neurosurg Psychiatr 1996; 60(2):185–187.

89. Barnett MH, Pollard JD, Davies L, McLeod JG. Cyclosporin A in resistant chronic inflammatory demyelinating polyradiculoneuropathy. Muscle Nerve 1998; 21:454–460.

90. Hodgkinson SJ, Pollard JD, McLeod JG. Cyclosporin A in the treatment of chronic demyelinating polyradiculoneuropathy. J Neurol Neurosurg Psychiatr 1990; 53(4):327–330.

91. Hess AD, Colombani PM. Mechanism of action of cyclosporine: a unifying hypothesis. Adv Exp Med Biol 1987; 213:309–330.

92. Levy GL. Long-term immunosuppression and drug interactions. Liver Transplant 2001; 11:S53–S59.

93. Lo A, Burckart GP. P-glycoprotein and drug therapy in organ transplantation. J Clin Pharm 1999; 39:995–1005.

94. Flechner SM, Katz AR, Rogers AJ, Van Buren C, Kahan BD. The presence of cyclosporine in body tissues and fluids during pregnancy. Am J Kidney Dis 1985; 5:60–63.

95. Rayes N, Neuhaus R, David M, SteinMuller T, Bechstein WO, Neuhaus P. Pregnancies following liver transplantation—how safe are they? A report of 19 cases under cyclosporine A and tacrolimus. Clin Transplant 1998; 12(5):396–400.

96. Wu A, Nathan B, Messner U et al. Outcome of 22 successful pregnancies after liver transplantation. Clin Transplant 1998; 12(5):454–464.

97. Levine TD, Pestronk A. IgM antibody-related polyneuropathies: treatment with B-cell depletion chemotherapy using rituximab. Neurology 1999; 52:1701–1704.

98. Pestronk A, Florence J, Miller T, Choksi R, Al-Lozi MT, Levine D. Treatment of IgM antibody associated polyneuropathies using rituximab. J Neurol Neurosurg Psychiatr 2003; 74:485–489.

99. Renaud S, Gregor M, Fuhr P et al. Rituximab in the treatment of polyneuropathy associated with anti-MAG antibodies. Muscle Nerve 2003; 27:611–615.

100. Johnson PW, Glennie MJ. Rituximab: mechanisms and applications. Br J Cancer 2001; 85:1619–1623.

101. Martina IS, van Doorn PA, Schmitz PI, Meulstee J, van der Meche FG. Chronic motor neuropathies: response to interferon-beta1a after failure of conventional therapies. J Neurol Neurosurg Psychiatr 1999; 66:197–201.
102. Hadden RD. Sharrack B, Bensa S, Soudain SE, Hughes RA. Randomized trial of interferon beta-1a in chronic inflammatory demyelinating polyradiculoneuropathy. Neurology 1999; 53:57–61.
103. Gorson KC, Allam G, Simovic D, Ropper AH. Improvement following interferon-alpha 2a in chronic inflammatory demyelinating polyneuropathy. Neurology 1997; 48:777–780.
104. Saperstein DS, Katz JS, Amato AA, Barohn RJ. Clinical spectrum of chronic acquired demyelinating polyneuropathies. Muscle Nerve 2001; 24:311–324.

37

Managing Joint and Skin Complications from Peripheral Neuropathy

M. Catherine Spires
University of Michigan, Ann Arbor, Michigan, USA

ABSTRACT

Peripheral neuropathy is frequently associated with skin and joint complications which can progress to lower extremity ulceration, Charcot arthropathy, and eventual limb loss. A classification of the complications is presented that is based on the sensorimotor peripheral neuropathy associated with diabetes mellitus. Medical management focuses on prevention of skin, soft tissue, and bone complication while preserving normal foot anatomy and function. Treatment interventions focus on orthoses, shoe modifications, and physical therapy.

1. INTRODUCTION

Peripheral neuropathy is a relatively common problem, and health care costs associated with neuropathy exceeds several billion dollars per year in the USA. Neuropathy from

657

diabetes mellitus is the most common form, and 50% of diabetics who have had the disease for >15 years are affected (1). Diabetic neuropathy is, therefore, used as the prototype for the nonsurgical management of the skin and joint complications of peripheral neuropathies. Goals are to provide a rational treatment plan for the complications of neuropathy that emphasizes interventions prior to foot ulceration or limb loss.

Control of locomotion is dependent not only upon efferent nerve activity, but also on the quality of afferent information reaching the central nervous system. The autonomic nervous system is also important in tissue homeostasis. In peripheral neuropathies, efferent, afferent, and autonomic dysfunction can occur. In diabetic neuropathy, sensory loss includes the modalities of pain, proprioception, and thermal perception and leads to the patient unknowingly subjecting their feet and lower extremities to repeated mechanic, chemical, or thermal trauma. In addition, the overall importance of the foot is often overlooked in primary care settings. The anatomy of the foot is complex, reflecting its biomechanical functions of weight bearing, sensory feedback, balance, shock absorption, and propulsion of the body during gait. Pertinent factors include:

1. The lateral foot, composed of the fourth and fifth metatarsal, toes, cuboid, and calcaneus, provides stability for stance and balance.
2. The medial foot includes the longitudinal arch, which is created by the cunieform bones, the navicular and talus, provides energy storing, torque, and energy transfer for forward propulsion for gait.
3. The ligaments of the foot passively support the arch of the foot.
4. The toes add balance and length to the foot's lever arm for forward propulsion.
5. Intrinsic and extrinsic foot muscles function to provide motor strength and control. Intrinsics muscles of the foot act to modulate the actions of larger and stronger extrinsics muscles to create a stable, but flexible weight bearing limb.

2. CLINICAL FEATURES AND TREATMENT

A clinical classification of soft tissue and joint complications that aids clinical decision making is presented in Table 37.1 and a treatment algorithm in Table 37.2.

2.1. Type I Foot

A type I foot includes impaired sensation when testing for large and small fiber nerve functions, but skin is intact and there is normal range of motion (ROM) and foot architecture. Some individuals have premorbid foot abnormalities such as pes planus and hallux valgus. The evidence of autonomic dysfunction is often present at this early stage, in the form of anhydrosis, leading to dry skin and progressive fissuring of the skin which can predispose to ulcers and other complications.

Clinical goals include soft tissue protection and maintenance of the normal shape and architecture of the foot. Management includes custom or off-the-shelf foot orthoses (FOs) to protect the skin from shear and stress forces. Patients with premorbid deformities often require custom orthoses. Orthoses made of soft materials, rather than rigid materials, are indicated.

Patients must be educated in foot care, including moisturizing skin, selecting appropriate shoe wear, and learning the risks associated with peripheral neuropathy. It has been reported that 70% of those with diabetic neuropathy had not had their feet measured for shoes in 10 years (2).

Table 37.1 Clinical Classification of Neuropathic Foot Pathology

Type I
  Impaired sensation
  Skin intact with normal architecture
Type II
  Soft tissue stiffness
  Joint contracture
  Impaired sensation
  Intact skin
Type III
  A Atrophy of soft tissue
      Callus formation
  B Biomechanical and bone deformities
  C Combination deformity
      Moderate skin, soft tissue, and bone
Type IV
  A Ulcer formation
      Wagner classification of ulcers
  B Acute Charcot joint deformity
  C End stage limb
      Severe deformity of skin, soft tissue, and bone

Table 37.2 Treatment of Neuropathic Foot Deformities

Type I foot
Goal: soft tissue protection and maintenance of the normal shape and architecture
 of the foot
Treatment
  Foot orthosis (FO) to correct or accommodate premorbid foot deformities
  Protect the skin
    Education regarding peripheral neuropathy
    FO with a soft bed
    Moisturizing and other foot hygiene
    Shoe wear
Type II foot
Goal: maintain normal foot and ankle range of motion (ROM) and strength
Treatment
  Physical therapy for exercise instruction in ROM, strengthening and balance
  Custom FOs may be needed
Type III foot
Goal: correct and normalize pressure distribution over the foot
  Accommodate bony abnormalities and abnormal biomechanics
  Reduce/eliminate callus and ulcer formation
  Prevent further deterioration of the foot function and architecture
Treatment
  Accommodative custom FOs
  Callus reduction and removal
  Shoe modifications or custom shoes

(*continued*)

Table 37.2 *Continued*

Type IV A foot
Goal: healing and prevention of further ulceration
    Eventual return to accommodative custom orthotics and shoes
Treatment: Meticulous wound care
    Sharp and mechanical debridement
    Antibiotics as needed
    Reducing pressure at the site of the ulcer to facilitate:
        Custom bivalved ambulatory ankle foot orthosis (AFO)
        Total contact cast (TCC)
        Other devices
Type IV B: acute Charcot deformity and/or fractures occur
Goal: osseous healing
    Maintaining foot architecture and function
    Return to ambulation
    Accommodative custom orthoses and foot wear
Treatment of acute phase
    Rest, nonweight bearing and immobilization of the foot
    Custom bivalved AFO
    Treat pain if present
Treatment of the sub acute reparative phase
    Begin weight bearing on limited basis
    Gradual weaning from AFO
    Wean to appropriate orthotics and shoe wear
    Custom shoe may be necessary
Type IV C: end stage deterioration of the foot
Goal: Amputation with functional residual limb
    Maximize remaining lower extremity function .
    Protection of the remaining foot and limb
Treatment
    Aggressive care of remaining lower extremity and foot
    Prosthetic restoration and rehabilitation

2.2. Type II Foot

Type II foot adds loss of normal ROM of the foot and ankle to sensory loss. Movement deficits include loss of dorsiflexion, great toe extension, and subtalar motion emerge. Early signs of foot intrinsic muscle wasting may be seen.

Loss of normal joint motion or abnormal motion increases the risk of soft tissue trauma. Contracture of the subtalar joint and the ankle increases plantar pressures. Limitations of the shock absorbing function of the ankle and subtalar joint can lead to inadequate dissipation of the vertical and shear forces of walking. As a result, reduction of ankle dorsiflexion to $<5°$ of neutral and subtalar motion to $<30°$ are associated with a significant increase in skin breakdown (3–5).

Another early finding is atrophy of the metatarsal fat pad and migration away from the metatarsal heads. The metatarsal heads are subsequently exposed to the forces of weight bearing. Increased pressure over the plantar surface of the metatarsal heads is highly correlated with foot ulcers (6), particularly at the first metatarsal (7,8).

In diabetics, biomechanical properties of the skin change (9). The stability of collagen and keratin in the stratum corneum, attributed to secondary nonenzymatic glycosylation, increases the stiffness and thickening of skin and other soft tissues, including tendon and joint structures. This is particularly notable in areas where the stratum corneum of the skin is thick, such as the plantar surface of feet.

Initial treatment goals are restoration of normal ROM and protection of soft tissues. Sensorimotor neuropathy affects static and dynamic balance. Physical therapy consultation is appropriate for ROM and for balance exercises to achieve unipedal stance of 10 s or greater to help prevent falls and foot and ankle injuries. Exercises are appropriate for stretching of the hind foot in subtalar neutral position to avoid abnormal stretching of ligaments of the medial foot as well as strengthening of the foot intrinsic muscles. These exercises must ultimately be performed at home on an ongoing basis.

Once ROM is normal or has plateaued, custom corrective FOs are indicated to preserve the ROM gained and protect soft tissues, ligamentous and bony architecture of the foot. The overall goal is to place and maintain the foot in a normal, or as normal as possible position, to avoid abnormal pressure distribution on the foot, particularly the plantar aspect, the most common site of ulcer formation. Areas of high-pressure sites are often precursors to ulcer formation, FOs should re-distribute the pressure to achieve even pressure distribution. In the case where normal dorsiflexion has been achieved but a persistent pes planus is present, the orthosis should position the foot with a medial longitudinal arch. The orthosis is made to facilitate the normal longitudinal arch by controlling the position of the sustentaculum tali rather than creating a mound of orthotic materials to lift the arch. If normal ROM cannot be achieved, orthoses which compensate for the fixed deformities are appropriate. For example, the patient with a fixed pes planus deformity requires that the orthosis be fabricated to the shape of their foot rather than trying to correct the deformity.

2.3. Type III and Type IV Feet

These are clinically more complicated and are subclassified. Subtype A reflects patients whose problems are primarily the result of muscle atrophy and loss of other soft tissue functions. Subtype B includes patients with predominantly bony architecture changes and complications. Subtype C combines soft tissue and bone involvement.

2.3.1. Type III A Foot

Damage is due to pressure and shear forces. Normal skin responds to chronic pressure and shear with hyperkeratosis and callus formation. Callus is associated with increased risk of ulceration and is more predictive of ulcer formation than increased plantar pressure alone. The first and fifth toes are the most common sites of callus and subsequent ulceration. Callus increases local pressure by 29% and increases ulceration risk by 11-fold (10).

Progressive intrinsic muscle leads to hammer and claw toe deformities. The dorsal surfaces of the toes, specifically the interphalangeal joints, are exposed to shear from the toe box of a shoe with inadequate toe box depth. Callus formation or evidence of shear requires prompt intervention as the soft tissue coverage of the interphalangeal joint is thin and a septic joint can readily occur resulting in toe loss. In addition to metatarsal plantar foot atrophy and migration, the imbalance of the pull of the extrinsic foot muscles over-power the foot intrinsic muscles causes disproportionate weight bearing on the plantar surface of the metatarsal heads. It is not surprising that the majority of plantar ulcers occur over the metatarsal joints (7,8).

Treatment involves decreasing abnormal stresses. This includes sharp debridement of callus, teaching patients to use pumice to reduce callus, and prescription for custom orthoses that evenly distribute plantar weight bearing pressure. Simple callus removal or reduction is associated with decreased pressure. At times, callus removal reveals an underlying ulcer referred to as a *malperforans ulcer*. Callus with hemosiderin staining also suggest an underlying ulcer (11).

Custom orthoses require meticulous fitting by the orthotist or pedorthotist. FOs need regular evaluation and inspection. Replacement may be required as often as every 6 months. To optimize custom FOs, the patient must be fitted with shoes that act synergistically with the FOs. For example, the patient experiencing too much pressure over the metatarsal heads may benefit from a rocker sole that decreases stance time over the metatarsal heads facilitating push off. As shoe needs become more specific, the orthotist or pedorthotist can order special shoes not available in typical shoe stores.

2.3.2. Type III B Foot

Deterioration of the bony architecture of the foot is typically seen first in the midfoot. The longitudinal arch begins to collapse and the navicula becomes increasingly prominent and descends. As the navicula descends, callus develops over the navicula. The keystone of the midfoot is the second metatarsal base recessed in the intercuneiform mortise. This is subject to deterioration, allowing the metatarsals to displace laterally precipitating cuboid and cuneiform collapse. The hind foot also becomes involved. With progression, the navicula drops further and becomes coplanar with the calcaneus and metatarsal heads. This causes the foot to be flat and rigid. Navicular changes can be very severe with the navicula descending below the plane of the foot creating a rocker foot deformity.

The key is to prevent further deterioration and architectural stabilization to prevent further bone disruption. Mild changes are managed with custom FOs and appropriate shoes. As the foot architecture deteriorates, regular follow up and monitoring for callus and ulcers become increasingly important. FOs may require more frequent replacement and custom made shoes may be required to prevent soft tissue and further bone changes.

2.3.3. Type III C Foot

Clinical changes affect both the soft and the bony tissues of the foot and ankle. The triad of increased plantar foot pressure, bony abnormalities, and impaired joint mobility are associated with ulceration and limb loss (12,13). Static plantar foot pressures can be measured using many devices, including the Harris mat or foot plate. Approximately 35% of the patients with foot pressures $>12.3\,\mathrm{kg/cm^2}$ (static pressure) developed foot ulcers (13).

Aggressive follow up is necessary to prevent further deterioration and limb loss. Custom FOs with creative use of thermoplastic materials to prevent ulceration are critical. Materials such as selective use of silicone can reduce shear. Socks with silicon between layers decreases shear, but many patients complain that the silicone layer further disrupts their balance.

2.3.4. Type IV A Foot

Foot ulcers distinguish a type IV A foot. A common classification system includes the following grades (14). Grade 1: ulcers are superficial and do not invade subcutaneous tissue. Grade 2: ulcers expose tendons, capsules, or bone, but there is no abscess or osteomyelitis. Grade 3: ulcers invade the joint space with abscess, tendon infection, or osteomyelitis present and are threatening to limb and life threatening. Grade 4: localized gangrene is present. Grade 5: wound severity precludes any possibility of limb salvage.

Meticulous wound management is essential. Blood glucose must be well controlled. Antibiotics are indicated for the infected ulcers. Local debridement of surrounding callus or devitalized tissue is needed on a regular basis and can be done in the clinic or after hydrotherapy. Hydrotherapy will mechanically debride loose tissues and soften other tissues to make debridement more effective. Trained physical therapists and nurse practitioners can provide wound care between physician visits in selected patients. Growth factors and specialized wound healing devices, such as the vacuum wound healing devices, are available, although scientific literature supporting their use is limited.

Reducing weight-bearing time on an ulcer facilitates wound healing. The time required for healing is related to high pressure at the site of the wound (3,15,16). There are limited studies to validate the effectiveness of the many and various offloading devices for ulcers, but clinical experience indicates that the most effective methods include bivalved ambulatory ankle foot orthosis (AFO) and total contact casts (TCCs). The bivalved ambulatory AFOs encase the entire lower leg and foot, with weight bearing distributed over the entire area of contact. This reduces the vertical and shear forces associated with ambulation. Areas of specific relief can be included in the design to off-load the ulcer. The bivalved AFO is durable, easily removed for wound care, and readily withstands the forces of ambulation over long periods. When fitting a patient with this type of AFO, one must make sure that the height of shoe on the other foot is corrected if a leg length discrepancy is created, because a leg length discrepancy may precipitate back pain or disrupt balance. Other disadvantages include cost and require an experienced orthotist to fit and fabricate. TCCs are based on the principles of decreasing motion and redistributing pressures. TCCs are relatively inexpensive but are effective for the patient who is not compliant. These need frequent removal for wound care. With use of the bivalved AFO or the TCCs, patients with impaired balance may require the use of a walker or cane until the devices are discontinued.

Commercial off the shelf devices are available, but it is difficult to achieve the control and off loading afforded by the bivalved AFO or the TCCs. However, these are valuable for interim use while a bivalved AFO is made. Additional temporizing options include commercially available shoes that do not allow weight bearing over affected areas of the foot. These shoes may have the sole designed such that it is open under the fore foot or heel.

Long-term studies indicate that once an ulcer has healed, the patient who returns to normal foot wear has a 90% chance of ulcer recurrence. Patients prescribed modified shoes and orthoses; however, have a recurrence rate of 19% (17,18). If ulcers are recurrent or protracted, the physician should prepare the patient for the possibility that the ulcer may not heal, may advance, and be life threatening. Patients need to be aware that surgery may be required, including major limb amputation.

2.3.5. Type IV B Foot

Charcot arthropathy or foot fractures characterize the type IV B foot. Charcot arthropathies occurs abruptly: the foot or ankle is erythematous, warm and swollen, and patients may or may not experience pain. Inexperienced clinicians may misdiagnoses this condition as cellutitis, osteomyelitis, acute inflammatory arthritis, or other infectious process, and patients may undergo bone biopsy when they do not respond to antibiotics leading to chronic deep nonhealing wounds. Blood studies demonstrate normal or slightly elevated white blood counts, but without a left shift. The sedimentation rate and acute phase reactants will be elevated. Bone scans are not often helpful in distinguishing between infection and Charcot arthropathy. X-ray, MRI, or CT imaging studies reveal osteopenia, joint destruction, and/or subluxation. Bone or cartilage debris is often seen. The acute process of bone fracturing is associated with bone resorption, increasing the risk of further bone destruction by weight bearing or minimal trauma.

Management is similar to that for an acute fracture, with rest and immobilization. Continued weight bearing leads to further foot destruction. A custom bivalved ambulatory orthosis should be prescribed to immobilize the foot, control edema, and maintain the bony structures in a normal architecture as possible. For the patient with pain, fitting with the AFO or off loading the limb often brings significant relief. If not, analgesics are indicated. Patients will need a cane (ergonomically designed grips are preferred to avoid median mononeuropathy at the wrist) or crutches for nonweight bearing, and physical therapy should be consulted for proper use.

During the reparative subacute phase of Charcot arthropathy, bone repair and remodeling are occurring. Bone scan can be used to follow the repair and will show decreasing activity in the affected areas. As the bones of the foot or ankle heal, edema resolves and the foot begins to take its final shape. During this period, frequent follow up is necessary to modify the AFO to minimize foot and ankle motion within the AFO and to correct for limb volume loss from the resolution of edema and development of muscle atrophy. The patient can resume activity, including ambulation, once in the subacute phase is well underway, but activity should be increased incrementally. The patient should be prescribed foot and ankle strengthening and balance exercises to regain strength and control resulting from immobilization.

Once healed, the bone scan will be normal. The foot will no longer be warm, edematous, or erythematous. However, healing may have resulted in an abnormally shaped joint. The patient should be weaned to a custom FO, and custom shoes will be needed for significant deformities when they cannot be accommodated with standard commercial therapeutic shoes.

2.3.6. Type IV C Foot

This is characterized by chronic ulcers and severe bone deformities. Despite aggressive care, limb loss is typically unavoidable. Meticulous wound care and foot protection taken time until amputation is needed. At this stage, the physician should have already introduced the concept of amputation, prosthetic limb restoration, and rehabilitation.

REFERENCES

1. Dyck PJ, Kratz KM, Karnes JL et al. The prevalence by staged severity of various types of diabetic neuropathy, retinopathy, and nephropathy in a population-based cohort: the Rochester Diabetic Neuropathy Study. Neurology 1993; 43(4):817–824.
2. Masson EA, Angle S, Roseman P, Soper D, Wilson I et al. Diabetic foot ulcers: Do patients know how to protect themselves. Pract Diabetes 1989; 6:22–23.
3. Mueller MJ, Diamond JE, Sinacore DR et al. Total contact casting in treatment of diabetic plantar ulcers. Controlled clinical trial. Diabetes Care 1989; 12(6):384–388.
4. Fernando DJ, Masson EA, Veves A, Boulton AJ. Relationship of limited joint mobility to abnormal foot pressures and diabetic foot ulceration. Diabetes Care 1991; 14(1):8–11.
5. Birke JA, Franks BD, Foto JG. First ray joint limitation, pressure, and ulceration of the first metatarsal head in diabetes mellitus. Foot Ankle Int 1995; 16(5):277–284.
6. Gooding GA, Stess RM, Graf PM, Moss KM, Louie KS, Grunfeld C. Sonography of the sole of the foot. Evidence for loss of foot pad thickness in diabetes and its relationship to ulceration of the foot. Invest Radiol 1986; 21(1):45–48.

7. Apelqvist J, Larsson J, Agardh CD. The influence of external precipitating factors and peripheral neuropathy on the development and outcome of diabetic foot ulcers. J Diabet Complications 1990; 4(1):21–25.

8. Birke JA, Sims DS. Plantar sensory threshold in the ulcerative foot. Lepr Rev 1986; 57(3):261–267.

9. Delbridge L, Ellis CS, Robertson K, Lequesne LP. Non-enzymatic glycosylation of keratin from the stratum corneum of the diabetic foot. Br J Dermatol 1985; 112(5):547–554.

10. Murray HJ, Young MJ, Hollis S, Boulton AJ. The association between callus formation, high pressures and neuropathy in diabetic foot ulceration. Diabet Med 1996; 13(11):979–982.

11. Young MJ, Cavanagh PR, Thomas G, Johnson MM, Murray H, Boulton AJ. The effect of callus removal on dynamic plantar foot pressures in diabetic patients. Diabet Med 1992; 9(1):55–57.

12. Ctercteko GC, Dhanendran M, Hutton WC, Le Quesne LP. Vertical forces acting on the feet of diabetic patients with neuropathic ulceration. Br J Surg 1981; 68(9):608–614.

13. Veves A, Murray HJ, Young MJ, Boulton AJ. The risk of foot ulceration in diabetic patients with high foot pressure: a prospective study. Diabetologia 1992; 35(7):660–663.

14. Wagner FW Jr. The dysvascular foot: a system for diagnosis and treatment. Foot Ankle 1981; 2(2):64–122.

15. Armstrong DG, Lavery LA, Bushman TR. Peak foot pressures influence the healing time of diabetic foot ulcers treated with total contact casts. J Rehabil Res Dev 1998; 35(1):1–5.

16. Boninger ML, Leonard JA Jr. Use of bivalved ankle-foot orthosis in neuropathic foot and ankle lesions. J Rehabil Res Dev 1996; 33(1):16–22.

17. Dyck PJ, Karnes JL, Daube J, O'Brien P, Service FJ. Clinical and neuropathological criteria for the diagnosis and staging of diabetic polyneuropathy. Brain 1985; 108(Pt 4):861–880.

18. Rubin G, Cohen E, Rzonca EC. Prostheses and orthoses for the foot and ankle. In: Frykberg RG, ed. The High Risk Foot in Diabetes Mellitus. New York: Churchill Livingstone, 1991.

38
West Nile Virus

Patrick Luedtke and John E. Greenlee
University of Utah, Salt Lake City, Utah, USA

ABSTRACT

West Nile virus is a mosquito-borne flavivirus initially identified in Africa and associated with recurring epidemics in Eastern Europe, Africa, and Israel. The virus first appeared in the United States in 1999 and has spread to 47 states. Among infected patients, 80% will be asymptomatic and 20% will be symptomatic, but neurological complications occur in ~1%. Three major neurological syndromes are described, which may occur individually or in combination: (i) lymphocytic meningitis; (ii) encephalitis; and (iii) myelitis with destruction of anterior horn cells. Prognosis for complete recovery from meningitis is excellent, is guarded with encephalitis, and poor for recovery of motor function following significant infection of anterior horn cells.

1. INTRODUCTION

West Nile virus (WNV) is a single-stranded RNA virus first isolated from a febrile woman in the West Nile district of Uganda in 1937 (1). The virus belongs to the Japanese encephalitis virus (JEV) antigenic complex of the family Flaviviridae (2,3). WNV is not primarily a human agent but is maintained in a "bird–mosquito–bird" cycle (4). Surveillance work revealed that WNV infects 36 species of mosquitoes, 27 mammalian species, and over 160 species of birds. The avian family most severely affected is *Corvidae* (crows, jays, magpies, ravens), and large "die-offs" of Corvids have been reported to precede some WNV outbreaks in humans. *Culex* species mosquitoes (predominantly *Culex tarsalis* and *Culex pipiens*) serve as the primary vector for human infection, and the virus is capable of vertical transmission within its mosquito host (4,5). Although a large volume of scientific work exists on WNV infection, many aspects of transmission and spread remain poorly understood. Despite the lack of detailed information, it is clear that humans are a "dead-end host," incapable of maintaining the life cycle of WNV (6).

The ancestral home of WNV is believed to be the tripartite region of Eastern Africa, Southwestern Asia, and the Middle East. The apparent long-standing endemicity of WNV in this area resulted in occasional reports of human outbreaks. Israel in particular, for reasons not clearly understood, though perhaps related to its location on a major bird migration route, has reported eight large WNV outbreaks between 1941 and 2000 (7–11).

The first large outbreak of WNV in Europe occurred in Romania in 1996. Between July and October of that year, 393 cases of WNV infection requiring hospitalization were reported (12). Following this outbreak, the Volgograd region of Russia reported an outbreak in 1999 during which 480 persons with WNV were hospitalized (13). These two outbreaks, coupled with the 1999 New York City outbreak and the large Israeli outbreak of 2000, highlight an apparent change in the tropism or virulence of WNV. In prior outbreaks, there was a mild flu-like illness with only a rare case of neuroinvasive disease, in contrast to recent outbreaks which have a marked increase in both the occurrence and the severity of neuroinvasive disease (10,14–16).

WNV first appeared in the United States in 1999, with infection appearing in birds, exotic animals in zoos, and humans in close temporal proximity (10,14,17). Since arriving in North America, WNV has marched inexorably across the continent. In the United States, after first appearing in humans in New York state in 1999, WNV caused human disease in three states in 2000, 10 states in 2001, 41 states in 2002, and 47 states by the end of 2004 (Alaska, Hawaii, and Washington had not reported human WNV disease as of mid-2005). In Canada, a similar pattern has emerged, with WNV first appearing in the province of Ontario in 2001, then marching progressively westward to affect six of the 10 provinces by the end of 2004 (18). Data from Mexico are less complete, and although no confirmed human cases of WNV (i.e., without a travel history to an affected area) have been reported in Mexico, evidence exists for widespread circulation of the virus in horses since at least 2002 (19,20).

WNV is most commonly acquired from the bite of an infected mosquito. However, transmission has been documented from organ transplantation, transfusion (blood, stem cell, and bone marrow), and breast-feeding (21–24). Intrauterine WNV infection has occurred in isolated cases, resulting in severe congenital disease (25,26). In most instances, however, WNV infection during pregnancy does not appear to result in fetal illness (27,28).

2. CLINICAL FEATURES

The incubation period for WNV human infection is 2–14 days. Present data suggest that 80% of all human WNV infections are clinically silent (29). Symptomatic human WNV infection usually presents as one of four clinical syndromes: West Nile fever (WNF), West Nile meningitis (WNM), West Nile encephalitis (WNE), and acute flaccid paralysis. These syndromes may occur individually or in combination. A fifth category, which encompasses a wide variety of neurological presentations, will be discussed separately. Approximately 20% of symptomatic WNV cases present as WNF. Less than 1% of WNV infections manifest as neuroinvasive disease (e.g., meningitis, encephalitis, acute flaccid paralysis). The CDC case definition for WNV infection is found in Table 38.1. Clinical features of each of the neurological syndromes associated with WNV infection are as follows.

2.1. West Nile Fever

WNF is an acute flu-like illness manifested by the sudden onset of malaise, fatigue, anorexia, headache, nausea, vomiting, myalgia, fever, eye pain, and a nonspecific maculopapular rash. Typically, these symptoms last <7 days, although recent reports have indicated that a minority of patients may remain symptomatic for as long as 6 weeks (2) (Ned Calonge, MD, MPH, Colorado State Epidemiologist, personal communications, 2003–2004).

2.2. West Nile Meningitis

WNM presents with meningismus (fever, headache, and nuchal rigidity), nausea, vomiting, and weakness. There are no unique clinical features that allow it to be distinguished from other viral meningitides (2,30).

2.3. West Nile Encephalitis

WNE typically presents as a diffuse encephalitis with fever, headache abnormal mental status, and in more severe cases, altered level of consciousness, abnormal mental state,

Table 38.1   CDC Diagnostic Criteria for WNV Infection

Case Classification
A clinically compatible illness, plus:
   Confirmed
   1. Fourfold or greater change in WNV-specific serum antibody titer.
   2. Isolation of WNV from or demonstration of specific WN viral antigen or genomic sequences in tissue, blood, CSF, or other bodily fluid.
   3. WNV-specific IgM antibodies demonstrated in serum by antibody-capture enzyme immunoassay and confirmed by demonstration of WNV-specific serum neutralizing antibodies in the same or a later specimen.
   Probable
   1. WNV-specific serum IgM antibodies detected by antibody-capture enzyme immunoassay but with no available results of a confirmatory test for WNV-specific serum neutralizing antibodies in the same or a later specimen.

Source: http://www.cdc.gov/ncidod/dvbid/westnile/clinicians/surveillance.htm#casedef.

and focal or diffuse neurological signs. WNE may present with focal neurological deficits including cerebellar ataxia and movement disorders indicative of basal ganglia involvement including tremor, myoclonus, and parkinsonian symptoms (30–33). Asthenia, fatigue, muscle pain, and weakness may persist for months (30). Severe weakness and gastrointestinal tract symptoms have been reported with WNE and may provide a clinical clue to WNV as the etiologic agent of the encephalitis (2,4,30).

2.4. Acute Flaccid Paralysis

Flaccid paralysis is a serious complication presenting as a neuromuscular rather than central nervous system syndrome. Infection of spinal motor neurons, resulting in a syndrome similar to poliovirus infection, have been reported in other flavivirus infections, in particular Japanese encephalitis (34). Soon after WNV appeared in this country, it was recognized that a minority of patients developed a flaccid paralysis suggestive of the Guillain–Barré syndrome (GBS) (35). Although the condition can mimic GBS syndrome, patients often present with flaccid paralysis involving a single extremity (36). Additionally, although lymphocytic infiltration of spinal nerve roots has been reported in a patient with WNV infection, axonal or demyelinating changes typical of GBS have not been identified, and the common pathology in patients with acute flaccid paralysis has been spinal cord infection with destruction of anterior horn cells (36–41).

2.5. Other Neurological Manifestations

Other neurological manifestations include encephalitis complicated by focal findings including movement disorders and cerebellar ataxia. WNV may also involve the eye to produce chorioretinitis or vitritis (39,42–45). Stiff-person syndrome with antibodies to glutamic acid decarboxylase has been described (46). A GenBank search revealed a 12 amino acid sequence in the NS1 protein of WNV which has extensive homology with the GAD65 region, suggesting immunological cross-reactivity between WNV and GAD (46).

3. LABORATORY EVALUATION

The diagnosis of WNV infection is dependent upon a compatible clinical presentation, occurring at the appropriate time of year, and confirmed by thoughtful laboratory testing. WNV infection should be suspected in any individual developing meningitis, encephalitis, or a syndrome of flaccid paralysis, especially in areas in which cases of WNV are being actively reported. In much of North America, the time period of greatest WNV transmission is from July to October. More temperate areas of the continent (e.g., Mexico and the southern United States) may have an extended WNV season owing to persistent mosquito activity, and WNV infection may occur throughout the year.

The laboratory evaluation of WNV infection involves three phases: (i) tests to document the presence of meningitis or encephalitis; (ii) tests to delineate areas of involvement within the central nervous system and to document the presence of CNS inflammation; and (iii) serological confirmation of WNV infection (which, currently, is accomplished by detection of antiviral antibodies).

3.1. Routine Laboratory Studies

Laboratory studies to detect CNS infection: a mild leukocytosis is frequently reported, but leukopenia with thrombocytopenia may also be seen, as well as a relative lymphopenia (3).

Blood chemistry may be normal, although a mild elevation in liver transaminases may be seen, and hyponatremia may be present in patients with inappropriate secretion of anti-diuretic hormone (47). Cerebrospinal fluid (CSF) examination typically shows a mild elevation in pressure (<250 mm CSF), lymphocytic pleocytosis, mild elevation of protein, and a normal ratio of blood glucose to CSF glucose. Cell count is usually 50–260 cells/mm^3, but may reach 2600 cells/mm^3. Cells may be polymorphonuclear leukocytes, and at presentation, these may account for the majority of cells (3,48). In one series of West Nile myelitis, cell count was normal in 20% of the patients (49). In occasional patients, oligoclonal bands may be present.

3.2. Neurologic Studies

Tests to delineate the extent and localization of neurological disease include imaging and electrodiagnosis. CT scans are not usually helpful. Experience with magnetic resonance imaging (MRI) changes is inconclusive, and there is a recommendation for an MRI registry of WNV cases (50) MRI may be normal, particularly early in the disease. In individual cases, areas of altered signal have been detected in the substantia nigra, basal ganglia, and thalamus (51,52). Other abnormalities include subcortical or leptomeningeal enhancement and abnormal signals in the cervical spinal cord (53–55). In cases with acute flaccid paralysis, nerve conduction studies show normal sensory nerve action potentials, whereas compound motor action potentials are normal or of reduced amplitude, but conduction velocities are normal. This pattern is distinct from that seen in GBS. Electromyography in acute flaccid paralysis shows fibrillation potentials and decreased motor unit recruitment (55,56).

3.3. Diagnosis of WNV Infection

A single, acute, CSF specimen positive for WNV-specific IgM antibodies is diagnostic of current WNV infection (2,57). Paired sera positive for WNV-specific IgM antibodies (fourfold or greater rise in titer in a convalescent serum sample obtained 14–21 days after illness onset compared with acute serum sample obtained 0–7 days after symptom onset) will also suffice as serological confirmation. Although serological testing is readily available in the private sector, it must be noted that acute and convalescent testing will not result in a timely diagnosis of WNV infection. There is a recent report detecting IgM antibodies to WNV in CSF up to 199 days after clinical presentation, indicating that detection of IgM antibodies in CSF is not invariably indicative of the acute phase of disease (58). WNV genomic sequences have been identified by polymerase chain reaction (PCR) in blood or in CSF (59–61). Standardized PCR methods are not uniformly available, however, and detection of IgM antibodies remains the diagnostic method of choice. Viral culture methods are not routinely available, and WNV may be inactivated during transportation at ambient temperature (62).

4. DIFFERENTIAL DIAGNOSIS

WNV infection should be suspected in any individual developing meningitis, encephalitis, or a syndrome of flaccid paralysis, especially in areas in which cases of WNV are being actively reported. In patients presenting with meningeal involvement, however, bacterial meningitis must be excluded. Enteroviral meningoencephalitis has the same seasonal predominance as WNV meningoencephalitis, as do the older arthropod-borne encephalitides in the United States, which include St. Louis encephalitis, Eastern equine encephalitis,

Western equine encephalitis, and California-LaCrosse encephalitis. Herpes simplex encephalitis, which has no seasonal predilection, may be indistinguishable from severe cases of WNV encephalitis. In patients with a history of travel outside the United States, consideration should be given to other arthropod-borne agents, whose likelihood will be dependent upon the region of travel (e.g. Japanese encephalitis or Murray Valley encephalitis in individuals traveling to Africa, Asia, or Australasia). Rapidly ascending weakness in a previously healthy patient may represent GBS rather than WNV myelitis. Rabies, which may also cause an ascending flaccid paralysis, should be considered with known exposure to potentially infected animals or with a history of travel to areas where rabies vaccination is not used. It should be kept in mind, however, that a history of animal bite is often absent. A wide range of potentially treatable agents may mimic viral meningoencephalitis, which includes a large number of bacterial agents, spirochetal agents such as Lyme disease, *Mycoplasma*, fungi, Rickettsial agents, and *Ehrlichia*, as well as postinfectious illnesses and a variety of noninfectious systemic disorders (3).

5. MANAGEMENT AND PROGNOSIS

Management is supportive. Specific therapy has not been developed. For the majority of West Nile fever cases, simple measures such as rest, analgesics, and antipyretic medications suffice. Cases of meningitis and, in particular encephalitis and acute flaccid paralysis, require hospitalization. In cases of flaccid paralysis, the possibility of respiratory failure must be considered. Ribavirin has not been proven effective in treatment of WNV encephalitis or flaccid paralysis. A multicenter study employing intravenous immunoglobulin G containing high titers of anti-WNV antibody is in progress. A vaccine is available for use in horses, but is not yet available for humans.

The prognosis of WNV infection is determined by the degree of involvement. Patients with WNF uniformly return to their baseline level of functioning, usually within a few weeks of presentation. Patients with WNM respond similarly, with return to baseline functioning within several months. Those patients with WNE appear to fare much worse, and in one study, only six of eight patients returned to their premorbid level of functioning at 6 months and five of the eight had significant postural or kinetic tremor at 8 months (30). Additionally, most had persistent fatigue and myalgias, and 50% had persistent cognitive deficits at 8 months from presentation. Data from the 1999 New York epidemic noted that only 37% of patients with CNS involvement had returned to baseline by 1 year. The prognosis for recovery is significantly worse in the elderly, and age of >75 is an independent risk factor for death from WNV (14). Prognosis for recovery in patients with acute flaccid paralysis is poor, similar to that in poliomyelitis, and is unlikely if significant numbers of motor neurons have been lost (30,55).

6. PATHOGENESIS

WNV infection in nature begins with introduction of the virus into its human host through the bite of a mosquito, but infection may also be transmitted by blood transfusion or breast milk. The virus is believed to replicate initially in the skin and regional lymph nodes. This replication produces a primary viremia that ultimately reaches the reticuloendothelial system (RES). A secondary viremia from this "seeding" of the RES may then lead to spread throughout the body, including the central nervous system (4). At the tissue level, the pathogenesis of WNV infection is poorly understood. Perivascular inflammatory infiltrates and microglial nodules have been observed in fatal cases of encephalitis (4,18,63). Cases of acute flaccid paralysis reveal anterior horn cell loss, gliosis, patchy neuronophagia, and infiltrates of lymphocytes and macrophages (4,40,64). The respective roles of humoral and cell-mediated immune response in control of WNV infection have not been fully defined. Animal models of WNV infection suggest that antibodies are essential in preventing dissemination to the central nervous system and that CD^{8+} lymphocytes play an important role in eradication of viral infection and prevention of viral persistence (65–67). The occurrence of severe WNV infection in transplant patients suggest that lymphocyte-mediated immune response may well be essential for successful eradication of the virus in man, as well.

REFERENCES

1. Smithburn KC, Hughes TP et al. A neurotropic virus isolated from the blood of a native of Uganda. Am J Trop Med Hyg 1940; 20:471–492.
2. Petersen LR, Marfin AA. West Nile virus: a primer for the clinician. Ann Intern Med 2002; 137(3):173–179.
3. Solomon T, Whitley RJ. Arthropod-borne viral encephalitides. In: Scheld WM, Whitley RJ, Marra CM, eds. Infections of the Central Nervous System. Philadelphia: Lippincott Williams & Wilkins, 2004:205–230.
4. Petersen LR, Marfin AA et al. West Nile virus. J Am Med Assoc 2003; 290(4):524–528.
5. Baqar S, Hayes CG et al. Vertical transmission of West Nile virus by *Culex* and *Aedes* species mosquitoes. Am J Trop Med Hyg 1993; 48(6):757–762.
6. Epidemic/Epizootic West Nile Virus in the United States: Guidelines for Surveillance, Prevention, and Control. August, 2003. 2003.
7. Goldblum N, Sterk VV et al. West Nile fever. The clinical features of the disease and the isolation of West Nile virus from the blood of nine human cases. Am J Trop Med Hyg 1954; 59:89–103.
8. Goldblum N, Jasinka-Klinberg W et al. The natural history of West Nile fever. I. Clinical observations during an epidemic in Israel. Am J Hyg 1956; 64(3):259–269.
9. Spigland W, Jacinska-Klinberg W et al. Clinical and laboratory observations in an outbreak of West Nile fever in Israel in 1957. Harefuah 1958; 54:275–281.
10. Giladi M, Metzkor-Cotter E et al. West Nile encephalitis in Israel, 1999: the New York connection. Emerg Infect Dis 2001; 7(4):659–661.
11. Chowers MY, Lang R et al. Clinical characteristics of the West Nile fever outbreak, Israel, 2000. Emerg Infect Dis 2001; 7(4):675–678.
12. Tsai TF, Popovici F et al. West Nile encephalitis epidemic in southeastern Romania. Lancet 1998; 352(9130):767–771.
13. Platonov AE, Shipulin GA et al. Outbreak of West Nile virus infection, Volgograd region, Russia, 1999. Emerg Infect Dis 2001; 7(1):128–132.
14. Nash D, Mostashari F et al. The outbreak of West Nile virus infection in the New York City area in 1999. N Engl J Med 2001; 344(24):1807–1814.
15. Briese T, Rambaut A et al. Phylogenetic analysis of a human isolate from the 2000 Israel West Nile virus epidemic. Emerg Infect Dis 2002; 8(5):528–531.
16. Klein C, Kimiagar I et al. Neurological features of West Nile virus infection during the 2000 outbreak in a regional hospital in Israel. J Neurol Sci 2002; 200(1–2):63–66.
17. Briese T, Jia XY et al. Identification of a Kunjin/West Nile-like flavivirus in brains of patients with New York encephalitis. Lancet 1999; 354(9186):1261–1262.
18. Pepperell C, Rau N et al. West Nile virus infection in 2002: morbidity and mortality among patients admitted to hospital in southcentral Ontario. CMAJ 2003; 168(11):1399–1405.
19. Blitvich BJ, Fernandez-Salas I et al. Serologic evidence of West Nile virus infection in horses, Coahuila State, Mexico. Emerg Infect Dis 2003; 9(7):853–856.

20. Lorono-Pino MA, Blitvich BJ et al. Serologic evidence of West Nile virus infection in horses, Yucatan State, Mexico. Emerg Infect Dis 2003; 9(7):857–859.

21. Pealer LN, Marfin AA et al. Transmission of West Nile virus through blood transfusion in the United States in 2002. N Engl J Med 2003; 349(13):1236–1245.

22. Kleinschmidt-DeMasters BK, Marder BA et al. Naturally acquired West Nile virus encephalomyelitis in transplant recipients: clinical, laboratory, diagnostic, and neuropathological features. Arch Neurol 2004; 61(8):1210–1220.

23. Williams K. Modes of transmission for West Nile virus. Clin Lab Sci 2004; 17(1):56.

24. From the Centers for Disease Control and Prevention. Possible West Nile virus transmission to an infant through breast-feeding—Michigan, 2002. J Am Med Assoc 2002; 288(16):1976–1977.

25. Intrauterine West Nile virus infection—New York, 2002. Morb Mortal Wkly Rep 2002; 51(50):1135–1136.

26. Alpert SG, Fergerson J et al. Intrauterine West Nile virus: ocular and systemic findings. Am J Ophthalmol 2003; 136(4):733–735.

27. Bruno J, Rabito FJ Jr et al. West Nile virus meningoencephalitis during pregnancy. J La State Med Soc 2004; 156(4):204–205.

28. Interim guidelines for the evaluation of infants born to mothers infected with West Nile virus during pregnancy. Morb Mortal Wkly Rep 2004; 53(7):154–157.

29. Mostashari F, Bunning ML et al. Epidemic West Nile encephalitis, New York, 1999: results of a household-based seroepidemiological survey. Lancet 2001; 358(9278):261–264.

30. Sejvar JJ, Haddad MB et al. Neurologic manifestations and outcome of West Nile virus infection. J Am Med Assoc 2003; 290(4):511–515.

31. Ceausu E, Erscoiu S et al. Clinical manifestations in the West Nile virus outbreak. Rom J Virol 1997; 48(1–4):3–11.

32. Kanagarajan K, Ganesh S et al. West Nile virus infection presenting as cerebellar ataxia and fever: case report. South Med J 2003; 96(6):600–601.

33. Sayao AL, Suchowersky O et al. Calgary experience with West Nile virus neurological syndrome during the late summer of 2003. Can J Neurol Sci 2004; 31(2):194–203.

34. Arya SC. Japanese encephalitis virus and poliomyelitis-like illness. Lancet 1998; 351(9120):1964.

35. Ahmed S, Libman R et al. Guillain–Barré syndrome: an unusual presentation of West Nile virus infection. Neurology 2000; 55(1):144–146.

36. Leis AA, Stokic DS et al. Clinical spectrum of muscle weakness in human West Nile virus infection. Muscle Nerve 2003; 28(3):302–308.

37. Fratkin JD, Leis AA et al. Spinal cord neuropathology in human West Nile virus infection. Arch Pathol Lab Med 2004; 128(5):533–537.

38. Omalu BI, Shakir AA et al. Fatal fulminant pan-meningo-polioencephalitis due to West Nile virus. Brain Pathol 2003; 13(4):465–472.

39. Doron SI, Dashe JF et al. Histopathologically proven poliomyelitis with quadriplegia and loss of brainstem function due to West Nile virus infection. Clin Infect Dis 2003; 37(5):e74–e77.

40. Sejvar JJ, Leis AA et al. Acute flaccid paralysis and West Nile virus infection. Emerg Infect Dis 2003; 9(7):788–793.

41. Bouffard JP, Riudavets MA et al. Neuropathology of the brain and spinal cord in human West Nile virus infection. Clin Neuropathol 2004; 23(2):59–61.

42. Anninger WV, Lomeo MD et al. West Nile virus-associated optic neuritis and chorioretinitis. Am J Ophthalmol 2003; 136(6):1183–1185.

43. Bains HS, Jampol LM et al. Vitritis and chorioretinitis in a patient with West Nile virus infection. Arch Ophthalmol 2003; 121(2):205–207.

44. Hershberger VS, Augsburger JJ et al. Chorioretinal lesions in nonfatal cases of West Nile virus infection. Ophthalmology 2003; 110(9):1732–1736.

45. Vandenbelt S, Shaikh S et al. Multifocal choroiditis associated with West Nile virus encephalitis. Retina 2003; 23(1):97–99.

46. Hassin-Baer S, Kirson ED et al. Stiff-person syndrome following West Nile fever. Arch Neurol 2004; 61(6):938–941.

47. Jeha LE, Sila CA et al. West Nile virus infection: a new acute paralytic illness. Neurology 2003; 61(1):55–59.

48. Tyler KL. Viral myelitis. In: Scheld WM, Whitley RJ, Marra CM, eds. Infections of the Central Nervous System. Philadelphia: Lippincott Williams & Wilkins, 2004:323–330.

49. Leis AA, Stokic DS et al. A poliomyelitis-like syndrome from West Nile virus infection. N Engl J Med 2002; 347(16):1279–1280.

50. Robertson HJ, Sejvar JJ. The need for a West Nile virus MRI registry. Am J Neuroradiol 2003; 24(9):1741–1742.

51. Rosas H, Wippold FJ. West Nile virus: case report with MR imaging findings. Am J Neuroradiol 2003; 24(7):1376–1378.

52. Bosanko CM, Gilroy J et al. West Nile virus encephalitis involving the substantia nigra: neuroimaging and pathologic findings with literature review. Arch Neurol 2003; 60(10):1448–1452.

53. Brilla R, Block M et al. Clinical and neuroradiologic features of 39 consecutive cases of West Nile virus meningoencephalitis. J Neurol Sci 2004; 220(1–2):37–40.

54. Olsan AD, Milburn JM et al. Leptomeningeal enhancement in a patient with proven West Nile virus infection. Am J Roentgenol 2003; 181(2):591–592.

55. Al Shekhlee A, Katirji B. Electrodiagnostic features of acute paralytic poliomyelitis associated with West Nile virus infection. Muscle Nerve 2004; 29(3):376–380.

56. Li J, Loeb JA et al. Asymmetric flaccid paralysis: a neuromuscular presentation of West Nile virus infection. Ann Neurol 2003; 53(6):703–710.

57. Shi PY, Wong SJ. Serologic diagnosis of West Nile virus infection. Expert Rev Mol Diagn 2003; 3(6):733–741.

58. Kapoor AH, Signs BK et al. Persistence of West Nile Virus (WNV) IgM antibodies in cerebrospinal fluid from patients with CNS disease. J Clin Virol 2004; 31(4):289–291.

59. Huang C, Slater B et al. First isolation of West Nile virus from a patient with encephalitis in the United States. Emerg Infect Dis 2002; 8(12):1367–1371.

60. Lanciotti RS, Kerst AJ et al. Rapid detection of West Nile virus from human clinical specimens, field-collected mosquitoes, and avian samples by a TaqMan reverse transcriptase–PCR assay. J Clin Microbiol 2000; 38(11):4066–4071.

61. Briese T, Glass WG et al. Detection of West Nile virus sequences in cerebrospinal fluid. Lancet 2000; 355(9215):1614–1615.

62. Mayo DR, Beckwith WH III. Inactivation of West Nile virus during serologic testing and transport. J Clin Microbiol 2002; 40(8):3044–3046.

63. Sampson BA, Armbrustmacher V. West Nile encephalitis: the neuropathology of four fatalities. Ann NY Acad Sci 2001; 951:172–178.

64. Kelley TW, Prayson RA et al. Spinal cord disease in West Nile virus infection. N Engl J Med 2003; 348(6):564–566.

65. Shrestha B, Diamond MS. Role of CD[8+] T cells in control of West Nile virus infection. J Virol 2004; 78(15):8312–8321.

66. Wang Y, Lobigs M et al. CD[8+] T cells mediate recovery and immunopathology in West Nile virus encephalitis. J Virol 2003; 77(24):13323–13334.

67. Diamond MS, Shrestha B et al. Innate and adaptive immune responses determine protection against disseminated infection by West Nile encephalitis virus. Viral Immunol 2003; 16(3):259–278.

39

Diagnostic Yield for Peripheral Neuropathy

A. Gordon Smith
University of Utah, Salt Lake City, Utah, USA

ABSTRACT

Accurate and efficient diagnosis of peripheral neuropathy requires an organized approach. Use of a standardized set of laboratory tests for all patients with suspected peripheral neuropathy is expensive, often misses the correct diagnosis, and frequently leads to false positive tests. Use of a rational diagnostic algorithm maximizes diagnostic yield and minimizes risk of misdiagnosis. Patients with chronic distal symmetric sensory predominant neuropathy require relatively few routine diagnostic tests.

1. INTRODUCTION

The diagnostic evaluation of peripheral neuropathy may provoke feelings of diagnostic nihilism if one is not familiar with peripheral nerve disease. There are hundreds of causes for peripheral neuropathy and the range of symptoms referable to peripheral nerve dysfunction is limited. Consequently, a "shotgun" diagnostic approach is often used, employing a standard set of diagnostic tests (Table 39.1). Such an approach may miss the diagnosis because the particular diagnostic test may not be on the "shotgun" panel. On the other hand, false positive diagnostic tests are not uncommon. Because of the large number of tests, several of which must be sent to specific reference laboratories,

Table 39.1 The "Shotgun" Approach to Peripheral
Neuropathy Consists of the Routine Measurement of a
Standardized Panel of Diagnostic Tests in all Patients

Vitamin B12
Folate
RPR
Thyroid stimulating hormone
Sedimentation rate
Rheumatoid factor
Antinuclear antibodies
Extractible nuclear antibodies
Serum protein electrophoresis
Antiganglioside antibody titers
Paraneoplastic antibody titers

Note: This is a list of tests often included in a shotgun panel. This
approach is expensive and inefficient, and it carries significant risk
of false positives.

this approach is expensive. However, although expensive, the sensitivity and specificity of
this panel are low. There are several tests that are only relevant for specific patient populations. For example, antiganglioside antibody panels may include anti-GM1 antibodies,
antimyelin associated glycoprotein antibodies, or both. The former is relevant only for
motor neuropathies, particularly multifocal motor neuropathy with conduction block,
and the later is relevant only for a subset of patients with chronic inflammatory demyelinating polyradiculoneuropathy (CIDP). These antibodies may be detectable in low levels
in normal subjects or patients with unrelated neuropathies, leading the unwary clinician to
wrongly associate the false positive laboratory test with the clinical syndrome.

Experienced clinicians often arrive at a diagnosis using a pattern recognition
approach. Particular patterns of disease are recognized and the diagnostic approach is
limited to few diagnostic tests. When successful, this diagnostic approach is very efficient
and cost effective. However, pattern recognition may only be employed by those with both
excellent clinical skills and a wealth of experience with peripheral nerve disease. If the
particular disorder has not been previously observed, if there is an atypical presentation,
or if the clinician (despite excellent skills) does not have a great deal of experience, the
pattern may not be recognized and the diagnosis missed.

For most clinicians, including experienced peripheral nerve experts encountering an
unusual disorder, a rational diagnostic approach is necessary. Several well-reasoned
approaches to the diagnosis of peripheral neuropathy have been suggested and each is
appropriate (1–5). This chapter will outline an organized approach to the classification
of peripheral neuropathies and will review the evidence for the routine use of commonly
ordered diagnostic tests in the evaluation of distal symmetric sensory predominant
neuropathy.

2. CONFIRMATION OF PERIPHERAL NEUROPATHY

The first step in the evaluation of a patient with a peripheral nerve disorder is confirmation
of the localization. The diagnosis of peripheral neuropathy is usually straightforward.
However, patients with isolated foot pain and numbness may present a diagnostic
challenge. There are many different causes for foot pain including orthopedic issues

and central nervous system dysfunction; differentiation from small fiber predominant neuropathy may be difficult on clinical grounds alone. Confirmation of a suspected diagnosis of peripheral neuropathy depends on one of several supportive diagnostic tests. Nerve conduction studies are the most commonly used test for peripheral neuropathy. Nerve conduction studies primarily reflect large fiber function and are therefore insensitive to small fiber injury. The sympathetic skin response may be used to assess small fiber function, but is relatively insensitive. Therefore, other tests must often be used to confirm the presence of a suspected small fiber predominant neuropathy.

Quantitative sensory testing (QST) is an accurate and reproducible method to determine the threshold for perceiving vibratory or cooling stimuli. Vibration threshold measures large fiber function and cooling reflects small, lightly myelinated nerve function. QST is abnormal in 57–72% of patients with small fiber neuropathy (6,7). QST is nonspecific in that other causes of sensory loss (e.g., radiculopathy, central nervous system processes) can increase perception thresholds. QST also requires patient cooperation and meticulous attention to the testing environment (e.g., temperature, noise, and other distractions). Unlike Nerve Conduction Studies (NCS), QST is a psychophysiologic measure, rather than a physiologic measure. As a result, QST is unable to differentiate between true sensory loss and simulated sensory loss (8). Therefore, QST should not be used as the primary means of differentiating functional sensory symptoms or signs from peripheral neuropathy.

Some degree of autonomic dysfunction is demonstrable in most patients with painful peripheral neuropathy. Autonomic testing provides a sensitive means of diagnosing small fiber nerve injury (Chapter 4). The most commonly available, and most sensitive tests measure sudomotor (sweat gland) function. Quantitative sudomotor axon reflex testing (QSART) is the easiest and most widely available procedure. A small circular chamber is placed on the skin. Acetylcholine is iontophoresed into the skin and stimulates terminal unmyelinated axons supplying sweat glands, resulting in reflex activation of surrounding sweat glands. The resulting sweat volume is measured quantitatively. QSART is abnormal in 70% of painful neuropathy patients (9). Unlike QST, QSART is specific for postganglionic adrenergic autonomic function. As with QST, special equipment is necessary, and careful attention must be paid to the testing protocol in order to obtain reliable results.

The only test that directly evaluates unmyelinated somatic sensory fibers is skin biopsy. A 3 mm punch biopsy is performed and the tissue stained with an antibody that stains peripheral nerve axons (Chapter 6). Unmeylinated axons subserving pain sensation may be easily observed coursing through the epidermis in normal subjects. In those with neuropathy, these fibers are depleted at distal sites. Like QSART, skin biopsy is both sensitive and specific (6). Skin biopsy of the distal leg is abnormal in subjects whose symptoms are limited to the feet. Unlike nerve biopsy, skin biopsy is minimally invasive, and often better tolerated than NCS. There is a minimal risk of infection, and no significant complications are reported in the literature. The biopsy site heals within 1–2 weeks in most subjects (similar to abrasion wounds) (10). The biopsy results in a scar that usually fades and may disappear after several months. The biopsy procedure is simple and rapidly performed (~10–15 min). When tissue processing and analysis require skill and time, the tissue may be easily shipped to a central processing laboratory.

The choice of which test to perform in a patient with suspected peripheral neuropathy and normal nerve conduction studies is based on patient symptoms and which equipment is available. If QST and QSART equipments are not available, a skin biopsy may be performed and shipped to a laboratory where the tissue can be processed. Overall, there is a poor correlation among QSART, QST and skin biopsy, suggesting that they measure separate functions (7). Patients may have an abnormality on one but not on the others.

Nerve biopsy is never indicated solely for the purpose of confirming a diagnosis of peripheral neuropathy. Even when electron microscopy is performed for analysis of small unmyelinated nerve fibers, nerve biopsy may be normal when other specific and less invasive tests, such as skin biopsy, are abnormal (11). Nerve biopsy should only be performed when there is suspicion of certain disorders, particularly amyloidosis, vasculitis, and tumor infiltration. Nerve biopsy is rarely necessary for the diagnosis of CIDP and should primarily be used to exclude other etiologies.

3. CLASSIFICATION OF PERIPHERAL NEUROPATHY

Most books of peripheral neuropathy (including this one) classify neuropathies based on underlying pathophysiology (inflammatory, metabolic, neoplastic, toxic etc.). This organization is useful for the reader interested in learning about a particular diagnosis. For the clinician attempting to diagnose an individual patient with an unknown peripheral neuropathy, this classification scheme is less useful. In the clinical setting, an algorithmic approach to the classification of individual peripheral neuropathies is necessary to limit the differential diagnosis and permit a reasoned and focused diagnostic evaluation.

Peripheral neuropathies can be classified based on system involvement (sensory, motor, and autonomic), anatomic pattern (distal, proximal, and asymmetric), temporal course (acute, subacute, and chronic), electrodiagnostic features (axonal, demyelinating, and mixed), or the presence of severe pain or positive family history (Table 39.2). Most patients with peripheral neuropathy have a chronic, distal predominant, sensory greater than motor neuropathy with positive sensory symptoms (tingling, prickling, and burning) and at least some degree of discomfort or pain. This prototypic pattern of neuropathy represents one of the most common problems seen by general neurologists and requires only a focused diagnostic evaluation that will be outlined suceedingly. However, recognition of the prototypic pattern necessitates a careful search for any atypical features suggestive of a different neuropathy pattern. These features, and selected disorders which characteristically cause them, are outlined in Table 39.2.

4. THE EVALUATION OF PROTOTYPIC NEUROPATHY

Patients with prototypic neuropathy comprise a relatively homogeneous group, presenting with numbness, positive sensory symptoms, and discomfort. Symptoms often develop over a period of months, then stabilize or progress slowly over years. Numbness and pain are distal predominant, primarily involving the feet and distal leg. While mild weakness of toe extension and ankle dorsiflexion may be observed, significant weakness is uncommon. Pain may be severe. Autonomic dysfunction is usually limited to sudomotor dysfunction in the feet, which often have a red or purple discoloration, and erectile dysfunction (9). The presence of bony abnormalities such as high arches, hammer toes, or neurogenic arthropathy (Charcot joint) should prompt an evaluation for an inherited neuropathy.

Once this pattern is recognized, the evaluation may be focused. All patients with suspected peripheral neuropathy should have a thorough medical history and require a careful general physical examination. Subtle historical details or examination findings may be very helpful in focusing the diagnostic evaluation, regardless of the neuropathy pattern. For example, several small angiokeratoma on a young male patient with a painful neuropathy suggest the diagnosis of Fabry disease. For patients with prototypic neuropathy, a careful search should be made for clinical evidence of toxic exposure, connective

Table 39.2   The Differential Diagnosis can be Focused by Recognizing Atypical Features

Prominent Motor Involvement	Prominent Sensory Involvement
Charcot Marie Tooth	Idiopathic
CIDP and variants (e.g., distal	Diabetes
acquired demyelinating	Vitamin B12 deficiency
peripheral neuropathy)	Pyridoxine toxicity
Lead	Drug toxicity (e.g., nucleoside analogs
Dapsone	Cisplatin
Porphyria	Dorsal root ganglionopathy
Multifocal motor neuropathy	Paraneoplastic
Motor neuron disease	Idiopathic
Prominent Autonomic Involvement	Sjogrens
Diabetes	HIV
Amyloidosis	Leprosy
Hereditary sensory autonomic	Hereditary sensory
neuropathy	autonomic neuropathy
Severe Pain	Amyloidosis
Idiopathic	Asymmetry
Diabetes	Vasculitis
HIV	Primary peripheral nerve
Amyloidosis	Systemic vasculitis
Fabry	Hereditary neuropathy with
Vasculitis	predisposition to pressure palsies
Proximal Involvement	Diabetic and non-diabetic lumbosacral
(non-length dependent)	radiculoplexus neuropathies
CIDP	("diabetic amyotrophy")
Diabetic and non-diabetic lumbosacral	CIDP ("Lewis Sumner" variant)
radiculoplexus neuropathies	Multifocal motor neuropathy
("diabetic amyotrophy")	Leprosy
Porphyria	Acute or Subacute Timecourse
Infiltrative or infectious polyradiculitis	Inflammatory
(e.g., carcinoma)	Guillain Barre Syndrome
Dorsal root ganglionopathy	Vasculitis
Paraneoplastic	Toxic Exposure
Idiopathic	Metals (e.g., arsenic)
	Solvents (e.g., n-Hexane)
	Porphyria
	Infectious neuropathies

Note: A selected list of diagnoses suggested by each atypical feature is provided.

tissue disease, or endocrine dysfunction. A differential diagnosis of prototypic neuropathy is displayed in Table 39.3, with symptoms or signs suggestive of each diagnosis.

While the differential diagnosis of prototypic neuropathy appears lengthy, in patients lacking clinical features suggestive of any particular disorder, the list of potential diagnostic possibilities is much shorter. The laboratory evaluation includes tests for disorders that directly cause nerve dysfunction or injury (e.g., vitamin B12 and diabetes) as well as tests for conditions that may be associated with neuropathy but are not necessarily causative (monoclonal gammopathy). Several studies have addressed the diagnostic yield of laboratory evaluation among this patient population. Among 93 patients with distal pain, numbness or tingling without symptoms of motor weakness, the only abnormality identified after

Table 39.3   The Differential Diagnosis of Prototypic
Peripheral Neuropathy

Idiopathic Neuropathy
Diabetes
Impaired Glucose Tolerance
Vitamin B12 Deficiency
Connective tissue disease
   Sjogren's Syndrome
   Rheumatoid Arthritis[a]
   Systemic Lupus Erythematosis[a]
Hypothyroidism[a]
Toxic Exposure
   Medications
      Chemotherapeutic agents (vincristine, taxol, platinum)
      Pyridoxine (high dose causes ganglionopathy)
      Macrodantin
      Metronidazole
      Amiodarone
   Solvents (chronic low level)
Familial

---

[a]Rarely the presenting symptom

extensive laboratory evaluation was a monoclonal gammopathy in 4/83 (5%) (12). The recommendation was that CBC, sedimentation rate, serum chemistry panel, serum protein electrophoresis (SPEP) and immunofixation (IFIX), and vitamin B12 levels be measured in all patients (1). In another study of 117 patients with sensory neuropathy, the only laboratory abnormalities were hypertryglyceridemia (34%), hypercholestoreamia (28%), monoclonal gammopathy in 4 (3.4%), positive extractible nuclear antigens (ENA) consistent with Sjögren's disease in 2 (0.2%), and positive antiribonucleoprotein (RNP) antibody consistent with mixed connective tissue disease in 1 (0.1%). Two patients had amyloidosis (one primary and one inherited) and both had symtpomatic orthostatic hypotension (7). Our data is consistent with these series. Among 138 consecutive patients with prototypic neuropathy, 1.6% had a low B12 level, and 2.8% had a monoclonal gammopathy of uncertain significance (MGUS). The most frequent abnormality was impaired glucose tolerance (IGT) defined as a serum glucose of 140–200, 2 h after a 75 g ahydrous dextrose oral load. Among 87 patients who underwent the recommended oral glucose tolerance test, 39 (45%) had IGT and 12 (13%) frank diabetes (13). This is consistent with retrospective data suggesting over one-third of patients with otherwise idiopathic neuropathy have IGT (14,15). The other neuropathy patient series described earlier did not include routine OGTT.

    The studies outlined earlier suggest only selected laboratory tests need to be routinely performed in patients with prototypic neuropathy who lack signs or symptoms suggesting a systemic disorder. All patients should undergo an oral glucose tolerance test to exclude diabetes or IGT. The Diabetes Control and Complications Trial demonstrated that glycemic control slows progression of diabetic neuropathy and the Diabetes Prevention Program demonstrated that diet and exercise intervention reduces the risk of progression of IGT to frank diabetes (16,17). Research is underway to determine if similar lifestyle intervention slows the rate of progression of neuropathy associated with IGT. Peripheral neuropathy caused by diabetes and IGT is reviewed in Chapter 11. IGT is part of the Metabolic Syndrome of insulin resistance, obesity, hyperlipidemia, and hypertension, and is associated with increased risk of large vessel atherosclerotic disease. The high incidence of hyperlipidemia in patients with painful sensory neuropathy suggests a high likelihood of insulin resistance (7). Because the Metabolic Syndrome may contribute to peripheral neuropathy and is a significant risk factor for coronary artery and cerebrovascular disease, all neuropathy patients should be have serum lipids and cholesterol measured.

A serum B12 level should be measured in all patients. Those with borderline serum levels (200–300 pg/mL) should also have methylmalonic acid and homocysteine levels tested to exclude a mild deficiency state (18).

Other tests are of less certain yield in the absence of clinical features suggesting a systemic disorder. Routine testing of thyroid function failed to reveal an abnormality in the neuropathy series reviewed. However, neuromuscular complaints are common among patients with hypothyroidism (19). Signs and symptoms of hypothyroidism should be carefully sought in all patients with peripheral neuropathy and diagnostic testing performed only when found.

Monoclonal gammopathy of unknown significance (MGUS) is associated with CIDP, but the relationship between MGUS and axonal neuropathy and is less certain. The population prevalence of MGUS rises to 3% among those over 70 years of age (20,21). In the neuropathy patient series described previously, the prevalence of MGUS ranged 1–5%, a rate not much higher than the population prevalence. There are no clinical differences between patients with idiopathic neuropathy and those with axonal neuropathy associated with MGUS (22). One argument in favor of screening neuropathy patients is that over 20 years of follow-up, ~20% of patients with MGUS develop a malignant lymphoproliferative disorder (21,23). However, the impact of early diagnosis of MGUS on ultimate outcome is unknown.

While systemic evidence of a connective tissue disease, such as rash, inflammatory arthritis, or keratoconjunctivitis sicca should prompt a careful serologic evaluation, routine testing for serum autoantibodies is of very low diagnostic yield. Up to 12% of healthy blood donors have a positive antinuclear antibody (ANA) at a low titer (24,25). Abnormal ANA tests in neuropathy subjects are usually of low titer and are of doubtful significance. A history of dry eyes or mouth raises the question of Sjögren's syndrome and serum SSA and SSB antibodies should be measured. While specific, these antibodies are absent in most patients with neuropathy due to Sjögren's syndrome and a minor salivary gland biopsy may be necessary to confirm the diagnosis (26).

There is significant commercial pressure to order antibody panels on patients with peripheral neuropathy. These panels typically include various combinations of antiganglioside and paraneoplastic antibodies. With the exception of antibodies associated with multifocal motor neuropathy (GM1), the Fisher variant of Guillain Barre Syndrome (GQ1b), defined paraneoplastic syndromes such as sensory ganglionopathy (Hu) and certain patients with CIDP (MAG), there is no benefit to the routine ordering of these tests. Antisulfatide antibodies in particular are of uncertain clinical significance (27). It is usually best to order only the specific antibody of clinical relevance, as the marketed panels may include several antibody tests that are not relevant. Panels may include antibodies associated with both motor (GM1) and sensory (MAG, Hu) neuropathies. Antibodies may be positive in a patient for whom the laboratory finding is clinically irrelevant, occasionally leading to inappropriate therapy.

5. IDIOPATHIC NEUROPATHY

The percentage of patients for whom no abnormality is found (e.g., idiopathic neuropathy) varies depending on the inclusion criteria of the particular study. In general, ~30% of patients with prototypic neuropathy have idiopathic neuropathy. Idiopathic neuropathy is more common among older patients, although it is not exclusively a disease of old age. The etiology of idiopathic neuropathy is unknown. Patients with idiopathic neuropathy share several characteristics in common with those who have glucose dysregulation. Both groups have a high prevalence of obesity and its complications. For example, the mean body-mass index of patients with idiopathic neuropathy is not different from that of patients with impaired glucose tolerance (14). Preliminary data suggest at least some patients with idiopathic neuropathy have abnormalities of microvascular reactivity similar to diabetes (28). These observations suggest obesity may be a common risk factor for diabetic, IGT, and idiopathic neuropathies.

While the diagnosis of idiopathic neuropathy may seem unsatisfying to the practitioner, it provides very useful prognostic information for the patient. Patients with neuropathy often have substantial fear of future disability and appropriate education is therefore very reassuring and often represents the most important therapeutic intervention. The natural history of idiopathic neuropathy is of very slow progression without disability beyond pain. Furthermore, the development of severe pain in patients who do not initially present with significant pain is rare.

Once a diagnosis of idiopathic neuropathy has been made, reevaluation is unnecessary unless the clinical scenario changes. Among 75 subjects with idiopathic neuropathy evaluated yearly for five years, no metabolic or toxic cause was identified and no patient developed a monoclonal gammopathy (29).

6. SUMMARY

The evaluation of patients with peripheral nerve disease can be efficient and informative when a rational and organized approach is used. One must first localize the neurologic lesion, confirm the presence of peripheral neuropathy, and characterize its features clinically and electrophysiologically. If nerve conduction studies are normal, QST, QSART, or skin biopsy are useful means of confirming the diagnosis. Patients with prototypic, distal, axonal sensorimotor neuropathy should undergo an OGTT and have their serum vitamin B12 level measured. Other tests should be performed if there are features suggesting another disorder. Those with atypical features (asymmetry, proximal involvement, pure motor or sensory, or autonomic involvement) should be evaluating for conditions known to cause the particular pattern. In patients with particularly confusing or unusual presentations, referral to a tertiary care neuromuscular center is frequently more useful than reverting to a shotgun diagnostic approach.

REFERENCES

1. Barohn R. Approach to peripheral neuropathy and neuronopathy. Sem Neurol 1998; 18:7–18.
2. Bromberg M, Smith A. Toward an efficient method to evaluate peripheral neuropathies. J Clin Neuromusc Dis 2002; 3:172–182.
3. Dyck P, Dyck J, Chalk C. The 10 P's: a mnemonic helpful in characterization of differential diagnosis of peripheral neuropathy. Neurology 1992; 41:14–18.
4. Dyck PJ, Dyck JB, Grant IA, Fealey RD. Ten steps in characterizing and diagnosing patients with peripheral neuropathy. Neurology 1996; 47:10–17.
5. Smith AG, Bromberg MB. A rational diagnostic approach to peripheral neuropathy. J Clin Neuormusc Dis 2003; 4:190–198.

6. Holland NR, Crawford TO, Hauer P, Cornblath DR, Griffin JW, McArthur JC. Small-Fiber sensory neuropathies: clinical course and neuropathology of idiopathic cases. Ann Neurol 1998; 44:47–59.

7. Periquet MI, Novak V, Collins MP et al. Painful sensory neuropathy prospective evaluation using skin biopsy. Neurology 1999; 53:1641–1647.

8. Freeman R, Chase K, Risk M. Quantitative sensory testing cannot differentiate simulated sensory loss from sensory neuropathy. Neurology 2003; 60:465–470.

9. Novak V, Freimer ML, Kissel JT et al. Autonomic impairment in painful neuropathy. Neurology 2001; 56(7):861–868.

10. Chien HF, Tseng TJ, Lin WM et al. Quantitative pathology of cutaneous nerve terminal degeneration in the human skin. Acta Neuropathol 2000; 102:455–461.

11. Herrmann D, Griffin J, Hauer P, Cornblath D, McArthur J. Epidermal nerve fiber density and sural nerve morphometry in peripheral neuropathies. Neurology 1999; 53:1634–1640.

12. Wolfe G, Baker N, Amato A et al. Chronic cryptogenic sensory polyneuropathy clinical and laboratory characteristics. Arch Neurol 1999; 56:540–547.

13. Smith AG, Singleton JR. The diagnostic yield of a standardized approach to idiopathic sensory-predominant neuropathy. Arch Intern Med 2004; 164(9):1021–1025.

14. Singleton JR, Smith AG, Bromberg MB. Increased prevalence of impaired glucose tolerance in patients with painful sensory neuropathy. Diab Care 2001; 24(8):1448–1453.

15. Novella SP, Inzucchi SE, Goldstein JM. The frequency of undiagnosed diabetes and impaired glucose tolerance in patients with idiopathic sensory neuropathy. Muscle Nerve 2001; 24:1229–1231.

16. Diabetes Control and Complications Research Group. The effect of intensive treatment of diabetes on the development and progression of long-term complications in insulin-dependent diabetes mellitus. New Engl J Med 1993; 329:977–986.

17. Diabetes Prevention Program Research Group. Reduction in the incidence of type 2 diabetes with lifestyle intervention or metformin. NEJM 2002; 346:393–403.

18. Saperstein DS, Barohn RJ. Peripheral Neuropathy Due to Cobalamin Deficiency. Curr Treat Options Neurol 2002; 4(3):197–201.

19. Duyff R, Van den Bosch J, Laman D, van Loon B, Linssen W. Neuromuscular findings in thyroid dysfunction a prospective clinical and electrodiagnostic study. J Neurol Neurosurg Psychiatry 2000; 68:750–755.

20. Kelly J, Kyle R, O'Brien P, Dyck P. Prevalence of monoclonal proteins in peripheral neuropathy. Neurology 1981; 31:1480–1483.

21. Kyle RA, Finkelstein S, Elveback LR, Kurland LT. Incidence of monoclonal proteins in a Minnesota community with a cluster of multiple myeloma. Blood 1972; 40:719–724.

22. Notermans N, Wokke J, Lokhorst H, Franssen H, van der Graaf Y. Polyneuropathy associated with monoclonal gammopathy of undetermined significance a prospective study of the prognostic value of clinical and laboratory abnormalities. Brain 1994; 117:1385–1393.

23. Kyle RA, Therneau TM, Rajkumar SV et al. A long-term study of prognosis in monoclonal gammopathy of undetermined significance. N Engl J Med 2002; 346(8):564–569.

24. Azizah MR, Azila MN, Zulkifli MN, Norita TY. The prevalence of antinuclear, anti-dsDNA and anti-RNP antibodies in a group of healthy blood donors. Asian Pac J Allergy Immunol 1996; 14:125–128.

25. de Vlam K, De Keyser F, Vergraggen G et al. Detection and identification of antinuclear antibodies in serum of normal blood donors. Clin Exp Rheumatol 1993; 11:393–397.

26. Grant IA, Hunder GG, Homburger HA, Dyck PJ. Peripheral neuropathy associated with sicca complex. Neurology 1997; 48(4):855–862.

27. Wolfe G, El-Feky W, Katz J, Brayan W, Wians F, Barohn R. Antibody panels in idiopathic polyneuropathy and motor neuron disease. Muscle and Nerve 1997; 20:1275–1283.

28. Smith A, Howard J, Kroll R, Singleton J. Microvascular dysfunction in diabetic and idiopathic peripheral neuropathy. Neurology 2003; 60:A386.

29. Notermans N, Wokke J, van der Graaf Y, Franssen H, van Dijk G, Jennekens F. Chronic idiopathic axonal polyneuropathy a five year follow up. J Neurol Neurosurg Psychiatry 1994; 57:1525–1527.

Index

About the Editors

MARK B. BROMBERG is Professor of Neurology and Director of the Neuromuscular and Motor Neuron Disease Programs, University of Utah, Salt Lake City. He received the M.D. degree, residency training in neurology, and fellowship training in electromyography and neuromuscular diseases from the University of Michigan, Ann Arbor. He received the Ph.D. degree in neurophysiology from the University of Vermont, Burlington, and completed postdoctoral research training in the field of motor control.

A. GORDON SMITH is Associate Professor of Neurology and Pathology, University of Utah, Salt Lake City, and the Salt Lake Veterans Administration Hospital, Utah. He is the Director of the University of Utah Peripheral Neuropathy and Therapeutic Botulinum Toxin Clinics and the Cutaneous Innervation Laboratory. He received the M.D. degree from the Mayo Medical School and completed a neurology residency and neuromuscular and clinical neurophysiology training at the University of Michigan.